# Dictionary of Optometry and Visual Science

*For Butterworth-Heinemann*

*Publishing Director:* Caroline Makepeace
*Development Editor:* Kim Benson
*Project Manager:* Ailsa Laing
*Designer:* George Ajayi
*Illustrations Manager:* Bruce Hogarth

# Dictionary of Optometry and Visual Science

SIXTH EDITION

**Michel Millodot**

OD PhD DOSc(Hon) FAAO FCOptom

*Professor Emeritus, Hong Kong Polytechnic University, Hong Kong*



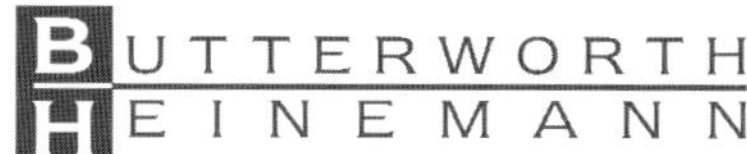


Edinburgh London New York Oxford Philadelphia St Louis Sydney Toronto 2004

BUTTERWORTH-HEINEMANN
An imprint of Elsevier Limited



First edition 1986
Second edition 1990
Third edition 1993
Fourth edition 1997
Fifth edition 2000
Sixth edition 2004

ISBN 0 7506 8808 4

**British Library Cataloguing in Publication Data**
A catalogue record for this book is available from the British Library

**Library of Congress Cataloging in Publication Data**
A catalog record for this book is available from the Library of Congress

**Note**
Knowledge and best practice in this field are constantly changing. As new research and experience broaden our knowledge, changes in practice, treatment and drug therapy may become necessary or appropriate. Readers are advised to check the most current information provided (i) on procedures featured or (ii) by the manufacturer of each product to be administered, to verify the recommended dose or formula, the method and duration of administration, and contraindications. It is the responsibility of the practitioner, relying on their own experience and knowledge of the patient, to make diagnoses, to determine dosages and the best treatment for each individual patient, and to take all appropriate safety precautions. To the fullest extent of the law, neither the Publisher nor the author assumes any liability for any injury and/or damage.

**The Publisher**

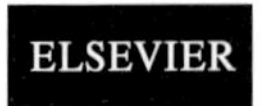

your source for books, journals and multimedia in the health sciences

**www.elsevierhealth.com**

The publisher's policy is to use **paper manufactured from sustainable forests**

Printed in China

# Contents

# Preface to the sixth edition

The continued acceptance of the *Dictionary of Optometry and Visual Science* has been very gratifying. It has now become a recommended text in most optometry courses around the world. I have felt compelled to devote much effort to the preparation of this new edition, to revise all the existing definitions, to expand many in order to include more relevant and up-to-date information and to improve the clarity wherever this was deemed necessary. The education and practice of optometry has been changing in the last few years as optometrists have become more involved in the management and co-management of some eye diseases, in addition to the traditional fields of practice. Therefore in this edition there are hundreds of new terms relating to ocular pathology, ocular pharmacology, ocular anatomy, optometric techniques, physiology and psychology of vision, contact lenses and optics.

Fifty-six new illustrations have been added and several older ones have been omitted or modified to improve their presentation. They enhance the understanding of the definitions and in many cases additional information is provided with the illustrations. 8 new tables have been added, while 5 older tables have been omitted as they were thought to have become obsolete. Tables not only summarize the written text but frequently supplement the definitions.

Overall the text now contains about 20% more material than in the last edition.

The aim of the *Dictionary of Optometry and Visual Science* remains to serve as a repository of all common terms used in this discipline and as a source of information for clinicians, students and researchers in optometry, ophthalmology, orthoptics, dispensing optics and visual science, as well as others searching for an answer to their query about the correction of visual anomalies, diseases, anatomy, physiology and optics of the eye and vision.

The entries are relatively brief and concise, although the foremost aim has been to provide the most relevant information in each definition. Thus a given disease will consist of a description of the condition including its aetiology, its main signs, symptoms and a note about its treatment. Busy practitioners and students would thus be spared the need to search through various sources for the desired information. Cross-references accompany most entries as they help the reader continue in the path of learning about a specific subject within the dictionary.

Synonyms appear at the end of many entries, as they are very common in the vocabulary of optometry. I have, however, retained the most common synonyms. They also vary from country to country. For example, stimulus deprivation amblyopia is the preferred term in the UK, whereas image degradation amblyopia is favoured in the USA.

The dictionary now contains more than 4900 terms, 83 tables and 192 illustrations and it is hoped that this new edition represents the most up-to-date and informative compilation of optometric and visual science terms available, yet in an approachable and affordable format.

I would like to thank the staff of Butterworth-Heinemann, especially Caroline Makepeace and Dr Kim Benson, for their continuous support over the years.

Tel Aviv 2004 — Michel Millodot

# About the dictionary

- The first dictionary of optometry and visual science
- More then 4900 terms
- Clear and comprehensive definitions
- 83 tables
- 192 illustrations
- Extensive cross-references
- The perfect tool for self-teaching and quick revision
- An invaluable companion to students and practitioners of optometry and all engaged in visual science

Over 4900 of the most commonly used terms in optometry and visual science are defined in this dictionary. The definitions are as clear and comprehensive as possible.

Many entries have *subentries*, in bold type letters, on subjects that are related to the main entry. In many instances they are defined there rather than repeat the definition elsewhere. The entries terminate often with the common *synonyms* (*Syn.*) and *abbreviations* and *symbols* and sometimes with a *Note*. In almost all instances there is a *cross-reference* (*See*) to help the reader continue in the path of self-teaching.

Subentries and synonyms are also given in alphabetical order as main terms but cross-referred to the entry where the definition is placed.

When a term is composed of *two or more words*, it is usually found under the noun. However, some discretion has been used and there are exceptions. These may occur when it is most likely that the reader will automatically look up the term under the adjective that appears more significant or almost generic (e.g. *base setting*, *Fresnel's formula*, *Landolt ring*, which are placed under *base*, *Fresnel's* and *Landolt* respectively). Similarly, when the noun is almost the only one of its type, while the adjective forms part of a large set of entries (e.g. *lens flare*, which is placed under *lens*). Also, when there are two or more adjectives and one of these is felt to be the most significant the term may be placed under the adjective (e.g. *Mallett fixation disparity unit* is placed under *Mallett*). However, at the alternative entry a cross-reference is given and therefore the reader knows immediately that there is a definition of that term in the dictionary.

*Abbreviations* and *symbols* are assembled in a table at the beginning of the dictionary. They have become very fashionable in the last few years, perhaps because of the widespread use of personal computers. Not all that exist are listed here; it has been necessary to try distinguishing between those that appear ephemeral and those that are destined to endure. And there is the added complication of existing differences between the common usage in different countries.

Prefixes and suffixes are frequently used in the formation of words. Thus a list of prefixes and suffixes employed in this dictionary appears at the beginning of the dictionary. It was also felt that the linguistic origin of a few of the most common terms used in the language of this discipline may be of interest. This is also given at the beginning of the dictionary.

*British spelling* has been used throughout this dictionary. However, when American spelling means that the first letter of the word is affected (e.g. *aesthesiometer*, *oedema*), both terms are noted, but the definition is placed with the British spelling.

# Abbreviations, acronyms and symbols

| | |
|---|---|
| A | ocular accommodation |
| Å | ångström unit = 0.1 nm |
| AACG | acute angle-closure glaucoma |
| AC | anterior chamber |
| AC/A | accommodative convergence/accommodation ratio |
| acc | accommodation |
| ACh | acetylcholine |
| ACG | angle-closure glaucoma |
| ACT | alternating cover test |
| add | addition for near vision |
| AFPP | apparent frontoparallel plane |
| AIDS | acquired immunodeficiency syndrome |
| AKC | atopic keratoconjunctivitis |
| AMD | age-related macular degeneration |
| amp acc | amplitude of accommodation |
| ARC | abnormal retinal correspondence |
| ARM | age-related maculopathy |
| ARMD | age-related macular degeneration |
| As | spectacle accommodation |
| Ast | astigmatism |
| A-V | arteriole–venule crossing |
| BAT | Brightness Acuity Tester |
| BC | base curve; back central radius |
| BCOD | back central optic diameter |
| BCOR | back central optic radius |
| BD | base-down (prism) |
| BE | both eyes |
| BI | base-in (prism) |
| BIO | binocular indirect ophthalmoscope |
| BO | base-out (prism) |
| BOZD | back optic zone diameter |
| BOZR | back optic zone radius |
| BP | blood pressure |
| BPR | back peripheral radius |
| BPZD | back peripheral zone diameter |
| BRAO | branch retinal arterial occlusion (*see* retinal arterial) |
| BRVO | branch retinal vein occlusion (*see* retinal vein) |
| BU | base-up (prism) |
| BUT | break-up time |
| BV | binocular vision |
| BVP | back vertex power |
| BVS | best vision sphere |
| CAB | cellulose acetate butyrate |
| CACG | chronic angle-closure glaucoma |
| CAG | closed-angle glaucoma |
| cc | chief complaint; concave; cum correctione (with correction) |
| cd | candela |
| CD | centration distance |
| C/D | cup–disc ratio |
| CDT | corneal damage threshold |
| CF | counting fingers |

| | |
|---|---|
| CFF | critical fusion frequency |
| CFT | corneal epithelial fragility threshold |
| CIE | Commission Internationale de l'Eclairage |
| CL | contact lens |
| CLAPC | contact lens-associated papillary conjunctivitis |
| CLARE | contact lens acute red eye |
| CLPC | contact lens papillary conjunctivitis |
| CMO | cystoid macular oedema |
| CNS | central nervous system |
| CNV | choroidal neovascularization |
| COR | critical oxygen requirement |
| CP | centration point |
| cpd | cycle per degree |
| CRAO | central retinal arterial occlusion |
| CRVO | central retinal vein occlusion |
| CR-39 | Columbia Resin 39 |
| CSCR | central serous chorioretinopathy |
| CSF | contrast sensitivity function |
| CSR | central serous retinopathy |
| CT | cover test |
| CTT | corneal touch threshold |
| CV | colour vision |
| CVS | computer vision syndrome |
| cyl | cylindrical power |
| cx | convex |
| D | dioptre; optical density |
| dB | decibel |
| DBL | distance between lenses |
| DBR | distance between rims |
| DCLP | Diploma in Contact Lens Practice |
| DDST | Denver Developmental Screening Test |
| dec | decentration |
| DEM | developmental eye movement test |
| *Dk* | oxygen permeability |
| *Dk/L* | oxygen transmissibility |
| *Dk/t* | oxygen transmissibility |
| DO | Diploma in Ophthalmology |
| DOMS | Diploma in Ophthalmic Medicine and Surgery |
| DOrth | Diploma in Orthoptics |
| DOS | Doctor of Ocular Science; Doctor of Optometric Science |
| DPA | diagnostic pharmaceutical agent |
| DR | diabetic retinopathy |
| DV | distance vision |
| DVD | dissociated vertical deviation |
| DVP | distance visual point |
| Dx | diagnosis |
| E | esophoria at distance; illumination |
| E′ | esophoria at near |
| ECCE | extracapsular cataract extraction (*see* cataract extraction) |
| EDTA | ethylenediamine tetraacetic acid |
| EF | eccentric fixation |
| EMG | electromyogram |
| EOG | electro-oculogram |
| EOP | equivalent oxygen pressure (*see* oxygen pressure) |
| ERG | electroretinogram |
| ERP | early receptor potential |
| eso | esophoria |
| ESOP | esophoria |
| esoT | esotropia |
| ET | esotropia at distance |
| ET′ | esotropia at near |

| | |
|---|---|
| exo | exophoria |
| exoT | exotropia |
| EW | extended wear contact lens |
| $F$ | focal power; refractive power; surface power; vergence power |
| $F_e$ | equivalent power; power of the eye |
| $F_v$ | front vertex power |
| $F'_v$ | back vertex power |
| $f$ | first focal length |
| $f'$ | second focal length |
| FAAO | Fellow of the American Academy of Optometry |
| FCOptom | Fellow of the College of Optometrists |
| fc | footcandle |
| FBOA | Fellow of the British Optical Association |
| FDP | frequency doubling perimetry |
| fL | footlambert |
| FM100 | Farnsworth-Munsell100 Hue test |
| FOH | familial ocular history |
| FOZD | front optic zone diameter |
| FCOptom | Fellow of the College of Optometrists |
| FVP | front vertex power |
| GH | general health |
| GP | gas permeable contact lens |
| GPC | giant papillary conjunctivitis |
| GPCL | gas permeable contact lens |
| GPL | gas permeable lens |
| $h$ | object height |
| $h'$ | image height |
| H | hypermetropia |
| HA | headache |
| HEMA | hydroxyethyl methacrylate |
| HGP | hard gas permeable contact lens |
| HIC | Humphriss immediate contrast test |
| HIV | human immunodeficiency virus |
| HM | hand movements |
| HRR | Hardy, Rand and Rittler colour vision test |
| Hz | hertz |
| I | luminous intensity |
| ICCE | intracapsular cataract extraction |
| ICE | iridocorneal endothelial syndrome |
| INO | internuclear ophthalmoplegia |
| IO | inferior oblique |
| IOL | intraocular lens implant |
| IOP | intraocular pressure |
| IOT | interocular transfer |
| IPD | interpupillary distance |
| IR | inferior rectus; infrared |
| J | Jaeger test type |
| K | centre corneal curvature of longest radius as measured with a keratometer; ocular refraction; spectacle refraction; degree kelvin |
| KC | keratoconus |
| KCS | keratoconjunctivitis sicca |
| KP | keratic precipitates |
| L | lambert; left; luminance; vergence |
| $l$ | object distance |
| $l'$ | image distance |
| LCA | longitudinal chromatic aberration |
| LE | left eye |
| LGB | lateral geniculate body (*see* geniculate bodies) |
| LGN | lateral geniculate nucleus |
| lm | lumen |
| LP | light perception |

| | |
|---|---|
| L/R | left hyperphoria |
| LR | lateral rectus; light reaction |
| LRK | laser refractive keratoplasty |
| LTG | low tension glaucoma |
| LVA | low vision aid |
| lx | lux |
| M | myopia; magnification |
| ma | metre angle |
| MAR | minimum angle of resolution |
| MBCO | Member of the British College of Optometrists |
| MGD | meibomian gland dysfunction |
| MPD | monocular pupillary distance |
| MR | medial rectus |
| MRI | magnetic resonance imaging |
| MS | multiple sclerosis |
| MTF | modulation transfer function |
| *n* | index of refraction |
| NAD | nothing abnormal discovered |
| NCD | near centration distance |
| NCT | Non-Contact Tonometer |
| ND | neutral density filter |
| NIBUT | non-invasive break-up time test |
| NLP | no light perception |
| nm | nanometre |
| NPC | near point of convergence |
| NPS | nearpoint stress |
| NRA | negative relative accommodation |
| NRC | normal retinal correspondence |
| NV | near vision |
| NVP | near visual point |
| OCA | Ophthalmological Congress Amsterdam notation |
| OD | Doctor of Optometry; oculus dexter; overall diameter |
| ODM | ophthalmodynamometer |
| OKN | optokinetic nystagmus |
| OS | oculus sinister; overall size |
| OU | oculus uterque |
| PAL | progressive addition lens |
| PAM | Potential Acuity Meter |
| PCCR | posterior central curve radius |
| PD | interpupillary distance; prism dioptre |
| PDR | proliferative diabetic retinopathy |
| PDT | photodynamic therapy (*see* maculopathy) |
| PHPV | persistent hyperplastic primary vitreous |
| PXF | pseudoexfoliation |
| PXS | pseudoexfoliation syndrome |
| PEK | photoelectric keratoscope; punctate epithelial keratitis |
| PERRLA | pupils equal, round and reactive to light and accommodation |
| ph | pinhole |
| pH | hydrogen ion concentration |
| PL | preferential looking |
| PMMA | polymethyl methacrylate |
| PNS | peripheral nervous system |
| POAG | primary open-angle glaucoma |
| POH | past ocular history |
| PRA | positive relative accommodation |
| PRK | photorefractive keratectomy |
| Px | patient |
| *r* | radius of curvature of a surface |
| R | right |
| RAPD | relative afferent pupillary defect (*see* pupil, Marcus Gunn) |
| RD | retinal detachment |

| | |
|---|---|
| RDS | random-dot stereogram |
| RE | right eye |
| REM | rapid eye movements |
| ret | retinoscopy |
| RGP | rigid gas permeable contact lens |
| RK | radial keratotomy |
| R/L | right hyperphoria |
| RP | retinitis pigmentosa |
| RPE | retinal pigment epithelium |
| RSM | relative spectacle magnification |
| $R_x$ | prescription |
| S | spherical power |
| SBV | single binocular vision |
| SCL | soft contact lens |
| SEAL | superior epithelial arcuate lesion (*see* staining, fluorescein) |
| SLK | superior limbic keratoconjunctivitis |
| SLO | scanning laser ophthalmoscope |
| SM | spectacle magnification |
| SMD | senile macular degeneration |
| SO | superior oblique |
| SOP | esophoria |
| SOT | esotropia |
| sph | spherical power |
| SPK | superficial punctate keratitis |
| SR | superior rectus |
| SWAP | short wavelength automated perimetry |
| TA | tonic accommodation |
| TABO | TechnischerAuschuss für Brillenoptik |
| TCA | transverse chromatic aberration |
| TD | total diameter |
| TIB | Turville Infinity Balance test |
| TNO | Technisch Natuurwetenschappelijk Onderzoek |
| $t_o$ | geometrical centre thickness (contact lens) |
| TPA | therapeutic pharmaceutical agent |
| TRIC | trachoma inclusion conjunctivitis (*see* conjunctivitis, adult inclusion) |
| TVAS | Test of Visual Analysis Skills |
| Tx | treatment |
| UV | ultraviolet |
| V | Abbé's number; constringence; vision; V-value |
| V1 | visual area 1 |
| VA | visual acuity |
| VDT | video display terminal |
| VDU | visual display unit |
| VECP | visual evoked cortical potential |
| VEP | visual evoked potential |
| VER | visual evoked response |
| VF | visual field |
| VKC | vernal keratoconjunctivitis |
| WD | working distance |
| X | exophoria at distance |
| X′ | exophoria at near |
| *x*-axis | transverse axis |
| XOP | exophoria |
| XOT | exotropia |
| XT | exotropia at distance |
| XT′ | exotropia at near |
| *y*-axis | anteroposterior axis |
| *z*-axis | vertical axis |
| $\alpha$ | angle alpha |
| $\Delta$ | prism dioptre |
| $\eta$ | stereoscopic visual acuity |

| | |
|---|---|
| θ | angle theta |
| κ | angle kappa |
| λ | angle lambda; wavelength |
| ν | frequency of light |
| ρ | reflection factor |
| ω | angle omega |
| ∞ | infinity (6 m (or 20 ft) or more) |

# Common prefixes and suffixes

| prefix | meaning | example |
|---|---|---|
| a- | not, without | aniridia (without an iris) |
| ab- | away from | abduct (turning away from midline) |
| ad- | to, towards | adduct (turning towards the midline) |
| ambi- | both | ambiocular (use either eye separately) |
| ana- | up, towards, apart | anatomy (to cut apart) |
| angi-, angio- | blood or lymph vessels | angioscotoma (scotoma due to blood vessels) |
| aniso- | unequal, dissimilar | anisophoria (variation in the amount of heterophoria) |
| anti- | against, opposed | antimetropia (opposite refraction in each eye) |
| bi- | twice, double | bifocal (two foci) |
| blephar-, blepharo- | eyelid | blepharitis (inflammation of the eyelids) |
| chrom- | colour | chromatic (pertaining to colour) |
| contra- | opposed, against | contralateral (opposite side) |
| cyano- | blue | cyanophobia (aversion to blue) |
| cycl-, cyclo- | circle | cycloduction (rotation of an eye) |
| de- | separation, reversal, deterioration | degeneration (worsening) |
| dextro- | right | dextroduction (rotation of an eye to the right) |
| deuter-, deutero- | two, second | deuteranopia (vision of two primary colours) |
| di- | two, apart | distichiasis (two rows of eyelashes) |
| dis- | apart, reversal, to separate | dispersion (separation of monochromatic components) |
| dys- | bad, difficult | dyslexia (difficulty with reading) |
| end-, endo- | within, inner | endothelium (the inner corneal layer) |
| epi- | upon, beside | episclera (upon the sclera) |
| exo- | from, out of, outside | exophthalmos (eye protruding out of the orbit) |
| extra- | outside of, beyond the scope of | extraocular (outside the eye) |
| gonio- | angle | gonioscopy (measurement of the anterior chamber angle) |
| haem- | blood | haematoma (tumour containing blood) |
| hemi- | half | hemianopsia (loss of vision in half of visual field) |
| hetero- | different, other | heterochromia (different coloured eyes) |
| hyper- | above, excessive | hyperaesthesia (above normal sensitivity) |
| hypo- | under, deficient, below | hypopyon (pus at the bottom of the anterior chamber) |
| infra- | below, under | infraduction (rotation of an eye downward) |
| inter- | between, among | interocular (between the eyes) |
| intra- | within, inside | intraocular (within the eye) |
| irid-, irido- | iris | iridoplegia (paralysis affecting the iris) |
| iso- | equal | isocoria (pupils of equal sizes) |
| kin-, kine- | movement | kinetic (pertaining to movement) |
| leuk-, leuko- | white, colourless | leukocoria (a white reflex within the pupil) |
| macro- | large, long | macropsia (large visual object) |
| meg-, mega- | large, oversize | megalophthalmos (abnormally large eye) |
| micro- | small, one millionth (1/100 000 or $10^{-6}$) | microphthalmia (very small eyeball)<br>micrometre (one millionth of a meter) |

| | | |
|---|---|---|
| milli- | one thousandth (1/1000 or $10^{-3}$) | millisecond (one thousandth of a second) |
| mono- | one, single | monocular (pertaining to one eye) |
| multi- | many | multifocal (many foci) |
| nano- | one billionth ($10^{-9}$) | nanometre (one billionth of a metre) |
| neur-, neuri-, neuro- | nerve, nervous system | neuropathy (disorder of nerves or the nervous system) |
| ocul- | eye | ocular (pertaining to the eye) |
| ophthalm- | | ophthalmia (inflammation of the eye) |
| ortho- | straight, correct, right | orthophoria (straight eyes) |
| pan- | all | panoramic vision (vision in all directions) |
| para- | beside, beyond, near, wrong | paraxial (near the axis) |
| peri- | around, near | perimetry (measurement of visual field 'around the centre') |
| phaco- | crystalline lens | phacoemulsification (a method of cataract removal) |
| phot-, photo- | light | photophobia (fear of light) |
| poly- | many | polyopia (many visual images) |
| post- | after, behind | postlenticular (behind the lens) |
| presby- | old | presbyopia (old eye) |
| pro- | before, in front of, in place of, forward | prophylaxis (prevention of a disease) projector (presentation of an image forward) |
| pseudo- | false | pseudoglaucoma (false glaucoma) |
| re- | again, backward | reflex (respond backward) |
| retro- | backward, behind | retrobulbar (behind the eye) |
| scot-, scoto- | darkness, shadow | scotoma (a dark area of the visual field) |
| sym-, syn- | together, with | symblepharon (adhesion of the bulbar and palpebral conjunctiva) |
| tele- | distant, far off | telescope (to view distant objects) |
| tono- | pressure, tension | tonometer (to measure intraocular pressure) |
| trans- | through, across | transmission (passage through) |
| tri- | three | trichromatic (three colours) |
| ultra- | beyond, extreme | ultraviolet (beyond the violet) |
| uni- | one | uniocular (one eye) |
| xanth-, xantho- | yellow | xanthelasma (yellow plaque on the eyelid) |
| xero- | dry | xerophthalmia (dryness of the cornea and conjunctiva) |

| **suffix** | **meaning** | **example** |
|---|---|---|
| -aemia | referring to blood | hyperaemia (excessive accumulation of blood) |
| -al | pertaining to, relating to | deuteranomal (pertaining to deuteranomaly) |
| -asis | condition, process | mydriasis (condition of an eye with a large pupil) |
| -cele | protrusion | descemetocele (bulging of Descemet's membrane) |
| -ectomy | excision of | iridectomy (excision of the iris) |
| -gram | recording | electro-oculogram (recording of eye movements) |
| -ia | state or condition | amblyopia (condition of reduced visual acuity) |
| -ic | pertaining to, relating to | chromatic (pertaining to colour) |
| -ism | condition, action | achromatism (being totally colour blind) |
| -ist | person or agent | orthoptist |
| -itis | inflammation | conjunctivitis (inflammation of the conjunctiva) |
| -lysis | separating, dissolution | iridodialysis (disinsertion of the iris from the ciliary body) |
| -malacia | softening | keratomalacia (an abnormally soft cornea) |
| -meter | measures | photometer (measures light) |
| -metry | process of measuring | keratometry (process of measuring the cornea) |
| -ogist | person or agent | ophthalmologist |
| -ology | science, study of, knowledge of | physiology (study of living organisms) |

| | | |
|---|---|---|
| -oma | tumour | retinoblastoma (tumour of the retina) |
| -opia | condition or defect | polyopia (many visual images) |
| -opsia | condition or defect | chromatopsia (objects appear falsely coloured) |
| -oxia | oxygen | hypoxia (state of decreased oxygen) |
| -pathy | disease | keratopathy (disease of the cornea) |
| -phobia | abnormal fear or intolerance | photophobia (abnormal fear or intolerance to light) |
| -plasty | surgical intervention | keratoplasty (corneal transplant) |
| -plegia | paralysis | ophthalmoplegia (paralysis of some ocular muscle/s) |
| -rrhaphy | suturing in place | tarsorrhaphy (suturing the eyelids) |
| -scope | instrument for examining | ophthalmoscope (examining inside the eye) |
| -scopy | act of examining | retinoscopy (process of measuring refraction) |
| -spasm | muscle contraction | blepharospasm (sudden contraction of the orbicularis muscle) |
| -tic | pertaining to | anaesthetic (pertaining to anaesthesia) |
| -tion | state or condition | perception (recognizing a percept) |
| -tomy | cutting, incision, division | keratotomy (incision of the cornea) |
| -tropia | to turn | exotropia (eye turning outward) |
| -trophy | nutrition, growth | hypertrophy (excessive growth of an organ) |

# Linguistic origin of common terms

**(G. Greek; L. Latin)**

| | |
|---|---|
| accommodation | L. *accommodatio*, adjustment |
| adaptation | L. *adaptatio*, process of adapting |
| amblyopia | G. *amblys*, dull + *ops*, eye |
| ametropia | G. *ametros*, irregular + *ops*, eye |
| aphakia | G. *a*, without + *phakos*, lens |
| asthenopia | G. *astheneia*, weakness + *ops*, eye |
| astigmatism | G. *a*, without + *stigma*, point |
| blindness | Anglo Saxon *blind* |
| cataract | L. *cataracta* or G. *katarrhaktes*, a waterfall |
| chromatism | G. *chroma*, colour |
| conjunctiva | L. *conjunctivus*, connecting |
| conjunctivitis | L. *conjunctivus* + G. *itis*, inflammation |
| cornea | L. *corneus*, horny |
| deuteranopia | G. *deuteros*, second + *a*, without + *ops*, eye |
| diplocoria | G. *diploos*, double + *kore*, pupil |
| diplopia | G. *diploos*, double + *ops*, eye |
| emmetropia | G. *emmetros*, proportioned + *ops*, eye |
| eye | Anglo Saxon *éage* |
| hemeralopia | G. *hemera*, day + *alaos*, obscure + *ops*, eye |
| heterophoria | G. *heteros*, different + *phora*, movement |
| hypermetropia | G. *hyper*, above + *metron*, measure + *ops*, eye |
| illusion | L. *illusio*, mock |
| keratitis | G. *keras*, horn + *itis*, inflammation |
| keratoplasty | G. *keras*, horn + *plasso*, to form |
| lens | L. *lentil* |
| macula | L. *a spot* |
| myopia | G. *myo*, to close + *ops*, eye |
| nyctalopia | G. *nyx*, night + *alaos*, obscure + *ops*, eye |
| nystagmus | G. *nystagmos*, a nodding |
| ophthalmic | G. *ophthalmos*, eyeball |
| ophthalmoscope | G. *ophthalmos*, eyeball + *skopeo*, to examine |
| optics | G. *optikos*, of sight |
| optometry | G. *optikos*, of sight + *metron*, measure |
| orthophoria | G. *orthos*, straight + *phora*, movement |
| orthoptics | G. *orthos*, straight + *optikos*, of sight |
| perimeter | G. *peri*, around + *metron*, measure |
| presbyopia | G. *presbys*, old man + *ops*, eye |
| pupil | L. *pupilla*, little doll |
| reflex | L. *reflecto*, to bend back |
| retina | L. *rete*, a net |
| sclera | G. *skleros*, hard |
| scotoma | G. *skotos*, darkness + *oma*, tumour |
| stereopsis | G. *stereos*, solid + *opsis*, vision |
| strabismus | G. *strabismos*, a squint |
| syndrome | G. *syn*, together + *dromos*, running |
| tritanopia | G. *tritos*, third + *a*, without + *ops*, eye |
| uvea | L. *uva*, grape |
| vision | L. *visio*, seeing |

# Acknowledgements

Many textbooks, journals, and dictionaries were used as sources for the writing of this *Dictionary of Optometry and Visual Science*. However, the following represent the primary references to which I am indebted:

D M Albert and F A Jakobiec, *Principles and Practice of Ophthalmology*, W B Saunders Co.; J F Amos, *Diagnosis and Management in Vision Care*, Butterworths; J D Bartlett and S D Jaanus, *Clinical Ocular Pharmacology*, Butterworths; W J Benjamin, *Borish's Clinical Refraction*, W B Saunders company; J Birch, *Diagnosis of Defective Color Vision*, Butterworth-Heinemann; A J Bron, R C Tripathi and B J Tripathi, *Wolff's Anatomy of the Eye and Orbit*, Chapman and Hall Medical; S E Caloroso and M W Rouse, *Clinical Management of Strabismus*, Butterworth-Heinemann; J Cronly-Dillon, *Vision and Visual Dysfunction*, 16 volumes, Macmillan Press; H Davson, *The Eye*, vols 1–4, Academic Press; C Dickinson, *Low Vision; Principles and Practice*, Butterworth-Heinemann; W A Douthwaite and M A Hurst, *Cataract*, Butterworth-Heinemann; K Edwards and R Llewellyn, *Optometry*, Butterworths; N Efron, *Contact Lens Complications*, Butterworth-Heinemann; J B Eskridge, J F Amos and J D Bartlett, *Clinical Procedures in Optometry*, J B Lippincott Company; D L Easty and J M Sparrow, *Oxford Textbook of Ophthalmology*, Oxford Medical Publications; B J W Evans, *Pickwell's Binocular Vision Anomalies*, Butterworth-Heinemann; T E Fannin and T Grosvenor, *Clinical Optics*, Butterworth-Heinemann; I Fatt and B A Weissman, *Physiology of the Eye*, Butterworth-Heinemann; E E Faye, *Clinical Low Vision*, Little Brown and Company; M H Freeman, *Optics*, Butterworth-Heinemann; B S Fine and M Yanoff, *Ocular Histology*, Harper and Row Publishers; K Gegenfurtner and L T Sharpe, *Color Vision, From Genes to Perception*, Cambridge University Press; R G Gilman, *Behavioral Optometry*, Paradox Publishing; J R Griffin and J D Grisham, *Binocular Anomalies*, Butterworth-Heinemann; T P Grosvenor, *Primary Care Optometry*, Butterworth-Heinemann; T P Grosvenor and M C Flom, *Refractive Anomalies: Research and Clinical Applications*, Butterworth-Heinemann; W M Hart, *Adler's Physiology of the Eye*, Mosby Year Book; D B Henson, *Optometric Instrumentation*, Butterworth-Heinemann; D B Henson, *Visual Fields*, Butterworth-Heinemann; M J Hogan, J A Alvarado and J E Weddell, *Histology of the Human Eye*, W B Saunders Co.; G Hopkins and R Pearson, *O'Connor Davies' Ophthalmic Drugs*, Butterworth-Heinemann; M Jalie, *The Principles of Ophthalmic Lenses*, The Association of Dispensing Opticians; J J Kanski, *Clinical Ophthalmology*, Butterworth-Heinemann; J R Larke, *The Eye in Contact Lens Wear*, Butterworth-Heinmann; S J Leat, R H Shute and C A Westall, *Assessing Children's Vision*, Butterworth-Heinemann; D D Michaels, *Visual Optics and Refraction*, The C V Mosby Co.; F W Newell, *Ophthalmology*, The C V Mosby Co.; G K von Noorden, *Binocular Vision and Ocular Motility*, The C V Mosby Co.; H Obstfeld, *Optics in Vision*, Butterworths; C W Oyster, *The Human Eye, Structure and Function*, Sinauer Associates Inc; D Pavan-Langston, *Manual of Ocular Diagnosis and Therapy*, Little, Brown and Company; A J Phillips and L Speedwell, *Contact Lenses*, Butterworth-Heinemann; R B Rabbetts, *Bennett and Rabbetts' Clinical Visual Optics*, Butterworth-Heinemann; H E Records, *Physiology of the Human Eye and Visual System*, Harper and Row, Publishers; R P Rutstein and K M Daum, *Anomalies of Binocular Vision*, The C V Mosby Co.; S H Schwartz, *Visual Perception*, Appleton and Lange; R S Snell and M A Lemp, *Clinical Anatomy of the Eye*, Blackwell Scientific Publications; W Tasman et al, *Duane's Clinical Ophthalmology*, 6 volumes, Lippincott Williams and Wilkins; D Vaughan, T Asbury and P Riordan-Eva, *General Ophthalmology*, Appleton and Lange; H J Wyatt, *Manual of Visual Anatomy and Physiology*, Professional Press Books; M Yanoff and J S Duker, *Ophthalmology*, Mosby.

I am most grateful to the following professional colleagues who have read some of the manuscript of this and earlier editions for their comments, suggestions and corrections: Dr Brian Brown, Mr Richard Earlam, Dr Daniel M Laby, Mrs Susan Millodot, Mr Len Morrison, Dr Rachel North, Mr Henri Obstfeld, Dr Ron Ofri, Ms Dinah Paritzky, Mr Ron Rabbetts, Prof Gordon Ruskell, Mr Jonathan Shapiro, Dr Avi Solomon, Dr Howard Solomons and Dr Yu Chun Pong.

Michel Millodot, 2004

# List of tables

# A



**A pattern** *See* **pattern, A.**

**abathic distance** *See* **plane, apparent frontoparallel.**

**Abbé's condenser** *See* **condenser, Abbé's.**

**Abbé's condition** *See* **sine condition.**

**Abbé's number** *See* **constringence.**

**Abbé's refractometer** *See* **refractometer.**

**abducens muscle** *See* **muscle, lateral rectus.**

**abducens nerve** *See* **nerve, abducens.**

**abducens nerve palsy** *See* **paralysis of the sixth nerve.**

**abduct** To turn away from the midline, as when the eye rotates outward.

**abduction** Outward rotation of an eye, that is away from the midline.
*See* **duction; syndrome, Duane's.**

**abductors** Extraocular muscles that move the eye outward, such as the lateral rectus, the inferior oblique and the superior oblique.
*See* **muscles, extraocular.**

**aberration** An optical defect in which the rays from a point object do not form a perfect point after passing through an optical system.
*See* **astigmatism, oblique; blur circle; coma; curvature of field; distortion.**

**aberration, axial chromatic** *See* **aberration, longitudinal chromatic.**

**aberration, lateral chromatic** Defect of an optical system (eye, lens, prism, etc.) in which the size of the image of a point object is extended by a coloured fringe, due to the unequal refraction of different wavelengths (dispersion). *Syn.* chromatic difference of magnification; transverse chromatic aberration (TCA).
*See* **dispersion; doublet.**

**aberration, longitudinal chromatic (LCA)** Defect of an optical system (eye, lens, prism, etc.) due to the unequal refraction of different wavelengths (dispersion) which results in an extended image along the optical axis. In the eye, blue rays are focused in front of the retina (by about 1 D) and red rays slightly behind the retina (0.25–0.5 D) when relaxed. When the eye is accommodated, blue rays tend to be focused near the retina and red rays are focused behind the retina (1 D). (Fig. A1) *Syn.* axial chromatic aberration.
*See* **chromoretinoscopy; chromostereopsis; constringence; dispersion; doublet; lens, achromatizing; pigment, macular; test, duochrome.**

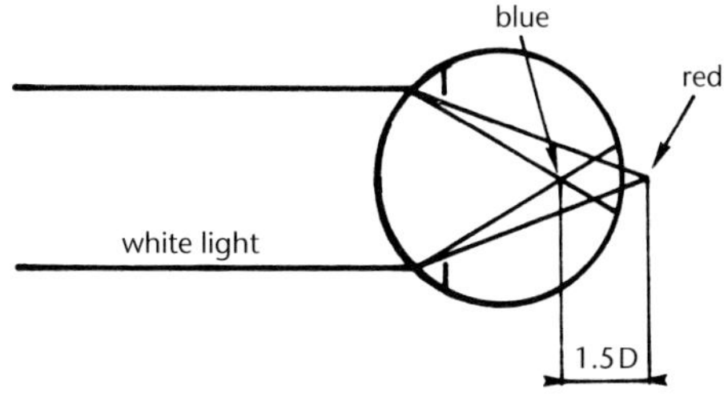


**Fig. A1** Longitudinal chromatic aberration of the eye

**aberration, monochromatic** Defect of an optical system (eye, lens, prism, etc.) occurring for a single wavelength of light. There are five such aberrations: spherical aberration, coma, curvature of field, oblique astigmatism and distortion. *Syn.* Seidel aberration.

**aberration, negative** *See* **aberration, spherical.**

**aberration, oblique** Aberration induced by a point object off the optical axis of the system. These comprise coma, curvature of field, distortion and oblique astigmatism.

**aberration, positive** *See* **aberration, spherical.**

**aberration prism** Additional effects of a prism on light, in addition to the expected change in direction of light. These effects include different magnifications, curvature of field and chromatic aberration.

**aberration, Seidel** *See* **aberration, monochromatic.**

**aberration, spherical** Defect of an optical system due to a variation in the focusing between peripheral and paraxial rays. The larger the pupil size, the greater the difference in focusing between the two rays. In the gaussian theory, the focus of the optical system is attributed to the paraxial rays. The distance, in dioptres, between the focus of the paraxial rays and the peripheral rays represents the amount of **longitudinal spherical aberration** of the system. When the peripheral rays are refracted more than the paraxial rays, the aberration is said to be **positive** or **undercorrected**. When the peripheral

rays are refracted less than the paraxial rays the aberration is said to be **negative** or **over-corrected**. The relaxed human eye has a small amount of positive spherical aberration (up to 1 D for a pupil of 8 mm diameter). (Fig. A2)
*See* **caustic; lens, aplanatic; theory, gaussian.**

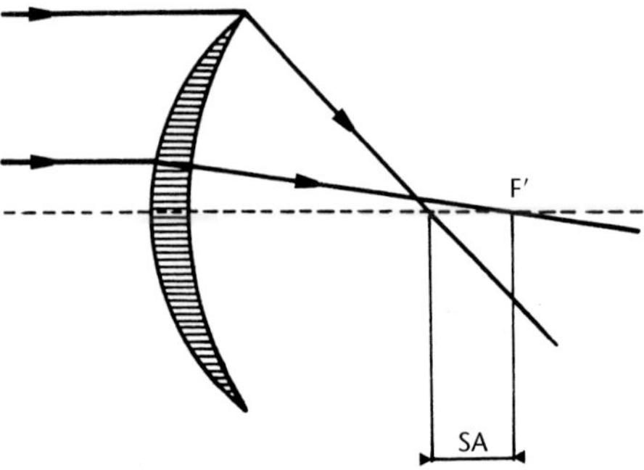


**Fig. A2** Spherical aberration of the eye. Two parallel rays coming from infinity are focused, one at F′ the secondary focal point corresponding to paraxial rays and the other peripheral ray in front or behind F′, depending on the type of spherical aberration. It is positive in this illustration (SA, longitudinal spherical aberration).

**aberration, transverse chromatic** *See* **aberration, lateral chromatic.**

**aberration, wavefront** The amount of deviation between an output wavefront emanating from an optical system and a conceptualized ideal (reference) wavefront. The specification of the deviation (or error) is usually fitted with a normalized Zernike expansion. The measurement of this aberration can be done subjectively or objectively (e.g. with an aberrometer based on the Hartmann-Shack principle). The method (called **aberrometry**) has been applied clinically to measure the aberrations displayed by optical systems, such as the eye, the eye with a correction, contact lenses (in vitro or in situ), intraocular lenses (in vitro or in situ), in corneal refractive surgery, cataract, etc. (Fig. A3). *Syn.* wavefront error.
*See* **wavefront.**

**Table A1** Aberrations of the eye

A Chromatic aberrations:
longitudinal (or axial): chromatic difference of focus
transverse (or lateral): chromatic difference of magnification

B Monochromatic aberrations (or Seidel aberrations):

| type | direction | stimulus |
|---|---|---|
| 1. spherical aberration | longitudinal transverse | light beam passing through large pupil |
| 2. coma | transverse | points objects off the optical axis |
| 3. oblique astigmatism | longitudinal | points objects off the optical axis |
| 4. curvature | longitudinal | extended objects of field |
| 5. distortion | transverse | extended objects |
| 6. wavefront aberration | transverse | extended objects |

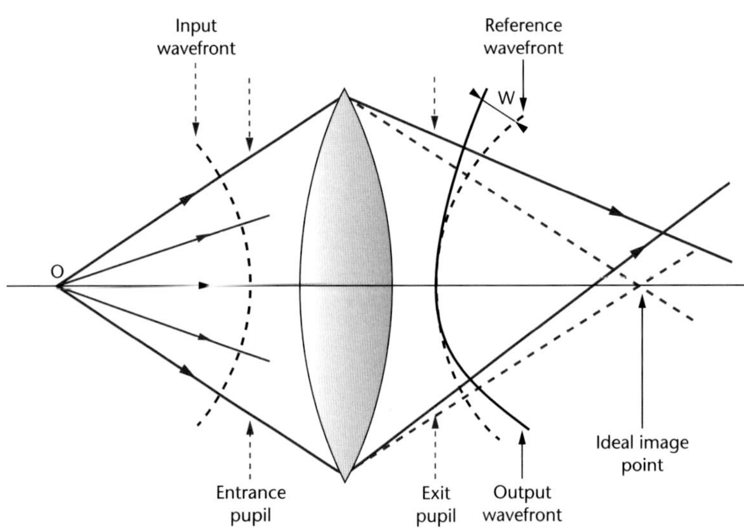


**Fig. A3** An input spherical wavefront of light is centred on object O. After emerging from a lens affected by monochromatic aberration, it is no longer spherical and the image-forming rays do not meet in the single ideal image point (the paraxial image). The wavefront aberration W is the distance between the ideal reference wavefront and the actual output wavefront at various distances from the optical axis

**aberrometry** *See* **aberration, wavefront.**

**aberroscope** Instrument for observing aberration. Such an instrument was designed by Tscherning to measure his own spherical aberration. It consists of a planoconvex lens with a grid made up of squares ruled on its plane surface.

**ablatio retinae** *See* **retinal detachment.**

**ablation** A procedure in which a tissue or body part is removed or destroyed by surgery, radiation or photocoagulation. *Example:* LASIK.
*See* **LASIK.**

**ablepharon** *See* **ablephary.**

**ablephary** Congenital absence, complete or partial, of the eyelids. *Syn.* ablepharon.

**ablepsia** *See* **blindness.**

**ablepsy** *See* **blindness.**

**Abney's law; phenomenon** *See* under the nouns.

**abnormal (anomalous) retinal correspondence** *See* **retinal correspondence, abnormal.**

**abrasion, corneal** *See* **corneal abrasion.**

**abscess** An accumulation of pus located in infected tissue.
*See* **ulcer.**

**absorbance** *See* **density, optical; factor, absorption.**

**absorption** Transformation of radiant energy into a different form of energy, usually heat, as it passes through a medium. Light that is absorbed is neither transmitted nor reflected. It may, however, be re-emitted as light of another wavelength as, for example, ultraviolet radiation is converted into visible radiation on absorption by a luminescent material. A substance that absorbs all radiations is called a black body.
*See* **body, black; density, optical; factor, absorption; fluorescence; transmission.**

**absorption factor** *See* **factor, absorption.**

**absorptive lens** *See* **lens, absorptive.**

**AC/A ratio** Ratio of the accommodative convergence AC (in prism dioptres) to the stimulus to accommodation A (in dioptres). The most common method of determining this ratio is by the **gradient method** (or **gradient test**) in which the phoria at near is measured after changing the accommodation with a spherical lens (usually +1.00 D or −1.00 D) placed in front of the two eyes. It is expressed as

$$\frac{AC}{A} = \frac{\alpha - \alpha'}{F}$$

where $\alpha$ is the phoria at near, and $\alpha'$ is the phoria at the same distance but through a lens of power F. The deviation is measured in prism dioptres, with + for esodeviation and − for exodeviation. *Example*: if the initial phoria is 4 Δ exo and 8 Δ exo when a lens of +1.00 D is placed in front of the eyes, the AC/A ratio is equal to $[-4 - (-8)]/1 = 4\,\Delta/D$. The average AC/A ratio is about 4 in young adults and tends to decline slightly with age. The gradient is not affected by proximal convergence, as the target distance and size are relatively constant. *Syn.* gradient.
Another method of determining the AC/A ratio (often called the heterophoria method) compares the phoria measured at distance and at near. It is expressed as

$$\frac{AC}{A} = PD + \frac{N - D}{K}$$

where PD is the interpupillary distance in cm, N the deviation at near, D the deviation at distance and K the near fixation distance in dioptres. *Example*: A patient has a PD of 70 mm, a distance phoria of 4 Δ eso and a near phoria of 8 Δ exo at 33.3 cm from the eyes, the AC/A ratio is equal to

$$7.0 + \frac{[-8 - (+4)]}{3} = \frac{3\,\Delta}{D}$$

*See* **convergence, accommodative; convergence, proximal; diopter, prism.**

**acanthamoeba keratitis** *See* **keratitis, acanthamoeba.**

**acanthocytosis** *See* **syndrome, Bassen–Kornzweig.**

**accessory lacrimal glands** *See* **glands, accessory lacrimal; glands of Krause; glands of Wolfring.**

**accommodation** Adjustment of the dioptric power of the eye. It is generally involuntary and made to see clearly objects at any distance. In man, this adjustment is brought about by a change in the shape of the crystalline lens.
*See* **aniso-accommodation; muscle, ciliary; reflex, accommodative; theory, Fincham's; theory, Helmholtz's of accommodation.**

**accommodation, amplitude of** The maximum amount of accommodation A which the eye can exert. It is expressed in dioptres, as the difference between the far point and the near point measured with respect either to the spectacle plane or the corneal apex or some other reference point. Thus,

$$A = K - B,$$

where B is the near point vergence and K is the far point vergence. A is always positive. In the emmetropic eye, A = −B, because the far point is at infinity and K = 0. So, if the near point of an emmetrope is at 25 cm from the spectacle plane, the amplitude of accommodation is equal to $-[-1/(25 \times 10^{-2})] = 4\,D$. The amplitude of accommodation declines from about 14 D at age 10 to about 0.5 D at age 60 (although the measured value is usually higher due to the depth of focus of the eye).

a

*See* **depth of focus; dioptre; method, minus lens; method, push-up; presbyopia; vergence.**

**Table A2** Mean amplitude of accommodation as a function of age, in Caucasians (the plane of reference is the spectacle plane)

| age (years) | Duane (*N* = 2000 subjects, push-up method) | Turner (*N* = 500 subjects, push-out method) |
|---|---|---|
| 10 | 13.5 | 13.0 |
| 15 | 12.5 | 10.6 |
| 20 | 11.5 | 9.5 |
| 25 | 10.5 | 7.9 |
| 30 | 8.9 | 6.6 |
| 35 | 7.3 | 5.75 |
| 40 | 5.9 | 4.4 |
| 45 | 3.7 | 2.5 |
| 50 | 2.0 | 1.6 |
| 55 | 1.3 | 1.1 |
| 60 | 1.2 | 0.7 |
| 65 | 1.1 | 0.6 |
| 70 | 1.0 | 0.6 |

**accommodation, astigmatic** Postulated unequal accommodation along different meridians of the eye attributed to a differential action of the ciliary muscle which would lead to a difference in the curvature of the surfaces of the crystalline lens along different meridians. *Syn.* meridional accommodation.

**accommodation, closed-loop** Accommodation response to visual stimuli in normal viewing conditions.
*See* **accommodation, open-loop.**

**accommodation, components of** The process of accommodation is assumed to involve four components: reflex, vergence, proximal and tonic accommodation (also called resting state of accommodation).
*See* **accommodation, convergence; accommodation, proximal; accommodation, reflex; accommodation, resting state of.**

**accommodation, consensual** Accommodation occurring in one eye when the other eye has received the dioptric stimulus.

**accommodation, convergence 1.** Accommodation induced directly by a change in convergence. **2.** That component of accommodation induced by the binocular disparity of the retinal images. *Syn.* vergence accommodation.
*See* **disparity, retinal.**

**accommodation, correction induced** Ocular accommodation induced when changing from spectacles to contact lenses in near vision. Spectacles induce less accommodation in myopes and more accommodation in hyperopes than that exerted by an emmetrope fixating at a given distance. Contact lenses do not induce any different accommodation than that required for a given distance. Consequently, myopes require more accommodation and hyperopes less accommodation when they transfer from spectacles to contact lenses. However, this change in accommodation is accompanied by a similar change in convergence, so that a myope transferring to contact lenses accommodates and converges more than with spectacles and the reverse applies for a hyperope.
*See* **convergence, correction induced.**

**accommodation, far point of** A point in space conjugate with the retina (more specifically the foveola) when the accommodation is relaxed. In emmetropia, the far point is at infinity; in myopia, it is at a finite distance in front of the eye; in hypermetropia, it is a virtual point behind the eye (Fig. A4). *Syn.* far point of the eye; punctum remotum.
*See* **sphere, far point.**

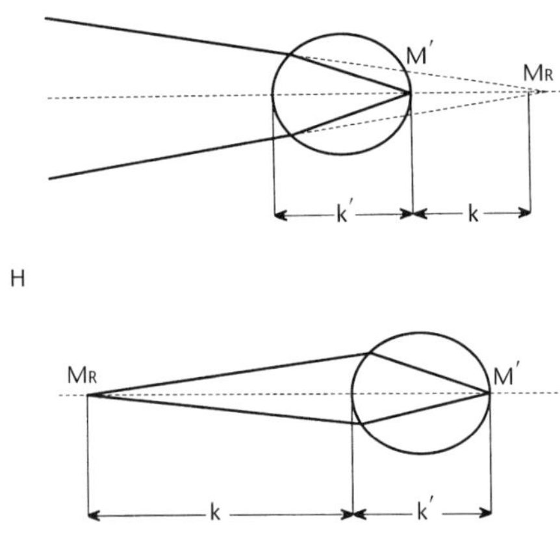


**Fig. A4** A hypermetropic eye H and a myopic eye M, fixating an object at the far point $M_R$

**accommodation, ill-sustained** *See* **accommodative insufficiency.**

**accommodation, insufficiency of** *See* **accommodative insufficiency.**

**accommodation, lag of 1.** The amount by which the accommodative response of the eye is less than the dioptric stimulus to accommodation. *Syn.* lazy lag of accommodation. **2.** The condition occurring in dynamic retinoscopy in which the neutral point is situated further from the eyes than is the retinoscopic target.
*See* **muscle, ciliary; retinoscopy, dynamic.**

**accommodation, lead of** The amount by which the accommodative response of the eye is greater than the dioptric stimulus to accommodation.
*See* **accommodation, lag of.**

**accommodation, mechanism of** Process by which the eye focuses onto an object. It does so by contracting the ciliary muscle which releases the tension on the zonular fibres allowing the elastic lens capsule to increase its curvature, especially that of the front surface. Along with these changes are an increase in the thickness of the lens, a decrease in its equatorial diameter and a reduction in pupil size. The ciliary muscle is controlled by the parasympathetic system which is triggered by an out of focus retinal image.
*See* **accommodation, convergence; accommodation, proximal; accommodative response; muscle, ciliary; reflex, accommodative.**

**accommodation, meridional** *See* **accommodation, astigmatic.**

**accommodation, microfluctuations of** Involuntary variations in the contraction of the intraocular muscles responsible for accommodation and resulting in changes of about 0.1–0.5 D with a frequency of 0.5–2.5 Hz.

**accommodation, near point of** The nearest point in space which is conjugate with the foveola when exerting the maximum accommodative effort. *Syn.* punctum proximum.
*See* **method, push-up; rule, near point; sphere, near point; test, Scheiner's.**

**accommodation, negative 1.** A relaxation of accommodation below the apparent zero level or when shifting from near to distance vision. **2.** *See* **accommodation, relative amplitude of.**

**accommodation, objective** Accommodation measured without the subject's judgement. This is accomplished by dynamic retinoscopy, by autorefractors or by visually evoked cortical potentials. The term is sometimes used incorrectly to refer to the amplitude of accommodation without the influence of the depth of focus (e.g. as measured by stigmatoscopy).
*See* **accommodation, subjective; optometer; potential, evoked cortical; retinoscopy, dynamic; stigmatoscopy.**

**accommodation, ocular** The amplitude of accommodation referred to the front surface of the cornea. *Symbol:* A.
*See* **accommodation, spectacle.**

**accommodation, open-loop** Accommodative response occurring without the usual stimulus to accommodation, such as a blurred retinal image. In these conditions, the accommodative system of the eye tends to return to its position of rest (or tonic accommodation). *Examples*: looking at an empty field; looking through a very small artificial pupil (0.5 mm or less).
*See* **accommodation, closed-loop.**

**accommodation, paralysis of** Total or partial loss of accommodation due to paralysis of the ciliary muscle.
*See* **muscle, ciliary.**

**accommodation, positive** Normal accommodation that occurs when looking from a distant to a near object.

**accommodation, proximal** That component of accommodation initiated by the awareness of a near object. *Syn.* psychic accommodation.
*See* **accommodation, reflex; accommodation, resting state of; accommodation, vergence; convergence, proximal.**

**accommodation, psychic** *See* **accommodation, proximal.**

**accommodation, range of** The linear distance between the far point and the near point. Part of the range of accommodation is virtual in the case of the hypermetrope.

**accommodation, relative amplitude of** The total amount of accommodation which the eye can exert while the convergence of the eyes is fixed. It can be **positive** (using concave lenses until the image blurs). This is called positive relative accommodation (PRA). It can be **negative** (using convex lenses until the image blurs). This is negative relative accommodation (NRA).
*See* **zone of clear, single, binocular vision.**

**accommodation, reserve** *See* **addition, near.**

**accommodation, resting state of** The passive state of accommodation of the eye in the absence of a stimulus, i.e. when the eye is either in complete darkness, or looking at a bright empty field. In this condition, the pre-presbyopic eye is usually focused at an intermediate point (about 80 cm on average, although there are large variations), that is, the emmetropic eye becomes myopic. This is presumably due to a balance between a parasympathetic innervation to the circular fibres of the ciliary muscle and a sympathetic innervation to the longitudinal fibres of the ciliary muscle. Thus, the resting state of accommodation would correspond to a position of equilibrium between the two systems. Accommodation from this state to the near point of accommodation would be the response to parasympathetic stimulation; and accommodation from this state to the far point of accommodation would be the response to sympathetic stimulation. *Syn.* dark accommodation; dark focus (these terms are not strictly synonymous but as they have been found to correlate well,

they have been adopted as synonyms); tonic accommodation (TA).
*See* **hysteresis, accommodative; muscle, ciliary; myopia, instrument; myopia, night; myopia, space; tonus; vergence, tonic.**

**accommodation, spasm of** Involuntary contraction of the ciliary muscle producing excess accommodation. It may be constant, intermittent, unilateral or bilateral. Patients typically complain of blurred distance vision and sometimes changes in perceived size of objects, and discomfort. If the patient is a low hyperope or emmetrope, it will give rise to **pseudomyopia** (or **false myopia** or **hypertonic myopia** or **spurious myopia**). Diagnosis is facilitated by cycloplegic refraction. Management includes removal of the primary cause, if possible (e.g. uveitis, or patient taking parasympathomimetic drugs), correction of the underlying refraction, if any, changes in the visual working conditions, positive lenses, accommodative facility exercises and only rarely cycloplegics.
*See* **accommodative facility; metamorphopsia.**

**accommodation, spectacle** The amplitude of accommodation referred to the spectacle plane. *Symbol*: $A_s$.
*See* **accommodation, ocular.**

**accommodation, subjective** Measurement of the accommodation based on the subject's judgements, such as the push-up or push-out method or the minus lens method.
*See* **accommodation, objective; method, minus lens; method, push-up.**

**accommodation, tonic** *See* **accommodation, resting state of.**

**accommodation, vergence** *See* **accommodation, convergence.**

**accommodative astigmatism** *See* **astigmatism, accommodative.**

**accommodative convergence** *See* **convergence, accommodative.**

**accommodative convergence/accommodation ratio** *See* **AC/A ratio.**

**accommodative excess** A condition in which the subject exerts more accommodation than required for the visual stimulus, or is unable to relax accommodation. It may be due to uncorrected hypermetropia, very prolonged near work, emotional problems, spasm of accommodation, uveitis, trigeminal neuralgia, syphilis, meningitis, head trauma, or the side effect of some pharmaceutical agent (e.g. a miotic drug). It is usually associated with convergence excess. The subject reports blurred vision at distance, asthenopia and often headaches. Treatment commonly includes plus lenses and facility exercises, besides therapy of the underlying cause. *Syn.* hyperaccommodation. *Note*: spasm of accommodation is one aspect of the general condition of accommodative excess, although some authors consider this term a synonym.
*See* **accommodation, spasm of; accommodative facility; convergence excess.**

**accommodative esotropia** A form of convergence of the visual axes (esodeviation) related to the process of accommodation. It is usually an acquired ocular deviation first presenting in the first decade of life. Children usually do not notice diplopia, but instead develop suppression, and later amblyopia. There may be a genetic predisposition to this condition. It is generally subdivided into four types: those associated with high hyperopia (refractive accommodative esotropia), those caused by an increased accommodative convergence to accommodation ratio (AC/A ratio), those presenting as a mixture of an accommodative esodeviation and a basic esodeviation and finally, those cases of previously controlled esodeviations which have deteriorated to constant esotropia.
*See* **refraction, cycloplegic.**

**accommodative facility** Ability of the eye/s to focus on stimuli at various distances and in different sequences in a given period of time. Clinically, this is measured either monocularly or binocularly usually by having the subject fixate a small target alternately through plus and minus lenses which are interchanged as soon as the target appears clear. The operation is repeated many times and the results are commonly presented in cycles per minute (one cycle indicates that both plus and minus lenses have been cleared). *Syn.* accommodative rock.
*See* **accommodative insufficiency; lens flippers.**

**accommodative inertia** Difficulty in altering the accommodative response, such that the latency and completion time of the process are delayed. It may occur as a result of prolonged near vision tasks. Orthoptic exercises may help in this condition.

**accommodative hysteresis** *See* **hysteresis, accommodative.**

**accommodative infacility** A condition in which there is a slowness in changing from one level of accommodation to another. Patients may complain of transitory blur. It may be due to diabetes, Graves' disease, measles or the side effects of some drugs. It is commonly associated with asthenopia. Treatment is aimed at the primary cause, but plus lenses and, especially, accommodative facility exercises are usually prescribed.
*See* **accommodative facility.**

a

**Table A3** Relationship between viewing distance and spectacle and ocular accommodation of a contact lens wearer and of 4 corrected hypermetropes (with thin spectacle lenses). The vertex distance was 14 mm and ocular accommodation was calculated using the formula A = K − B. The ocular accommodation exerted by a contact lens wearer is the same for all refractive errors and equal to that of an emmetrope

| distance from spectacle lens (cm) | spectacle accom. (D) | ocular accom. (D) of contact lens wearer | ocular accom. (D) of hypermetropes | | | |
|---|---|---|---|---|---|---|
| | | | +2 | +4 | +6 | +8 |
| 100 | 1.00 | 0.99 | 1.04 | 1.11 | 1.17 | 1.25 |
| 67 | 1.49 | 1.46 | 1.55 | 1.64 | 1.74 | 1.86 |
| 50 | 2.00 | 1.95 | 2.06 | 2.18 | 2.31 | 2.46 |
| 40 | 2.50 | 2.42 | 2.55 | 2.71 | 2.87 | 3.05 |
| 33 | 3.03 | 2.91 | 3.07 | 3.25 | 3.45 | 3.67 |
| 25 | 4.00 | 3.79 | 4.00 | 4.24 | 4.49 | 4.77 |
| 20 | 5.00 | 4.67 | 4.94 | 5.22 | 5.54 | 5.88 |
| 16 | 6.25 | 5.75 | 6.07 | 6.42 | 6.80 | 7.22 |
| 14 | 7.14 | 6.49 | 6.86 | 7.25 | 7.68 | 8.14 |
| 12 | 8.33 | 7.46 | 7.88 | 8.32 | 8.81 | 9.34 |
| 10 | 10.00 | 8.77 | 9.25 | 9.77 | 10.34 | 10.95 |

**Table A4** Relationship between viewing distance and spectacle and ocular accommodation of a contact lens wearer and of 5 corrected myopes (with thin spectacle lenses). The vertex distance was 14 mm and ocular accommodation was calculated using the formula A = K − B. The ocular accommodation exerted by a contact lens wearer is the same for all refractive errors and equal to that of an emmetrope

| distance from spectacle lens (cm) | spectacle accom. (D) | ocular accom. (D) of contact lens wearer | ocular accom. (D) of myopes | | | | |
|---|---|---|---|---|---|---|---|
| | | | −4 | −6 | −8 | −10 | −12 |
| 100 | 1.00 | 0.99 | 0.89 | 0.84 | 0.80 | 0.76 | 0.72 |
| 67 | 1.49 | 1.46 | 1.31 | 1.25 | 1.18 | 1.13 | 1.07 |
| 50 | 2.00 | 1.95 | 1.75 | 1.66 | 1.58 | 1.50 | 1.43 |
| 40 | 2.50 | 2.42 | 2.17 | 2.06 | 1.96 | 1.87 | 1.78 |
| 33 | 3.03 | 2.91 | 2.61 | 2.48 | 2.36 | 2.25 | 2.14 |
| 25 | 4.00 | 3.79 | 3.41 | 3.24 | 3.08 | 2.93 | 2.80 |
| 20 | 5.00 | 4.67 | 4.21 | 4.00 | 3.80 | 3.62 | 3.46 |
| 16 | 6.25 | 5.75 | 5.18 | 4.92 | 4.69 | 4.47 | 4.26 |
| 14 | 7.14 | 6.49 | 5.85 | 5.57 | 5.30 | 5.05 | 4.82 |
| 12 | 8.33 | 7.46 | 6.73 | 6.40 | 6.10 | 5.82 | 5.55 |
| 10 | 10.00 | 8.77 | 7.92 | 7.54 | 7.18 | 6.85 | 6.55 |

**accommodative insufficiency** Insufficient amplitude of accommodation which is unequivocally below the appropriate level for the age. It may be due to extreme fatigue, influenza, high stress, systemic medication, ocular inflammation, head trauma, thyroid disease or the juvenile form of diabetes mellitus. The condition is often associated with convergence insufficiency, general fatigue, measles, multiple sclerosis, or myotonic dystrophy, etc. It is the most common accommodative dysfunction. Patients complain of blurred vision, or difficulty in sustaining clear vision at near; this is often accompanied by a frontal headache and even sometimes by pain in the eye. A mild form of convergence insufficiency is often referred to as **ill-sustained accommodation** in which the response may be initially normal but cannot be maintained. It is easily discovered with accommodative facility exercises. Ill-sustained accommodation may be a precursor of accommodative insufficiency. Treatment is aimed at the primary cause, but plus lens correction, and in some cases exercises such as accommodative facility training are prescribed. *Syn.* premature presbyopia.
*See* **accommodative facility; convergence insufficiency; headache, ocular; ophthalmopathy, thyroid; presbyopia.**

**accommodative reflex** *See* **reflex, accommodative.**

**accommodative response** The response of the accommodative system when the eye changes fixation from one point in space to another. The reaction time for the accommodative response is

about 370 ms. Clinically it can be estimated by measuring the accommodative lag or accommodative lead.
*See* **accommodation, lag of; accommodation, mechanism of; effect, Mandelbaum; reflex, accommodative.**

**accommodative rock** *See* **accommodative facility.**

**accommodometer** Instrument used to measure accommodation such as the near point rule.
*See* **rule, near point.**

**acetazolamide** *See* **carbonic anhydrase inhibitors; glaucoma, open-angle.**

**acetone** Liquid ketone (dimethyl ketone and propanone) used as a solvent for many organic compounds (e.g. cellulose acetate) and for repairing spectacle frames.

**acetylcholine (ACh)** Neurohumoral transmitter with special excitatory properties of all preganglionic autonomic nerve fibres, all parasympathetic post-ganglionic fibres, a few post-ganglionic sympathetic fibres and motor fibres to skeletal muscles. Acetylcholine is synthesized and liberated by the action of the enzyme choline acetylase which occurs in all cholinergic nerves. Acetylcholine exists only momentarily after its formation, being hydrolysed by the enzyme **acetylcholinesterase** which is present in the neurons of cholinergic nerves throughout their entire lengths and at neuromuscular junctions. The alkaloid **muscarine** has pharmacological actions that are similar to many of the actions of acetylcholine at the parasympathetic neuroeffector sites only. **Antimuscarinic drugs** (also referred to as **anticholinergics** or **parasympatholytics**) such as atropine, cyclopentolate, homatropine, hyoscine and tropicamide antagonize this muscarinic action.
*See* **atropine; cholinergic; cyclopentolate; cycloplegia; homatropine; hyoscine; miotics; mydriatic; nicotine; pilocarpine; synapse.**

**acetylcholinesterase** An enzyme that degrades and inactivates acetylcholine. This compound is mainly found in neurons and at neuro-muscular junctions. Drugs that inhibit this enzyme (e.g. diisopropyl fluorophosphate, physostigmine, edrophonium, echothiophate, DFP) can be used in the diagnosis and possible treatment of myasthenia gravis as well as certain forms of esotropia and glaucoma. *Syn.* specific cholinesterase.
*See* **acetylcholine.**

**achromasia** *See* **achromatopsia.**

**achromat** *See* **lens, achromatic.**

**achromatic 1.** *See* **lens, achromatic. 2.** The condition of being totally colour blind.
*See* **achromatopsia; light, white; spectrum, equal energy.**

**achromatic axis; colour; interval; lens** *See* under the nouns.

**achromatic light stimulus, specified** Any specified illuminant capable of being accepted as white under usual conditions of observation. *Note*: This includes the CIE standard illuminants (CIE).
*See* **illuminants, CIE standard.**

**achromatic prism** *See* **prism, achromatic.**

**achromatism 1.** The condition of being totally colour blind. *Syn.* achromatopsia. **2.** Absence of colour. **3.** Condition of a lens or an optical system corrected for, or free from, chromatic aberration.
*See* **monochromat.**

**achromatizing lens** *See* **lens, achromatizing.**

**achromatopsia** Total colour blindness. *Syn.* achromasia; achromatic vision; achromatism; acritochromacy; monochromatism.
*See* **colour vision, defective; monochromat.**

**acinar cell** *See* **cell, acinar.**

**acne rosacea** A chronic inflammatory disease of the sebaceous glands of the skin of the face. It usually appears in middle-aged individuals. Nearly a third of these patients have blepharoconjunctivitis with staphylococcal infection and a few per cent will develop rosacea keratitis. The patient presents with papules, pustules, erythema, telangiectasia and in some cases, rhinophyma, as well as facial erythema. Treatment includes lid hygiene with hot compresses, removal of crusts from the lid margins, and topical and systemic antibiotics.
*See* **blepharitis, marginal; keratitis, rosacea.**

**Acquired Immune Deficiency Syndrome (AIDS)** *See* **syndrome, acquired immune deficiency.**

**acorea** Absence of the pupil of the eye.

**acritochromacy** *See* **achromatopsia.**

**actinic** Pertaining to the chemical activity of radiant energy (especially ultraviolet) on absorption by certain substances. In the eye, the cornea, in particular, but also the lens and retina are most susceptible.
*See* **blindness, eclipse; retinopathy, solar.**

**actinic keratoconjunctivitis; keratopathy** *See* under the nouns.

**action spectrum** *See* **spectrum, action.**

**active position; transport** *See* under the nouns.

**acuity, angular visual** *See* **acuity, monotype visual.**

**acuity cards, Teller** Test cards used to assess the visual acuity of infants. The set consists of 16 rectangular grey cards, each approximately 26 by 56 cm. Fifteen of the cards contain a high contrast square-wave grating, 12 by 12 cm, each of a given spatial frequency, and located either on the left or the right of a central peephole in the card. The average luminance of the grating is approximately equal to that of the grey background. The spatial frequencies of the gratings range from 0.3 to 38 cpd when viewed from 55 cm. The procedure consists in starting with the card with the lowest spatial frequency (or coarser grating) and proceeding to cards with finer gratings. The observer watches the infant through the central peephole and his or her task is to make a subjective judgement, based on the infant's head and eye movements, of which is the finest grating card that the child can just resolve. The spatial frequency of this last card represents the estimate of the visual acuity. The procedure using these cards is based on the method of preferential looking but it is simpler, quicker and equally reliable.
*See* **cycle per degree; method, preferential looking.**

**Table A5** Average relative visual acuity in the central region of the retina

| eccentricity (degrees) | acuity (%) | Snellen fraction (m) | Snellen fraction (ft) |
|---|---|---|---|
| 0 | 100 | 6/6 | 20/20 |
| 0.5 | 80 | 6/7.5 | 20/25 |
| 1 | 66 | 6/9 | 20/30 |
| 1.5 | 57 | 6/11 | 20/37 |
| 2 | 49 | 6/12 | 20/40 |
| 2.5 | 41 | 6/14.5 | 20/48 |
| 3 | 39 | 6/15 | 20/50 |
| 3.5 | 37 | 6/16 | 20/53 |
| 4 | 35 | 6/17 | 20/57 |
| 4.5 | 33 | 6/18 | 20/60 |
| 5 | 32 | 6/19 | 20/63 |
| 6 | 29 | 6/21 | 20/70 |
| 7 | 27 | 6/22 | 20/73 |

**acuity, central visual** Visual acuity of the fovea and the macular area.
*See* **fixation, eccentric; macula lutea.**

**acuity, decimal visual** Visual acuity expressed as a decimal. The Snellen fraction is reduced, e.g. 6/18 (or 20/60 in feet) = 0.33. If the acuity is given in visual angle, decimal acuity is the reciprocal, e.g. 1/(3 minutes of arc) = 0.33.
*See* **acuity, visual; Snellen fraction.**

**acuity, dynamic visual** Capacity to see distinctly moving objects. *Syn.* kinetic visual acuity.

**acuity, kinetic visual** *See* **acuity, dynamic visual.**

**acuity, letter visual 1.** Visual acuity determined with letters on a chart. **2.** Visual acuity determined with single isolated letters.
*See* **acuity, morphoscopic visual.**

**acuity, line visual** *See* **acuity, morphoscopic visual.**

**acuity, minimum separable visual** *See* **acuity, visual.**

**acuity, monotype visual** Visual acuity determined with single isolated optotypes and therefore uninfluenced by neighbouring contours. *Syn.* acuity, angular visual.
*See* **acuity, morphoscopic visual; optotype.**

**acuity, morphoscopic visual** Visual acuity determined with a group of optotypes such as, for example, a line of letters or Landolt rings. The result may thus be influenced by neighbouring contours. *Syn.* line visual acuity.
*See* **acuity, letter visual; acuity, monotype visual; acuity, visual; phenomenon, crowding.**

**acuity, near visual** Capacity for seeing distinctly the details of an object at near. It is specified in various ways: (1) As the angle of resolution of the smallest resolvable print (in minutes of arc) at a given near distance. (2) As a Snellen fraction, either as one which is equivalent to the distance visual acuity (**Snellen equivalent**) or more correctly as one which indicates the actual distance (e.g. 16/32 if the distance is 16 inches). (3) As an arbitrary Jaeger notation (e.g. J6). (4) As **N notation** (using Times Roman typeface) or **Points** (using any typeface), such as N8 at 40 cm (or simply 8-point), where N refers to near and the number to the amount of points (a point is a unit used by printers to specify print size and is equal to 1/72 of an inch). Thus N8 indicates that the overall height is 8/72 inch (or 2.82 mm) or about 4/72 inch (or 1.41 mm) for lower-case letters. (5) As **M Units**. For the usual font styles (e.g. Times Roman, Century) used in newsprint, 8-point print is usually considered to be approximately equal to 1M Unit, so M units = points/8 or 1M = N8, 2M = N16, etc.
*See* **acuity, visual; chart, Bailey–Lovie; Jaeger test types.**

**acuity, objective visual** Visual acuity measured without the subject's judgement.
*See* **potential, visual evoked cortical; method, preferential looking; test, optokinetic nystagmus.**

**acuity, peripheral visual** Visual acuity of the peripheral regions of the retina, outside the macula.

a

Table A6 Relationship between several near visual acuity notations

| Snellen equivalent in metres (feet) | | | |
|---|---|---|---|
| 25 cm | 40 cm | Points | M units |
| 6/240 (20/800) | 6/144 (20/480) | 80 | 10.0 |
| 6/192 (20/640) | 6/120 (20/400) | 64 | 8.0 |
| 6/144 (20/480) | 6/96 (20/320) | 48 | 6.4 |
| 6/120 (20/400) | 6/72 (20/240) | 40 | 4.8 |
| 6/96 (20/320) | 6/60 (20/200) | 32 | 4.0 |
| 6/72 (20/240) | 6/48 (20/160) | 24 | 3.2 |
| 6/60 (20/200) | 6/36 (20/120) | 20 | 2.4 |
| 6/48 (20/160) | 6/30 (20/100) | 16 | 2.0 |
| 6/36 (20/120) | 6/24 (20/80) | 12 | 1.6 |
| 6/30 (20/100) | 6/18 (20/60) | 10 | 1.2 |
| 6/24 (20/80) | 6/15 (20/50) | 8 | 1.0 |
| 6/18 (20/60) | 6/12 (20/40) | 6 | 0.8 |
| 6/15 (20/50) | 6/9 (20/30) | 5 | 0.6 |
| 6/12 (20/40) | 6/7.5 (20/25) | 4 | 0.5 |
| 6/9 (20/30) | 6/6 (20/20) | 3 | 0.4 |
| 6/6 (20/20) | 6/3.6 (20/12) | 2 | 0.25 |

**acuity, resolution visual** *See* **acuity, visual.**

**acuity, Snellen** Visual acuity as measured with Snellen letters.

**acuity, static visual** Acuity determined with stationary test types or test objects.
*See* **acuity, dynamic visual; test type.**

**acuity, stereoscopic visual** The ability to detect the smallest difference in depth between two objects. It is expressed as the difference η between the two angles subtended at any two objects in the field of view by the base line (or interpupillary distance). This threshold angle η (eta) is given by the approximate relationship, in radians

$$\eta = \frac{\text{PD} \times \Delta\text{D}}{\text{d}^2}$$

where PD is the interpupillary distance, d the test distance of the reference object and ΔD the distance between the two objects. (To convert the result into seconds of arc it should be multiplied by $180/\pi \times 60 \times 60 = 206\,265$). The difference between the two angles $u_1 - u_2$ (the difference between the two retinal images) is called **binocular disparity** or **retinal disparity** and the difference between the two angles $\beta - \alpha$ is called the **relative binocular parallax** (Fig. A5). Stereoscopic visual acuity is extremely fine, varying between 5 and 15 seconds of arc. It tends to decrease with age and it is positively correlated with Snellen visual acuity. *Example*: suppose ΔD is equal to 2 mm, d is 827 mm and the PD is 64 mm

$$n = \frac{64(2)}{(827)^2}(206\,265) = 38 \text{ seconds of arc}$$

*Syn.* stereo-acuity; stereo-threshold.
*See* **angle of stereopsis; disparity, retinal; stereopsis; test, Howard–Dolman; test, three needle; vectogram.**

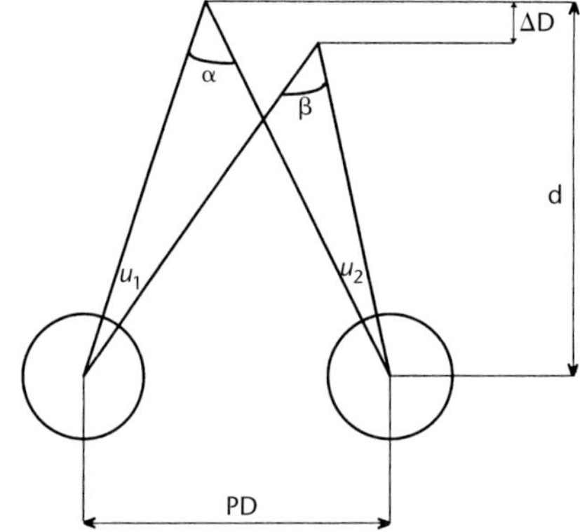


**Fig. A5** Stereoscopic visual acuity, $\eta = u_1 - u_2 = \beta - \alpha$

**acuity, unaided visual** Visual acuity without any correction. *Syn.* vision; unaided vision.

**acuity, vernier visual** The ability to detect the alignment or otherwise of two lines as in the reading of a vernier scale. This is the finest acuity being of the order of 1–5 seconds of arc depending on the length of the line; the longer the line, the more acute the detection. *Syn.* aligning power.
*See* **hyperacuity.**

**acuity, visual (VA)** Capacity for seeing distinctly the details of an object. Quantitatively, it is represented in two ways:

1. As the reciprocal of the minimum angle of resolution (in minutes of arc). This is the **resolution visual acuity**. *Syn.* minimum separable visual acuity.
2. As the Snellen fraction. This is measured using letters or Landolt rings or equivalent objects.

Average clinical visual acuity varies between 6/4 and 6/6 (or 20/15 and 20/20 in feet). Visual acuity varies with the region of the retina (being maximum in the foveola), with general illumination, contrast, colour and type of test, time of exposure, the refractive error of the eye, etc. *See* **angle of resolution, minimum; cycle per degree; hyperacuity; isoacuity; optotype; sensitivity, contrast; Snellen fraction; test, Cardiff acuity; test, photostress; test, Sheridan-Gardiner; visual efficiency scale, Snell-Sterling.**

**Table A7** Relationship between several distance visual acuity notations

| Snellen fraction (m) | Snellen fraction (ft) | min. angle of resolution (min. of arc) | Decimal |
|---|---|---|---|
| 6/180 | 20/600 | 30.0 | 0.03 |
| 6/150 | 20/500 | 25.0 | 0.04 |
| 6/120 | 20/400 | 20.0 | 0.05 |
| 6/90 | 20/300 | 15.0 | 0.07 |
| 6/60 | 20/200 | 10.0 | 0.10 |
| 6/30 | 20/100 | 5.0 | 0.20 |
| 6/24 | 20/80 | 4.0 | 0.25 |
| 6/21 | 20/70 | 3.5 | 0.29 |
| 6/18 | 20/60 | 3.0 | 0.33 |
| 6/15 | 20/50 | 2.5 | 0.40 |
| 6/12 | 20/40 | 2.0 | 0.50 |
| 6/9 | 20/30 | 1.5 | 0.67 |
| 6/7.5 | 20/25 | 1.3 | 0.80 |
| 6/6 | 20/20 | 1.0 | 1.0 |
| 6/4.5 | 20/15 | 0.75 | 1.33 |
| 6/3 | 20/10 | 0.5 | 2.0 |

**acute angle-closure glaucoma; stromal keratitis** *See* under the nouns.

**acyanopsia** Inability to recognize blue tints. *See* **chromatopsia.**

**acyclovir** *See* **antiviral agents.**

**Adams desaturated D-15 test** *See* **test, Farnsworth.**

**adaptation** **1.** Process by which a sensory organ (e.g. the eye) adjusts to its environment (e.g. to luminance, colour or contact lens wear). **2.** The reduction in sensitivity to continuous sensory stimulation. The neurophysiological correlate corresponds to a decrease in the frequency of action potentials fired by a neuron, despite a stimulus of constant magnitude. Visual adaptation is prevented from occurring by the continuous involuntary movements of the eyes. *See* **movements, fixation; potential, action; stabilized retinal image.**

**adaptation, chromatic** Apparent changes in hue and saturation after prolonged exposure to a field of a specific colour.

**adaptation, dark** Adjustment of the eye (particularly regeneration of visual pigments and dilatation of the pupil), such that, after observation in the dark, the sensitivity to light is greatly increased, i.e. the threshold response to light is decreased. This is a much slower process than light adaptation. Older people usually take longer to adapt to darkness and only reach a higher threshold than young people. *See* **adaptometer; glare tester; hemeralopia; pigment, visual.**

**adaptation, light** Adjustment of the eye (particularly bleaching of visual pigments and constriction of the pupil), such that, after observation of a bright field, the sensitivity to light is diminished, i.e. the threshold of luminance is increased.

**adaptation, prism** *See* **adaptation, vergence.**

**adaptation, sensory** Mechanism by which the visual system adjusts to avoid confusion and diplopia of the perceptual impression due to an abnormal motor condition (e.g. strabismus). *See* **strabismus.**

**adaptation, vergence** A process by which the eyes return to their condition of habitual heterophoria or orthophoria after a heterophoria has been induced by prisms (**prism adaptation**) in front of one or both eyes (as, for example, when lens centration does not coincide with the interpupillary distance), or by spherical lenses, or due to changes in the orbital contents with increasing age. This adaptation process may be related to the phenomenon of orthophorization. People who have symptomatic binocular vision anomalies do not, or only partially, show vergence adaptation to prisms. Vergence adaptation decreases with increasing age. *See* **heterophoria; orthophorization.**

**adaptometer** An instrument for measuring the variations in threshold of luminance. The most common is that of **Goldmann–Weekers.**

**add** *See* **addition, near.**

**addition, near** The difference in spherical power between the distance and near corrections. *Abbreviated*: add. A common method of arriving at the power of the addition is to measure the patient's working distance and the amplitude of accommodation. The add is obtained as follows

$$\text{add} = (1 \text{ metre/working distance in metre}) - x\,(\text{amplitude})$$

where $x$ is the percentage of the total amplitude of accommodation which is to be used: two-thirds is usually more appropriate for young presbyopes (below about 52 years of age), while one-half is more appropriate for older

a

presbyopes. Thus, this formula allows for a certain amount of the amplitude of accommodation to be left in **reserve** (usually one-third or one-half). *Syn.* reading addition.
*See* **distance, reading; presbyopia.**

**adduct** To turn towards the midline.

**adduction** Rotation of an eye towards the midline (Fig. A6).
*See* **duction; paralysis of the third nerve; syndrome, Duane's.**

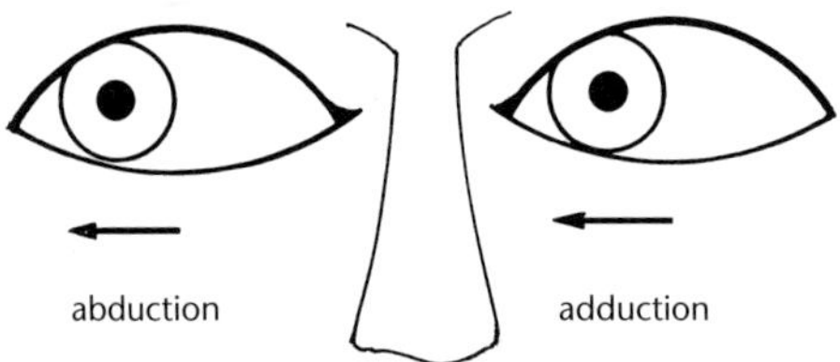


Fig. A6 Abduction of the right eye and adduction of the left eye in this right gaze

**adductors** Extraocular muscles that move the eye inward, such as the medial rectus, the inferior rectus and the superior rectus.
*See* **muscles, extraocular.**

**adenopathy** *See* **lymphadenopathy.**

**adequate stimulus** *See* **stimulus, adequate.**

**adhesion** *See* **synechia.**

**Adie's pupil; syndrome** *See* under the nouns.

**adipose tissue** A type of fatty tissue that is present in large amounts in the orbit. The fat surrounds the orbit and acts as a cushion for the globe. The fat is divided by fibrous septae and is kept posteriorly by Tenon's capsule.

**adnexa oculi** *See* **appendages of the eye.**

**adrenaline (epinephrine)** A hormone of the adrenal medulla which, instilled in the eye, causes a constriction of the conjunctival vessels, dilates the pupil and diminishes the intraocular pressure.
*See* **adrenergic receptors; decongestant, ocular; glaucoma, open-angle; naphazoline; noradrenaline (norepinephrine).**

**adrenergic agonist** *See* **sympathomimetic drugs.**

**adrenergic blocking agents** *See* **sympatholytic drugs.**

**adrenergic receptors** Receptors which are stimulated by adrenaline (epinephrine) and noradrenaline (norepinephrine) and other catecholamines. There are two types of adrenergic receptors: (1) **a-receptors** which are mainly excitatory to smooth muscles and gland cells but cause relaxation of intestinal smooth muscles; (2) **b-receptors** of which there are (at least) two types, $\beta_1$ and $\beta_2$. Generally, stimulation of β-receptors produces an inhibitory response, although in some cases the effect is excitatory (e.g. in the heart). *Example*: the dilator pupillae muscle contains mainly α-adrenergic receptors and stimulation (e.g. with adrenaline) produces mydriasis. On the other hand, there are drugs that block the effect of catecholamines on α- or β-adrenergic receptors and are called α- or β-blockers (or sympatholytic drugs or adrenergic receptor agonists). *Example*: the ciliary epithelium contains mainly β-receptors and a β-blocker such as timolol inhibits the secretion of aqueous humour thus reducing intraocular pressure. *Syn.* adrenoceptor.
*See* **alpha-adrenergic agonists; alpha-adrenergic antagonists; beta-blocker; glaucoma, open-angle; miotics; mydriatic; sympatholytic drugs; sympathomimetic drugs.**

**adrenocorticosteroids** Compounds created by the adrenal cortex that have distant metabolic effects. There are three types of compounds created by the adrenal cortex: glucocorticoids, mineralocorticoids, and androgens. Of these, the glucocorticoids are most important to the visual system due to their antiinflammatory effects. The antiinflammatory effect is thought to be mediated by inhibition of prostaglandin synthesis.
*See* **antiinflammatory drug; steroid.**

**adult inclusion conjunctivitis** *See* **conjunctivitis, adult inclusion.**

**aerial image** *See* **image, aerial.**

**aerial perspective** *See* **perspective, aerial.**

**aerobic** Needing oxygen to sustain life.
*See* **anaerobic.**

**aesthesiometer** Instrument for the measurement of sensitivity, especially tactile. The cornea and eyelid margins are the ocular structures measured. There are many types of aesthesiometers. The most common is that of **Cochet–Bonnet** (Fig. A7). It consists of a nylon monofilament of constant diameter which, depending upon its length, can exert more or less pressure. The length at which the subject responds to, say, 50% of the number of stimulations represents the corneal touch threshold. That length is converted into pressure using a calibration curve. *Note*: also spelt esthesiometer.
*See* **corneal fragility; corneal touch threshold; hyperaesthesia, corneal; sensitivity, corneal.**

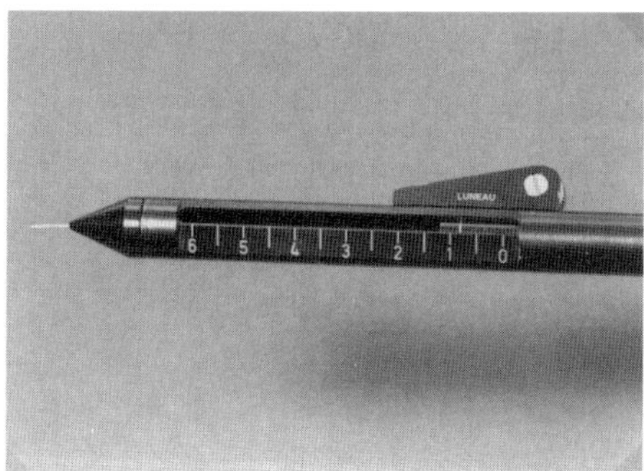


Fig. A7 Cochet–Bonnet aesthesiometer

**aetiology** The cause or origin of a disease. *Note*: also spelt etiology.
*See* **diagnosis; epidemiology.**

**afferent** Carrying from the periphery to the central or the main structure.
*See* **efferent.**

**afferent limb, of pupillary pathway** Section of the visual pathway originating in the rods and cones of the retina and terminating in the brainstem. The fibres follow the visual pathway, decussating in the optic chiasma, and continuing in the optic tracts. The fibres exit the optic tracts before reaching the lateral geniculate body, and project to the brainstem. After synapsing in the brainstem, the fibres then project to the ipsilateral and contralateral Edinger–Westphal nuclei.
*See* **reflex, pupil light.**

**afferent pupillary defect** *See* **pupil, Marcus Gunn.**

**afocal** Refers to a lens or an optical system with zero focal power, i.e. in which incident rays entering parallel emerge parallel.
*See* **aniseikonia; lens, afocal; lens, aniseikonic.**

**after-cataract** An opacity in the capsule of the crystalline lens which recurs after extracapsular extraction. *Syn.* secondary cataract.
*See* **cataract; cataract extraction, extracapsular.**

**after-effect, motion** *See* **after-effect, waterfall.**

**after-effect, tilt** Observation of a temporary change in the perceived orientation of lines after having adapted to lines tilted in another direction. If, for example, you stare at white and black bars tilted to the left for a minute or so, then look at vertical bars these will now appear to tilt slightly to the right. This is an example of the adaptation of orientation-specific cells in the visual system which become fatigued and therefore temporarily less responsive.
*See* **adaptation; after-effect, waterfall; cell, orientation-specific.**

**after-effect, waterfall** Observation of a movement in the opposite direction when fixating a stationary object, after having looked at a waterfall for some time. This is an example of phenomena which are used to infer the existence of channels in the visual system. It is suggested that there are two opposed directionally-sensitive neural channels (or neurons) which are normally in balance for stationary stimuli, but when the activity of one channel is fatigued by prolonged stimulation the other one becomes the active one. The waterfall after-effect is a special case of **motion or movement after-effect** (or **motion after-image**). *Syn.* waterfall effect; waterfall illusion.
*See* **channel; spiral, Plateau's.**

**after-image** Visual sensation persisting after the original stimulus has been removed. If observed in darkness following stimulation by a high intensity, brief duration light source, seven different after-image phases are frequently noted. The first phase, also called **Hering's after-image**, is a positive after-image and it is followed by a negative after-image. After a short interval (less than half a second) a second positive after-image, called **Purkinje after-image** or **Bidwell's ghost**, appears, the character of which depends upon the conditions of adaptation, the colour of the stimulus and the retinal region stimulated (best in the periphery). Afterwards, a second negative after-image is sometimes observed followed by a third positive after-image, called **Hess after-image**. After a long dark interval, a third negative after-image may appear followed after another long dark interval by a fourth positive after-image. If the light stimulus is of moderate intensity the last phases will be absent.
*See* **law, Emmert's; test, after-image.**

**after-image, complementary** An after-image in which the colour is complementary to the colour of the original stimulus.

**after-image, Hering's; Hess** *See* **after-image.**

**after-image, homochromatic** An after-image in which the colour appears the same as in the original stimulus.

**after-image, motion** *See* **after-effect, waterfall; spiral, Plateau's.**

**after-image, negative** An after-image in which the light areas of the original stimulus appear dark, the dark areas appear light and the coloured areas appear in a complementary colour.
*See* **after-image, positive.**

**after-image, positive** An after-image which appears the same as the original stimulus.
*See* **after-image, negative.**

**after-image, Purkinje** *See* **after-image.**

a

**after-image test** *See* **test, after-image.**

**after-image transfer test** *See* **test, after-image transfer.**

**against movement** *See* **movement, against.**

**agnosia** Inability to recognize the import of sensory stimuli (e.g. to recognize shape, faces and the orientation of objects), although the receptors and the sensory pathway are intact. The condition is attributed to a disturbance in the association area of the cortex. If the sense of sight is affected, it is called **visual agnosia** (or **perceptual** or **psychic blindness**).
*See* **alexia; apraxia, optical; areas, visual association; prosopagnosia.**

**agonist 1.** An agonistic muscle. **2.** A substance (e.g. a drug, hormone or neurotransmitter) that binds with a cell receptor to initiate a physiological response similar to that produced by the natural neurotransmitter or hormone. *Example*: pilocarpine which mimics the effect of acetylcholine acting on cholinergic receptors.
*See* **antagonist.**

**agonist drug** A drug that combines with the receptor to mimic or enhance the effect of a neurotransmitter.
*See* **alpha-adrenergic agonist.**

**agonistic muscle** *See* **muscle, agonistic.**

**agraphia** Inability to write, usually as a result of a brain lesion. If the person can write from dictation but not from copying, it is called **visual agraphia.**

**Aicardi's syndrome** *See* **syndrome, Aicardi's.**

**AIDS** *See* **syndrome, acquired immunodeficiency.**

**aids, low vision** Optical (e.g. loupe) or non-optical (e.g. large numeral telephone) appliances and devices designed to assist the partially sighted patient.
*See* **glass, magnifying; lamp, halogen; lens, telescopic; loupe; spectacles, pinhole; telescope, galilean; typoscope; vision, low.**

**air-puff tonometer** *See* **tonometer, non-contact.**

**Airy's disc** *See* **disc, Airy's.**

**akinaesthesia 1.** Inability to perceive moving objects. *Example*: as a glass is filling up with water the person cannot see the level moving, but only a succession of fixed images. **2.** Lack or loss of muscular sense.

**alacrima** Absence of secretion from the lacrimal gland. However, the typical picture is one of reduced tear secretion more correctly termed **hypolacrima**. It may occur as a result of occlusion of the orifices of the lacrimal gland due to trauma, cicatrization, diseases (e.g. trachoma); it may be congenital (e.g. Riley–Day syndrome) or it may be due to a neurogenic cause (secondary to brain damage) or to a systemic disease (e.g. Sjögren's syndrome). Treatment includes artificial tears, bland ointments, sealed scleral contact lenses and in very severe cases tarsorrhaphy.
*See* **gland, lacrimal; keratitis sicca; syndrome, Riley–Day; syndrome, Sjögren's; tarsorrhaphy; tears; tears, artificial.**

**Alagille syndrome** *See* **syndrome, Alagille.**

**albedo retinae** Oedema of the retina.

**albinism** Congenital anomaly characterized by an absence of pigment in the skin, hair, iris, retina and choroid. The iris is a pale, buff colour because of the absence of melanocytes, the fundus and the pupil are reddish and the eye transilluminates markedly. There is poor visual acuity, photophobia and nystagmus depending on the type of albinism. There are two main types of hereditary albinism: the **oculocutaneous** type (**tyrosinase-negative albinism**), an autosomal recessive trait which affects the skin, hair and eyes and the **ocular** type which is confined to the eyes and being X-linked affects males only.
*See* **fundus, ocular; inheritance; melanin; nystagmus; photophobia; transillumination.**

**Albright's syndrome** *See* **syndrome, Albright's.**

**alcohol** *See* **antiseptic.**

**alexia** Inability to recognize written or printed words due to a lesion in the brain. This is a form of visual agnosia. *Syn.* word blindness.
*See* **agnosia; dyslexia.**

**aligning power** *See* **acuity, vernier visual.**

**aligning prism** *See* **heterophoria, associated.**

**alignment fit** *See* **fitted on K.**

**alkaptonuria** A rare, hereditary, metabolic disorder characterized by dark urine. It is due to an error in the metabolism of the amino acids tyrosine and phenylalanine, which usually break down by oxidation to homogentisic acid. However, in this condition homogentisic acid is not broken down but stored in tissues, especially cartilage which it turns bluish-black, and excreted in the urine. Ocular signs are pigmentation of the sclera, most markedly near the insertions of the recti muscles, and of the cornea and conjunctiva.

**all or none law** *See* **law, all or none.**

**Allen–Thorpe gonioprism** *See* **gonioprism.**

**allergic conjunctivitis** *See* **conjunctivitis, allergic.**

**allergic reactions (type I hypersensitivity)** An abnormal reaction occurring when an antigen reacts with an antibody (e.g. immunoglobulin E, IgE) attached to a mast cell or basophil. This leads to the release of specific chemical mediators of allergy (e.g. histamine) that react with target organs throughout the body. Systemic signs include: itching, lacrimation, skin rash and possibly haemodynamic collapse and shock.
*See* **antihistamine; mast cell stabilizers.**

**allometropia** Refraction of the eye along any line except the visual axis (or line of sight) therefore representing the refraction of any extrafoveal region. *Example*: if an eye is emmetropic along the visual axis, at 40 degrees of temporal retinal eccentricity the allometropia will be about plano −2.50 × 90° and at 50 degrees, +0.50–3.50 × 90°.
*See* **astigmatism, oblique.**

**allowance** *See* **retinoscope.**

**allyl diglycol carbonate** *See* **CR-39 material.**

**all-trans** *See* **rhodopsin.**

**alpha-adrenergic agonist** An alpha-adrenergic agonist that reduces the production of aqueous humour. It is used topically in the treatment of glaucoma. Common agents include apraclonidine and brimonidine.
*See* **adrenergic receptor; sympathomimetic drugs.**

**alpha-adrenergic antagonist** An adrenergic blocking agent which produces miosis and a slight reduction in intraocular pressure. It is used mainly to reverse the mydriatic effect of sympathomimetic drugs (e.g. phenylephrine hydrochloride), or even some antimuscarinic drugs (e.g. tropicamide). Common agents include dapiprazole and moxisylyte (thymoxamine). *Syn.* alpha-blocker.
*See* **sympatholytic drugs.**

**alpha angle** *See* **angle, alpha.**

**alpha-blocker** *See* **alpha-adrenergic antagonist.**

**alpha waves** Rhythmic oscillation in electrical potential occurring in the cortex of the human brain when awake and at rest. The rate of oscillation is 8–13 Hz. *Syn.* alpha rhythm.
*See* **potential, resting membrane.**

**alternate cover test** *See* **test, cover.**

**alternating checkerboard stimulus** A type of light stimulus used in performing electrophysiological testing. Most often used in the pattern electroretinogram (PERG), it maintains constant luminance to the entire retina. The PERG measures ganglion cell function, in contrast to the ERG which measures the function of the photoreceptor and bipolar cell layers of the retina.
*See* **electroretinogram.**

**alternating hypertropia; strabismus** *See* under the nouns.

**altitudinal hemianopsia** *See* **hemianopsia, altitudinal.**

**Alvarez lens** *See* **lens, Alvarez.**

**amacrine cell** *See* **cell, amacrine.**

**amaurosis 1.** Partial or total loss of sight due to a lesion somewhere in the visual pathway, but not in the eye itself. **2.** Synonym for blindness.
*See* **blindness.**

**amaurosis fugax** Transient unilateral loss of vision. The visual loss varies from partial to total blindness and rarely lasts longer than 10 minutes. It is usually caused by a temporary occlusion in the internal carotid artery, which produces an insufficient blood flow to the ophthalmic artery and may lead to closure of the central retinal artery. *Syn.* blackout.
*See* **angiography, fluorescein; arteritis, temporal; blackout; bruit; plaques, Hollenhorst's; retinal arterial occlusion.**

**amaurosis, Leber's congenital** *See* **Leber's congenital amaurosis.**

**ambiocularity 1.** *See* **dominance, ocular. 2.** In strabismus, the condition in which the patient uses either eye.

**ambiguous figure** *See* **figure, Blivet; figure, Kanisza; Necker cube; Schroeder's staircase; vase, Rubin's.**

**amblyope** Person who has amblyopia.

**amblyopia** A condition characterized by reduced visual acuity due to a lesion in the eye or in the visual pathway, which hinders the normal development of vision, and which is not correctable by spectacles or contact lenses. The usual clinical criterion is 6/9 (or 20/30) or less in one eye, or a two-line difference or more, on the acuity chart between the two eyes. Amblyopia may occur as a result of: suppression in the deviated eye in strabismus (**strabismic amblyopia**; formerly called **amblyopia ex anopsia** which amounts to about 20% of all cases); a blurred image in the more ametropic eye in uncorrected anisometropia (**anisometropic amblyopia** which amounts to about 50% of all cases); bilateral blurred images in uncorrected refractive errors (**isoametropic amblyopia**); a blurred image in one of the meridians of high uncorrected astigmatism (**meridional amblyopia**); any of the above three is also called **refractive amblyopia**;

opacities in the ocular media (e.g. congenital cataract, severe ptosis) in infants (**stimulus deprivation amblyopia or visual deprivation amblyopia or image degradation amblyopia**) after the lesion has been removed; continuous occlusion of an eye as may occur in occlusion treatment (**occlusion amblyopia**); arsenic, lead or quinine poisoning (**toxic amblyopia**) or the more specific types of toxic amblyopia such as those caused by excessive use of alcohol (**alcohol amblyopia**), methanol (**methanol amblyopia**), quinine (**quinine amblyopia**) or tobacco (**tobacco amblyopia**), although the latter three may actually be due to nutritional deficiencies (**nutritional amblyopia**); psychological origin (**hysterical amblyopia**) or of unknown origin (**idiopathic amblyopia**).

Many of these amblyopias are **functional**, i.e. in which no organic lesion exists as in hysterical, refractive, isoametropic, strabismic or stimulus deprivation amblyopia. Others are organic, i.e. they are due to some pathological (e.g. congenital cataract) or anatomical anomalies (e.g. malorientation of retinal receptors), as in nutritional, toxic or visual deprivation amblyopia. Amblyopia occurs in 2–4% of the population. There is usually a reduction in the amplitude of accommodation in amblyopic eyes. Treatment of amblyopia depends on the type. However, the younger the patient, the more likely that the treatment will be successful. Typically, the principal treatment is occlusion of the fixating eye (or the eye with the best acuity) by patching or blurring with atropine sulfate to force the other eye to take up fixation, after full refractive correction. Other procedures (alternatives or supplemental to patching) include penalization, kicking a ball towards a specific target, playing catch a ball, bar reading, pleoptics (when there is eccentric fixation as well), and any other procedures which require fixation like drawing, duplicating letter sequences on a typewriter, cutting out patterns, etc.

*See* **cheiroscope; disc, pinhole; eye, amblyopic; fixation, eccentric; nystagmus; occlusion treatment; penalization; period, critical; phenomenon, crowding; pleoptics; strabismus; suppression; test, bar reading; test, neutral density filter.**

**amblyopia, hysterical** Apparent loss of vision due to a psychological disorder. The patient really believes that he or she cannot see although this is not supported by physiological impairment. The condition is often characterized by a constricted visual field or tunnel vision.
*See* **vision, tunnel.**

**amblyopia, meridional** Amblyopia in one of the two principal meridians of an astigmatic eye. The amblyopia usually affects the most defocused meridian and its severity tends to vary with the amount of astigmatism. This amblyopia is of neural origin. Optical correction of the patient as young as possible usually prevents this condition. *Syn.* astigmatic amblyopia.

**amblyopic eye** *See* **eye, amblyopic.**

**amblyopic nystagmus** *See* **nystagmus.**

**amblyoscope, major** *See* **amblyoscope, Worth.**

**amblyoscope, Wheatstone** Amblyoscope using mirrors to change the angle of convergence or divergence. *Syn.* Wheatstone stereoscope.

**amblyoscope, Worth** A modified haploscope introduced by Worth consisting of two angled tubes held in front of the eyes which present a different image to each eye, and which can be turned to any degree of convergence or divergence. If the instrument is incorporated into a table, it is called a **major amblyoscope** of which there are various types called **Synoptiscope** or **Synoptophore.**
*See* **haploscope.**

**Ames room** *See* **room, Ames.**

**amethocaine hydrochloride** *See* **tetracaine.**

**ametrope** Person who has ametropia.

**ametropia** Anomaly of the refractive state of the eye in which, with relaxed accommodation, the image of objects at infinity is not formed on the retina. Thus vision may be blurred. The ametropias are: **astigmatism, hypermetropia** and **myopia**. The absence of ametropia is called **emmetropia**. *Syn.* refractive error; error of refraction; refraction (although not strictly correct since this term may also refer to the lack of ametropia).
*See* **emmetropia; refraction; refractive error; theory, biological–statistical; theory, emmetropization; theory, nativistic.**

**ametropia, axial** Ametropia due primarily to an abnormal length of the eye while the refractive power is approximately normal.

**ametropia, refractive** Ametropia due primarily to an abnormal refractive power of the eye while the length is approximately normal. Refractive ametropias can be attributed to either an abnormal radius of curvature of the surfaces of the cornea, or the crystalline lens (**curvature ametropia**) or to an abnormal index of refraction of one or more of the ocular media (**index ametropia**).

**Ammann's test** *See* **test, neutral density filter.**

**amphotericin B** *See* **antifungal agent.**

**amplitude of accommodation** *See* **accommodation, amplitude of.**

**amplitude of convergence** *See* **convergence, amplitude of.**

**Amsler chart; grid** *See* **chart, Amsler.**

**anaerobic** Ability to sustain life in an atmosphere devoid of oxygen.
*See* **aerobic.**

**anaesthesia 1.** A loss of sensation in a part, or in the whole body, induced by the administration of a drug (an **anaesthetic agent**). **2.** A loss of sensation, usually touch, in a part of the body as a result of some nervous lesion. *Example*: corneal anaesthesia. *Note*: also spelt anesthesia.

**anaesthesia, topical** Application of a local anaesthetic agent to an area of the skin or mucous membrane (e.g. conjunctiva) to produce anaesthesia. The application may be via direct instillation, soaked swabs, ointments or sprays. *Syn.* surface anaesthesia.
*See* **anaesthesia; anaesthetic.**

**anaesthetic** Any substance used to produce a loss of pain sensation either in the whole of the body when unconscious (**general anaesthetic**) or to some part of the body when awake (**local anaesthetic**). *Note*: also spelt anesthetic.

**anaesthetic agent, local** *See* **benoxinate; cocaine; lidocaine; proxymetacaine; tetracaine.**

**anaglyph** Stereogram consisting of two superimposed and laterally displaced drawings or photographs of the same scene but taken from two directions and in complementary colours (usually red and green). If the anaglyphs are viewed through filters of the same colour, one to each eye, and induce retinal disparity (of a fixed amount) they give rise to the perception of depth or stereopsis. A set of cards, or targets on the same card, to induce various amounts of retinal disparity can be used to detect and train fusion and stereopsis (e.g. Tranaglyphs).
*See* **colour, complementary; disparity, retinal; fusion, sensory; perception, depth; stereogram, random-dot; stereopsis.**

**analgesic** A remedy or agent which relieves pain.

**analyser 1.** Polarizing device used to determine the plane of vibration of a beam of light. *Examples*: Nicol prism, polaroid sheet, tourmaline crystal. **2.** In a polariscope, the second of the two polarizing elements, the first being the polarizer.
*See* **light, polarized; polariscope; polarizer.**

**analyser, Friedmann visual field** Instrument designed to examine the central visual field. It utilizes a single xenon discharge tube placed within an integrating bowl, in front of which are fenestrated plates which can present 15 different patterns composed of either two, three or four stimuli of variable intensity and brief duration. Mark II has two programmes with 18 and 31 patterns each.
*See* **perimeter; perimeter, computerized; screener, Harrington–Flocks visual field.**

**Analyser, Humphrey Vision** Subjective refractometer utilizing continuously variable-power lenses developed by Alvarez. The image of a target is formed by this variable-power lens and is reflected by a concave mirror situated 3 m away from the patient. The vergence of light entering the eye can be changed by changing the power of the Alvarez lens: spherical, as well as astigmatic, errors of refraction and binocular vision tests can be made. The spherocylinder correction is automatically computed.
*See* **lens, Alvarez; optometer.**

**anaphoria** *See* **hypertropia, alternating.**

**anastigmatic lens** *See* **lens, anastigmatic.**

**anastomosis** A natural communication between two blood vessels or other tubular structures. *Example*: the long posterior ciliary artery divides into two branches as it enters the posterior part of the ciliary muscle and at its anterior end these branches anastomose with each other and with the anterior ciliary arteries to form the major or arterial circle of the iris.
*See* **arterial circle of the iris, major.**

**anatomical position of rest** *See* **position of rest, anatomical.**

**anatropia** *See* **hypertropia, alternating.**

**aneurysm** A localized dilatation of the walls of a blood vessel, usually an artery, as a result of infection, injury or degeneration. It is filled with fluid or clotted blood. Aneurysms occur in diabetic retinopathy leading to haemorrhages and oedema.
*See* **paralysis of the third nerve; retinopathy, diabetic.**

**angiogram** The photographic image obtained in fluorescein angiography.

**angiography, fluorescein** A technique aimed at observing the vessels of the fundus of the eye and iris by using photography following the intravenous injection of fluorescein. It is a useful technique which facilitates the diagnosis of various retinal (e.g. diabetic retinopathy, retinal artery occlusion, retinal vein occlusion, age-related maculopathy), choroidal (e.g. tumour of the choroid) and iris disorders. However, those of the choroid and iris are more difficult to observe.
*See* **flush, choroidal; retinopathy, diabetic.**

a

**angioid streaks** Degeneration of Bruch's membrane of the choroid characterized by brown or reddish lines or streaks in the fundus of the eye. The condition is bilateral, although one eye may be affected more than the other. Patients may occasionally be aware of some visual impairment in the visual field depending on the location of the streaks. The membrane is very fragile and liable to rupture in the case of ocular trauma, which may lead to macular haemorrhage and visual loss. Angioid streaks are often found in association with **pseudoxanthoma elasticum** (an eruption of small, superficial, solid elevation of the skin of the neck and other areas), Paget's disease or sickle-cell anaemia.
*See* **choroid; disease, Paget's; membrane, Bruch's; syndrome, Ehlers–Danlos.**

**angioma** Tumour of the blood vessels.

**angiomatosis retinae** *See* **disease, von Hippel's.**

**angioscotoma** A scotoma produced by the shadow cast by the retinal blood vessels. It looks like the branches of a tree which extend from the blind spot. It is seen only in special conditions of illumination as when illuminating the fundus of the eye by gently moving a penlight over the closed eyelid, or when illuminating the fundus through the sclera, or when plotting the visual field. This phenomenon is sometimes used as a test to predict gross macular function in a patient with dense cataract where visualization of the fundus is impossible, although better results are obtained with the blue field entoptoscope. *Syn.* Purkinje figures; Purkinje shadows; Purkinje tree.
*See* **entoptoscope, blue field; image, entoptic.**

**angle alpha** Angle between the visual axis and the optical axis formed at the first nodal point of the eye. The visual axis usually lies nasal to the optical axis on the plane of the cornea (**positive** angle alpha). It is, on average, equal to about 5° in the adult eye. If it lies temporal to the optical axis, the angle is denoted **negative** (Fig. A8). *Symbol*: α.
*See* **angle lambda; axis, optical.**

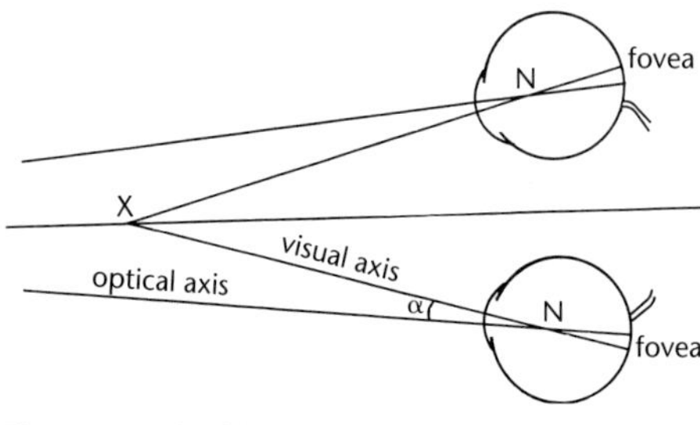


**Fig. A8** Angle alpha

**angle of altitude 1.** The angle through which the eyes have turned up or down from the primary position by a rotation about the transverse axis (*x*-axis). **2.** The angle between the plane of regard and the subjective horizontal plane. *Syn.* angle of elevation.

**angle of anomaly** Angle between the line of visual direction of the fovea and the line of visual direction of the abnormal corresponding point of the same deviated eye. It is usually represented by the difference between the objective and subjective angles of deviation in abnormal retinal correspondence.
*See* **angle of deviation; line of direction; retinal correspondence, abnormal.**

**angle of the anterior chamber** Angle at the periphery of the anterior chamber formed by the root of the iris, the front surface of the ciliary body and the trabecular meshwork. *Syn.* angle of filtration; drainage angle; irido-corneal angle.
*See* **chamber, anterior; glaucoma, neovascular; gonioscope; meshwork, trabecular; method, van Herick, Shaffer and Schwartz; test, shadow.**

**angle, apical** *See* **angle, prism.**

**angle of azimuth** The angle through which the eyes have turned right or left from the primary position by a rotation about the vertical axis.

**angle, Brewster's** *See* **angle of polarization.**

**angle-closure glaucoma** *See* **glaucoma, angle-closure.**

**angle, contact** Angle formed by a surface and a tangent to a sessile drop of fluid (usually water) at the point where the drop meets the surface. This angle indicates the degree of **wettability** of that surface. The more wettable (or hydrophilic) the material, the smaller the angle, being equal to 0° for a completely hydrophilic material when water spreads evenly over that surface. Hydrophobic surfaces can have contact angles greater than 90°, e.g. silicone rubber in which the angle is about 120° (Fig. A9). *Syn.* wetting angle.
*See* **silicone rubber; test, sessile drop.**

**angle of convergence** Angle between the lines of sight of the two eyes which are in a state of convergence. The angle is positive when the lines of sight intersect in front of the eyes, and negative when they intersect behind the eyes. *Note*: some authors regard the angle of convergence as the rotation of one eye only towards the fixation point, and refer to the angle of convergence of both eyes, defined above, as the **total angle of convergence** or the **total convergence**. The total angle of convergence required for binocular fixation of a target is equal to

$$\text{convergence (in } \Delta) = \frac{\text{PD (in cm)}}{d \text{ (in m)}}$$

or $\text{convergence (in } \Delta) = \text{convergence (in ma)} \times \text{PD (in cm)}$

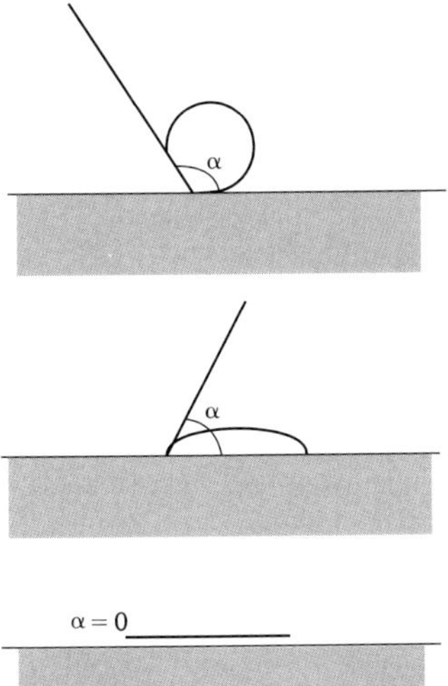


Fig. A9 Different contact angles α between a drop of fluid and a contact lens material

where *d* is the distance between the target and the midpoint of the base line and PD the interpupillary distance. *Syn.* angle of triangulation. *See* **angle, metre; dioptre, prism; distance, interpupillary; line, base; line of sight.**

**angle of convergence, total** *See* **angle of convergence.**

**angle, critical** That angle of incidence which results in the refracted ray travelling along the surface between the two media (angle of refraction equal to 90°). If the angle of incidence is greater than the critical angle, the ray is totally reflected. If, however, the angle of incidence is smaller than the critical angle, the ray is refracted (with some light reflected). The critical angle $i_c$ is given by the following formula

$$\sin i_c = \frac{n'}{n}$$

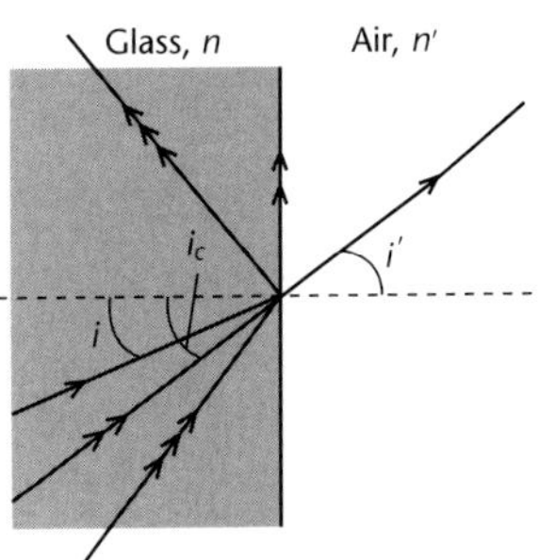


Fig. A10 Critical angle $i_c$ and total internal reflection ($i$, angle of incidence; $i'$, angle of refraction)

where $n$ and $n'$ are the indices of the media on each side of the surface, with the light travelling from the high index medium $n$ to the low index medium $n'$ (Fig. A10). *Syn.* limiting angle. *See* **optics, fibre; prism, reflecting; reflection, total; refractometer.**

**angle of deviation 1.** Angle through which a ray of light is deviated on reflection by a mirror, or refraction by a lens or prism. **2.** Angle between the visual axis (or line of sight) of the deviated eye in strabismus and the straight ahead position while the other eye fixates straight ahead. It can be assessed subjectively by having the patient report simultaneous perception (e.g. the lion in the cage seen in the amblyoscope) or objectively as measured by the practitioner either with the amblyoscope or using prisms and cover test, or by the Hirschberg test. *Syn.* angle of squint; angle of strabismus. *See* **amblyoscope, Worth; angle of anomaly; axis, visual; incomitance; method, Hirschberg's; method, Javal's; method, Krimsky's; prism; prism, minimum deviation of a.**

**angle of divergence** Angle between the lines of sight of the two eyes which are in a state of divergence. *See* **line of sight.**

**Table A8** Critical angle (in degrees) beyond which all the light is reflected at the surface separating various transparent substances from air or water

| | | critical angle $i_c$ | |
|---|---|---|---|
| **substance** | **refractive index $n$** | **in contact with air $n'$ = 1** | **in contact with water $n'$ = 1.333** |
| water | 1.333 | 48.6 | – |
| spectacle crown glass | 1.523 | 41.0 | 61.1 |
| flint glass (dense) | 1.62 | 38.1 | 55.4 |
| flint glass (extra dense) | 1.706 | 35.9 | 51.4 |
| PMMA | 1.49 | 42.2 | 63.5 |
| CR-39 | 1.498 | 41.9 | 62.9 |
| polycarbonate | 1.586 | 39.1 | 57.2 |
| diamond | 2.42 | 24.4 | 33.4 |

**angle, drainage** *See* **angle of the anterior chamber.**

**angle of elevation** *See* **angle of altitude.**

**angle eta** *See* **acuity, stereoscopic visual.**

**angle, external** *See* **canthus.**

**angle of filtration** *See* **angle of the anterior chamber.**

**angle gamma** The angle between the optical axis and the fixation axis.
*See* **axis, fixation; axis, optical.**

**angle of incidence** Angle between the incident ray and the normal to the surface at the point of incidence in either reflection or refraction at a surface separating two media.

**angle, irido-corneal** *See* **angle of the anterior chamber.**

**angle kappa** Angle between the pupillary axis and the visual axis, measured at the nodal point. *Symbol*: κ.
*See* **angle lambda; axis, pupillary; axis, visual; axis, optical; line of sight.**

**angle lambda** Angle between the pupillary axis and the line of sight formed at the centre of the entrance pupil. It is this angle which is measured clinically as it is almost equal to angle alpha. *Symbol*: λ.
*See* **axis, pupillary; line of sight.**

**angle, limiting** *See* **angle, critical.**

**angle, metre (ma)** Unit of convergence which is equal to the reciprocal of the distance (in metres) between the point of fixation assumed to lie on the median line and the base line of the eyes. Thus, if an object is located at 25 cm from the base line, each eye converges through 4 ma; at 1 metre, 1 ma, etc. Metre angles of convergence can be converted into prism dioptres of convergence by multiplying by the subject's interpupillary distance expressed in cm. *Example*: for a PD of 6.0 cm, a convergence of 5 ma = 30 Δ.
*See* **angle of convergence; dioptre, prism; line, median; line, base.**

**angle, palpebral** *See* **canthus.**

**angle, pantoscopic** Angle between the spectacle plane and the frontal plane of the face when the superior edge of the lens is farther away from the face than the inferior edge (Fig. A11). *Syn.* pantoscopic tilt.
*See* **angle, retroscopic; plane, frontal; plane, spectacle.**

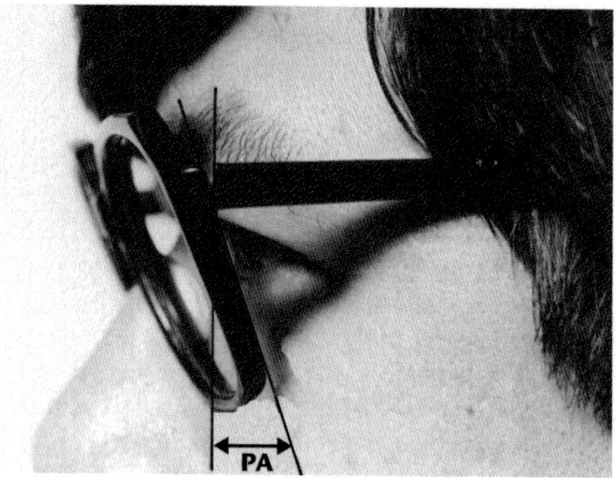


**Fig. A11** Pantoscopic angle PA

**angle of polarization** The angle of incidence at which the reflected light is maximally polarized. At this angle, the reflected and refracted rays are 90° apart (Fig. A12). This angle $i$ is given by the equation

$$\tan i = \frac{n_2}{n_1}$$

and measures 56.7° when the first medium $n_1$ is air and the second medium $n_2$ is a glass with an

**Table A9** Relationship between viewing distance and convergence in metre angles and prism dioptres (for both eyes) for 4 interpupillary distances (PD in cm)

| object distance from cornea (cm) | metre angle (ma) | convergence (in prism dioptres) PD: 6.0 | 6.4 | 6.8 | 7.0 |
|---|---|---|---|---|---|
| 200 | 0.5 | 3.0 | 3.2 | 3.4 | 3.5 |
| 100 | 1.0 | 6.0 | 6.4 | 6.8 | 7.0 |
| 67 | 1.5 | 9.0 | 9.6 | 10.2 | 10.5 |
| 50 | 2.0 | 12.0 | 12.8 | 13.6 | 14.0 |
| 40 | 2.5 | 15.0 | 16.0 | 17.0 | 17.5 |
| 33 | 3.0 | 18.0 | 19.2 | 20.4 | 21.0 |
| 25 | 4.0 | 24.0 | 25.6 | 27.2 | 28.0 |
| 20 | 5.0 | 30.0 | 32.0 | 34.0 | 35.0 |
| 16 | 6.25 | 37.5 | 40.0 | 42.5 | 43.7 |
| 14 | 7.14 | 42.8 | 45.7 | 48.5 | 50.0 |

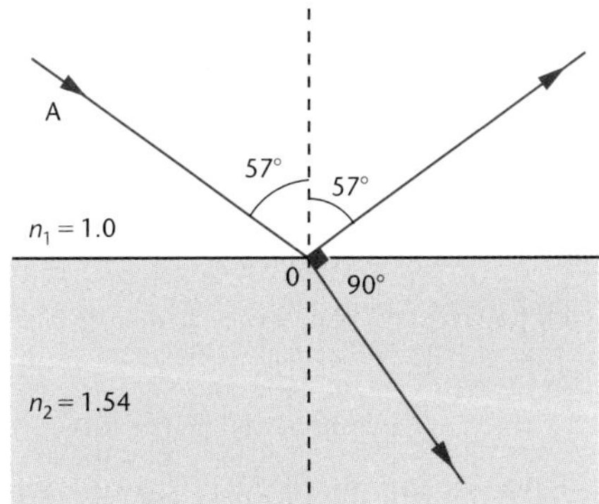


**Fig. A12** Ray of non-polarized light AO is incident to the surface at the polarizing angle. Most of the light is transmitted across the surface and partially polarized, the rest being reflected and polarized maximally (i.e. vibrating in one plane only)

index of refraction equal to 1.523. *Syn.* Brewster's angle.
*See* **light, polarized.**

**angle, prism** The angle between the two refracting surfaces of a prism. *Syn.* apical angle; refracting angle (this term is deprecated because of the confusion with 'angle of refraction').

**angle recession** A tear between the longitudinal and circular muscles of the ciliary body. It is most often noted following blunt trauma to the anterior segment. It is typically followed by hyphaemia. This form of injury predisposes the individual to elevated intraocular pressure (i.e. increased risk of glaucoma) in the future. With a gonioscope, angle recession appears with an abnormally wide ciliary body band with a prominent scleral spur and some torn iris processes. There are also marked variations in the width and depth of the angle in different quadrants of the eye.
*See* **angle of the anterior chamber; ciliary body; cyclodialysis; hyphaemia; iridodialysis; muscle, ciliary.**

**angle of reflection** Angle between the reflected ray and the normal to the surface at the point of incidence.

**angle, refracting** *See* **angle, prism.**

**angle of refraction** Angle between the refracted ray and the normal to the surface at the point of emergence.

**angle of resolution, minimum (MAR)** The angle subtended at the nodal point of the eye (or the centre of the entrance pupil) by two points or two lines which can just be distinguished as separate.
*See* **acuity, visual; chart, log MAR.**

**angle, retroscopic** Angle between the spectacle plane and the frontal plane of the face when the superior edge of the lens is closer to the face than the inferior edge. *Syn.* retroscopic tilt.
*See* **angle, pantoscopic; plane, frontal; plane, spectacle.**

**angle of squint** *See* **angle of deviation.**

**angle of stereopsis** The difference between the angles subtended at the centres of the entrance pupils of the two eyes by two points located in space at different distances from the eyes.
*See* **acuity, stereoscopic visual; stereopsis; test, Howard–Dolman; test, three-needle.**

**angle of strabismus** *See* **angle of deviation.**

**angle of triangulation** *See* **angle of convergence.**

**angle, viewing** *See* **angle, visual.**

**angle, visual** The angle subtended by the extremities of an object at the anterior nodal point of the eye. If the object is far away, the point of reference can be the centre of the entrance pupil or even the anterior pole of the cornea. *Syn.* viewing angle.

**angle, wetting** *See* **angle, contact.**

**angling** Adjusting the angle which the sides of a spectacle frame make with the plane of its front.

**ångström unit** Unit of wavelength of radiant energy. One unit is equal to one ten thousand millionth of a metre ($10^{-10}$m). *Symbol*: A or Å. It is preferable to use the nanometre which is an SI unit.
*See* **nanometre.**

**aniridia** Complete, or almost complete, absence of the iris of the eye. It can be acquired, due to trauma, or inherited as an autosomal dominant trait. The patient is photophobic and in congenital cases there is usually amblyopia and sometimes nystagmus. Contact lenses incorporating an artificial iris, or tinted spectacle lenses, help in this condition.
*See* **irideremia; lens, cosmetic contact.**

**aniseikometer** *See* **eikonometer.**

**aniseikonia** A difference in size and/or shape of the visual images of the two eyes. This may be due either to unequal axial lengths of the two eyes, to an unequal distribution of the retinal elements or an inequality of the cortical representation of the two ocular images (**basic** or **intrinsic aniseikonia**). It is most frequently induced by lenses of different power used in the correction of anisometropia (**refractive aniseikonia**). Symptoms include visual discomfort, visual distortion of space and sometimes difficulty in achieving binocular vision, as for example in spectacle corrected unilateral aphakia. Aniseikonia is measured with an eikonometer,

a

although a simple test consists of separating the retinal images of a large target (e.g. a test chart) with prisms and comparing them: placing size lenses in front of one eye until the images appear equal will give an indication of the amount of aniseikonia.
*See* **anisometropia; eikonometer; image, visual; lens, aniseikonic; magnification, shape; magnification, spectacle; test, New Aniseikonia; test, Turville infinity balance.**

**aniso-accommodation** Unequal accommodative response in the two eyes when fixating an object binocularly. It may result from a disease (e.g. glaucoma, ophthalmoplegia, paralysis of the third nerve, unilateral cataract), uncorrected anisometropia, viewing a near object to the side, toxins affecting one eye more than the other, or trauma.

**anisochromatic** Not of uniform colour.

**anisochromatopsia** Deficiency of colour vision in one eye only, or of unequal severity in the two eyes.

**anisochromia** *See* **heterochromia.**

**anisocoria** Condition in which the pupils of the eyes are not of equal size. Typically one pupil is abnormal and cannot either dilate or constrict. It may be physiological (e.g. in antimetropia) or it may be part of a syndrome, the most common being those of Adie's and Horner's. Physiological anisocoria remains constant irrespective of the level of illumination. Anisocoria can occur as a result of injury (e.g. to the iris sphincter muscle), inflammation (e.g. iridocyclitis), diseases of the iris, paralysis of the third nerve, angle-closure glaucoma, systemic diseases (e.g. diabetes, syphilis) or accidental drug instillation into the eye (if the drug or substance has anticholinergic properties the condition is then referred to as **anticholinergic mydriasis** or **'atropine' mydriasis**). The search for the cause of anisocoria is facilitated by testing the pupil light reflexes and responses to locally instilled drugs (Fig. A13).
*See* **pupil; reflex, pupil light; pupillometer.**

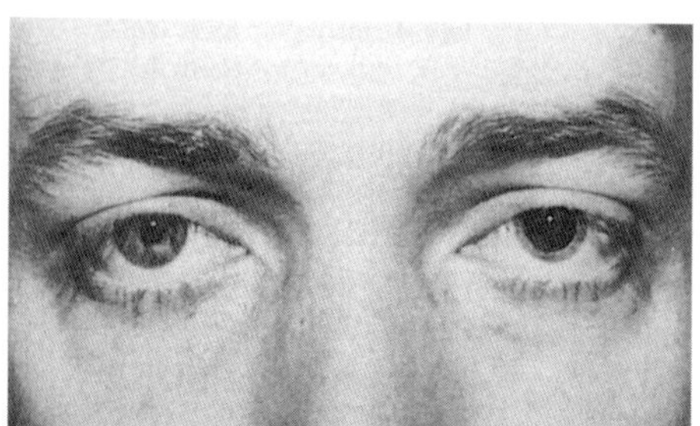

**Fig. A13** Anisocoria

**anisocycloplegia** Unequal responses following the binocular instillation of a cycloplegic.

**anisohypermetropia** Unequal amount of hypermetropia in the two eyes. *Syn.* compound hypermetropic anisometropia.

**anisometrope** A person who has anisometropia.

**anisometropia** Condition in which the refractive state of a pair of eyes differs and therefore one eye requires a different lens correction from the other. Correction may induce aniseikonia and when the eyes deviate from the optical axes of the lenses, anisophoria. Uncorrected anisometropia of low amounts may cause eyestrain or diplopia. Large amounts rarely cause symptoms as one of the retinal images is typically suppressed or there is amblyopia. *Syn.* asymmetropia; heterometropia; heteropsia.
*See* **aniso-accommodation; antimetropia; aniseikonia; anisophoria; effect, differential prismatic; isometropia.**

**anisometropia, compound hypermetropic** *See* **anisohypermetropia.**

**anisometropia, compound myopic** *See* **anisomyopia.**

**anisometropia, mixed** *See* **antimetropia.**

**anisometropia, simple** Anisometropia in which one eye is emmetropic and the other either hypermetropic (**simple hypermetropic anisometropia**) or myopic (**simple myopic anisometropia**).

**anisomyopia** Unequal amount of myopia in the two eyes. *Syn.* compound myopic anisometropia.

**anisophoria 1.** A type of heterophoria in which the amount varies with the direction of gaze. It may be due to: (a) a paresis or spasm of one or more of the extraocular muscles, or (b) an anisometropic spectacle correction in which different prismatic effects induce different phorias when the eyes look in different directions of gaze (this type is called **optical anisophoria**). **2.** A latent deviation in which the angular relationship between the visual axes of the two eyes is not equal depending upon which eye is fixating. This is a form of incomitance.
*See* **aniseikonia; anisometropia; effect, differential, prismatic; heterophoria; incomitance.**

**anisopia** Unequal vision in the two eyes.

**anisotropic** State of an optical medium in which the optical properties are not the same in all directions, due to the fact that the refractive index is not the same for all directions. An incident ray will be divided, within a uniaxial anisotropic medium, into two refracted rays; an ordinary ray which obeys Snell's law and an extraordinary

**Table A10** Approximate retinal image size differences (in %) for various anisometropias corrected by spectacles (vertex distance = 12 mm)

| anisometropia difference (D) | axial anisometropia (%)* | refractive anisometropia† | |
|---|---|---|---|
| | | hypermetropic (%) | myopic (%) |
| 1.0 | 0.25 | 1.50 | 1.25 |
| 1.5 | 0.37 | 2.25 | 1.88 |
| 2.0 | 0.50 | 3.00 | 2.50 |
| 2.5 | 0.62 | 3.75 | 3.12 |
| 3.0 | 0.75 | 4.50 | 3.75 |
| 3.5 | 0.87 | 5.25 | 4.38 |
| 4.0 | 1.00 | 6.00 | 5.00 |
| 4.5 | 1.12 | 6.75 | 5.62 |
| 5.0 | 1.25 | 7.50 | 6.25 |
| 5.5 | 1.37 | 8.25 | 6.88 |
| 6.0 | 1.50 | 9.00 | 7.50 |

*The two eyes are assumed to be of the same refractive power but of different lengths.
†The two eyes are assumed to be of the same length but of different refractive powers.

ray which follows a different law. Most crystals are anisotropic.
*See* **birefringence; dichroism; isotropic.**

**ankyloblepharon** Partial or complete adhesion of the edge of one eyelid to that of the other. It may occasionally result from a cicatrizing lesion of the eyelid margins or following tarsorrhaphy. It may also be congenital in which case the eyelids are joined together by bands of tissue and this condition is called **ankyblepharon filiform adnatum.**
*See* **tarsorrhaphy.**

**ankylosing spondylitis** *See* **iridocyclitis; uveitis.**

**annular synechia** *See* **synechia, annular.**

**annulus ciliaris** The ring-line structure between the iris and the choroid. *Syn.* ciliary ring.

**annulus of Zinn** The common tendon from which arise the four recti muscles of the eye. It surrounds the optic foramen and a part of the medial end of the superior orbital fissure. *Syn.* tendon of Zinn.

**anomaloscope** An instrument for testing colour vision in which the observer is required to match one-half of a circular field which is illuminated with yellow with a mixture of green and red in the other half. The yellow half can be varied in brightness, while the other may be varied continuously from red to green. A certain combination of the red and green mixture is considered normal and variations from that mixture indicate anomalous colour vision. With this instrument one can distinguish between a protanope and a protanomal and between a deuteranope and a deuteranomal. *Syn.* Nagel anomaloscope. Some anomaloscopes also test for blue-yellow colour vision deficiencies, e.g. **Pickford–Nicholson anomaloscope.**
*See* **colour vision, defective; Rayleigh equation.**

**anomalous retinal correspondence** *See* **retinal correspondence, abnormal.**

**anomalous trichromatism** *See* **trichromatism, anomalous.**

**anophthalmia** Congenital absence of all tissues of the eyes. It is due to a failure of the outgrowth of the optic vesicle to form the optic cup. However, in many cases some development occurs and there is a rudimentary presence of one or both eyes, such as extreme microphthalmia. *Syn.* anophthalmos; anophthalmus; anopia.
*See* **cup, optic; microphthalmia; monophthalmia; vesicle, optic.**

**anophthalmia, unilateral** *See* **monophthalmia.**

**anophthalmos; anophthalmus** *See* **anophthalmia.**

**anopia** *See* **anophthalmia.**

**anopsia, quadrantic** *See* **quadrantanopsia.**

**anorthoscope** An apparatus for producing and studying **anorthoscopic perception** which is the veridical perception of an image viewed under very uncommon conditions. It consists of a pair of circular discs mounted one behind the other. A figure is drawn on the rear disc and viewed through a slit in the front disc rotating at a different speed. The shape of the image will be clearly perceived.

**anoxia** Complete absence of oxygen.
*See* **hypoxia.**

a

**antagonism, lateral** *See* **inhibition, lateral.**

**antagonist 1.** An antagonistic muscle. **2.** A substance (e.g. a drug, hormone or neurotransmitter) that depresses the action of an agonist or binds to a cell receptor without eliciting a physiological response (e.g. excitation or inhibition). *Examples*: atropine and hyoscine which block the effect of acetylcholine acting on cholinergic receptors and timolol which blocks adrenergic receptors.
*See* **agonist.**

**antagonist drug** A drug that blocks or reduces the effect of a neurotransmitter.
*See* **beta-blocker.**

**antagonistic muscle** *See* **muscle, antagonistic.**

**antazoline phosphate** *See* **antihistamine.**

**anterior chamber** *See* **chamber, anterior.**

**anterior chamber angle** *See* **angle of the anterior chamber.**

**anterior chamber cleavage syndrome** *See* **Peter's anomaly.**

**anterior ciliary arteries** *See* **arteries, ciliary.**

**anterior pole** *See* **poles of the eyeball.**

**anterior segment of the eye** Portion of the eye comprising all the structures situated between the front surface of the cornea and the front surface of the vitreous. The eyelids are sometimes included in this definition.

**anterior synechia; uveitis** *See* under the nouns.

**antibacterial** *See* **antibiotic.**

**antibiotic 1.** Pertaining to the ability to destroy or inhibit other living organisms. **2.** A substance derived from a mould or bacterium, or produced synthetically, that destroys or inhibits the growth of other microorganisms and is thus used to treat infections. Some substances have a narrow spectrum of activity whereas others act against a wide range of both gram-positive and gram-negative organisms (**broad-spectrum antibiotics**). Antibiotics can be classified into several groups according to their mode of action on or within bacteria:
(1) Drugs inhibiting bacterial cell wall synthesis, such as the β-lactams (e.g. penicillin, cephalosporins), bacitracin and vancomycin. (2) Drugs affecting the bacterial cytoplasmic membrane, such as polymyxin B and gramicidin. (3) Drugs inhibiting bacterial protein synthesis, such as aminoglycosides (e.g. framycetin, neomycin, gentamicin and tobramycin), tetracyclines, macrolides (e.g. erythromycin and azithromycin) and chloramphenicol. (4) Drugs inhibiting the intermediate metabolism of bacteria, such as sulfonamides (e.g. sulfacetamide sodium) and trimethoprim. (5) Drugs inhibiting bacterial DNA synthesis, such as nalixidic acid (e.g. ciprofloxacin, lomefloxacin, norfloxacin and ofloxacin) and fluoroquinolones. (6) Other antibiotics such as fusidic acid, the diamidines, such as propamidine and dibropropamidine. *Syn.* antibacterial.

**anticholinergic** *See* **acetylcholine.**

**anticholinergic mydriasis** *See* **anisocoria.**

**anticholinesterase drugs** Parasympathetic drugs that inhibit or inactivate the enzyme acetylcholinesterase, allowing prolonged activity of acetylcholine. They cause miosis and ciliary muscle contraction. There are two groups: reversible which are of short duration (up to 12 hours or so), such as neostigmine, physostigmine and edrophonium chloride, and irreversible which lasts for days or weeks, such as demecarium bromide and diisopropyl fluorophosphate (DFP).
*See* **acetylcholine; miotics.**

**antifungal agent** Any substance which destroys or prevents the growth of fungi. It is one of the antibiotic groups. *Examples*: amphotericin B; miconazole; natamycin; nystatin. *Syn.* antimycotic agent.
*See* **antibiotic.**

**antihistamine** Any substance that reduces the effect of histamine or blocks histamine receptors, usually the histamine 1 (H1) receptor. It is used in the treatment of allergic conjunctivitis and also in the temporary relief of minor allergic symptoms of the eye. Common agents include antazoline, cetirizine, chlorpheniramine, emedastine, levocabastine, and loratidine.
*See* **allergic reactions; mast cell stabilizers.**

**anti-infective drug** A general term indicating either an antibiotic (or antibacterial), an antifungal or an antiviral agent, as well as the sulfonamides.

**antiinflammatory drug** A drug which inhibits or suppresses most inflammatory responses of an allergic, bacterial, traumatic or anaphylactic origin, as well as being immunosuppressant. They include the corticosteroids (e.g. betamethasone, dexamethasone, fluorometholone, hydrocortisone, loteprednol etabonate, prednisolone, rimexolone, triamcinolone). They are sometimes combined with an anti-infective drug (e.g. betamethasone combined with neomycin or sulfacetamide). Corticosteroids have side effects, such as enhancing the activity of herpes simplex virus, fungal overgrowth, raising intraocular pressure or cataract formation.
There are other antiinflammatory drugs which are non-steroidal (NSAID) and have little toxicity.

They act mainly by blocking prostaglandin synthesis. These include diclofenac sodium, flurbiprofen, indomethacin, ketorolac and oxyphenbutazone.
*See* **steroid.**

**antimetropia** A condition in which one eye is myopic and the other hypermetropic. *Syn.* mixed anisometropia.
*See* **anisocoria; anisometropia.**

**antimuscarinic drugs** *See* **acetylcholine; mydriatic.**

**antimycotic agent** *See* **antifungal agent.**

**anti-reflection coating** A thin film of transparent material, usually a metallic fluoride (e.g. magnesium fluoride), deposited on the surface of a lens which increases transmission and reduces surface reflection. *Abbreviated*: AR coating. *Syn.* anti-reflection film.
*See* **coating; Fresnel's formula; image, ghost; lens, coated.**

**antiseptic** An agent which kills or prevents the growth of bacteria. This term is generally restricted to agents that are sufficiently non-toxic for superficial application to living tissues. These include the **preservatives** for eye drops and contact lens solutions. Examples of antiseptics are alcohol, benzalkonium chloride, cetrimide, chlorbutanol, chlorhexidine, hydrogen peroxide, thimerosal (or thiomersalate). Other agents, which are too toxic to be applied to living tissues are called **disinfectants** and are used to sterilize instruments and apparatus.
*See* **disinfection by boiling; ethylenediamine tetraacetic acid; neutralization; sterilization.**

**antiviral agents** Substances which inhibit the growth of a virus (e.g. herpes) by inhibiting DNA or RNA synthesis. Common agents include acyclovir, idoxuridine, ganciclovir sodium, trifluridine (or trifluorothymidine) and vidarabine.
*See* **keratitis; keratitis, herpetic.**

**Anton's syndrome** *See* **syndrome, Anton's.**

**aperture** An opening, or the area of a lens, through which light can pass.
*See* **pupil.**

**aperture, angular** Half of the maximum plane subtended by a lens at the axial point of an object or image. (Sometimes the full plane angle is taken as the angular aperture but this is not convenient in optical calculations.)
*See* **sine condition.**

**aperture of a lenticular lens** That portion of a lenticular lens which has the prescribed power (British Standard).
*See* **lens, lenticular.**

**aperture, numerical** An expression designating the light-gathering power of microscope objectives. It is equal to the product of the index of refraction $n$ of the object space and the sine of the angle $u$ subtended by a radius of the entrance pupil at the axial point on the object, i.e. $n \sin u$.

**aperture, palpebral** The gap between the margins of the eyelids when the eye is open. An abnormal increase in the aperture occurs in some conditions, including Graves' disease, buphthalmos, Parinaud's syndrome and retrobulbar tumour. An abnormal decrease in the aperture occurs in some conditions, including ptosis, microphthalmos and ophthalmoplegia (Fig. A14 and Fig. A15). *Syn.* interpalpebral fissure (this term is more accurate although used infrequently); palpebral fissure.
*See* **exophthalmos; eyelids.**

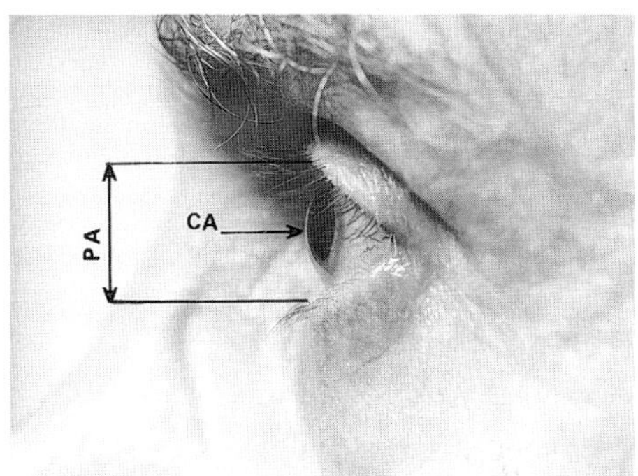


**Fig. A14** Palpebral aperture PA and corneal apex CA

**aperture plane** *See* **plane, aperture.**

**aperture ratio** *See* **aperture, relative.**

**aperture, relative** The reciprocal of the f number. It is therefore equal to the ratio of the diameter of the entrance pupil to the primary focal length of an optical system. *Syn.* aperture ratio. *Note*: the definition of this term is not universally accepted; some authors define it as the reverse of the above.
*See* **f number.**

**aperture-stop** *See* **diaphragm.**

**apex, corneal** The most anterior point of the cornea when the eye is in the primary position (Fig. A14). It does not automatically coincide with any common reference point (e.g. line of sight).
*See* **bearing, apical; clearance, apical; optical zone of cornea; position, primary.**

**apex of a prism** The thinnest part of the prism where the two faces intersect.
*See* **base of a prism; prism.**

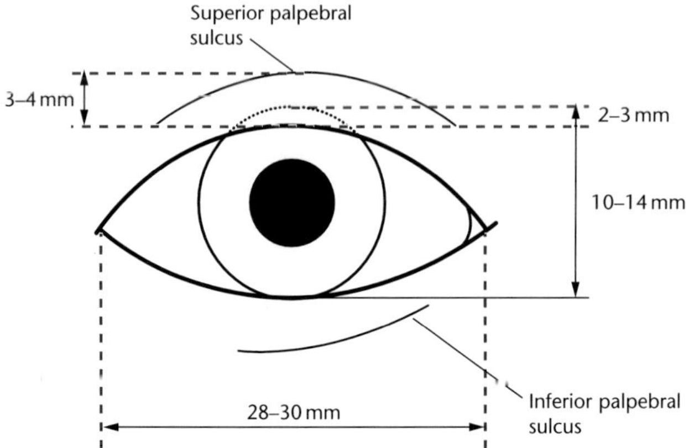


**Fig. A15** Average dimensions of the normal palpebral aperture of a Caucasian eye

**aphake** Person who is aphakic.

**aphakia** Ocular condition in which the crystalline lens is absent. It may be congenital but usually it is due to surgical removal of a cataract. As a result the eye has no accommodative power and is usually highly hypermetropic.
*See* **aniseikonia; cataract; eye, pseudophakic; lens, aphakic; phakic; phenomenon, jack-in-the-box; vitreous detachment.**

**aphakic eye; lens** *See* under the nouns.

**aphakic pupillary block** *See* **pupillary block.**

**apical bearing** *See* **bearing, apical.**

**apical clearance** *See* **clearance, apical.**

**aplanatic** Pertains to an optical system which is free from spherical aberration and coma.
*See* **lens, aplanatic.**

**aplanatic lens** *See* **lens, aplanatic.**

**apochromatic lens** *See* **lens, apochromatic.**

**aponeurosis** *See* **muscle, levator palpebrae superioris.**

**apoptosis** A fragmentation of a cell into membrane-bound particles that are phagocytosed by other cells. It is believed to be genetically programmed.
*See* **neuroprotection.**

**apostilb** The luminance of a perfectly diffusing surface that reflects 1 lumen per square metre. This measure is often used in visual field analysis, where the luminance of the background and targets is measured in apostilb.

**apparent frontoparallel plane** *See* **plane, apparent frontoparallel.**

**apparent pupil** *See* **pupil of the eye, entrance.**

**apparent size** *See* **size, apparent.**

**apparent strabismus** *See* **strabismus, apparent.**

**appendages of the eye** The adjacent structures of the eye such as the lacrimal apparatus, the extraocular muscles and the eyelids, eyelashes, eyebrows and the conjunctiva. *Syn.* adnexa oculi.

**apperception** The ability to perceive and interpret fully any psychic content or sensory stimuli. *Example*: the apperception aroused by new objects in the visual field which are noticed when entering an unfamiliar room.

**applanation tonometer** *See* **tonometer, applanation.**

**appliance, optical** Any optical system which is used in conjunction with the eye. Optical appliances include spectacles, contact lenses to correct sight and/or anomalies of binocular vision and also telescopes or microscopes to magnify an object. *Syn.* optical aid.
*See* **dispensing, optical; optometry; ptosis.**

**apraclonidine hydrochloride** *See* **alpha-adrenergic agonist.**

**apraxia** A disorder of voluntary movement, characterized by the inability to accomplish a skilled or purposeful movement, in the absence of motor paralysis, sensory loss or of a general lack of coordination. It is due to a cerebellar disease.

**apraxia, ocular motor** A congenital inability to perform some voluntary ocular movements. Children with this condition often use head thrusts to move their eyes to the left or to the right.

**apraxia, optical** Apraxia in which there is an inability to copy or to draw in proper spatial orientation. It is usually associated with visual agnosia. *Syn.* visual apraxia.
*See* **agnosia.**

**apraxia, visual** *See* **apraxia, optical.**

**aqueduct of Sylvius** A canal in the midbrain connecting the third and fourth ventricles. *Syn.* cerebral aqueduct.

**aqueous flare** Scattering of light seen when a slit-lamp beam is directed, obliquely to the plane of the iris, into the anterior chamber. It occurs as a result of increased protein content, and usually inflammatory cells, in the aqueous humour. Visual impairment depends on the intensity of the flare. It is a sign of intraocular inflammation. *See* **effect, Tyndall; iritis; uveitis.**

**aqueous humour** *See* **humour, aqueous.**

**AR coating** *See* **anti-reflection coating.**

**arachnoid** The middle member of the three meninges covering the brain, the spinal cord and the optic nerve. From the optic nerve it becomes continuous with the sclera.
*See* **sclera.**

**arc eye** *See* **keratoconjunctivitis, actinic.**

**arc perimeter** *See* **perimeter, arc.**

**arc, pupillary reflex** *See* **reflex, pupil light.**

**arc of contact** That portion of an extraocular muscle which wraps around the surface of the globe prior to the insertion of its tendon into the sclera. The point where the muscle first comes into contact with the globe is called the **contact point**. The arc of contact continually alters its length as the eye rotates. *Syn.* contact arc.

**Archambault's loop** *See* **loop, Meyer's.**

**arcs, blue** Entoptic phenomenon appearing as two bands of blue light arching from above and below the source towards the blind spot. This phenomenon is induced by a small source of light (preferably red) stimulating the temporal side of the retina near the fovea.
*See* **image, entoptic.**

**arcuate nerve fibre bundle** *See* **fibres, arcuate.**

**arcuate scotoma** *See* **scotoma, arcuate.**

**arcus juvenilis** *See* **arcus, corneal.**

**arcus marginale** *See* **orbital septum.**

**arcus, corneal** A greyish-white ring (or part of a ring) opacity occurring in the periphery of the cornea, in middle and old age. It is due to a lipid infiltration of the corneal stroma. With age the condition progresses to form a complete ring. That ring is separated from the limbus by a zone of clear cornea. The condition can also appear in early or middle life and is referred to as **arcus juvenilis** (or **anterior embryotoxon**): it is somewhat whiter than corneal arcus. Arcus juvenilis is often associated with heart disease in men. *Syn.* arcus senilis; gerontoxon.

**arcus senilis** *See* **arcus, corneal.**

**Arden gratings; plates** *See* **test, Arden grating.**

**Arden index; ratio** *See* **electro-oculogram.**

**area centralis** *See* **macula lutea.**

**area of comfort** Zone of comfort.
*See* **criterion, Percival.**

**area, extrastriate visual** *See* **areas, visual association.**

**area, fusion** *See* **area, Panum's.**

**area, Panum's** An area in the retina of one eye, any point of which, when stimulated simultaneously with a single point in the retina of the other eye, will give rise to a single percept. Its diameter in the fovea is about 5 minutes of arc and increases towards the periphery (Fig. A16). *Syn.* fusion area.
*See* **disparity, retinal; horopter; Panum's fusional space; retinal corresponding points.**

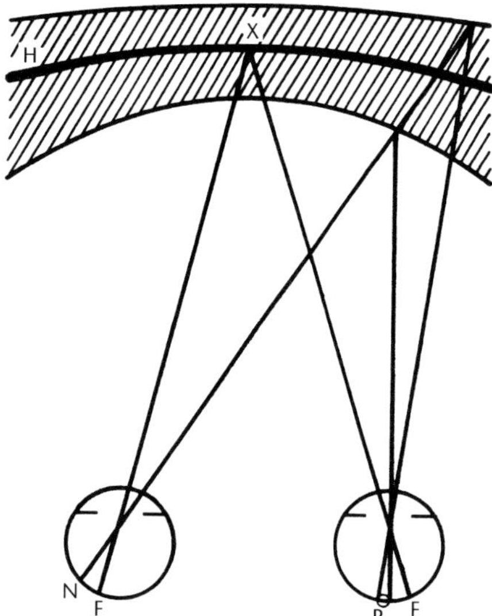


**Fig. A16** The eyes are fixating X on the horopter H. Stimulation of point N in the left retina and of any point within Panum's area P of the right retina gives rise to a perception of singleness and stereopsis. Visual lines extrapolated from the limits of Panum's area P indicate the far and near limits of Panum's fusional space (shaded) by their intersection with the visual line of point N in the left eye (F, fovea)

**area, rod-free** *See* **foveola.**

**area, striate** *See* **area, visual.**

**area, visual 1.** Any region of the brain in which visual information is processed. **2.** This is Brodmann's area 17 in each occipital lobe. It contains six layers of cells numbered 1 to 6 from top, layer 4 being subdivided into three sublayers

a

4A, 4B and 4C. Layer 4C receives inputs from the photoreceptors in the retina via the lateral geniculate bodies. There are also some afferents to layers 1 and 6. The primary visual area is identified by a white striation (**line of Gennari**) on each side of the calcarine fissure. This white line appears in the middle of the fourth layer of the visual cortex and is composed of fibres from the optic radiations. *Syn.* primary visual area; primary visual cortex; striate area; striate cortex; V1; visual cortex. **3.** It also refers to all parts of each occipital lobe related to visual functions. *Syn.* prestriate cortex.
*See* **column, cortical; cortex, occipital; geniculate bodies, lateral; magnification, cortical; pathway, visual.**

**areas, Brodmann's** Areas of the cerebral cortex defined by Brodmann and numbered from 1 to 52. Areas 17, 18 and 19 represent the visual area and visual association areas in each cerebral cortex.
*See* **area, visual; areas, visual association; cortex, occipital.**

**areas, visual association** They are the **parastriate area** (or **Brodmann's area 18**) and the **peristriate area** (or **Brodmann's area 19**) of the occipital cortex surrounding the visual area. Areas 18 and 19 are subdivided into multiple zones (called V2, V3, V4, V5, V6, etc.). They receive projections from the striate cortex. They are also connected to other areas of the cortex and via the corpus callosum with areas 18 and 19 of the opposite hemisphere and receive feedback information. It has been shown that V4 and the inferotemporal cortex or IT (components of the ventral or temporal cortex) receive substantial input from the parvocellular pathway. V5 (also called middle temporal cortex or MT, a component of dorsal or parietal cortex) receives input from the magnocellular pathway. Processing which occurs in the visual association areas helps to interpret the message that reaches the visual area and to recall memories of previous visual experiences. *Syn.* extrastriate visual area; extrastriate cortex; prestriate cortex (these terms actually represent all the regions outside the striate cortex where visual processing takes place); secondary visual cortex.

**argon laser** *See* **laser, argon.**

**Argyll Robertson pupil** *See* **pupil, Argyll Robertson.**

**argyrosis** The presence of silver in the deep corneal stroma or Descemet's membrane.

**Arlt's line** *See* **trachoma.**

**arterial circle of the iris, major** A vascular circle located in the anterior part of the ciliary body near the root of the iris. It is formed by the anastomosis of the two long posterior ciliary arteries and the seven anterior ciliary arteries. It supplies the iris, the ciliary processes and the anterior choroid.
*See* **arteries, ciliary.**

**arterial circle of the iris, minor** An incomplete vascular circle located in the region of the collarette of the iris. It is formed by arterial and venous anastomoses. It supplies the pupillary zone of the iris.
*See* **arterial circle of the iris, major; collarette.**

**arteries, ciliary** Branches of the ophthalmic artery which supply the whole of the uveal tract, the sclera and the edge of the cornea with its neighbouring conjunctiva. The ciliary arteries comprise: (1) The short posterior ciliary arteries. (2) The long posterior ciliary arteries. (3) The anterior ciliary arteries.
The **short posterior ciliary arteries** (s.p.c.a.) are some 10–20 branches of the ophthalmic artery which pierce the eyeball around the optic nerve to supply the posterior choroid, the optic disc, the circle of Zinn, the cilioretinal and episcleral arteries. The **long posterior ciliary arteries** (l.p.c.a.) are two branches from the ophthalmic artery which pierce the sclera on either side of the optic nerve, further anteriorly than the s.p.c.a., and course in the perichoroidal space. They form, with the anterior ciliary arteries, the **major arterial** (or **iridic**) **circle of the iris**, which supplies the ciliary body, the anterior choroid and the iris. The **anterior ciliary arteries** are derived from the arteries to the four recti muscles and they anastomose in the ciliary muscle with the l.p.c.a. to form the major arterial circle of the iris. They also give branches that supply the episclera (**episcleral arteries**), sclera, limbus and conjunctiva (**anterior and posterior conjunctival arteries**).
*See* **anastomosis; arterial circle of the iris, major.**

**arteries, conjunctival** *See* **arteries, ciliary.**

**arteriosclerosis** Thickening and hardening of the walls of arteries which results in an obstruction of the blood flow. In the retina, the branches of the central retinal artery may become straightened at first, later they become lengthened and tortuous, the arteriolevenule (A-V) crossings are abnormal. Arteries resemble '**copper wire**' as they become infiltrated with lipid deposits and eventually as '**silver wire**' as the deposits increase and the whole thickness of the artery appears as a bright white reflex. Some retinal oedema may be present and as the disease progresses there are retinal haemorrhages and small sharp-edged exudates without surrounding oedema. This retinal condition is called arteriosclerotic retinopathy.
*See* **atherosclerosis; neuropathy, ischaemic optic; retinopathy, hypertensive; sphygmomanometer.**

**arteritis, giant cell** *See* **arteritis, temporal.**

**arteritis, temporal** An inflammatory disease of the wall of arteries, mainly of the extracranial vessels, which occurs in people who are over 60 years of age. The condition is characterized by headache and pain in muscles and joints, such as those of the jaws, and sometimes fever. A sudden loss of vision in one eye (amaurosis fugax) may occur in the first few weeks after the onset of the disease due to an occlusion of either the central retinal artery or of the short posterior ciliary arteries that supply the optic nerve. Prompt administration of systemic corticosteroids (e.g. hydrocortisone) has been found to be of great value in the management of this condition. *Syn.* giant cell arteritis (strictly speaking this term is usually reserved for a more generalized condition).
*See* **amaurosis fugax; neuropathy, ischaemic optic; pupil, Adie's.**

**artery** A tubular, elastic vessel which carries blood away from the heart. Its walls are thicker than those of veins in order to withstand the greater pressure of blood on the arterial side of the circulation.
*See* **vein.**

**artery, central retinal** A branch of the ophthalmic artery entering the optic nerve some 6–12 mm from the eyeball. It enters the eye through the optic disc and divides into superior and inferior branches and both these branches subdivide into nasal and temporal branches which course in the nerve fibre layer, supplying the capillaries feeding the bipolar and the ganglion cell layers of the retina (except for the fovea).
*See* **arteritis, temporal; cherry-red spot; retinal arterial occlusion; vein, central retinal.**

**artery, carotid** *See* **amaurosis fugax.**

**artery, cilioretinal** A small artery running from the temporal side of the optic disc to the macular area. It originates from the circle of Zinn and supplies the retina between the macula and the disc. This artery is present in only about a fifth, or less, of human eyes. If a patient possesses this artery central vision will be spared in case of occlusion of the central retinal artery. In some other eyes the cilioretinal artery supplies some other region of the retina.
*See* **circle of Zinn.**

**artery, copper wire** *See* **arteriosclerosis.**

**artery, hyaloid** An artery that is present during the embryological period. It arises from the ophthalmic artery, runs forward from the optic disc to the lens where it spreads over the posterior lenticular surface as a capillary net which in turn anastomoses with a capillary net located on the anterior lens surface. Thus the lens becomes enveloped by an anastomosing vascular network called the **tunica vasculosa lentis**. The hyaloid artery also gives rise to a large number of branches, the **vasa hyaloidea propria**, which at times almost fills the vitreous cavity. The hyaloid artery degenerates by the 8th month of gestation to become the central retinal artery.
*See* **canal, hyaloid; fissure, optic; hyaloid remnant.**

**artery, infraorbital** A terminal branch of the internal maxillary artery which enters the orbit through the inferior orbital fissure and leaves via the infraorbital canal. It supplies the inferior rectus and inferior oblique muscles, the lacrimal sac, and the lower eyelid and sometimes the lacrimal gland.
*See* **fissure, inferior orbital.**

**artery, internal carotid** A branch of the common carotid artery. The internal carotid artery gives rise to many branches and in particular the ophthalmic artery after it passes through the cavernous sinus. It terminates in the anterior and middle cerebral arteries.
*See* **amaurosis fugax; circle of Willis; plaques, Hollenhorst's; sinus, cavernous.**

**artery, lacrimal** It arises from the ophthalmic artery to the outer side of the optic nerve. It supplies the lacrimal gland, the conjunctiva and eyelids giving origin to the lateral palpebral arteries.

**artery, ophthalmic** Vessel arising from the internal carotid artery and which enters the orbit through the optic canal. It gives rise to numerous branches: (1) Central retinal artery. (2) Posterior ciliary arteries. (3) Lacrimal artery (and lateral palpebral and zygomatic branches). (4) Muscular branches. (5) Supraorbital artery. (6) Anterior and posterior ethmoidal arteries. (7) Recurrent meningeal artery. (8) Supratrochlear artery. (9) Medial palpebral arteries. (10) Dorsal nasal artery.
Thus, the ophthalmic artery supplies all the tunics of the eyeball, most of the structures in the orbit, the lacrimal sac, the paranasal sinuses, and the nose (Fig. A17).

**artery, silver wire** *See* **arteriosclerosis.**

**artery, supraorbital** Branch of the ophthalmic artery which supplies the upper eyelid, the scalp and also sends branches to the levator palpebrae superioris muscle and the periorbita.

**arthritis, rheumatoid** *See* **rheumatoid arthritis.**

**artificial daylight; eye; pupil; tears** *See* under the nouns.

**artifact** Anything made or introduced artificially which misleads the results of an investigation, image or test. *Example*: in visual evoked cortical potentials, any wave that has its origin elsewhere than in the visual area.

**A-scan** *See* **ultrasonography.**

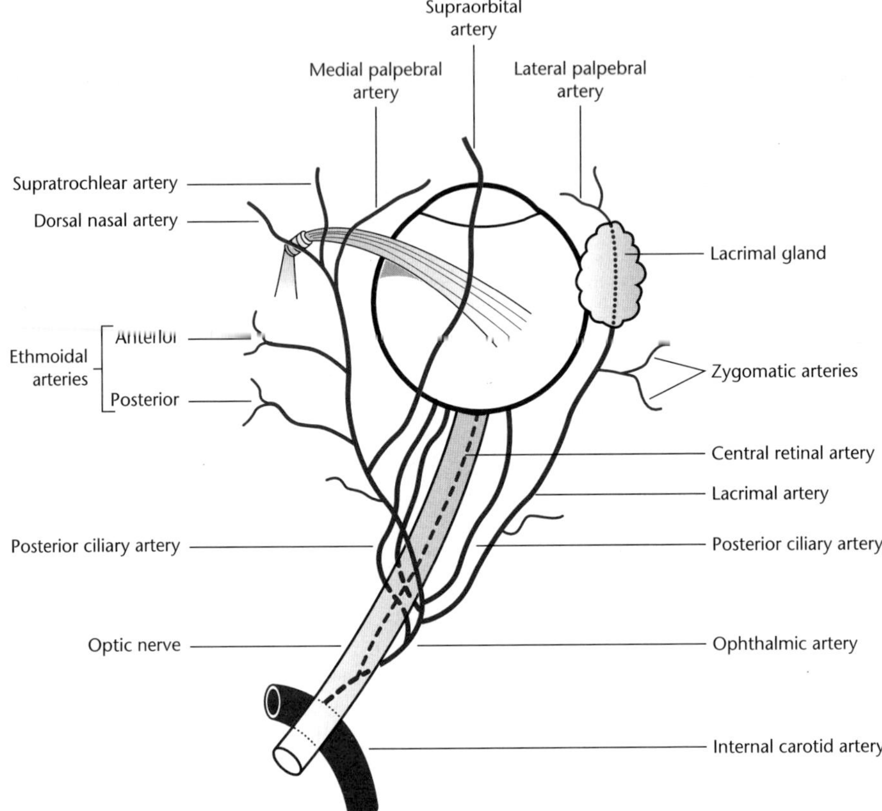


**Fig. A17** The ophthalmic artery and its branches. The meningeal and muscular branches are not indicated in the diagram

**aspheric lens** *See* **lens, aspheric.**

**aspherical** Literally 'not spherical' but this term is usually restricted to surfaces of revolution having identical but non-circular (e.g. parabolic) sections in all meridians (British Standard).
*See* **lens, aspherical.**

**asteroid hyalosis** Degenerative changes occurring more commonly in males and mainly in one eye. It consists of numerous small stellate or discoid opacities (called **asteroid bodies**) suspended in the vitreous humour. These opacities appear creamy white when viewed by ophthalmoscopy. They rarely affect vision. *Syn.* Benson's disease.
*See* **humour, vitreous; ophthalmoscope; synchisis scintillans.**

**asthenopia** Term used to describe any symptoms associated with the use of the eyes. The causes of asthenopia are numerous: sustained near vision, either when the accommodation amplitude is low or hypermetropia is uncorrected (**accommodative asthenopia**), aniseikonia (**aniseikonic a.**), astigmatism (**astigmatic a.**), pain in the eye (**asthenopia dolens**), heterophoria (**heterophoric a.**), ocular inflammation (**asthenopia irritans**), hysteria (**nervous a.**), uncorrected presbyopia (**presbyopic a.**), improper illumination (**photogenous a.**) or retinal disease (**retinal a.**). *Syn.* eyestrain; near point stress (NPS) (although this term is restricted to any symptoms arising from near vision).
*See* **convergence excess; convergence insufficiency; divergence insufficiency; fatigue, visual; headache, ocular.**

**astigmat** A person who has astigmatism.

**astigmatic** Pertaining to astigmatism.

**astigmatic dial; fan chart** *See* **chart, astigmatic fan.**

**astigmatic interval** *See* **Sturm, interval of.**

**astigmatic lens** *See* **lens, astigmatic.**

**astigmatism** A condition of refraction in which the image of a point object is not a single point but two focal lines at different distances from

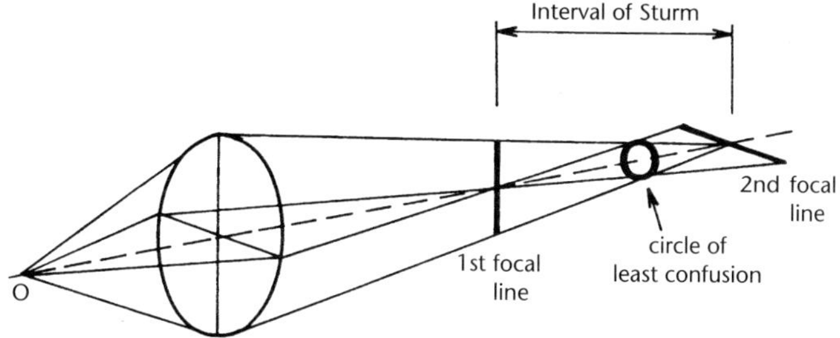


Fig. A18 Astigmatic beam of light (O, object)

**Table A11** Approximate relationship between uncorrected astigmatism and visual acuity

| | Snellen visual acuity | |
|---|---|---|
| **astigmatism (D)** | **(m)** | **(ft)** |
| 4.50 | 6/60 | 20/200 |
| 3.50 | 6/36 | 20/120 |
| 2.50 | 6/24 | 20/80 |
| 1.75 | 6/18 | 20/60 |
| 1.25 | 6/12 | 20/40 |
| 0.75 | 6/9 | 20/30 |
| 0.25 | 6/6 | 20/20 |
| 0.00 | 6/5 | 20/16 |

the optical system. The two focal lines are generally perpendicular to each other. In the eye, it is a refractive error which is generally caused by one or several toroidal shapes of the refracting surfaces, or by the obliquity of the light entering the eye, but it can also develop as a result of subluxation of the lens, diabetes, cataract, keratoconus or trauma (**acquired astigmatism**) (Fig. A18).
*See* **amblyopia, meridional; chalazion; chart, astigmatic fan; circle of least confusion; headache, ocular; Javal's rule; lens, cross-cylinder; line, focal; method, fogging; stigmatism; Sturm, interval of; test for astigmatism, cross-cylinder; test, fan and block.**

**astigmatism, accommodative** Astigmatism induced by accommodation. It is not known whether this is caused by a tilt of the crystalline lens or unequal alterations of the curvatures of the crystalline lens.
*See* **accommodation.**

**astigmatism, against the rule** Ocular astigmatism in which the refractive power of the horizontal (or near horizontal) meridian is the greatest (Fig. A19). The percentage of people with against the rule astigmatism increases beyond the age of about 45 and becomes more common than with the rule astigmatism in people beyond the age of about 55. Corneal

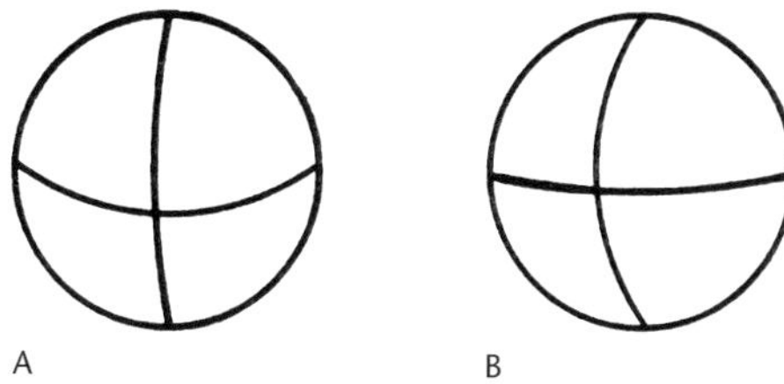


Fig. A19 Types of astigmatism (A, against the rule; B, with the rule)

astigmatism is the main cause of this shift. *Syn.* indirect or inverse astigmatism.
*See* **astigmatism, with the rule.**

**astigmatism, compound** Astigmatism in which the two principal meridians of an eye are either both hypermetropic (**compound hypermetropic astigmatism**) or both myopic (**compound myopic astigmatism**) (Fig. A20).
*See* **hypermetropia; myopia.**

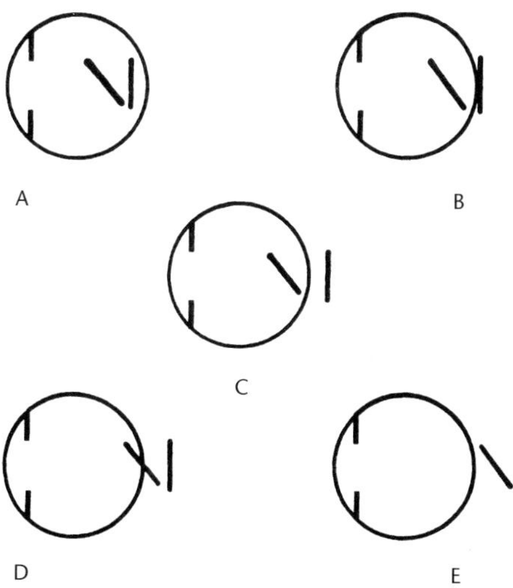


Fig. A20 Clinical types of astigmatism (A, compound myopic; B, simple myopic; C, mixed; D, simple hyperopic; E, compound hyperopic)

**astigmatism, direct** *See* **astigmatism, with the rule.**

**astigmatism, indirect** *See* **astigmatism, against the rule.**

**astigmatism, induced 1.** Astigmatism introduced when using contact lenses with toroidal back optic zones. This astigmatism is due to the fact that a toroidal back optic surface separates two media of different refractive indices (the contact lens and tears) and this occurs principally with rigid toric surfaces. Using contact lenses of lower refractive index reduces the amount of induced astigmatism (such as gas permeable rather than PMMA). **2.** Astigmatism introduced when a contact lens slips or tilts on the eye. This is due to the fact that the chief ray is deviated and is no longer normal to the front surface of the lens. The amount thus produced is small (about 0.50 D for a slip of 3 mm) but increases if the lens tilts as well as slips.
*See* **astigmatism, residual.**

**astigmatism, internal** *See* **astigmatism, total.**

**astigmatism, inverse** *See* **astigmatism, against the rule.**

**astigmatism, irregular** Ocular astigmatism in which the two principal meridians are not at right angles to each other. This condition is often the result of injury or disease (e.g. keratoconus), but can also exist in an eye with irregularities in the refractive power in different meridians of the crystalline lens.
*See* **lens, combination; lens, piggyback.**

**astigmatism, lenticular** Astigmatism of the crystalline lens. It is usually due to variations in the curvature of one or both surfaces and much less commonly to irregularities in its refractive index. Lenticular astigmatism is typically against the rule.
*See* **astigmatism, total.**

**astigmatism, mixed** Ocular astigmatism in which one principal meridian is hypermetropic and the other myopic (Fig. A20).
*See* **hypermetropia; myopia.**

**Table A12** Average amount of oblique astigmatism (in dioptres) at different angles to the visual axis

| angle (deg) | nasal retina | temporal retina |
|---|---|---|
| 0 | 0 | 0 |
| 10 | 0.28 | 0.29 |
| 20 | 0.55 | 0.74 |
| 30 | 1.0 | 1.58 |
| 40 | 1.7 | 2.45 |
| 50 | 2.7 | 3.6 |
| 60 | 3.9 | 4.75 |

**astigmatism, oblique 1.** Astigmatism in which the two principal meridians are neither approximately horizontal nor approximately vertical. **2.** Aberration of an optical system which occurs when the incident light rays form an angle with the optical axis which exceeds the conditions of gaussian optics. It gives rise to separate **tangential** and **sagittal** line foci instead of a single image point.
*See* **allometropia; lens, anastigmatic; Petzval surface; ray, paraxial; Sturm, interval of.**

**astigmatism, physiological** Astigmatism not exceeding 0.5–0.75 D in the normal eye.

**astigmatism, refractive** *See* **astigmatism, total.**

**astigmatism, residual** Astigmatism still present after correction of a refractive error.
*See* **astigmatism, induced.**

**astigmatism, simple** Ocular astigmatism in which one principal meridian of the eye is emmetropic and the other myopic (**simple myopic astigmatism**) or hypermetropic (**simple hypermetropic astigmatism**) (Fig. A20).
*See* **emmetropia; hypermetropia; myopia.**

**astigmatism, total** Astigmatism of the eye comprising both anterior corneal and internal astigmatism (i.e. **lenticular astigmatism**) and astigmatism of the posterior surface of the cornea. *Syn.* refractive astigmatism.
*See* **Javal's rule.**

**astigmatism, with the rule** Astigmatism in which the refractive power of the vertical (or near vertical) meridian is the greatest (Fig. A19). *Syn.* direct astigmatism.
*See* **astigmatism, against the rule.**

**astigmatoscope** Instrument for observing and measuring the astigmatism of an eye. *Syn.* astigmometer; astigmoscope.

**astrocytes** Neuroglial cells with many processes found in the central nervous system, the retina (especially the ganglion cells, the inner plexiform layers and the nerve fibre layer) and the optic nerve. Their function is believed to be nutritional and structural. *Syn.* Cajal's cells.
*See* **retina.**

**astronomical telescope** *See* **telescope.**

**asymmetropia** *See* **anisometropia.**

**A syndrome** *See* **pattern, A.**

**ataxia** An inability to coordinate muscular activity during voluntary movements.

**ataxia, Friedreich's** *See* **ataxia, hereditary spinal.**

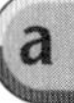

**ataxia, hereditary spinal** A hereditary degeneration of the posterior and lateral columns of the spinal cord occurring in childhood. It is characterized by general ataxia, nystagmus and, sometimes, ptosis and external ophthalmoplegia. *Syn.* Friedreich's ataxia.

**atheroma** Fatty deposits which lead to the formation of plaques in the blood vessels.
*See* **arteriosclerosis; plaques, Hollenhorst's.**

**atherosclerosis** A form of arteriosclerosis in which fatty deposits occur in the middle coat of arteries. The deposits or plaques, which form at the site of arterial damage, often block or shut off the blood flow. Atherosclerosis occurs usually in elderly people.
*See* **arteriosclerosis; atheroma.**

**atopic reactions** *See* **keratoconjunctivitis, atopic.**

**atrophy choroidal** A group of ocular degenerations of the choroid. These lesions have been grouped according to the area involved and the topographical pattern noted. Classical disease states include gyrate atrophy as well as choroideraemia. These lesions are often inherited, demonstrating both autosomal recessive and dominant inheritance patterns.
*See* **choroideraemia.**

**atrophy, optic** Degeneration of the optic nerve fibres characterized by a pallor of the optic disc which may appear greyish, yellowish or white. This condition leads to a loss of visual acuity or changes in the visual fields or both. The change in colour of the disc is due to a loss of the normal capillarity of the disc and to a deposition of fibrin or glial tissue which replaces the nerve fibres. **1. Primary** or **simple optic atrophy**. The disc margins are well defined and usually the lamina cribrosa is unobscured. The colour is pale pink to white. Glaucoma is the chief cause of primary optic atrophy. **2. Secondary optic atrophy**. The difference with the former is that in this condition there is evidence of preceding oedema or inflammation. The margins of the disc appear blurred and glial proliferation is present over the surface of the disc, thus obscuring the lamina cribrosa. The colour is yellowish to grey. Papilloedema gives rise to secondary optic atrophy.
*See* **glaucoma, open-angle; Leber's hereditary optic atrophy; papilloedema; syndrome, Foster Kennedy.**

**atropine** An alkaloid obtained from the belladonna plant. It is an antimuscarinic drug. In the eye it acts as a mydriatic and as a cycloplegic. It paralyses the pupillary sphincter and the ciliary muscle by preventing the action of acetylcholine at the parasympathetic nerve endings.
*See* **acetylcholine; cycloplegia; mydriatic.**

**atropine-like drug** *See* **mydriatic.**

**atropine mydriasis** *See* **anisocoria.**

**attenuation 1.** A reduction of intensity of a radiation as it passes through an absorbing or scattering medium. **2.** Narrowing of a blood vessel. **3.** *See* **penalization.**

**Aubert's phenomenon** *See* **phenomenon, Aubert's.**

**aura, visual** Visual sensations which precede an epileptic attack or a migraine. These sensations may appear as light flashes, scintillating scotomata, etc.

**auscultation** *See* **bruit.**

**auto keratometer** *See* **keratometer, auto.**

**autokinesis, visual** *See* **illusion, autokinetic visual.**

**autorefraction 1.** A procedure of refraction in which the patient adjusts the controls of the instrument. **2.** Refraction carried out with an electronic optometer which is fully objective, generally using infrared light and which can be operated by a non-specialist.
*See* **optometer, infrared; refractive error.**

**autorefractor** *See* **optometer.**

**autorefractometer** *See* **optometer.**

**A-V crossing** *See* **arteriosclerosis.**

**automated perimeter** *See* **perimeter, automated.**

**avascular zone** *See* **foveola.**

**avulsion** The forcible separation of two parts, or tearing away of a part or of an organ. *Examples*: avulsion of the retina at the ora serrata; avulsion of the eyelid at its insertion.

**axanthopsia** Yellow blindness.
*See* **chromatopsia.**

**Axenfeld's intrascleral nerve loop** *See* **loop, Axenfeld's intrascleral nerve.**

**Axenfeld's anomaly; syndrome** *See* **syndrome, Axenfeld's.**

**axes of Fick** Three mutually perpendicular axes which intersect at the centre of rotation of the eye. They are the *x*-, *y*-, and *z*-axes. *Syn.* primary axes of Fick.
*See* **axis, anteroposterior; axis, transverse; axis, vertical.**

**axial length of the eye** *See* **length of the eye, axial.**

**axial magnification** *See* **magnification, axial.**

a

**axial ray** *See* **ray, axial.**

**axis, achromatic** A line in the eye along which light passes through all the optical elements and emerges without chromatic dispersion. Although it may lie close to the optical axis it does not necessarily coincide with it.
*See* **chromostereopsis; dispersion; parallax, chromatic.**

**axis, anteroposterior** A line passing through the anterior and posterior poles and the centre of rotation of the eye. It is perpendicular to the transverse (or *x*-axis) and the vertical (or *z*-axis). *Syn.* sagittal axis; *y*-axis.
*See* **centre of rotation of the eye; poles of the eyeball.**

**axis, cylinder 1.** A line of zero curvature on a cylindrical surface. **2.** That principal meridian of a planocylinder in which the power is zero.
*See* **lens, astigmatic.**

**axis, fixation** The line joining the object of regard to the centre of rotation of the eye. *Syn.* line of fixation.

**axis, geometrical** The line passing through the anterior and posterior poles of the eye. If the refractive surfaces are symmetrical about that axis, it will then coincide with the optical axis.
*See* **axis, optical; poles of the eyeball.**

**axis notation** *See* **axis notation, standard.**

**axis notation, standard** The accepted axis notation for cylinders, the same for each eye, whereby the specified axis direction denotes the angle of the cylinder axis with the horizontal measured anti-clockwise from 0° to 180°, the front surface of the lens being viewed (British Standard). (Fig. A21) *Syn.* TABO notation (although the TABO notation specifies the axis direction from 0° to 360°); OCA notation.

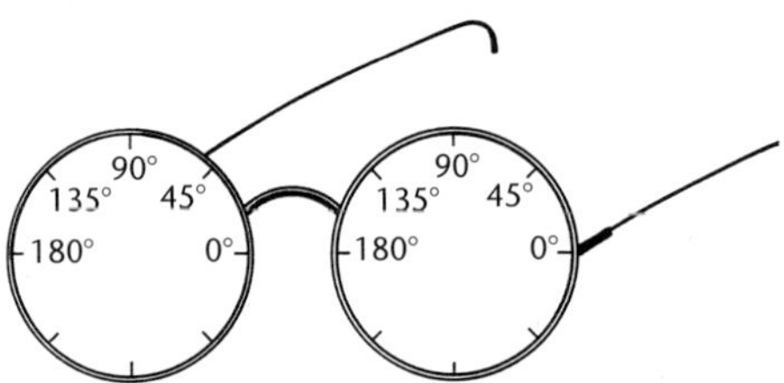


**Fig. A21** Illustration of the standard cylinder axis notation

**axis, optical 1.** The line joining the optical centres of the refractive surfaces of the eye (a theoretical concept in the eye). A close approximation of this axis is represented by aligning the Purkinje images of a test object (Fig. P10, page 243). **2.** The line normal to the surfaces of a lens along which light passes undeviated.
*See* **images, Purkinje–Sanson.**

**axis, orbital** The line from the middle of the orbital opening to the centre of the optic foramen. The orbital axes of a normal adult make an angle of approximately 45° with each other.
*See* **orbit.**

**axis, principal** A line passing through the centre of curvature of a surface and through its vertex.
*See* **vertex.**

**axis, pupillary** The line passing through the centre of the entrance pupil of the eye and the pole of the cornea. *Syn.* pupillary line.
*See* **poles of the eyeball.**

**axis, sagittal** *See* **axis, anteroposterior.**

**axis, transverse** A horizontal line passing through the centre of rotation of the eye and lying in Listing's plane. *Syn.* *x*-axis.
*See* **axis, anteroposterior; plane, Listing's.**

**axis, vertical** A vertical line passing through the centre of rotation of the eye. *Syn.* *z*-axis.
*See* **axis, anteroposterior.**

**axis, visual** The line joining the object of regard to the foveola and passing through the nodal points which are often considered as coincident, as they are very close to each other. Strictly, this axis is not a single straight line as it consists of two parts: one line connecting the object of regard to the first nodal point and the other line parallel and connecting the second nodal point to the foveola. *Syn.* visual line.
*See* **line of sight.**

**axis, x-** *See* **axis, transverse.**

**axis, y-** *See* **axis, anteroposterior.**

**axis, z-** *See* **axis, vertical.**

**axometer 1.** Instrument for determining the axis of a cylindrical lens and the optical centre of a lens. **2.** Instrument used in the subjective determination of the principal meridians of an astigmatic eye. *Syn.* axonometer.

**axon** *See* **neuron.**

# B



**bacitracin** An antibiotic drug with similar properties to penicillin and effective principally against gram-positive bacteria, such as Staphylococci and Streptococci. It is mainly used in combination with other agents (e.g. polymyxin B) for treating external eye infections (e.g. blepharoconjunctivitis).
*See* **antibiotic.**

**back haptic size** *See* **haptic size, back.**

**back of a lens** Relating to that surface nearer to the eye (British Standard).

**back optic zone diameter** *See* **optic zone diameter.**

**back optic zone radius** *See* **optic zone radius, back.**

**back vertex focal length** *See* **vertex focal length.**

**back vertex power** *See* **power, back vertex.**

**backward masking** *See* **metacontrast.**

**baclofen** An analogue of gamma-aminobutyric acid (GABA) used orally to treat skeletal muscle spasm and in the management of nystagmus, particularly periodic alternating nystagmus.

**bacterial conjunctivitis** *See* **conjunctivitis, acute.**

**bacteriostatic** A term describing substances such as sulfonamides and tetracycline which inhibit the growth and propagation of bacteria, but do not actually destroy bacteria.
*See* **antibiotic.**

**Badal's optometer** *See* **optometer, Badal's.**

**'bag', capsular** A sack-like structure remaining within the eye following extracapsular cataract extraction or phacoemulsification. The implanted intraocular lens is placed within this structure to re-create the usual phakic state.
*See* **cataract extraction; phacoemulsification.**

**Bagolini's glass; test** *See* **glass, Bagolini's.**

**Bailey–Lovie acuity chart** *See* **chart, Bailey–Lovie.**

**Bailliart's ophthalmodynanometer** *See* **ophthalmodynanometer.**

**balance, binocular** Condition characterized by the two eyes being simultaneously in focus or equally out of focus.
*See* **test, balancing.**

**balance, muscle** The status of the eye muscle function as represented by the phoria measurement.
*See* **heterophoria.**

**balancing lens; test** *See* **lens, balancing.**

**Baldwin's illusion** *See* **illusion, Baldwin's visual.**

**Balint's syndrome** *See* **syndrome, Balint's.**

**ballast** Additional weight of material incorporated in a part of a contact lens to maintain it in a given orientation (Fig. B1). This is often provided by giving prismatic power to the lens (**prism ballast lens**).

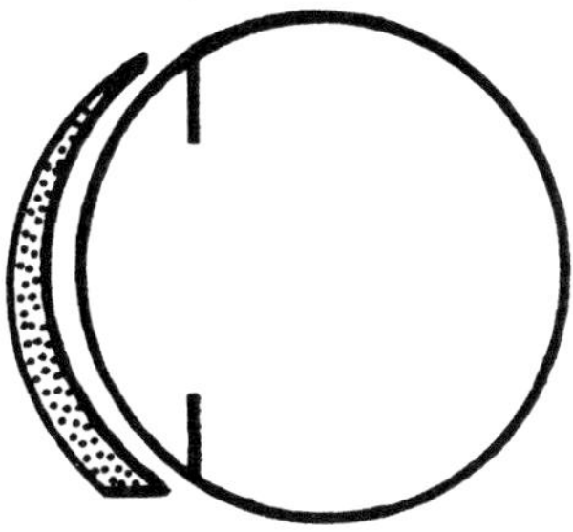

**Fig. B1** Truncated and prism-ballasted toric contact lens

**band keratopathy** *See* **keratopathy, band.**

**band, retinoscopic** A strip of light seen in the retinoscopic reflex of an astigmatic eye, especially when neutralizing one of the principal meridians.
*See* **retinoscope.**

**band-shaped corneal dystrophy** *See* **keratopathy, band.**

**bandage lens** *See* **lens, therapeutic soft contact.**

**bar reader** *See* **grid, Javal's.**

**bar reading** *See* **test, bar reading.**

**Barany's nystagmus** *See* **nystagmus.**

**Bardet–Biedl syndrome** *See* **syndrome, Laurence–Moon–Bardet–Biedl.**

**baring of the blind spot** *See* **blind spot, baring of the.**

**barrel-shaped distortion** *See* **distortion.**

**Barrer** A unit of oxygen permeability of a contact lens material. *Symbol*: *Dk*. It is equal to the product of the diffusion coefficient *D* of oxygen through the material (i.e. the speed at which oxygen molecules pass through the material) and the solubility *k* of oxygen in the material (i.e. the

number of oxygen molecules that can be absorbed in a given volume of material).
*See* **oxygen permeability; oxygen transmissibility.**

**base–apex direction** *See* **base setting.**

**base–apex line** *See* **base setting.**

**base curve** *See* **curve, base.**

**base line** *See* **line, base.**

**base of prism** The edge of a prism at which the faces are separated by a maximum distance.
*See* **base setting; prism.**

**base setting** The direction of the line from apex to base of a prism in a principal section (a section lying in a plane perpendicular to the refracting edge). The setting position for the base of a prism is normally specified by the direction 'base-up' (or base-down, in or out as the case may be) in which 'up' and 'down' have their ordinary meanings, 'in' means towards the nose and 'out' towards the temple. Base–apex line, base–apex meridian and base–apex direction are deprecated terms (British Standard). Alternatively, the TABO notation is used. Abbreviations for the placement of the base of the prism are **BD** (for base down), **BI** (for base towards the nose), **BO** (for base towards the temple) and **BU** (for base up).
*See* **axis notation, standard; base of prism.**

**base of vitreous** *See* **humour, vitreous.**

**Basedow's disease** *See* **disease, Graves'.**

**Bassen–Kornzweig syndrome** *See* **syndrome, Bassen–Kornzweig.**

**Batten–Mayou disease** *See* **disease, Batten–Mayou.**

**beam of light** *See* **light, beam of.**

**beamsplitter** An optical system which separates an incident beam of light into two beams of lesser intensity, one reflected and the other transmitted, e.g. a semi-silvered mirror.

**bearing, apical** An area of contact between the back surface of a rigid contact lens and the apex of the cornea. It is observed with the fluorescein test.
*See* **apex, corneal; test, fluorescein.**

**bedewing, endothelial** A cluster of inflammatory cells deposited on the posterior surface of the corneal endothelium. They have been noted with anterior eye inflammation and contact lens wear. The symptoms may include slight stinging sensation, some interference with vision and intolerance to contact lens wear. Reduction of wearing time is usually indicated and in severe cases contact lens wear must be ceased.
*See* **blebs, endothelial; corneal endothelium.**

**Behçet's disease** *See* **disease, Behçet's.**

**belladonna** *See* **atropine.**

**Bell's palsy** *See* **palsy, Bell's.**

**Bell's phenomenon** *See* **phenomenon, Bell's.**

**Benedikt's syndrome** *See* **syndrome, Benedikt's.**

**Benham's top** A disc, half black and half white with a number of concentric black bars on the white half which when rotated evokes a sensation of colour (Fig. B2). *Syn.* Benham–Fechner top.

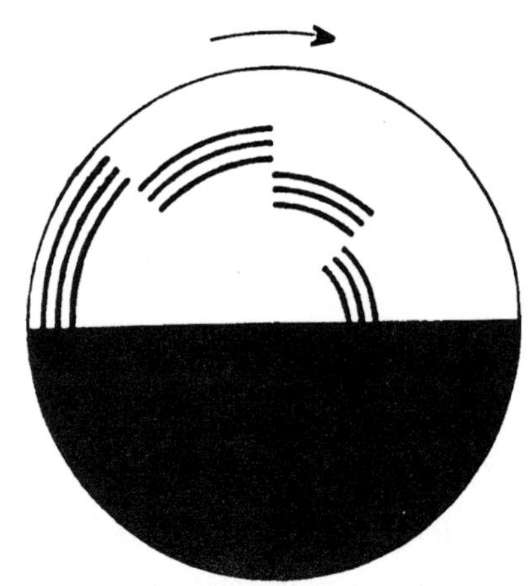

Fig. B2 Benham's top

**benoxinate hydrochloride** A topical corneal anaesthetic, generally used in 0.4% solution. It may be used to carry out tonometry, gonioscopy, to remove a foreign body, etc. *Syn.* oxybuprocaine hydrochloride. When used for applanation tonometry it is combined with 0.25% sodium fluorescein.
*See* **anaesthetic.**

**Benson's disease** *See* **asteroid hyalosis.**

**benzalkonium chloride** *See* **antiseptic.**

**Berger's loupe** *See* **loupe, Berger's.**

**Berger's postlenticular space** *See* **postlenticular space.**

**Bergmeister's papilla** *See* **glial veil.**

**Berlin's disease** *See* **disease, Berlin's.**

**Bernell clip** *See* **clipover.**

**Best's disease** *See* **disease, Best's.**

**best vision sphere** *See* **method, fogging.**

**Best's vitelliform macular dystrophy** *See* **disease, Best's.**

**best-form lens** *See* **lens, best-form.**

**beta-adrenergic blocking agent** *See* **beta-blocker.**

**beta-blocker** A drug that blocks or reduces the action of neurotransmitters on beta adrenergic receptors. It reduces secretion of aqueous humour and consequently intraocular pressure and it is used in the treatment of glaucoma. Common beta-blockers include timolol maleate, betaxolol, carteolol, levobunolol and metipranolol. *Syn.* beta-adrenergic blocking agent.
*See* **adrenergic receptors; miotics.**

**betamethasone** *See* **antiinflammatory drugs.**

**betaxolol hydrochloride** *See* **adrenergic receptors; beta-blocker.**

**bethanechol chloride** *See* **pilocarpine.**

**Bezold–Brücke phenomenon** *See* **phenomenon, Bezold–Brücke.**

**Bianchi's valve** *See* **lacrimal apparatus; valve of Hasner.**

**bichrome test** *See* **test, duochrome.**

**biconcave lens** *See* **lens, biconcave.**

**biconvex lens** *See* **lens, biconvex.**

**Bidwell's experiment** *See* **experiment, Bidwell's.**

**Bidwell's ghost** **1.** A special case of a moving positive after-image occurring behind a moving spot of light. This after-image seems like a ghost light trailing behind. **2.** *See* **after-image.**

**Bielschowsky's head tilt test** *See* **test, Bielschowsky's head tilt.**

**Bielschowsky's phenomenon** *See* **phenomenon, Bielschowsky's.**

**Bietti's band-shaped corneal dystrophy** *See* **keratopathy, actinic.**

**bifixation** Imaging of an object on the fovea of each eye simultaneously. *Syn.* bifoveal fixation.

**billiards spectacles** *See* **spectacles, billiards.**

**bimatoprost** *See* **prostaglandin analogues.**

**binasal hemianopsia** *See* **hemianopsia, binasal.**

**binocular** Pertaining to both eyes.

**binocular balance** *See* **balance, binocular.**

**binocular disparity** *See* **acuity, stereoscopic visual; disparity, retinal; perception, depth.**

**binocular fusion** *See* **fusion, sensory.**

**binocular indirect ophthalmoscope** *See* **ophthalmoscope, binocular indirect.**

**binocular lock** *See* **heterophoria, associated.**

**binocular lustre; parallax; rivalry** *See* under the nouns.

**binocular single vision** *See* **vision, binocular single.**

**binocular vision** *See* **vision, binocular.**

**binocular visual field** *See* **field, binocular visual.**

**binoculars** A set of two identical telescopes, one for each eye, which gives binocular vision of magnified distant objects. The images are erected using either an eyepiece of negative power, or prisms, or very occasionally, an additional lens system placed between objective and eyepiece. On binoculars, the magnification $M$ and the diameter $D$ of the objective or entrance pupil are shown as $M \times D$ (e.g. $8 \times 30$). *Syn.* field glasses; prism binoculars (for those which use prisms as erectors).
*See* **erector; telescope, galilean; telescope, terrestrial.**

**binoculars, prism** *See* **binoculars.**

**biocular** Pertaining to the use of the two eyes but without fusion or stereopsis. The term is primarily used in clinical testing and vision therapy in which different prisms are placed in front of each eye.

**biofeedback** A technique whereby visual (or bodily) processes normally under involuntary control (e.g. accommodation) are displayed to the subject, enabling voluntary control to be learnt. It has been used in myopia control and in acuity improvement but the value of the technique in these conditions is still unproven.
*See* **response, SILO.**

**biological–statistical theory** *See* **theory, biological–statistical.**

**bioluminescence** Emission of light by living organisms, e.g. firefly, certain fungi, etc.
*See* **luminescence.**

**biometry of the eye** The measurement of the various dimensions of the eye and of its components and their interrelationships.
*See* **constants of the eye; images, Purkinje–Sanson; keratometer; ophthalmophakometer; optometer; pachometer; ultrasonography.**

**biomicroscope** **1.** An instrument designed for detailed examination of ocular tissues containing a magnifying system and usually used in conjunction with a slit-lamp. **2.** Term commonly used

to describe a slit-lamp (although this is not strictly correct).
*See* **slit-lamp; lens, Hruby.**



**bioptic telescope** *See* **telescope, bioptic.**

**bipolar cell** *See* **cell, bipolar.**

**bi-prism, Fresnel's** Optical device consisting of two prisms of very small refracting power, set base to base and which forms two images of a single source. It is often used to produce interference fringes, double prism.
*See* **interference fringes, test, double prism.**

**birefringence** Property of anisotropic media such as crystals, whereby an incident light beam is split up into two beams, each plane polarized at right angles to the other. One beam, called **ordinary**, obeys Snell's law, while the other, called **extraordinary**, does not. *Syn.* double refraction.
*See* **anisotropic; law of refraction; prism, Nicol; prism, Wollaston.**

**bitemporal hemianopsia** *See* **hemianopsia, bitemporal.**

**Bitot's spot** Foamy patch found on the bulbar conjunctiva near the limbus in xerophthalmia and due to vitamin A deficiency. *Syn.* Bitot's patch.
*See* **xerophthalmia.**

**Bjerrum screen** *See* **screen, tangent.**

**Bjerrum's scotoma; sign** *See* **scotoma, Bjerrum's.**

**black** A visual sensation having no colour and being of extremely low luminosity.

**black body; eye** *See* under the nouns.

**blackout** Synonym for amaurosis fugax. It also includes the temporary loss of vision and consciousness occurring in unprotected pilots, due to a reduction of blood supply to the eye and brain at high acceleration.
*See* **amaurosis fugax.**

**blanching, limbal** A whitening of the limbal area due to pressure from the edge of a soft lens which fits too tightly.
*See* **lens, steep; limbus; test, push-up.**

**bleaching 1.** The process of changing colour from the pink of a dark-adapted retina to a pale yellow colour after it has been exposed to light. This is due to the reaction of the rhodopsin pigment. The process is reversible if the healthy retina is allowed to remain in the dark. **2.** Process to remove a tint from organic lenses.
*See* **pigment, visual; rhodopsin.**

**bleary eye** *See* **eye, bleary.**

**blebs, endothelial** Oedema of some cells of the corneal endothelium which bulge towards the aqueous humour. With specular microscopy or with high magnification biomicroscopy the cells appear as black areas as they do not reflect light towards the observer. Blebs occur within minutes of inserting a contact lens on the eye and disappear within hours after insertion. They may result from a local acidic pH shift at the endothelium.
*See* **bedewing, endothelial; corneal endothelium; illumination, specular reflection; oedema; pH.**

**blending** The process by which the different curvatures of a contact lens or of a bifocal lens are made to merge in a transition zone, with the purpose of eliminating the dividing line.
*See* **optic zone diameter; transition.**

**blennorrhoea neonatorum** *See* **ophthalmia neonatorum.**

**blephara** The eyelids. *Singular*: blepharon.

**blepharitis** Inflammation of the eyelids. The most common of these is marginal blepharitis.
*See* **blepharitis, marginal; eyelids; glands, meibomian; hordeolum, external.**

**blepharitis, angular** Inflammation of the canthi, affecting especially the inner canthus.

**blepharitis, marginal** Chronic inflammation of the eyelid margin accompanied by crusts or scales usually due to a bacterial infection (e.g. *Staphylococcus aureus*), an allergy, or to excessive secretion of lipid by the meibomian glands and the glands of Zeis (**seborrhoeic blepharitis**). The condition is commonly associated with keratoconjunctivitis sicca. Symptoms include dryness, itching and burning and are usually worse in the morning. Treatment consists mainly of frequent cleaning of the lid margins with a cotton-tipped applicator (or face cloth or cotton ball) dipped in a diluted solution of baby shampoo; warm compresses and an antibiotic ointment (e.g. erythromycin) and occasionally systemic antibiotics such as tetracycline, especially in seborrhoeic blepharitis. In complicated cases, corticosteroids will also be used.
*See* **acne rosacea; glands, meibomian; glands of Zeis; meibomianitis; trichiasis.**

**blepharitis, seborrhoeic** *See* **blepharitis, marginal.**

**blepharitis, ulcerative** Inflammation of the eyelid margin characterized by small ulcers.

**blepharochalasis** An atrophy of the upper eyelids causing a fold of tissue which often hangs over the eyelid margins. The condition follows recurrent episodes of oedema and inflammation, usually in young people. Treatment is surgical.
*See* **dermatochalasis; epiblepharon.**

**blepharo-conjunctivitis** Inflammation of the conjunctiva and eyelids.

**blepharon** *See* **blephara.**

**blepharoncus** Tumour of the eyelids.

**blepharophimosis** A congenital condition characterized by a generalized narrowing of the palpebral fissure. It produces a pseudoptosis but it commonly forms part of the blepharophimosis syndrome.
*See* **pseudoptosis; syndrome, blepharophimosis.**

**blepharoplasty** Any operation of the eyelid. It may be done for cosmetic reasons (e.g. to erase the signs of ageing) or for medical reasons (e.g. ptosis, entropion, ectropion).
*See* **blepharochalasis; dermatochalasis.**

**blepharoplegia** Paralysis of an eyelid.

**blepharoptosis** *See* **ptosis.**

**blepharospasm** Tonic or chronic spasm of the orbicularis oculi muscle which involves involuntary closure of the eyelids. It is often provoked by a foreign body in the eye, an abrasion or inflammation of the cornea or conjunctiva, or by excessive exposure to ultraviolet light (e.g. actinic keratoconjunctivitis). Treatment consists chiefly of injection into the muscles around the eyelids of botulinum toxin.
*See* **botulinum toxin; chemodenervation; keratoconjunctivitis, actinic; muscle, orbicularis.**

**blepharostat** *See* **eye speculum.**

**blepharosynechia** Adhesion of the eyelids to each other or to the eyeball.

**blind sight** A term used to indicate someone who is totally blind but yet is able, unconsciously, to locate an object on the basis of visual cues. It indicates a lesion which has destroyed the visual cortex but in which the retinotectal pathway to the superior colliculus remains unaffected. This pathway is not involved in conscious vision but receives some information from the retina.
*See* **pathway, retinotectal.**

**blind spot, baring of the** A visual field defect in which there is such a marked contraction of the peripheral temporal visual field that it lies on, or nasal to, the blind spot. Although it may occur in open-angle glaucoma, it is not indicative of the disease as it occurs in other conditions (e.g. miosis).
*See* **scotoma, Bjerrum's.**

**blind spot** Physiological negative scotoma in the visual field corresponding to the head of the optic nerve. It is not seen in binocular vision as the two blind spots do not correspond in the field. In monocular vision it is usually not noticed. It has the shape of an ellipse with its long axis vertical and measuring approximately 7.5° whereas its shorter axis along the horizontal measures approximately 5.5°. Its centre is located 15.5° to the temporal side of the centre of the visual field and 1.5° below the horizontal meridian. *Syn.* blind spot of Mariotte; physiological blind spot; punctum caecum (Fig. B3).
*See* **fibres, myelinated nerve; image, retinal; scotoma, negative.**

+

**Fig. B3** Demonstration of the blind spot. Looking at the cross with the right eye at about 20 cm, one sees the black circle disappear

**blind spot esotropia; syndrome** *See* **syndrome, Swann's.**

**blindness 1.** Inability to see. **2.** Absence or severe loss of vision so as to be unable to perform any work for which eyesight is essential. *Syn.* ablepsia; ablepsy; amaurosis.

**blindness, blue** *See* **tritanopia.**

**blindness, colour** Sometimes this term is incorrectly used to cover all forms of colour vision deficiency, however mild or severe.
*See* **achromatopsia; colour vision, defective; deuteranopia; monochromat; protanopia; tritanopia.**

**blindness, congenital stationary night** A non-progressive retinal disorder due to a presumed defect in neural transmission between the rods and the bipolars in the retina. It is characterized by night blindness, but normal daylight visual acuity and visual fields. It may be inherited as an autosomal dominant, autosomal recessive or X-linked trait.

**blindness, cortical** Loss of vision due to a lesion in the areas of the occipital lobes of the brain associated with visual functions. It may result from trauma or from a vascular disease (e.g. a circulatory occlusion caused by a stroke).

**blindness, day** *See* **hemeralopia.**

**blindness, eclipse** Partial or complete loss of central vision due to a foveal lesion caused by fixating the sun without adequate eye protection. This condition is caused mainly by the infrared radiations from the sun.
*See* **actinic.**

**blindness, flash** *See* **keratoconjunctivitis, actinic.**

**blindness, green** *See* **deuteranopia.**

**blindness, legal** The definition varies from country to country. In the UK it is equal to either 3/60 (20/400) or worse; or 6/60 (20/200) or worse, with markedly restricted fields.

**blindness, night** *See* **hemeralopia.**

**blindness, perceptual** *See* **agnosia.**

**blindness, red** *See* **protanopia.**

**blindness, river** *See* **onchocerciasis.**

**blindness, snow** *See* **keratoconjunctivitis, actinic.**

**blindness, word** *See* **alexia.**

**blink** A temporary closure of the eyelids (usually of both eyes). Blinks are usually involuntary but may be voluntary. The frequency of blinking is conditioned by a number of external and internal factors, e.g. glare, wind, emotion, attention, tiredness, etc. Normal blink rate is about 10 blinks per minute, although there are wide variations. The duration of a full blink is approximately 0.3–0.4 s. Blink rates are often altered with contact lens wear and in some diseased states (e.g. chalazion, Graves' disease).
*See* **reflex, corneal; tears; wink.**

**Blivet figure** *See* **figure, Blivet.**

**blobs** Areas of the primary visual cortex containing neurons responsive to colour stimulation. These areas appear as spots of colour (blobs) when they are stained with the enzyme cytochrome oxidase as brain cells derive energy from the oxidase metabolism. Lighter-staining areas appear in between called **'interblobs'**.

**Bloch's law** *See* **law, Bloch's.**

**blood pressure** *See* **sphygmomanometer.**

**bloomed lens** *See* **lens, coated.**

**blooming** *See* **coating.**

**blot haemorrhage** *See* **haemorrhage, blot.**

**blue** Visual sensation evoked by radiations within the waveband 450–490 nm. It is a primary colour and the complementary of yellow.
*See* **colour, complementary; colours, primary.**

**blue arcs** *See* **arcs, blue.**

**blue blindness** *See* **tritanopia.**

**blue field entoptoscope** *See* **entoptoscope, blue field.**

**blue-yellow blindness** *See* **tritanopia.**

**blue sclera** *See* **sclera, blue.**

**blur 1.** Degradation of an image formed by an optical system as a result of lack of focusing, aberrations, diffusion of light, etc. **2.** A pattern in which the border is indistinct.
*See* **lens flare; vision, blurred.**

**blur back test** *See* **test, plus 1.00 D blur.**

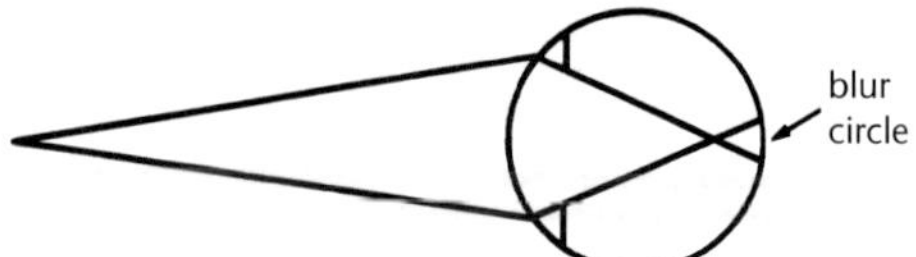


**Fig. B4** Blur circle corresponding to an image formed in front of the retina

**blur circle** A circular patch of light formed on the retina resulting from a point object whose image is focused either in front of, or behind the retina, or due to excessive aberrations of the optical system of the eye. The size of the blur circle increases with the distance of the ocular image from the retina and with the diameter of the pupil. Its diameter can be expressed in angular terms (in min arc) as,

$$\alpha = 3.48 \times \Delta F \times d$$

where $\Delta F$ is the defocus (in dioptres) with respect to the object point, and $d$ the pupil diameter (in mm). *Example*: An object at infinity is viewed by a 2 D uncorrected myope with a 4.0 mm pupil diameter, i.e. $\alpha = 3.48 \times 2 \times 4 = 28$ min arc (Fig. B4). *Syn.* circle of confusion; circle of diffusion.
*See* **aberration; depth of field.**

**blur point** The point at which the fixation target appears blurred on the introduction of increasing prisms and/or lens power, as for example in a test for relative convergence.
*See* **convergence, relative; zone of clear, single, binocular vision.**

**blur, spectacle** Reduction in visual acuity noticed with spectacles after removal of hard contact lenses (PMMA). This may be due to corneal oedema, alteration of the corneal index of refraction, surface distortion of the cornea, etc. Refitting the patient with lenses of greater oxygen transmissibility (e.g. gas permeable) often relieves this symptom.
*See* **oedema; oxygen.**

**blur test, plus 1.00 D** *See* **test, plus 1.00 D blur.**

**blurred vision** *See* **vision, blurred.**

**bobbing, ocular** Spontaneous, rapid downward movements of both eyes followed by a slow drift to the straight ahead position. It occurs in patients, usually comatose, who have lesions of the brainstem.

**bodies, colloid** *See* **drusen.**

**bodies, cytoid** Small, swollen white spots found on the retina resembling cells. They are due to degenerated retinal nerve fibres in which cellular components become trapped in the peripheral

axons of the optic nerve blocking axonal flow. Collection of cytoid bodies are thought to represent the 'cotton-wool' spots found on or around the optic disc in papilloedema, retinal trauma, diabetic retinopathy, AIDS, systemic lupus erythematosus, etc.
*See* **exudate.**

**bodies, lateral geniculate** *See* **geniculate bodies, lateral.**

**body, black** Thermal radiator which absorbs completely all incident radiation, whatever the wavelength, the direction of incidence or the polarization. This radiator has, for any wavelength, the maximum spectral concentration of radiant flux at a given temperature (CIE). *Syn.* full radiator; planckian radiator.
*See* **absorption; colour temperature; law, Planck's.**

**body, vitreous** *See* **humour, vitreous.**

**body, white** A sample exhibiting diffuse reflection and having a reflectance of approximately 100%. *Examples*: coating of magnesium oxide; sand-blasted opal glass surface; plaster of Paris.
*See* **coating; diffusion.**

**Bommarito clip** *See* **clipover.**

**bones of the orbit** *See* **orbit.**

**book retinoscopy** *See* **retinoscopy, dynamic.**

**botulinum toxin** A poisonous substance which paralyses muscles and leads to inhibition of the release of acetylcholine from presynaptic neuromuscular terminals. The effect can last for weeks after being injected into a muscle. It is used as an alternative or addition to extraocular muscle surgery in the management of strabismus. It is also sometimes used in the management of blepharospasm.
*See* **blepharospasm; chemodenervation; strabismus.**

**Bowen's disease** *See* **disease, Bowen's.**

**Bowman's membrane** *See* **membrane, Bowman's.**

**boxing centre; system** *See* under the nouns.

**brachium of the superior colliculus** A bundle of nerve fibres that leaves the optic tract below the pulvinar of the thalamus to enter the pretectal nucleus near the superior colliculus. Damage to the brachium results in a reduced pupil reflex to light, but not to near objects.
*See* **colliculi, superior; nucleus, pretectal; reflex, pupil light.**

**brachymetropia** Term proposed by Donders for myopia.

**bracketing** A procedure used in subjective refraction in which large and equal steps of dioptric changes are made above and below the presumed correct answer and then reducing the size of the dioptric changes and shifting the centre of the range, until the finest and just detectable blur is induced by equal steps above and below the refractive error. It is commonly used with patients with low vision.

**Braille** System of printing for blind persons, consisting of points raised above the surface of the paper used as symbols to indicate the letters of the alphabet. Reading is accomplished by touching the points with the fingertips.

**break point** *See* **point, break.**

**break-up time test** *See* **test, break-up time.**

**Brewster's angle** *See* **angle of polarization.**

**Brewster's stereoscope** *See* **stereoscope, Brewster's.**

**bridge** That part of a spectacle frame which forms the main connection between the lenses or rims. The bridge assembly is generally taken to include the pads, if any (British Standard).
*See* **spectacles.**

**bridge, flush** The bridge of a spectacle frame with zero projection.

**bridge, inset** A spectacle frame so shaped that the bearing surface of the bridge is behind the plane of the lenses.

**bridge, keyhole** Bridge of a spectacle frame with pads, looking like the outline of the upper part of a keyhole.

**bridge, pad** A bridge of a spectacle frame with two pads acting as the resting surface on the nose.

**bridge, saddle** A bridge so shaped as to rest on the nose over a continuous area, but in which the ends of the bearing surface are extended to lie behind the back plane of the front (British Standard).

**brightness** Attribute of visual sensation according to which an area appears to emit more or less light. *Syn.* luminosity. *Note 1*: In British recommended practice, the term brightness is now reserved to describe brightness of colour (i.e. the opposite of dullness) as used in the dyeing industry. *Note 2*: This attribute is the psychosensorial correlate, or nearly so, of the photometric quantity luminance (CIE).
*See* **luminance.**

**brightness constancy** *See* **constancy, brightness.**

**brimonidine tartrate** *See* **alpha-adrenergic agonist.**

b

**brinzolamide** *See* **carbonic anhydrase inhibitors.**

**Broca's pupillometer** *See* **pupillometer, Broca's.**

**Broca–Sulzer phenomenon** *See* **effect, Broca–Sulzer.**

**Brock's after-image test** *See* **test, after-image transfer.**

**Brock's string** A white string used to demonstrate physiological diplopia. One end of the string is placed against the bridge of the nose and the other end against a distant object (e.g. a doorknob). The subject should see two strings intersecting wherever the horizontal components of the visual axes meet. Red and green filters, one before each eye, enhance or facilitate the observation of the two strings. Several beads, each of a different colour, are usually threaded on the string so that they can be moved at will. One bead may be used for fixation while the other/s appear double; in crossed diplopia for the one closer to the eyes than the fixation bead, and in uncrossed diplopia for the one further away than the fixation bead. Brock's string is commonly used in visual training. The observation of physiological diplopia with Brock's string is often referred to as **Brock's string test**. *Syn.* bead on string.
*See* **diplopia, physiological.**

**Brodmann's areas** *See* **areas, Brodmann's.**

**Brown's superior oblique tendon sheath syndrome** *See* **syndrome, Brown's superior oblique tendon sheath.**

**Bruch's membrane** *See* **membrane, Bruch's.**

**Brücke's muscle** *See* **muscle, ciliary.**

**Brücke–Bartley effect** *See* **effect, Brücke–Bartley.**

**Bruckner's method** *See* **method, Bruckner's.**

**bruit** A sound heard on auscultation of the heart, lungs, large arteries or veins, or any large cavity (e.g. the orbit). The auscultation is carried out with a stethoscope. *Example*: An occlusive disease of the carotid artery caused by atherosclerosis leads to a reduction in blood flow through the carotid arteries (and a concomitant reduction in blood flow through vessels of the eye and orbit). It gives rise to a swishing sound with the chest-piece of the stethoscope on the neck over the carotid artery.
*See* **amaurosis fugax.**

**brunescent, cataract** *See* **cataract, nuclear.**

**brushes, Haidinger's** *See* **Haidinger's brushes.**

**B-scan** *See* **ultrasonography.**

**bulbar** Pertaining to the eyeball.

**bulbar conjunctiva** *See* **conjunctiva.**

**bull's eye maculopathy** *See* **maculopathy, bull's eye.**

**bulla** A fluid-filled blister appearing on the surface of the cornea when it is severely oedematous (increased thickness of more than 25%). It gives rise to a reduction of visual acuity and pain on rupturing. *Example*: bullous keratopathy. *Plural*: bullae.
*See* **keratopathy, bullous.**

**bullous keratopathy** *See* **keratopathy, bullous.**

**bundle of light** *See* **light, beam of.**

**Bunsen–Roscoe law** *See* **law, Bunsen–Roscoe.**

**buphthalmos** *See* **glaucoma, congenital.**

**bupivacaine hydrochloride** A local anaesthetic of the amide type used in eye surgery. It is used in 0.25–0.75% solution. It is often mixed with lidocaine hydrochloride. Its action starts after about 5 minutes and lasts for about 10 hours.
*See* **anaesthetics; lidocaine; procaine.**

**Burton lamp** *See* **lamp, Burton.**

**Busacca's nodules** *See* **Koeppe's nodules.**

**button** The preformed piece of glass which will become the segment of a fused bifocal or multifocal lens. It is ground and polished on one side to the appropriate curvature for fusing to the main lens (British Standard).
*See* **lens, bifocal.**

# C

**CAB** Cellulose acetate butyrate is a transparent thermoplastic material which is used in the manufacture of gas permeable contact lenses as it transmits some oxygen. It is a copolymer with varying percentages of cellulose, butyryl and acetyl. CAB lenses vary in their characteristics depending on the percentages of the three components. It is also used to make spectacle frames. *See* oxygen permeability; spectacle frame, plastic.

**calcarine fissure** *See* **fissure, calcarine.**

**caliper** A device used to measure distances between structures or surfaces. It usually comprises a scale at one end, while at the other end are two legs which can be adjusted to the appropriate measurement. *Example*: lens thickness caliper. *See* **lens measure.**

**caloric nystagmus** *See* **caloric testing.**

**caloric testing** A neuro-ophthalmic technique in which cold and warm water is used to stimulate the vestibular system creating horizontal nystagmus (called **caloric nystagmus** or **Barany's nystagmus**). Cold water placed in the ear induces a fast beating vestibular nystagmus with the fast phase moving away from the stimulated ear, while warm water causes the fast phase to move in the direction of the stimulated ear. The mnemonic COWS (cold – opposite, warm – same) is used to describe this effect. By placing the subject at a 30 degree upright position, heated or cooled water stimulates the now vertical horizontal semicircular canals.
*See* **nystagmus.**

**camera, fundus** A camera attached to an indirect ophthalmoscope aimed at photographing the image of the fundus of the eye. This image is produced by the objective of the ophthalmoscope at the first focal point of the objective of the viewing microscope (and of the camera) which forms an image on the film. A flip mirror within the optical path of the viewing microscope allows the observer to view the image of the fundus and focus it, thus ensuring that the image being photographed is as clear as that being viewed. Fundus cameras usually require a dilated pupil of about 4 mm and their fields of view extend up to 45°. They provide an objective photographic record of any condition in the fundus. They can also be used to take photographs of the anterior segment of the eye.
*See* **fundus, ocular; ophthalmoscope, indirect; ophthalmoscope, scanning laser.**

**camera obscura** *See* **camera, pinhole.**

**camera, pinhole** A camera in which the lens is replaced by a pinhole (e.g. **the camera obscura**).

**campimeter** An instrument for the measurement of the visual field, especially the central region (usually within a radius of 30°).
*See* **analyser, Friedmann visual field; chart, Amsler; perimeter; screen, tangent.**

**campimetry** Measurement of the visual field with a campimeter.

**canal, Cloquet's** *See* **canal, hyaloid.**

**canal, Hannover's** A space about the equator of the crystalline lens made up between the anterior and posterior parts of the zonule of Zinn and containing aqueous humour and zonular fibres (Fig. C1).
*See* **Zinn, zonule of.**

**canal, hyaloid** A channel in the vitreous humour, running from the optic disc to the crystalline lens. In fetal life this canal contains the hyaloid artery which nourishes the lens but it usually disappears prior to birth. *Syn.* central canal; Cloquet's canal; Stilling's canal.
*See* **artery, hyaloid; humour, vitreous.**

**canal, infraorbital** A channel beginning at the infraorbital groove in the floor of the orbit and ending at the infraorbital foramen of the maxillary bone opening onto the face below the inferior orbital margin. It is a channel for the infraorbital artery and the infraorbital nerve.

**canal, optic** A canal leading from the middle cranial fossa to the apex of the orbit in the small wing of the sphenoid bone through which pass the optic nerve and the ophthalmic artery. *Syn.* optic foramen.
*See* **artery, ophthalmic; nerve, optic; orbit.**

**canal of Petit** A space between the posterior fibres of the zonule of Zinn and the anterior surface of the vitreous humour (Fig. C1).
*See* **humour, vitreous; Zinn, zonule of.**

**canal, Schlemm's** A circular venous sinus located in the corneoscleral junction, anterior to the scleral spur and receiving aqueous humour from the anterior chamber and discharging into the aqueous and the anterior ciliary veins (Fig. C1). *Syn.* scleral sinus; sinus circularis iridis; sinus venosus sclerae; venous circle of Leber.

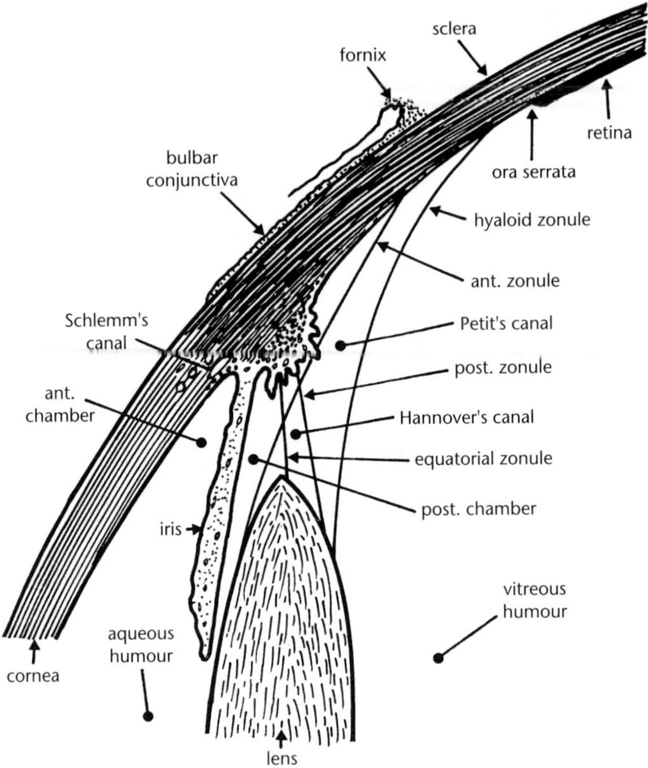


**Fig. C1** Section diagram through the anterior portion of the eye

*See* **humour, aqueous; meshwork, trabecular; scleral spur; vein, aqueous.**

**canal, Stilling's** *See* **canal, hyaloid.**

**canaliculi** *See* **lacrimal apparatus.**

**canaliculitis** Inflammation of a lacrimal canaliculus, most frequently the lower one. The patient presents with a red, irritated eye with 'pouting' of the punctum and a slight discharge which can be expressed by compressing the canaliculus.

**candela** The candela is the luminous intensity in a given direction of a source emitting monochromatic radiation of frequency $540 \times 10^{12}$ Hz and the radiant intensity of which in that direction is 1/683 watt per steradian. The candela so defined is the base unit applying to photopic quantities. *Symbol*: cd.

**candela per square metre** SI unit of luminance. *Syn.* nit. *Symbol*: $cd/m^2$.
*See* **luminance; SI unit.**

**candelpower** Designates a luminous intensity expressed in candelas.

**canthal tendon** *See* **ligament, palpebral.**

**canthus** The angle formed by the upper and lower eyelids at the nasal (**inner canthus** or **medial canthus**) or temporal (**outer canthus** or **external angle**) end. *Plural*: canthi. *Syn.* palpebral angle. *See* **caruncle, lacrimal; conjunctivitis, angular; epicanthus; eyelids.**

**capsular fixation** Process of inserting an intraocular lens implant into the capsular bag following cataract extraction.
*See* **capsulectomy; phacoemulsification.**

**Capsule, Bonnet's** *See* **Tenon's capsule.**

**capsule, crystalline lens** Transparent elastic capsule covering the crystalline lens. The thickness of the capsule varies; the anterior portion is thicker than the posterior and it is also thicker towards the periphery (or equator). This variation in thickness plays a role in moulding the lens substance, contributing to an increase in the curvature of the front surface, in particular, during accommodation. The capsule increases in thickness with age, and its modulus of elasticity decreases with age, which (besides flattening of the lens, and a hardening of the lens substance) contributes to presbyopia. Under electron microscopy the capsule appears to have a lamellar structure

that disappears with age. The capsule receives the insertion of the zonular fibres.
*See* **fibres, lens; lens, crystalline; modulus of elasticity; presbyopia; shagreen of the crystalline lens; theory, Fincham's; Zinn, zonule of.**

**capsule, Tenon's** *See* **Tenon's capsule.**

**capsulectomy** The surgical removal of a capsule, such as that of the crystalline lens.

**carbachol** *See* **parasympathomimetic drug.**

**carbonic anhydrase inhibitors** Drugs which are used to reduce the secretion of aqueous humour and consequently decrease the intraocular pressure. Those in use are sulfonamide derivatives. *Examples*: acetazolamide, brinzolamide, dichlorphenamide, dorzolamide. They are administered systemically or topically in the treatment of glaucoma.

**carboxymethylcellulose** *See* **tears, artificial.**

**carcinoma** A malignant tumour of the epithelium, the tissue that lines the skin and internal organs of the body. It tends to invade surrounding tissues and to metastasize to distant regions of the body via the lymphatic vessels or the blood vessels. It is a form of cancer. *Example*: carcinoma of the skin.
*See* **epithelioma; keratosis, seborrhoeic.**

**carcinoma, sebaceous gland** A malignant tumour arising from the meibomian gland or occasionally from the gland of Zeis. It frequently affects the upper eyelids of old people. Initially the tumour resembles a chalazion or a chronic blepharitis. However, this tumour is aggressive and may invade the orbit. It may metastasize. Treatment usually consists of thorough surgical excision.
*See* **blepharitis; chalazion.**

**carcinoma, squamous cell** A malignant skin cancer that affects the eyelids and conjunctiva. It is aggressive and may metastasize. It occurs most commonly in old people who have had extensive sun exposure. Treatment consists mainly of surgical excision.
*See* **xeroderma pigmentosum.**

**Cardiff acuity test** *See* **test, Cardiff acuity.**

**cardinal planes; points** *See* under the nouns.

**cardinal positions of gaze** These are the following six version movements of the eyes: dextroversion (to the right), laevoversion (to the left), dextroelevation (up to the right), laevoelevation (up to the left), dextrodepression (down to the right), and laevodepression (down to the left).
*See* **test, motility; version.**

**cardinal rotation** A rotation of the eye from the primary position to a secondary position about either the *x*-axis or the *z*-axis.
*See* **axis, transverse; axis, vertical; position, primary; position, secondary.**

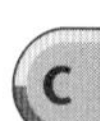


**carrier** *See* **lens, lenticular.**

**carteolol hydrochloride** *See* **sympatholytic drugs.**

**caruncle, lacrimal** A small pink fleshy structure situated in the inner canthus.
*See* **canthus.**

**case history** *See* **history, case.**

**Cassegrain telescope** *See* **telescope.**

**cast** *See* **impression, eye.**

**cat's eye syndrome** *See* **syndrome, cat's eye.**

**catadioptric system** An optical system employing both reflecting and refracting components as used, for example, in a lighthouse. This design makes long focal length more compact and mirrors, unlike lenses or prisms, are free of chromatic aberration.
*See* **image, catadioptric.**

**cataphoria** *See* **kataphoria.**

**cataract** Partial or complete loss of transparency of the crystalline lens substance or its capsule. Cataract may occur as a result of age, trauma, systemic diseases (e.g. diabetes), ocular diseases (e.g. anterior uveitis), high myopia, long-term steroid therapy, excessive exposure to infrared and ultraviolet light, heredity, maternal infections, Down's syndrome, etc. The incidence of cataract increases with age, amounting to more than 50% in the population over 82 years. It is also more prevalent in Africa, Asia and South America than in Europe and North America. The main symptom is a gradual loss of vision, often described as 'misty'. Some patients may also notice transient monocular diplopia, others fixed spots (not floaters) in the visual field and others better vision in dim illumination. Cataracts can easily be seen with the retinoscope, the ophthalmoscope and especially with the slit-lamp, although depending on the type, one instrument may be better than the other. At present the main treatment is surgical. Extraction is performed for one of three reasons: visual improvement, medical or cosmetic.
*See* **after-cataract; capsule, crystalline lens; disease, Wilson's; entoptoscope, blue field; glare tester; hyperacuity; implant, intraocular lens; lens, crystalline; leukocoria; maxwellian view system, clinical; myopia, lenticular; phacoemulsification; rheumatoid arthritis; syndrome, Down's; ultrasonography; ultraviolet; vitreous, persistent hyperplastic primary.**

C

**cataract, after-** *See* **cataract, secondary.**

**cataract, anterior capsular** A small central opacity located on the anterior lens capsule, either of congenital origin or due to a perforating ulcer of the cornea.
*See* **sign, Vogt's.**

**cataract, axial** Cataract situated along the antero-posterior axis of the crystalline lens (Fig. C2).

**cataract, bipolar** Lens opacity involving both the anterior and the posterior poles of the lens (Fig. C2).
*See* **cataract, polar.**

**cataract, blue** *See* **cataract, blue-dot.**

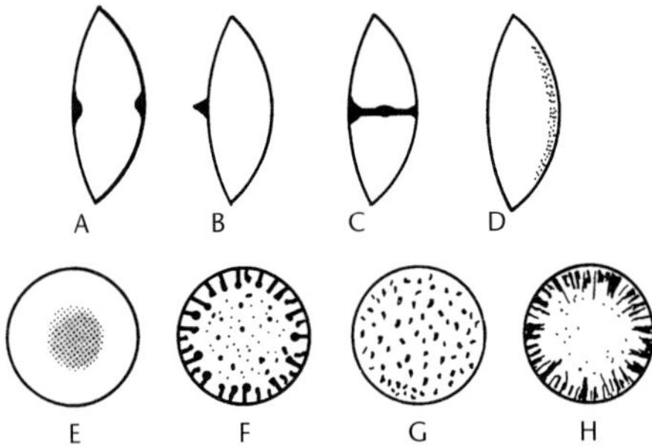


**Fig. C2** Examples of cataracts (A, bipolar; B, pyramidal; C, axial; D, cupuliform (or subcapsular); E, nuclear; F, coronary; G, snowflake; H, cuneiform)

**cataract, blue-dot** A developmental anomaly of the crystalline lens characterized by numerous small opacities in the outer nucleus and cortex which appear as translucent bluish dots. The condition is very common and does not usually affect acuity. *Syn.* blue cataract; punctate cataract.

**cataract, brown; brunescent** *See* **cataract, nuclear.**

**cataract, capsular** An opacity affecting only the capsule of the crystalline lens.
*See* **capsule, crystalline lens.**

**cataract, central** *See* **cataract, nuclear.**

**cataract, chalky** A cataract characterized by the presence of lime salt deposits.

**cataract, complicated** A cataract caused by or accompanying another intraocular disease, such as glaucoma, cyclitis, anterior uveitis or a hereditary retinal disorder such as retinitis pigmentosa or Leber's disease. *Syn.* secondary cataract.
*See* **cataract, cuneiform; Leber's hereditary optic atrophy; retinitis pigmentosa; syndrome, Down's; syndrome, Fuchs'; syndrome, rubella.**

**cataract, congenital** Cataract occurring as a result of faults in the early development of the lens. This type is often associated with mental handicap, Down's syndrome, maternal rubella, galactosaemia, etc.
*See* **cataract, anterior capsular; cataract, nuclear; syndrome, Down's; syndrome, rubella.**

**cataract, coronary** A cataract characterized by a series of opacities having the shape of a crown or ring near the periphery of the lens (Fig. C2).

**cataract, cortical** Cataract affecting the cortex of the lens. The opacities often begin as spokes or isolated dots or clusters forming the cuneiform or subcapsular types of cataract, but eventually the opacity spreads through the entire cortex.
*See* **cataract, cuneiform; cataract, senile.**

**cataract, cuneiform** Senile cataract characterized by opacities distributed within the periphery of the cortex of the lens in a radial manner, like spokes on a wheel. The opacities are sometimes distributed more uniformly in the posterior or anterior cortex, but directly under the capsule. The condition is then called **cupuliform** (or **subcapsular**) **cataract**. Subcapsular cataracts are often the result of radiation exposure or secondary to other eye diseases (e.g. uveitis, retinitis pigmentosa) or toxic damage such as by corticosteroid drugs, besides age. Cuneiform cataracts are the most common type of cortical cataract (Fig. C2).
*See* **cataract, senile; lens, crystalline.**

**cataract, cupuliform** *See* **cataract, cuneiform.**

**cataract, diabetic** Cataract associated with diabetes. In old eyes this type is similar to that of a non-diabetic person but in young eyes it is typically of the snowflake type.
*See* **cataract, snowflake; diabetes.**

**cataract, electric** Cataract caused by an electric shock.

**cataract extraction, extracapsular (ECCE)** Surgical procedure for the removal of a cataractous crystalline lens. The anterior capsule is excised, the lens nucleus is removed and the residual equatorial cortex is aspirated. The posterior capsule may be polished. An intraocular lens implant may then be inserted.
*See* **capsule, crystalline lens; capsulectomy; implant, intraocular lens; phacoemulsification.**

**cataract extraction, intracapsular (ICCE)** Surgical procedure for the removal of a cataractous crystalline lens. The entire lens, together with its capsule, is removed. This procedure is rarely performed nowadays.
*See* **vitreous detachment.**

**cataract, fluid** Hypermature cataract in which the lens substance has degenerated into milky fluid.

**cataract, glassblower's** *See* **cataract, heat-ray.**

**cataract, heat-ray** Cataract due to excessive exposure to heat and infrared radiation. *Syn.* glass-blower's cataract; thermal cataract.
*See* **exfoliation of the lens; infrared.**

**cataract, hypermature** The last stage in the development of senile cataract in which the lens substance has disintegrated.
*See* **cataract, incipient; cataract, intumescent cortical; cataract, mature; glaucoma, phacolytic.**

**cataract, incipient** The first stage in the development of senile cataract characterized by streaks similar to the spokes of a wheel or with an increased density of the nucleus.
*See* **cataract, hypermature; cataract, intumescent cortical; cataract, mature; lens, crystalline; sight, second.**

**cataract, intumescent cortical** A stage of development of a cataract in which the lens, especially the cortex, absorbs fluid and swells. It may lead to secondary angle-closure glaucoma. The cataract can progress to the hypermature stage in which case the fluid leaks out resulting in shrinkage of the lens and wrinkling of the anterior capsule leaving the harder nucleus free within the capsule.
*See* **cataract, hypermature; cataract, morgagnian.**

**cataract, lamellar** *See* **cataract, zonular.**

**cataract, mature** The middle stage in the development of senile cataract characterized by a completely opaque lens and considerable loss of vision.
*See* **cataract, hypermature; cataract, incipient; cataract, senile.**

**cataract, morgagnian** A hypermature cataract in which the cortex has shrunk and liquefied and the nucleus floats within the lens capsule. Degraded lens proteins may leak into the aqueous humour and cause phacolytic glaucoma. *Syn.* cystic cataract; sedimentary cataract.
*See* **cataract, intumescent cortical; glaucoma, phacolytic.**

**cataract, nuclear** Cataract affecting the lens nucleus. It can be either congenital or senescent in origin. It frequently leads to an increase in myopia (or decrease in hyperopia). In some cases it reaches such a brown colour that it is called **brunescent cataract** (or **brown cataract**). *Syn.* central cataract (Fig. C2).
*See* **cataract, senile; lens, crystalline.**

**cataract, punctate** *See* **cataract, blue-dot.**

**cataract, pyramidal** Congenital cataract consisting of an opacity located at the anterior pole of the crystalline lens and protruding forward into the anterior chamber (Fig. C2).

**cataract, secondary 1.** *Syn.* for complicated cataract. **2.** *Syn.* for after-cataract.
*See* **after-cataract; cataract, complicated.**

**cataract, senescent** Cataract affecting older persons. It is the most common type of cataract and may take several forms: cortical, cuneiform, cupuliform, nuclear or mature. *Syn.* senile cataract.
*See* **cataract, cortical; cataract, cuneiform; cataract, nuclear; cataract, mature.**

**cataract, snowflake** A cataract characterized by greyish or whitish flakelike opacities. It is usually found in young diabetics or severe cases of diabetes (Fig. C2).
*See* **cataract, diabetic; diabetes.**

**cataract, soft** Cataract in which the lens nucleus is soft.
*See* **lens, crystalline.**

**cataract, subcapsular** *See* **cataract, cuneiform.**

**cataract, sunflower** *See* **chalcosis lentis.**

**cataract, thermal** *See* **cataract, heat-ray.**

**cataract, traumatic** Cataract following injury to the lens, its capsule, or to the eyeball itself.

**cataract, zonular** Cataract affecting one layer of the crystalline lens only. *Syn.* lamellar cataract.

**catoptric image** *See* **image, catoptric.**

**catoptrics** The branch of optics which deals with reflection and reflectors.

**caustic** The concentration of light in the caustic surface of a bundle of converging light rays which represents the focal image in an optical system uncorrected for spherical aberration. It appears as a hollow luminous cusp with its apex at the paraxial focus.
*See* **aberration, spherical.**

**cavernous sinus** *See* **sinus, cavernous.**

**cecocentral** *See* **centrocecal.**

**cell, A** *See* **cell, Y.**

**cell, acinar** A type of cell found within the body of the lacrimal gland. This cell lines the lumens of glands in a lobular pattern and produces a serous secretion.

**cell, amacrine** Retinal cell located in the inner nuclear layer connecting ganglion cells with bipolar cells. Some have an ascending axon synapsing with receptors.

**cell, B** *See* **cell, X.**

**cell, basal** *See* **corneal epithelium.**

**cell, binocular** A cell in the visual cortex which responds to stimulation from both eyes. It may, however, show an ocular dominance for either eye. It responds more strongly when corresponding regions of each eye are stimulated by targets of similar size and orientation.
*See* **column, cortical; hypercolumn.**

**cell, bipolar** Retinal cell located in the inner nuclear layer connecting the photoreceptors with amacrine and ganglion cells.

**cell, C** *See* **cell, W.**

**cell, Cajal's** *See* **astrocytes.**

**cell, clump** Large, pigmented round cells found in the pupillary zone of the iris stroma. They are considered to be macrophages containing mainly melanin granules. The number of these cells increases with age.

**cell, complex** A cell in the visual cortex whose receptive field consists of a large responsive area, approximately rectangular in shape, surrounded by an inhibitory region. The stimulus which is usually a slit or a straight line gives an optimum response if appropriately orientated but falling anywhere within the excitatory area. These cells tend to respond optimally to the movement of a specifically orientated slit. Many complex cells also respond better when the optimally orientated slit is moved in one direction rather than in the opposite direction. In general, complex cells show non-linear spatial summation properties.
*See* **area, visual; cell, hypercomplex; cell, simple; field, receptive; summation.**

**cell, cone** Photoreceptor of the retina which connects with a bipolar cell and is involved in colour vision and high visual acuity and which functions in photopic vision. The outer segment of the cell is conical in shape, except in the fovea centralis where it is rod-like. In the **outer segment** (i.e. the part closest to the pigment epithelium) are contained hollow discs (or lamellae), the membranes of which are joined together and are also continuous with the boundary membrane of the cone cell. The visual pigments are contained in these discs. There are three types of cones, each containing a different pigment sensitive to a different part of the light spectrum. They are referred to as long-wave-sensitive (or **L-cones**), medium-wave-sensitive (or **M-cones**) and short-wave-sensitive (or **S-cones**). There are about six million cones in the retina, with the greatest concentration in the macular area (Fig. C3).
*See* **effect, Stiles–Crawford; ellipsoid; foveola; macula; pedicle, cone; pigment, visual; retina; theory, duplicity; vision, photopic.**

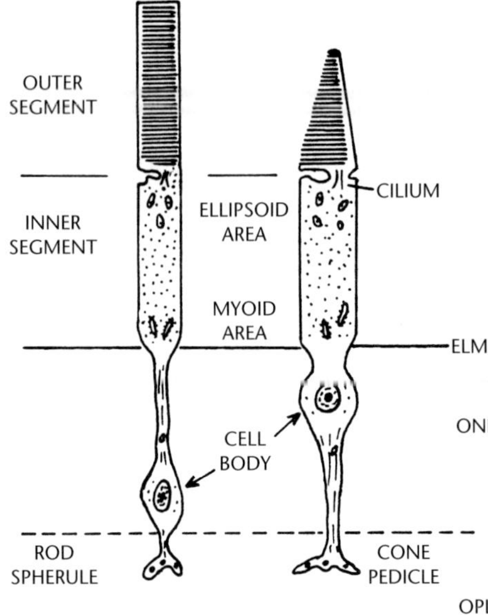


**Fig. C3** Structures of a rod and a cone cell of the retina (ELM, external limiting membrane; ONL, outer nuclear layer; OPL, outer plexiform layer)

**cell, fixed** *See* **corneal corpuscle.**

**cell, ganglion 1.** Retinal cell which connects the bipolars and other cells in the inner plexiform layer with the lateral geniculate body. The axons of the ganglion cells constitute the optic nerve fibres. There are many types of ganglion cells. The two major types are: the **magno** (or **M** or **parasol**) **ganglion cells** which project mainly to the magnocellular layers of the lateral geniculate bodies; and the **parvo** (or **P** or **midget**) **ganglion cells** which project to the parvocellular layers. They comprise about 10% and 80% of the ganglion cells respectively. **2.** One of a collection of nerve cell bodies found in a ganglion.
*See* **cell, W; cell, X; cell, Y; retina.**

**cell, goblet** Cell of the conjunctival epithelium which secretes mucin.
*See* **conjunctiva; glands of Henle; mucin; xerophthalmia.**

**cell, horizontal** Retinal cell located in the inner nuclear layer which connects several cones and rods together.

**cell, hypercomplex** A cell in the visual cortex that receives inputs from several simple and complex cells and therefore has an even more elaborate receptive field than a complex cell. It is most effectively stimulated by a stimulus of a specific size and of a specific orientation and which is moved in a specific direction.
*See* **cell, complex; cell, simple.**

**Table C1** Main distinguishing features of the two principal types of ganglion cells of the retina

| properties | P cell (or X cell) | M cell (or Y cell) |
|---|---|---|
| size of cell body | small | large |
| dendritic spread | small | medium/large |
| receptive field size | small | medium/large |
| retinal distribution | 90% of these at the macula | 5% of these at the macula; about 13% overall |
| projection | LGN parvocellular layers | LGN magnocellular layers |
| type of response | sustained | transient |
| light sensitivity | low | high |
| wavelength response | selective (except X cells) | non-selective |
| spatial sensitivity | fine target detail | large target detail |
| temporal sensitivity | low target velocity | high target velocity |

C

**cell, M** *See* **cell, ganglion; cell, Y.**

**cell, magno** *See* **geniculate bodies, lateral.**

**cell, midget** *See* **cell, ganglion.**

**cell, Mueller's** Neuroglial cell in the retina with its nucleus in the inner nuclear layer and with fibres extending from the external to the internal limiting membrane. These cells support the neurons of the retina and possibly assist in their metabolism. *Syn.* Müller cell.
*See* **membrane of the retina, external limiting.**

**cell, orientation-specific** A cell that responds best to specifically orientated lines. This is the case for almost all cells in the visual cortex. *Examples*: complex cell; simple cell.
*See* **cell, complex; cell, simple; field, receptive.**

**cell, P** *See* **cell, ganglion; cell, X.**

**cell, parasol** *See* **cell, ganglion.**

**cell, parvo** *See* **geniculate bodies, lateral.**

**cell, rod** Photoreceptor cell of the retina which connects with a bipolar cell. It contains rhodopsin and is involved in scotopic vision. The molecules of rhodopsin are contained in about 1000 hollow discs (double lamellae or membranes) which are isolated from each other and from the boundary membrane of the rod cell. These discs are found in the **outer segment** (i.e. the part closest to the pigment epithelium) of the cell. There are about 100 million rod cells throughout the retina; only a small area, the foveola, is free of rods (Fig. C3).
*See* **eccentricity; ellipsoid; foveola; retina; rhodopsin; spherule, rod; theory, duplicity; vision, scotopic.**

**cell, simple** A cell in the visual cortex whose receptive field consists of an excitatory and an inhibitory area separated by a straight line, or by a long narrow strip of one response flanked on both sides by larger regions of the opposite response. Responses occur only to a straight line or a narrow strip orientated approximately parallel to the boundary/ies between the two areas. In general, simple cells show linear spatial summation properties. They are presumably the first cells where the nervous impulses are processed as they enter the visual cortex.
*See* **area, visual; cell, complex; field, receptive.**

**cell, squamous** *See* **corneal epithelium.**

**cell, W** A retinal ganglion cell in the cat, with slow axonal conduction which sends information to the superior colliculus and to the centre involved in the control of pupillary diameter, rather than to the lateral geniculate body. There are very few such cells. In primates, this retinal ganglion cell is usually referred to as C (or Pγ) cell.
*See* **cell, X; cell, Y.**

**cell, wing** *See* **corneal epithelium.**

**cell, X** A retinal ganglion cell in the cat, mainly located in the central region of the retina and which assists in high acuity and colour vision. X cells tend to give **sustained** responses to stimuli and to have linear spatial summation properties. This is the most common type of ganglion cells (about 82%). This cell transmits information principally to the parvo cells of the lateral geniculate bodies. In primates, this retinal ganglion cell is usually referred to as **P** (or B or Pβ) cell.
*See* **cell, ganglion; cell, Y; cell, W; geniculate bodies, lateral.**

**cell, Y** A retinal ganglion cell in the cat, mainly located in the periphery of the retina and which assists in movement perception. Y cells tend to give **transient** responses to stimuli and to have non-linear spatial summation properties. This cell transmits information principally to the magno cells of the lateral geniculate bodies. In primates, this retinal ganglion cell is usually referred to as **M** (or A or Pα) cell.
*See* **cell, ganglion; cell, X; cell, W; geniculate bodies, lateral.**

**cells, colour-opponent** Cells which respond by increasing response to light of some wavelengths

and decreasing their response to others (usually complementary). If the light stimulus contains both sets of wavelengths the two responses tend to cancel each other. Two types of cells have been identified: red-green cells and blue-yellow cells. These cells are found mainly in the lateral geniculate bodies but also among retinal ganglion cells. The responses of these cells support Hering's theory of colour vision. *Syn.* opponent-process cell (although this term also includes a cell which increases its response to white light and decreases its response to dark).
*See* **theory, Hering's of colour vision.**

**cells, Langerhans'** Dendritic cells located mainly in the epidermis, mucous membranes and lymph nodes. They have surface receptors for immunoglobulin (Fc), complement (C3) and surface HLA-DR (Ia) antigen. Langerhans' cells are also found in the conjunctival epithelium and among the basal cells, mainly of the peripheral, corneal epithelium. They have antigenic functions, stimulate T lymphocytes, prostaglandin production and participate in cutaneous delayed hypersensitivity and corneal graft rejection. Extended wear of contact lenses tends to induce an increase of these cells. They are also found in histiocytic tumours.

**cellulose acetate butyrate** *See* **CAB.**

**cellulitis, preseptal** Swelling or infection of the eyelid tissue in front of the orbital septum. There is redness, swelling and tenderness of the eyelid. The condition is treated with systemic antibiotics.
*See* **orbital septum.**

**cellulitis, orbital** Infection of the orbital contents caused by *Staphylococcus aureus*, *Streptococcus* and *Haemophilus influenzae*. It is often caused by the spread of infection from adjacent structures, especially the sinuses. The clinical signs are fever, pain, proptosis, redness, swelling of the lid and orbital tissue and restricted eye movements which may occasionally lead to diplopia and as the condition worsens visual acuity decreases. Initial management consists of parenteral antibiotics but surgery may become necessary.
*See* **lamina papyracea.**

**central corneal optical zone** *See* **optical zone of cornea.**

**central fusion** *See* **fusion, sensory.**

**central retinal artery; vein** *See* under the nouns.

**central retinal artery occlusion** *See* **retinal arterial occlusion.**

**central retinal vein occlusion** *See* **retinal vein occlusion.**

**central serous retinopathy** *See* **retinopathy, central serous.**

**central vision; visual acuity** *See* under the nouns.

**centration distance (CD)** The specified horizontal distance between the right and left centration points of a pair of ophthalmic lenses.
*See* **centration point; distance, near centration.**

**centration distance, near (NCD)** The horizontal distance between the right and left centration points used for near vision.

**centration point** The point at which the optical centre (of a lens) is to be located in the absence of a prescribed prism, or after any prescribed prism has been neutralized. If the centration point is not specified, it is located at the standard optical centre position (British Standard).

**centre, boxing** The point midway between the two horizontal and the two vertical sides of the rectangle enclosing the lens, in the boxing system. *Syn.* geometric centre of a cut lens.
*See* **system, boxing.**

**centre, optical** That point (real or virtual) on the optical axis of a lens which is, or appears to be, traversed by rays emerging parallel to their original direction. Applied to an ophthalmic lens, it is commonly regarded as coinciding with the vertex of either surface (British Standard).
*See* **points, nodal; vertex.**

**centre of rotation of the eye** When the eye rotates in its orbit, there is a point within the eyeball which is more or less fixed relative to the orbit. This is the centre of rotation of the eye. In reality, the centre of rotation is constantly shifting but by a small amount. It is considered, for convenience, that the centre of rotation of an emmetropic eye lies on the line of sight of the eye 13.5 mm behind the anterior pole of the cornea when the eye is in the **straight ahead position** (or **straightforward position**), that is when the line of sight is perpendicular to both the base line and the frontal plane.
*See* **axis, anteroposterior; line, base; line of sight; plane, frontal.**

**centre, standard optical position** A reference point specific to each spectacle lens shape. The standard optical position is on the vertical line passing through the boxed centre, and is at the boxed centre.
*See* **centre, boxing; system, boxing.**

**centre, visual** Centre of the brain concerned with vision.
*See* **area, visual; fissure, calcarine.**

**centrocecal** An area of the retina which includes the macula, the optic disc and the area in between. *Note*: also spelt centrocaecal. *Syn.* cecocentral.

**cephalosporin** *See* **antibiotic.**

**cerium oxide** A pink powder derived from the metallic element cerium. It is used to polish lenses and it is also added to ophthalmic glass to absorb ultraviolet radiations.
*See* **polishing.**

**cetirizine** *See* **antihistamine.**

**cetrimide** *See* **antiseptic.**

**chalazion** A chronic inflammatory lipogranuloma due to retention of the secretion (such as blocked ducts) of a meibomian gland in the tarsus of an eyelid. It is characterized by a gradual painless swelling of the gland without marked inflammatory signs and sometimes astigmatism which is induced by the cyst pressing on the cornea. Small chalazia may disappear spontaneously but large ones usually have to be incised and **curetted** (i.e. removal of the pus with a scraper) through a tarsal incision. Resolution may also occur after local injection of a corticosteroid drug (e.g. dexamethasone or triamcinolone). *Syn.* meibomian cyst (although it is not a true cyst because its walls are made of granulomatous tissue and not lined by epithelium).
*See* **antiinflammatory drug; eyelids; glands, meibomian; hordeolum, internal.**

**chalcosis lentis** A cataract caused by excessive amount of copper in the eye. It appears as small yellowish-brown opacities in the subcapsular cortex of the lens and pupillary zone with petal-like spokes that extend towards the equator. It may be due to an intraocular foreign body containing copper, or from eyedrops that contain copper sulfate, or as part of Wilson' s disease. Management consists mainly of removal of the foreign body. *Syn.* sunflower cataract.
*See* **disease, Wilson's.**

**chamber, anterior (AC)** Space within the eye filled with aqueous humour and bounded anteriorly by the cornea and posteriorly by the iris and the part of the anterior surface of the lens which appears through the pupil. Its average axial length is 3.1 mm.
*See* **angle of the anterior chamber; gonioscope; iris; method, van Herick, Shaffer and Schwartz; test, shadow.**

**chamber, posterior** Space within the eye filled with aqueous humour and bounded by the posterior surface of the iris, the ciliary processes, the zonule and the anterior surface of the lens.

**chamber, vitreous** Space within the eye filled with vitreous humour and bounded by the retina, ciliary body, canal of Petit and the postlenticular space of Berger.
*See* **canal of Petit; humour, vitreous; postlenticular space, Berger's.**

**chambers of the eye** The anterior, posterior and vitreous chambers of the eye.

**Chandler's syndrome** *See* **syndrome, Chandler's.**

**channel** A concept relating to the evidence that information about a particular feature of an image is transmitted and processed in the visual pathway approximately independently of information about other domains. The evidence was obtained from various experiments: matching, threshold elevation, after-effect, etc. *Examples*: the three channels of colour vision theory; the spatial frequency channels.
*See* **after-effect, waterfall.**

**chaos, light** *See* **light, idioretinal.**

**chart, Amsler** One of a set of charts used to detect abnormalities in the central visual field which are so slight that they are undetected by the usual methods of perimetry. There are various patterns, each on a different chart, 10 cm square. One commonly used chart consists of a white grid of 5 mm squares on a black background. Each pattern has a dot in the centre which the patient fixates. When fixated at a distance of 30 cm the entire chart subtends an angle of 20°. If there is any visual impairment (usually as a result of macular disease) it is demonstrated by the absence or irregularities of the lines (Fig. C4). *Syn.* Amsler grid.
*See* **maculopathy, age-related; metamorphopsia.**

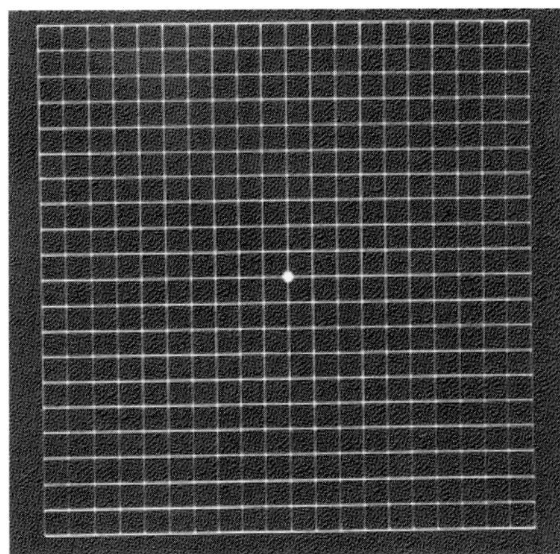

**Fig. C4** Amsler chart

**chart, astigmatic fan** A test pattern consisting of a semicircle of radiating black lines on a white background for determining the presence and the amount, as well as the axis of ocular astigmatism. If the chart resembles the 'clock face' type it is called an **astigmatic dial** or **clock dial chart** (Fig. C5).

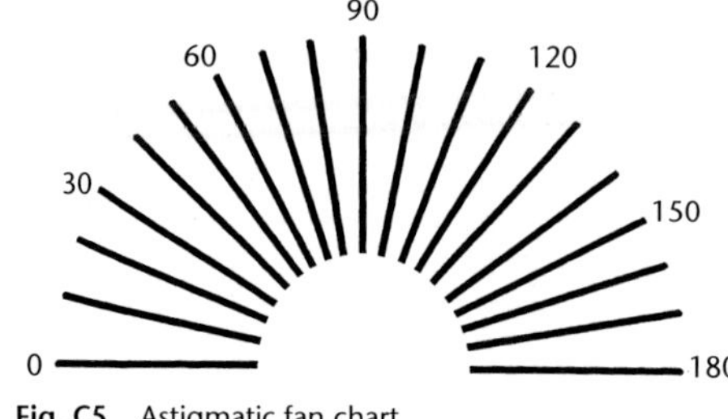


Fig. C5 Astigmatic fan chart

**chart, Bailey–Lovie** A visual acuity chart with letter sizes ranging from 6/60 (20/200) to 6/3 (20/10) in 14 rows of 5 letters. Each row has letters which are approximately 4/5 the size of the next larger letters and the letters in each row have approximately the same legibility (within ±10%). It is most useful with low vision patients. This is the most commonly used type of log MAR charts (Fig. C6). There is also a **Bailey–Lovie Word Reading Chart** for near vision. It is composed of words rather than letters. The size progression of each line is logarithmic. The typeface used is the lower case Times Roman customarily used in newspapers and books, and the range of sizes varies between 80-point and 2-point print (or the Snellen equivalent at 40 cm of 6/144 or 20/480 to 6/3.6 or 20/12, respectively). There are 20 such charts, each with a different set of words.
*See* **acuity, near visual; chart, contrast sensitivity; chart, log MAR; chart, reduced contrast Bailey–Lovie near log MAR letter; vision, low.**

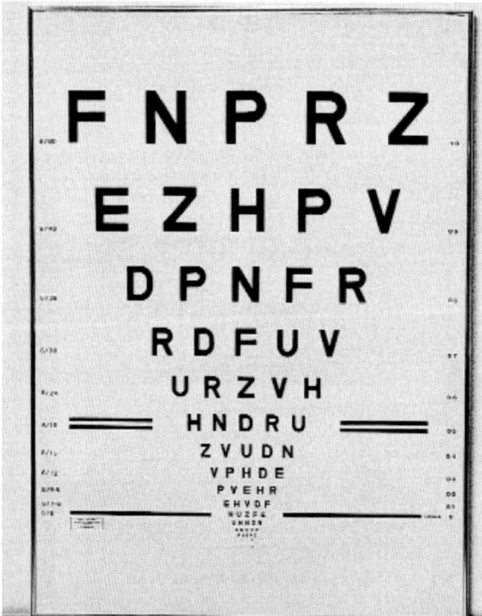


Fig. C6 Bailey–Lovie chart

**chart, clock dial** *See* **chart, astigmatic fan.**

**chart, contrast sensitivity** A chart designed to test contrast sensitivity. Such a test is useful with patients having low vision and in the early detection of diseases. *Examples*: Pelli–Robson chart; reduced contrast Bailey–Lovie near log MAR letter chart.
*See* **acuity cards, Teller; chart, Pelli–Robson; chart, reduced contrast Bailey–Lovie near log MAR letter; sensitivity, contrast; test, Arden grating; Vistech.**

**chart, illiterate E** Chart for carrying out a subjective visual acuity test on a person who cannot read. It consists of a graduated series of the Snellen letter E orientated in various directions which the subject must recognize. This procedure is sometimes called the **'E' test** or **'E' game.**
*See* **acuity cards, Teller; chart, Snellen; 'E' game.**

**chart, Landolt broken ring** A visual acuity chart using a graduated series of Landolt rings in which the target thicknesses and gaps are equal to one-fifth of the outer diameter. The subject must indicate the orientation of the gap which usually appears in either of four directions: right, left, up or down. This test is less subjective than the Snellen chart. *Syn.* Landolt C chart.
*See* **chart, Snellen; Landolt ring.**

**chart, log MAR** A visual acuity chart in which the rows of optotypes vary in a logarithmic progression. The multiplier of the geometric progression is usually equal to 1.2589 or 0.1 log unit. On one side of such a chart the rows of optotypes are usually labelled with the traditional Snellen notation. On the other side of each row visual acuity is labelled as the logarithm of the minimum angle of resolution (log MAR) which is the logarithm to the base 10 of the angular subtense of the stroke widths of the optotypes at a standard distance.
*See* **chart, Bailey–Lovie.**

**chart, Pelli–Robson** A contrast sensitivity chart consisting of eight lines of letters, all of the same size, subtending 3 degrees at a viewing distance of 1 m. On each line there are two groups, each containing three different letters; the letters in each group have the same contrast. The contrast of the different letters in each group decreases by a factor of $1/\sqrt{2}$ and the range of contrast varies between 100 and 0.6% in 16 steps. The subject is asked to read the letters starting with those of high contrast and continuing until two or three letters in one group are incorrectly named. The contrast threshold is represented by that of the previous group of letters. The chart gives the results in log contrast sensitivity. This test provides a measurement of contrast sensitivity at low to intermediate spatial frequencies depending

**Table C2** Relationship between the Snellen fraction and the log MAR notation for distance visual acuity

| Snellen fraction (m) | (ft) | log MAR |
|---|---|---|
| 6/150 | 20/500 | 1.4 |
| 6/120 | 20/400 | 1.3 |
| 6/95 | 20/320 | 1.2 |
| 6/75 | 20/250 | 1.1 |
| 6/60 | 20/200 | 1.0 |
| 6/48 | 20/160 | 0.9 |
| 6/38 | 20/125 | 0.8 |
| 6/30 | 20/100 | 0.7 |
| 6/24 | 20/80 | 0.6 |
| 6/19 | 20/63 | 0.5 |
| 6/15 | 20/50 | 0.4 |
| 6/12 | 20/40 | 0.3 |
| 6/9.5 | 20/32 | 0.2 |
| 6/7.5 | 20/25 | 0.1 |
| 6/6 | 20/20 | 0 |
| 6/4.75 | 20/16 | −0.1 |
| 6/3.75 | 20/12.5 | −0.2 |
| 6/3 | 20/10 | −0.3 |

upon the viewing distance. *Syn.* Pelli–Robson contrast sensitivity test.
*See* **sensitivity, contrast.**

**chart, Raubitschek** A test target for determining the axis and the amount of astigmatism of the eye. It consists of two parabolic lines (known as wings) in an arrowhead pattern, parallel and closely spaced at one end, and each diverging from each other through a 90° angle at the other end. There are several methods of using this test. *Syn.* Raubitschek arrows; Raubitschek dial.
*See* **chart, astigmatic fan.**

**chart, reduced contrast Bailey–Lovie near log MAR letter** A set of 30 Bailey–Lovie charts designed to measure contrast sensitivity. Each chart has a different contrast, half of the charts contains the letters of the distance Bailey–Lovie chart and the other half contains the letters of the near Bailey–Lovie chart. All the charts have the same average reflectance and the contrast of the charts ranges from 0.95 to 0.0013%. The charts are presented to the subject in order of increasing contrast and the subject reads the letters from the largest to the smallest lines that they are able to. Threshold resolution in log min arc is determined for each of the 30 charts and a contrast sensitivity curve can thus be determined.
*See* **chart, Bailey–Lovie; chart, contrast sensitivity; sensitivity, contrast.**

**chart, Snellen** A visual acuity test using a graduated series of **Snellen letters** (or Snellen test types), in which the limbs and the spaces between them subtend an angle of one minute of arc at a specified distance. The letters are usually constructed so that they are 5 units high and 4 units wide, although some charts use letters which fit within a square subtending 5 minutes of arc at that distance.
*See* **acuity, Snellen; chart, Landolt broken ring; Snellen fraction.**

**chart, test** A board externally illuminated, an internally illuminated transparent plastic or glass sheet, or slide for projection on which are printed optotypes or other tests used in the subjective determination of refraction. *Syn.* letter chart.
*See* **legibility; optotype.**

**Table C3** Relationship between Snellen visual acuity and letter height at two viewing distances (the letter corresponding to an acuity of 6/6 subtends 5′ and the gap in the letter 1′)

| Snellen acuity (m) | (ft) | letter height (mm) 4 m | 6 m |
|---|---|---|---|
| 6/3 | 20/10 | 2.9 | 4.4 |
| 6/4.5 | 20/15 | 4.4 | 6.5 |
| 6/6 | 20/20 | 5.8 | 8.7 |
| 6/7.5 | 20/25 | 7.3 | 10.9 |
| 6/9 | 20/30 | 8.7 | 13.1 |
| 6/12 | 20/40 | 11.6 | 17.5 |
| 6/15 | 20/50 | 14.5 | 21.8 |
| 6/18 | 20/60 | 17.5 | 26.2 |
| 6/24 | 20/80 | 23.3 | 34.9 |
| 6/30 | 20/100 | 29.1 | 43.6 |
| 6/36 | 20/120 | 34.9 | 52.4 |
| 6/48 | 20/160 | 46.5 | 69.8 |
| 6/60 | 20/200 | 58.1 | 87.3 |
| 6/120 | 20/400 | 116.4 | 174.5 |

**Chavasse lens** *See* **lens, Chavasse.**

**check ligament** *See* **ligament, check.**

**checkerboard pattern** *See* **pattern, checkerboard.**

**cheiroscope** An instrument used in the management of amblyopia, suppression and hand and eye coordination. It consists of presenting a line drawing to one eye (usually the dominant one) which is traced by a pencil or crayon in the field of view of the other eye. The two fields of view are separated by a septum and a small mirror is used to reflect the line drawing. Stereoscopes can easily be adapted into cheiroscopes.

**chemodenervation** A technique in which a pharmacologic compound (e.g. atropine, botulinum toxin) is used to paralyse a muscle or group of muscles. This technique is most often used in

the treatment of certain forms of strabismus as well as blepharospasm.
*See* **blepharospasm; botulinum toxin; strabismus.**

**chemosis** Severe oedema of the conjunctiva.
*See* **conjunctiva; ophthalmopathy, thyroid.**

**cherry-red spot** Bright red appearance of the macular area in an eye with occlusion of the central retinal artery, Tay–Sachs disease or Niemann–Pick disease. In the case of central retinal artery occlusion the surrounding area is white due to ischaemia but the reddish reflex from the intact choroidal vessels beneath the fovea shows at that spot since the retina is thinnest there. There is a very marked, if not complete, loss of vision which appears suddenly. In cases of storage disease (i.e. Niemann–Pick or Tay–Sachs), the area surrounding the fovea is artificially whitened and opaque, offsetting the normal pinkish colour of the fovea.
*See* **disease, Niemann–Pick; disease, Tay–Sachs; retinal arterial occlusion.**

**Cheshire cat effect** *See* **effect, Cheshire cat.**

**chiasma, optic** A structure located above the pituitary gland and formed by the junction and partial decussation (crossing-over) of the optic nerves. The fibres from the nasal half of the retina of the left eye cross over to join the fibres from the temporal half of the right retina to make up the right optic tract and vice versa. About 53% of the axons of the optic nerves cross to the opposite tract (Fig. C7). A lesion of the chiasma produces a typical field defect (heteronymous hemianopsia).
*See* **circle of Willis; decussation; hemianopsia, heteronymous; nerve, optic; pathway, visual; stereo-blindness; tracts, optic.**

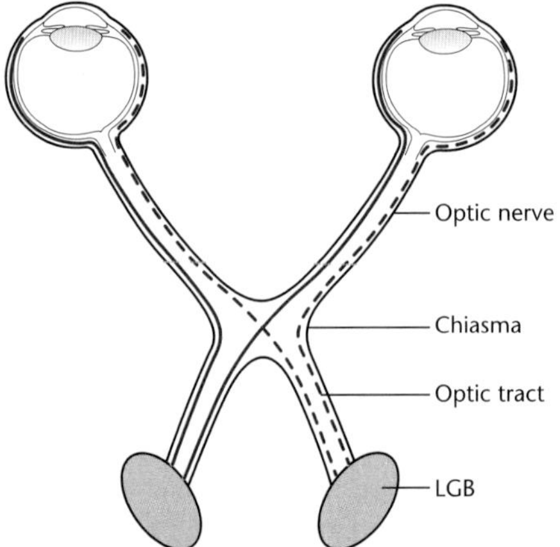


**Fig. C7** An illustration of the decussation of the optic nerve fibres occurring in the optic chiasma. Information from one side of the visual field is transmitted to the contralateral, lateral geniculate body (LGB)

**chiastopic fusion** *See* **fusion, chiastopic.**

**chlamydial infection** *See* **conjunctivitis, adult inclusion; keratitis, epithelial; ophthalmia neonatorum; trachoma.**

**chloramphenicol** *See* **antibiotic.**

**chlorbutanol** *See* **antiseptic.**

**chlorhexidine** *See* **antiseptic.**

**chlorolabe** *See* **pigment, visual.**

**chlorpheniramine** *See* **antihistamine.**

**chlorophobia** An abnormal aversion to green.
*See* **chromatophobia.**

**chlortetracycline** *See* **antibiotic.**

**chloropsia** *See* **chromatopsia.**

**choked disc** *See* **papilloedema.**

**cholinergic** Relates to those structures (e.g. nerve fibres, receptors) that have actions similar to those caused by acetylcholine. Cholinergic receptors are of two types: **nicotinic** receptors which are situated in striated muscles (e.g. the extraocular muscles) and **muscarinic** receptors which are situated in parasympathetically innervated structures (e.g. the iris and ciliary body).
*See* **acetylcholine; muscles, extraocular; muscles, intraocular; mydriatic; nicotine; parasympathomimetic drug.**

**choriocapillaris** Layer of the choroid adjacent to the membrane of Bruch and consisting of a network of capillaries which supplies nutrients to the retina.
*See* **choroid; membrane, Bruch's.**

**chorioretinitis** Inflammation of the retina and the choroid.
*See* **nystagmus.**

**chorioretinopathy, central serous** *See* **retinopathy, central serous.**

**choroid** The highly vascular tunic of the eye lying between the retina and sclera. Its main function is to nourish the retina. It is a thin membrane extending from the optic nerve to the ora serrata. It consists of five main layers from without inward: the suprachoroid (or lamina fusca), the layers of vessels (Haller's layer and Sattler's layer), the choriocapillaris and the membrane of Bruch (or lamina vitrea).
*See* **choriocapillaris; choroiditis; epichoroid; fuscin; membrane, Bruch's; naevus, choroidal.**

**choroidal flush; melanoma** *See* under the nouns.

**choroidal naevus** *See* **naevus, choroidal.**

**choroideraemia** A bilateral, X-linked, recessive inherited degeneration of the choroid and retinal

pigment epithelium characterized by night blindness which begins in early youth. Most males are myopic. The condition is mild and non-progressive in females. Both males and females display a salt and pepper appearance of the fundus, but in males it advances to complete atrophy and eventually blindness. *Note*: also spelt choroideremia. *Syn.* progressive choroidal atrophy; progressive tapetochoroidal atrophy.
*See* **inheritance.**

**choroiditis** Inflammation of the choroid. The ophthalmoscopic appearance is a whitish yellow area stippled with pigment. However, it is most often associated with an inflammation of the retina (chorioretinitis) and of the other tissues of the uvea.
*See* **iritis; uveitis.**

**choroiditis, Tay's** *See* **drusen, familial dominant.**

**chroma** *See* **Munsell colour system.**

**chromatic** Pertaining to colour.

**chromatic aberration** *See* **aberration, lateral chromatic; aberration, longitudinal chromatic.**

**chromatic adaptation; dispersion; parallax** *See* under the nouns.

**chromatic stereopsis** *See* **chromostereopsis.**

**chromatic vision** *See* **vision, colour.**

**chromaticity** Colour quality of a colour stimulus definable by its chromaticity coordinates, or by its dominant (or complementary) wavelength and its purity taken together (CIE).
*See* **dominant wavelength; saturation; wavelength.**

**chromaticity diagram** Plane diagram showing the results of mixtures of colour stimuli, each chromaticity being represented by a single point on the diagram (Fig. C8). *Syn.* colour triangle.
*See* **illuminants, CIE standard; light, white; purple; spectrum locus.**

**chromatophobia** An abnormal aversion to colours or to certain colours (e.g. **erythrophobia**, an abnormal aversion to red). It may be psychological or physiological, such as an abnormal sensitivity to some short wavelengths following cataract extraction. *Syn.* chromophobia.
*See* **chlorophobia; cyanophobia.**

**chromatopsia** Abnormal condition in which objects appear falsely coloured. Depending upon the colour seen, the chromatopsia is called **xanthopsia** (yellow vision), **erythropsia** (red vision), **chloropsia** (green vision) or **cyanopsia** (blue vision). This condition may appear after a cataract operation (blue and red vision) or following exposure to an intense illumination (red vision)

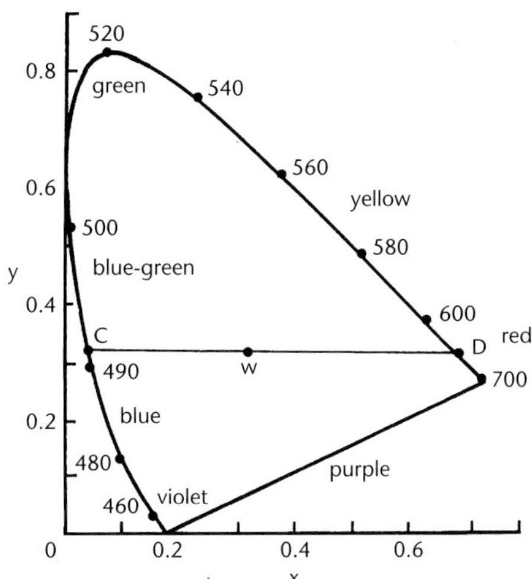


**Fig. C8** The CIE chromaticity diagram (1931) (W, white light illuminant C; C and D, complementary wavelengths). Spectral colours are shown on the curved wavelength (or spectral) locus and non-spectral purples are shown along the straight line joining the spectral limits, 400–700 nm

or in people suffering from carbon monoxide poisoning and oxygen deprivation. This may cause some damage to the areas of the visual cortex involved in the processing of colour perception, because these areas are supplied with more blood vessels than other areas of the visual cortex. *Syn.* chromopsia.
*See* **euchromatopsia; xanthopsia.**

**chromophobia** *See* **chromatophobia.**

**chromoretinoscopy** An objective method of measuring the longitudinal chromatic aberration of the eye by carrying out retinoscopy through various coloured filters (usually a red and a green filter). However, it is necessary to use a retinoscope source of high luminance (e.g. halogen). The difference in the retinoscopic value obtained with the two coloured filters represents the longitudinal chromatic aberration of the eye between these two dominant wavelengths.
*See* **aberration, longitudinal chromatic.**

**chromostereopsis** A sensation of apparent depth among coloured objects placed at the same distance from the subject and viewed binocularly, when the pupils are eccentric to the achromatic axes or the visual axes do not coincide with the achromatic axes. This phenomenon is attributed to the retinal disparity created by the chromatic aberration of the eye. If the objects are red and blue (or green), the red appears closer than the blue (or green) in many people. Other people see the reverse impression and a few others do not see any apparent depth at all. The phenomenon can be enhanced, eliminated or

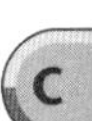

reversed by using prisms or pinhole pupils placed in different regions of the pupil. If the pinhole pupils are decentred symmetrically temporally in front of the natural pupils the red object will appear closer than the blue (**positive chromostereopsis**) and if they are decentred nasally the blue object appears closer than the red (**negative chromostereopsis**). Apparent depth is eliminated when the pinholes are centred on the achromatic axes or when using prisms of appropriate power and direction. *Syn.* chromatic stereopsis; colour stereoscopy.
*See* **aberration, longitudinal chromatic; axis, achromatic; parallax, chromatic; stereopsis.**

**chrysiasis** A deposition of gold in tissues, especially the cornea and conjunctiva and the lens leading to cataract. It occurs as a result of prolonged gold therapy (e.g. gold tablets which are occasionally used in the treatment of rheumatoid arthritis).

**cicatricial ectropion; entropion; pemphigoid** *See* under the nouns.

**CIE standard illuminants** *See* **illuminants, CIE standard.**

**cilia** The eyelashes (*singular*: cilium).

**ciliares, striae** *See* **stria.**

**ciliary arteries** *See* **arteries, ciliary.**

**ciliary block glaucoma** *See* **glaucoma, ciliary block.**

**ciliary body** Part of the uvea, anterior to the ora serrata and extending to the root of the iris where it is attached to the scleral spur. It comprises the ciliary muscle and the ciliary processes and is roughly triangular in sagittal section. The whole ciliary body forms a ring. The part just beyond the ora serrata is smooth and is thus known as **pars plana** (or **orbiculus ciliaris**). Anterior to this lies a region of ridges which are the ciliary processes; this region is called the **pars plicata** (or **corona ciliaris**).
*See* **angle recession; ciliary processes; cyclitis; iridodialysis; muscle, ciliary; scleral spur; stria.**

**ciliary flush** *See* **injection, ciliary.**

**ciliary ganglion; injection** *See* under the nouns.

**ciliary margin** *See* **iris, plateau.**

**ciliary muscle** *See* **muscle, ciliary.**

**ciliary nerve** *See* **nerve, long ciliary.**

**ciliary processes** About 70 ridges, some 2 mm long and 0.5 mm high arranged meridionally and forming the corona ciliaris of the ciliary body. The ciliary processes consist essentially of blood vessels which are the continuation forward of those of the choroid. The region of the ciliary processes is the most vascular of the whole eye. The processes are involved in the secretion of aqueous humour.
*See* **ciliary body; humour, aqueous; stria.**

**ciliary ring** *See* **annulus ciliaris.**

**ciliosis** Spasmodic twitching of the eyelids.

**cilium** An eyelash (*plural*: cilia).

**circadian rhythm** *See* **rhythm, circadian.**

**circle, blur; of confusion** *See* **blur circle.**

**circle of Haller** *See* **circle of Zinn.**

**circle of least confusion** The smallest cross-section of a circular bundle of an astigmatic pencil formed by an astigmatic lens and situated between the two focal lines.
*See* **astigmatism; lens, astigmatic; line, focal; Sturm, conoid of.**

**circle of Vieth–Müller** *See* **horopter, Vieth–Müller.**

**circle of Willis** An arterial ring surrounding the optic chiasma and hypothalamus. It is formed anteriorly by the anterior cerebral arteries which are linked by the anterior communicating artery; posteriorly, by the division of the basilar artery into the posterior cerebral arteries and, laterally the latter are united by the posterior communicating arteries to the internal carotid arteries. An aneurysm in one part of the circle of Willis may compress the optic chiasma resulting in a visual field loss. As the terminal branches of the internal carotid arteries are called the middle cerebral arteries, the circle of Willis is sometimes considered to be formed laterally by the latter (Fig. C9).
*See* **artery, internal carotid; chiasma, optic; haemorrhage, preretinal; hemianopsia, heteronymous.**

**circle of Zinn** Anastomosing circle of short ciliary arteries which have pierced the sclera about the optic nerve. Branches pass forward to the choroid, inward to the optic nerve and backward to the pial network. *Syn.* circle of Haller.

**citric acid cycle** *See* **cycle, Krebs.**

**City University test** *See* **plates, pseudoisochromatic.**

**CLARE** *See* **contact lens acute red eye.**

**clearance, apical** The distance between the posterior surface of a contact lens and the apex of the cornea.
*See* **apex, corneal; bearing, apical.**

**cliff, visual** A device for testing depth perception. It consists of two identically patterned horizontal surfaces, one well below the other; the upper is extended over the lower by means of a sheet of transparent glass. A subject (usually a newborn

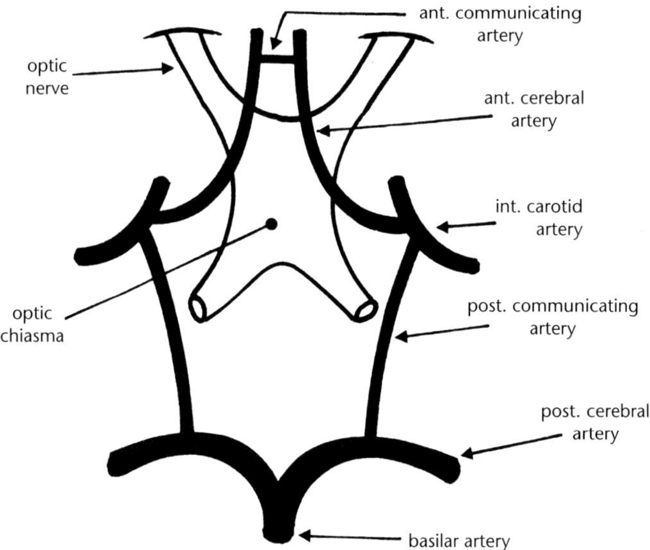


**Fig. C9** Diagram showing the circle of Willis and the optic chiasma

of a species) placed in the centre of the upper surface and who is unwilling to move onto the transparent glass that projects over the lower surface is assumed to possess depth perception. Many species have been found to possess depth perception at birth, indicating an innate sense, unaffected by learning experience.
*See* **perception, depth.**

**clinical interferometer** *See* **maxwellian view system, clinical.**

**clinometer** Apparatus used to measure ocular torsion.

**clip, Halberg** Tradename for a plastic device with two cells used for holding trial lenses which is clipped over a lens of a pair of spectacles (Fig. C10).
*See* **clipover.**

**clip-on** *See* **clipover.**

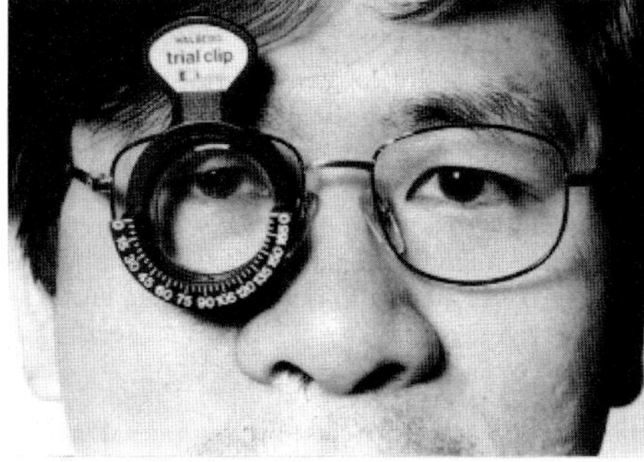


**Fig. C10** Halberg clip

**clipover** An attachment holding an auxiliary lens or lenses (an add, a prism or a tint) in front of spectacles by spring action. There are many (albeit similar) types of clips which fit over one lens of a pair of spectacles (e.g. Bernell clip, Bommarito clip, Halberg clip, Jannelli clip). They are used extensively in the refraction of low vision patients. *Syn.* clip-on; fit-over; trial lens clip.
*See* **clip, Halberg.**

**clip, trial lens** *See* **clipover.**

**clobetasone** *See* **antiinflammatory drug.**

**clock dial chart** *See* **chart, astigmatic fan.**

**Cloquet's canal** *See* **canal, hyaloid.**

**closed-angle glaucoma** *See* **glaucoma, angle-closure.**

**clouding, central corneal** Diffuse, hazy appearance of the cornea due to oedema of the central region of the cornea, usually associated with the wearing of hard contact lenses (mainly PMMA), but it may also occur in keratoconus, Fuch's endothelial dystrophy or disciform keratitis. It is most easily seen with a slit-lamp using retro-illumination against the pupil margin or sclerotic scatter illumination. This condition may give rise to Sattler's veil.
*See* **cornea; cornea guttata; illumination, retro-, sclerotic scatter; keratitis, disciform; keratoconus; lens, contact; oedema; Sattler's veil; slit-lamp.**

**coated lens** *See* **lens, coated.**

tests, e.g. anomaloscope, pseudoisochromatic plates, Farnsworth test. The following types of defective colour vision are usually recognized: **anomalous trichromatic vision** or **anomalous trichromatism; dichromatic vision** or **dichromatism; monochromatic vision** or **monochromatism** (total colour blindness), anomaly of vision in which there is perception of luminance but not of colour. Both anomalous trichromatism and dichromatism occur in three distinct forms called respectively **protanomalous vision** and **protanopia, deuteranomalous vision** and **deuteranopia, tritanomalous vision** and **tritanopia.** The causes of defective colour vision may be an impairment of a cone pigment or a reduced number of cone cells. The majority of cases of defective colour vision are inherited. Acquired defects are rare and mostly tritanopic. They may be due to glaucoma, retinal or optic nerve disease, drug or chemical toxicity, diabetes, retinitis pigmentosa, etc. The inherited type occurs as a sex-linked disorder in which the defective gene is on the X chromosome. Since men have only one X chromosome while women have two, sex-linked disorders (most being X-linked recessive) affect mainly males who inherit the genetic defect from their mother. For women to show the defect, both of their X chromosomes have to carry the defective gene, a rare occurrence. Defective colour vision occurs in about 8% of the male population and 0.5% of the female population. *Syn.* daltonism.
*See* **achromatopsia; anomaloscope; deuteranomaly; deuteranopia; Edridge–Green lantern; lens, X-Chrom; monochromat; nystagmus; pigment, visual; plates, pseudoisochromatic; protanomaly; protanopia; rule, Kollner's; test, Farnsworth; test, lantern; test, wool; tritanomaly; tritanopia.**

**colours, confusion** Colours that are confused by a dichromat. The colours confused by a deuteranope, a protanope and a tritanope are not the same. For example, the deuteranope will confuse reds, greens and greys, whereas the protanope will confuse reds, oranges, blue-greens and greys. *See* **deuteranopia; plates, pseudoisochromatic; protanopia; tritanopia.**

**colours, fundamental** *See* **colours, primary.**

**colours, primary** Any sets of three colours such as, for example, red, green and blue which, by additive colour mixture of the stimuli in varying proportions, can produce any colour sensation. *Syn.* fundamental colours.
*See* **colour mixture.**

**colours, spectral** The colours produced by the various radiations of the visible spectrum.
*See* **light.**

**column, cortical** In the visual cortex, neurons with similar properties are arranged in columns (about 2 mm high) perpendicular to the surface of the cortex. The columns traverse the six cortical layers until they reach the white matter. Neurons throughout this column respond to the same orientation (**orientation column**) and to the same ocular dominance (**ocular dominance column**). A neighbouring column will then have neurons responding to a slightly different orientation from the one next to it and perhaps the same ocular dominance. Neurons in layer 4 represent an exception as they may respond to any orientation or to one eye only.
*See* **area, visual; hypercolumn.**

**coma** Monochromatic aberration of an optical system produced when the incident light beam makes an angle with the optical axis. The image

**Table C6** Classification of defective colour vision

| type | anomalous trichromats | | |
|---|---|---|---|
| **frequency:** | **deuteranomal** | **protanomal** | **tritanomal** |
| male | 4.6% | 1% | 0.0001% |
| female | 0.35% | 0.03% | unknown |
| colour response | slight green deficiency | red deficiency | blue deficiency |
| | **dichromats** | | |
| **frequency:** | **deuteranope** | **protanope** | **tritanope** |
| male | 1% | 1.1% | 0.005% |
| female | 0.01% | 0.01% | 0.003% |
| colour response | green deficiency | insensitive to red | blue deficiency |
| neutral point | 498 nm | 493 nm | 570 nm |
| | **monochromats** | | |
| **frequency** | **cone monochromat** | **rod monochromat** | |
| | unknown | 0.003% | |

appears like a comet with the tail pointing towards the axis.
*See* **aberration; aberration, monochromatic; lens, aplanatic; sine condition.**

**combination lens** *See* **lens, combination.**

**combination system** *See* **lens, piggy-back.**

**comitance** *See* **concomitance.**

**commissure** Band of nerve fibres connecting corresponding structures in the brain or spinal cord.
*See* **corpus callosum.**

**commotio retinae** *See* **disease, Berlin's.**

**compensated heterophoria** *See* **heterophoria, compensated.**

**compensating prism** *See* **prism, relieving.**

**compensatory eye movements** *See* **reflex, static eye.**

**complementary after-image; colour** *See* under the nouns.

**complex cell** *See* **cell, complex.**

**compliance** The willingness to strictly follow the instructions given by a clinician. *Example*: following the cleaning instructions and wearing schedule given after contact lens fitting.

**compound astigmatism; eye; optical system** *See* under the nouns.

**computer vision syndrome** *See* **syndrome, computer vision.**

**computerized perimeter; tomography** *See* under the nouns.

**concave** Pertaining to a surface shaped like the inside of a sphere.
*See* **lens, diverging; mirror, concave.**

**concomitance** The condition in which the two eyes move as a unit, that is maintaining a constant angle between them for all directions of gaze when fixating at a fixed distance. *Syn.* comitance.
*See* **incomitance; muscles, extraocular; strabismus, concomitant.**

**concretions, conjunctival** Minute, hard, whitish spots of calcium present in the palpebral conjunctiva due to cellular degeneration. This condition occurs most commonly in the elderly or in people with prolonged conjunctivitis. They are asymptomatic but may be removed with a needle. *Syn.* conjunctival lithiasis.
*See* **conjunctiva.**

**condenser** An optical system with a large aperture and small focal length used in microscopes and projectors in order to concentrate as much light as possible onto an object. *Syn.* condensing lens.

**condenser, Abbés** Microscope substage condenser consisting of a doublet with a high numerical aperture.
*See* **aperture, numerical; doublet; microscope; triplet.**

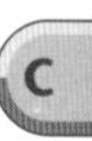

**condensing lens** *See* **condenser.**

**cone cell** *See* **cell, cone.**

**cone degeneration; dystrophy** *See* **dystrophy, cone.**

**cone monochromat** *See* **monochromat.**

**cone-rod dystrophy** *See* **dystrophy, cone-rod.**

**confocal** Having the same focus. *Example*: in a slit-lamp, the microscope and the illumination system have the same focus, i.e. they are confocal.

**confocal microscope** *See* **microscope, confocal.**

**confrontation test** *See* **test, confrontation.**

**confusion, circle of** *See* **blur circle.**

**confusion colours** *See* **colours, confusion.**

**congenital** Refers to a condition that dates from the time of birth. It may or may not be hereditary.

**congruous scotomas** *See* **scotomas, congruous.**

**conical cornea** *See* **keratoconus.**

**conjugate distances** *See* **distances, conjugate.**

**conjugate movements** *See* **version.**

**conjugate points** *See* **distances, conjugate.**

**conjunctiva** A thin transparent mucous membrane lining the posterior surface of the eyelids from the eyelid margin and reflected forward onto the anterior part of the eyeball where it merges with the corneal epithelium at the limbus. It thus forms a sac, the **conjunctival sac** which is open at the palpebral fissure and closed when the eyes are shut. The depths of the unextended sac are 14–16 mm superiorly and 9–11 mm inferiorly. The conjunctiva is divided into three portions: **1.** The portion that lines the posterior surface of the eyelids is called the **palpebral conjunctiva**. It is itself composed of the **marginal conjunctiva** which extends from the eyelid margin to the **tarsal conjunctiva**; the tarsal conjunctiva which extends from the marginal conjunctiva to the **orbital conjunctiva**; and the orbital conjunctiva which extends from the tarsal conjunctiva to the fornix. **2.** That lining the eyeball is the **bulbar conjunctiva**. It is itself composed of the **limbal conjunctiva** which is fused with the episclera at the limbus and the **scleral conjunctiva** which extends from the

limbal conjunctiva to the fornix. **3.** The intermediate part forming the bottom of the conjunctival sac, unattached to the eyelids or the eyeball and joining the bulbar and the palpebral portion is called the **fornix** (or **conjunctival fold**, or **cul-de-sac**).
*See* **dyskeratosis; eversion, lid; eyelids; gland, conjunctival; Krause's end bulbs; sulcus, subtarsal; syndrome, Stevens–Johnson.**

**conjunctiva, corneal** The stratified squamous epithelium of the cornea.

**conjunctival injection** *See* **injection, conjunctival.**

**conjunctival lithiasis** *See* **concretions, conjunctival.**

**conjunctival naevus** *See* **naevus, conjunctival.**

**conjunctival sac** *See* **conjunctiva.**

**conjunctivitis** Inflammation of the conjunctiva. It may be acute, subacute or chronic. It may be due to an allergy, an infection (e.g. *Staphylococcus, Streptococcus, Haemophilus*, etc.), a virus inflammation, an irritant (dust, wind, chemical fumes, ultraviolet radiation or contact lenses), or as a complication of gonorrhoea, syphilis, influenza, hay fever, measles, etc. Conjunctivitis is characterized by various signs and symptoms which may include conjunctival injection, oedema, small follicles or papillae, secretions (purulent, mucopurulent, membranous, pseudomembranous or catarrhal), pain, itching, grittiness and blepharospasm. The most common type of conjunctivitis is that due to a bacterium and in many cases is self-limiting and subsides without treatment. Treatment of that type includes irrigation of the lid and the use of topical antibiotics.
*See* **concretions, conjunctival; injection, conjunctival; ophthalmia neonatorum; syndrome, Stevens–Johnson; trachoma.**

**conjunctivitis, actinic** *See* **keratoconjunctivitis, actinic.**

**conjunctivitis, acute** Conjunctivitis characterized by an onset of hyperaemia (most intense near the fornices), purulent or mucopurulent discharge and symptoms of irritation, grittiness and sticking together of the eyelids on waking. In severe cases there will be chemosis, eyelid oedema, subconjunctival haemorrhages and photophobia. The bacterial type is caused by *Staphylococcus epidermidis, Staph. aureus, Haemophilus influenzae* (*H. aegyptius*, Koch–Weeks bacillus), *Streptococcus pneumoniae* (pneumococcus). A rare form of acute conjunctivitis is caused by the *Neisseria* species (gonococcus, meningococcus, e.g. **gonococcal conjunctivitis**) which produce a more severe form of the disease referred to as **hyperacute bacterial conjunctivitis** or **acute purulent conjunctivitis**. These require immediate treatment with systemic and topical antibiotics. Acute conjunctivitis is also caused by viruses, such as herpes simplex or adenoviruses. All forms of acute conjunctivitis occasionally spread to the cornea. **Bacterial conjunctivitis** often resolves without treatment within two weeks. Treatment consists of topical antibiotic therapy (e.g. chloramphenicol, erythromycin) and warm wet compresses. **Acute allergic conjunctivitis** most typically resolves spontaneously, otherwise treatment includes sodium cromoglycate. **Acute follicular conjunctivitis** is treated by antiviral agents (e.g. acycloguanosine), although in many cases the condition is self-limiting.
*See* **antibiotic; antiviral agents.**

**conjunctivitis, acute haemorrhagic** A highly contagious viral infection of the anterior segment resulting in haemorrhage of the bulbar conjunctiva. The infection is caused by a picornavirus, often associated with pre-auricular adenopathy and a follicular conjunctivitis. The infection is self-limited and lasts 7–10 days. No specific treatment is presently available.

**conjunctivitis, adult inclusion** An acute conjunctivitis caused by the serotypes D to K of *Chlamydia trachomatis* and typically occurring in sexually active adults in whom the genitourinary tract is infected. Signs in the eye usually appear 1 week following sexual exposure. It may also occur after using contaminated eye cosmetics or soon after having been in a public swimming pool, or in newborn infants (called **neonatal inclusion conjunctivitis** or **neonatal chlamydial conjunctivitis**) which is transmitted from the mother during delivery and appears some 5 to 14 days after birth. The conjunctivitis is mucopurulent with follicles in the fornices which often spread to the limbal region. The condition is commonly associated with punctate epithelial keratitis, preauricular lymphadenopathy, marginal infiltrates and, in long-standing infection, micropannus in the superior corneal region may also appear. Differentiation from viral follicular conjunctivitis is made through culture, serological and cytological studies. Treatment consists of using both systemic and topical tetracyclines, although in pregnant or lactating women erythromycin is preferable.
*Syn.* trachoma-inclusion conjunctivitis (TRIC).
*See* **conjunctivitis, follicular; follicle, conjunctival; keratitis, punctate epithelial; lymphadenopathy; ophthalmia neonatorum; trachoma.**

**conjunctivitis, allergic** Conjunctivitis caused by an allergy. Common allergens are pollens associated with hay fever, grass (seasonal **allergic conjunctivitis**) and air pollutants, house dust mites, smoke (**perennial allergic conjunctivitis**). It is characterized by hyperaemia, itching, burning,

swelling, tearing, discharge and photophobia. Conjunctival scrapings contain a large number of eosinophils and serum IgE is elevated. The condition is often associated with rhinitis (**allergic rhinoconjunctivitis**). Treatment commonly includes decongestants, oral antihistamines, mast cell stabilizers (e.g. lodoxamine, sodium cromoglycate) and if severe, topical corticosteroid eyedrops.
*See* **antihistamine; conjunctivitis, vernal; decongestants; mast cell stabilizer.**

**conjunctivitis, angular** Subacute bilateral inflammation of the conjunctiva due to the diplobacillus of Morax–Axenfeld. It involves the conjunctiva in the region of the canthi.
*See* **canthus.**

**conjunctivitis, bacterial** *See* **conjunctivitis, acute.**

**conjunctivitis, catarrhal** Type of conjunctivitis associated with the common cold or catarrhal irritation. It can appear in the acute or chronic form.

**conjunctivitis, contagious** Acute conjunctivitis caused by Koch–Weeks bacillus, adenovirus types 3 and 7 or 8 and 19, or a pneumococcus infection. It may be transmitted by respiratory or ocular infections, contaminated towels or equipment (e.g. tonometer heads). It is characterized by acute onset, redness, tearing, discomfort and photophobia. The condition is often self-limiting but keratitis is a common complication. *Syn.* epidemic conjunctivitis; epidemic keratoconjunctivitis; pink eye (colloquial).
*See* **conjunctivitis, acute.**

**conjunctivitis, eczematous** *See* **conjunctivitis, phlyctenular.**

**conjunctivitis, egyptian** *See* **trachoma.**

**conjunctivitis, epidemic** *See* **conjunctivitis, contagious.**

**conjunctivitis, flash** Conjunctivitis due to exposure to an electric arc, as from a welder's torch.

**conjunctivitis, follicular** Conjunctivitis characterized by follicles (usually in one eye only) caused by adenoviruses or chemical or toxic irritation and frequently associated with lymphadenopathy.
*See* **conjunctivitis, adult inclusion; follicle, conjunctival; lymphadenopathy; zinc sulphate.**

**conjunctivitis, giant papillary (GPC)** Conjunctivitis, characterized by the appearance of 'cobblestones' (large papillae of 0.5 mm or more) on the tarsal conjunctiva of the upper eyelid (and sometimes the lower eyelid). Symptoms include itching, discomfort, mucous discharge and poor vision due to the presence of mucus. The condition may be induced by contact lens wear, ocular prosthesis, or exposed sutures following surgery. This conjunctivitis closely resembles vernal conjunctivitis and is also believed to be an allergic condition. In its early stages as a contact lens-induced condition, it is often referred to as **contact lens papillary conjunctivitis** or **contact lens associated papillary conjunctivitis** (CLPC, CLAPC). In these cases the regular use of surfactant and protein removal tablets as well as frequent lens replacement reduce the incidence of this condition which is less prevalent with the wear of rigid gas permeable than soft contact lenses. Management may also include mast cell stabilizers (e.g. sodium cromoglycate) or antihistamine (e.g. levocabastine) and cessation of lens wear.
*See* **conjunctivitis, vernal; deposits, contact lens; enzyme; surfactant.**

**conjunctivitis, gonococcal** *See* **conjunctivitis, acute.**

**conjunctivitis, granular** *See* **trachoma.**

**conjunctivitis, lacrimal** Chronic conjunctivitis caused by an infection of the lacrimal passages.
*See* **lacrimal apparatus.**

**conjunctivitis, ligneous** A rare, chronic conjunctivitis characterized by the formation of a firm, whitish membrane or pseudomembrane on the tarsal conjunctiva, usually of the upper eyelid. It is typically bilateral, begins in childhood although it may present in patients up to age 85, is more common in females than in males and may persist for months or years. Its cause is unknown but the predisposing factors include bacterial and viral infections, trauma, hypersensitivity reactions and increased vascular permeability and it is often associated with inflammations of other mucous membranes. The most effective treatment is surgical excision followed by topical cyclosporine drops, but the condition has a tendency to recur.
*See* **conjunctivitis, pseudomembranous.**

**conjunctivitis, membranous** *See* **conjunctivitis, pseudomembranous.**

**conjunctivitis, neonatal** *See* **ophthalmia neonatorum.**

**conjunctivitis, phlyctenular** Conjunctivitis characterized by the presence of nodules on the bulbar conjunctiva and which sometimes may spread to the cornea. It is due to an allergic reaction to an antigen (e.g. *Staphylococcus aureus, Candida albicans*). Symptoms are soreness, and photophobia when the cornea is involved. It is associated with superficial vascularization. Treatment is generally with topical corticosteroids. *Syn.* eczematous conjunctivitis; phlyctenulosis.
*See* **conjunctiva; keratitis, phlyctenular.**

**conjunctivitis, pseudomembranous** A nonspecific inflammatory reaction characterized by the formation on the conjunctiva of a coagulated fibrinous plaque consisting of inflammatory cells and an exudate containing mucus and proteins. This plaque forms either a membrane or a pseudomembrane. The latter is loosely adherent to the conjunctival epithelium and can be peeled off without bleeding or damage to the underlying epithelium. A true membrane on the other hand, usually occurs with intense inflammation (**membranous conjunctivitis**). In this case the conjunctival epithelium becomes necrotic and adheres firmly to the overlying membrane which, when peeled leaves a raw, bleeding surface. The cause of either condition may be an infection of which the common sources are herpes simplex virus, adenovirus, beta-haemolytic *Streptococcus*, *Neisseria gonorrhoeae* or as a result of the Stevens–Johnson syndrome, ligneous conjunctivitis, ocular cicatricial pemphigoid, atopic keratoconjunctivitis, chemical burns (especially alkali burns), radiation injury or post-surgical complications.
*See* **conjunctivitis, ligneous; pemphigoid, cicatricial; syndrome, Stevens–Johnson.**

**conjunctivitis, sun lamp** *See* **keratoconjunctivitis, actinic.**

**conjunctivitis, swimming pool** *See* **conjunctivitis, adult inclusion.**

**conjunctivitis, vernal** Chronic, bilateral conjunctivitis which recurs in the spring and summer and is more often seen in boys than girls. Its origin is probably due to an allergy. It is characterized by hard flattened papillae of a bluish-white colour separated by furrows and having the appearance of 'cobblestones' located in the upper palpebral portion of the conjunctiva. A second type of vernal conjunctivitis exists which affects the limbal region of the bulbar conjunctiva, characterized by the formation of small, gelatinous white dots called **Trantas' dots** or **Horner–Trantas' dots**. The chief symptom of the disease is intense itching. Treatment consists mainly of cold compresses and limited (because of side effects) use of topical corticosteroids (e.g. dexamethasone, prednisolone). Sodium cromoglycate or lodoxamide have also been found to be very successful in treating this condition and with fewer side effects than corticosteroids. *Syn.* vernal keratoconjunctivitis (VKC) (although this is not strictly speaking a synonym since the condition often involves the cornea; spring catarrh; vernal catarrh.
*See* **antihistamine; mast cell stabilizers.**

**conjunctivitis, viral** Conjunctivitis caused by a virus. A variety of viruses can produce the disease.

**conoid of Sturm** *See* **Sturm, conoid of.**

**consecutive esotropia; exotropia; strabismus** *See* **strabismus, consecutive.**

**consensual** *See* **reflex, pupil light.**

**constancy** Perceptual phenomenon whereby the properties of certain objects appear to remain relatively constant, despite changes in the stimulus characteristics which induced the perception. All constancies occur only within a limited range.

**constancy, brightness** Perceptual phenomenon whereby the brightness of an object appears to remain relatively constant, despite changes in the level of its illumination. *Example*: white paper appears white whether it is seen in sunlight or in the weaker or yellower illumination of a light bulb. *Syn.* lightness constancy.

**constancy, colour** Perceptual phenomenon whereby the colour of an object appears to remain relatively constant, despite changes in the spectral composition of the incident light.

**constancy, shape** Perceptual phenomenon whereby the shape of an object appears to remain relatively constant, despite changes in the viewing angle. *Example*: A circle held obliquely to the line of sight appears more circular than it should due to shape constancy although its retinal projection is oval.

**constancy, size** Perceptual phenomenon whereby the size of an object appears to remain relatively constant, despite changes in the viewing distance (and therefore of its retinal image size).

**constants of the eye** Average dimensions of the various parameters of the eye adopted to represent a typical eye. These vary slightly depending upon the authors, such as Donders, Gullstrand, Bennett–Rabbetts, etc.
*See* **eye, reduced; eye, schematic; power.**

**constant, Planck's** *See* **photon.**

**constringence** A positive number (*symbol*: V) which specifies any transparent medium. It is equal to

$$V = \frac{n_D - 1}{n_F - n_C}$$

where $n_D$, $n_F$ and $n_C$ are the refractive indices for the Fraunhofer spectral lines D (589.3 nm), F (486.1 nm) and C (656.3 nm). A material with a high constringence (e.g. V = 50) produces less chromatic aberration than one with a low constringence (e.g. V = 30). The reciprocal of the constringence is called the dispersive power. *Syn.* Abbé's number; V-value.
*See* **aberration, longitudinal chromatic; dispersion; glass, crown; glass, flint; index of refraction; lines, Fraunhofer's.**

**Table C7** Optical constants of an average adult Caucasian eye

| structure or surface | refractive index | radius of curvature (mm) | distance from ant. surface of cornea (mm) |
|---|---|---|---|
| cornea | 1.376 | – | – |
| aqueous humour | 1.336 | – | – |
| lens (total) | 1.42 | – | – |
| vitreous humour | 1.336 | – | – |
| ant. corneal surface | – | 7.8 | 0 |
| post. corneal surface | – | 6.7 | 0.5 |
| ant. lens surface | – | 10.6 | 3.6 |
| accommodated | – | 6.1 | 3.2 |
| post. lens surface | – | −6.2 | 7.2 |
| accommodated | – | −5.3 | 7.2 |
| retina | 1.363 | – | 24.1 |

**Table C8** Constringence (V) of some transparent media (index of refraction *n*)

| | *n* | V |
|---|---|---|
| **glass** | | |
| spectacle crown | 1.523 | 59 |
| dense barium crown | 1.620 | 60 |
| lanthana crown | 1.713 | 54 |
| zinc crown | 1.508 | 61 |
| light flint | 1.581 | 41 |
| dense flint | 1.620 | 36 |
| extra dense flint | 1.706 | 30 |
| titanium oxide | 1.701 | 31 |
| **polymer** | | |
| PMMA | 1.492 | 57 |
| CR-39 | 1.498 | 58 |
| Polycarbonate | 1.586 | 30 |
| Polystyrene | 1.590 | 31 |
| Water (at 37°C) | 1.331 | 56 |
| Aqueous and vitreous (at 37°C) | 1.334 | 56 |

**contact arc** *See* **arc of contact.**

**contact lens** *See* **lens, contact.**

**contact lens acute red eye (CLARE)** An acute corneal inflammation caused by overnight wear of soft contact lenses. It is characterized by pain, usually unilateral, redness, tearing, photophobia, corneal infiltrates and blurred vision that suddenly appears upon waking. The lens is, in most cases, tight or immobile and it is the breakdown of debris which accumulated behind the lens which caused the inflammatory reaction. The lens must be removed immediately and patching of the eye and antiinflammatory therapy may be necessary. *Syn.* immobile lens syndrome; non-ulcerative keratitis; tight lens syndrome.
*See* **lens, steep.**

**contour** The outline of a part of a retinal image where the light intensity changes abruptly.

**contraindication** The presence of a condition or disease which renders some particular type of treatment undesirable. *Example*: contact lenses are contraindicated in very dusty, dry and smoky atmospheres.

**contralateral** A term relating to the opposite side. *See* **geniculate bodies, lateral; ipsilateral.**

**contraocular** Pertaining to the opposite eye.

**contrast 1.** Subjective sense: subjective assessment of the difference in appearance of two parts of a field of view seen simultaneously or successively. Hence, **luminosity contrast, lightness contrast, colour contrast, simultaneous contrast, successive contrast. 2.** Objective sense: quantities defined by the formulae for **luminance contrast**

$$\text{(a)}\ \frac{L_2 - L_1}{L_1} \quad \text{(b)}\ \frac{L_2 - L_1}{L_2 + L_1} \quad \text{(c)}\ \frac{L_2}{L_1}$$

*Note*: Example (c) is better known as luminance ratio (CIE). $L_2$ is the maximum luminance and $L_1$ is the minimum luminance.
*See* **frequency, spatial; sensitivity, contrast; threshold, differential.**

**contrast sensitivity test** *See* **chart, contrast sensitivity; sensitivity, contrast.**

**contrast threshold** *See* **sensitivity, contrast; threshold, differential.**

**conus** *See* **crescent, myopic.**

**convention, sign** *See* **sign convention.**

**convergence 1.** Movement of the eyes turning inward or towards each other (Fig. C12). **2.** Characteristic of a pencil of light rays directed towards a real image point.
*See* **angle of convergence; vergence.**

**convergence accommodation** *See* **accommodation, convergence.**

**convergence, accommodative** That component of convergence which occurs reflexly in response to a change in accommodation. It is easily

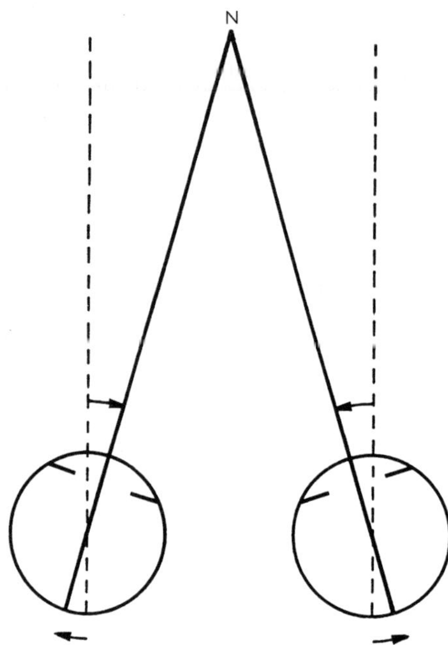


Fig. C12 Convergence from a distant to a near object N

demonstrated by having one eye fixate from a far point to a near point along its line of sight, while the other eye is occluded. The occluded eye will be seen to make a convergence movement in response to the accommodation. Alternatively, one eye fixates while the other is occluded. If a minus lens is placed in front of the fixating eye, the occluded eye will be seen to converge. *Syn.* accommodative vergence; associative convergence.
*See* **convergence, fusional; convergence, initial; convergence, proximal; convergence, tonic; fusion, motor.**

**convergence, amplitude of** The angle through which each eye is turned from the far to the near point of convergence. *Syn.* amplitude of triangulation.
*See* **angle, metre; convergence, far point of; convergence, near point of.**

**convergence, angle of** *See* **angle of convergence.**

**convergence, correction induced** Convergence induced when changing from spectacles to contact lenses in near vision. Spectacles centred for distance vision induce base-in prisms in myopes and base-out prisms in hyperopes, in near vision. Thus, a spectacle-wearing myope converges less and a spectacle-wearing hyperope converges more than an emmetrope fixating at a given distance (Fig. C13). Optically centred contact lenses do not induce any prismatic effect and the amount of convergence remains the same for all refractive errors. Consequently, myopes require more convergence and hyperopes less convergence when they transfer from spectacles to contact lenses. However, this change in convergence is accompanied by a similar change in accommodation, so that a myope transferring to contact lenses converges and accommodates more than with spectacles and the reverse applies for a hyperope.
*See* **accommodation, correction induced; prism, induced.**

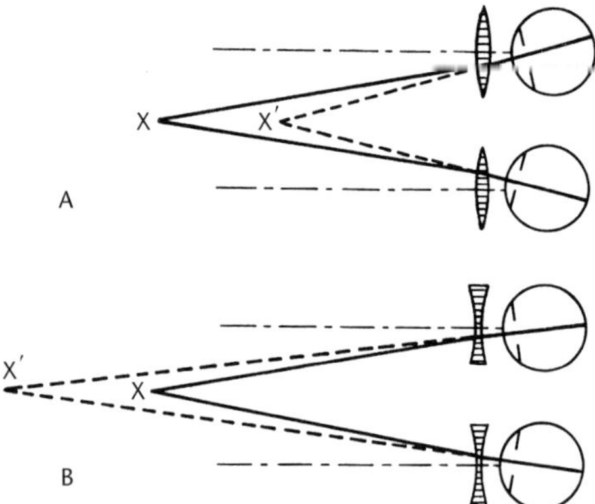


Fig. C13 Prismatic effects induced when an observer fixates a near object X wearing lenses centred for distance vision (A, plus lenses induce base-out prismatic effects and the hyperope overconverges to X′; B, minus lenses induce base-in prismatic effects and the myope underconverges to X′)

**convergence excess** A high esophoria at near, associated with a relatively orthophoric condition at distance. It usually gives rise to complaints of headaches and other symptoms of asthenopia accompanying prolonged close work.
*See* **accommodative excess; esophoria.**

**convergence, far point of** The farthest point where the lines of sight intersect when the eyes diverge to the maximum.

**convergence, fusional** That component of convergence which is induced by fusional stimuli or which is available in excess of that required to overcome the heterophoria. It is usually a **positive fusional convergence**, but in some cases the eyes need to diverge to obtain fusion and this is called **negative fusional convergence**. An example is the movement of the eyes from the passive (one eye covered, the other fixating an object) to the active (both eyes fixating foveally the same object) position. However, as disparate retinal stimuli are a more powerful component of convergence than fusion, the concept of fusional convergence is being substituted by motor fusion (or disparity vergence).
*See* **convergence, accommodative; convergence, initial; convergence, proximal; convergence,**

relative; convergence, tonic; fusion, chiastopic; fusion, motor; fusion, orthopic; vergence facility.**

**convergence, fusional reserve** *See* **convergence, relative.**

**convergence, initial** Movement of the eyes from the physiological position of rest to the position of single binocular fixation of a distant object in the median plane and on the same level as the eyes. Initial convergence is triggered by the fixation reflex.
*See* **convergence, accommodative; convergence, fusional; convergence, tonic; position of rest, physiological.**

**convergence, instrument** *See* **convergence, proximal.**

**convergence insufficiency** An inability to converge, or to maintain convergence, usually associated with a high exophoria at near and a relatively orthophoric condition at distance. It results in complaints of fatigue or even diplopia due to the inability to maintain (and sometimes even to obtain) adequate convergence for prolonged close work. Treatment includes orthoptic exercises (e.g. **the pencil-to-nose exercise** or **pencil push-up** in which the tip of a pencil is moved slowly towards the eyes while it is maintained singly for as long as possible and this procedure is repeated until the pencil can be brought within 10 cm before doubling occurs), or a reading addition sometimes with BI prisms.
*See* **accommodative insufficiency; convergence, near point of; exophoria.**

**convergence, near point of (NPC)** The nearest point where the lines of sight intersect when the eyes converge to the maximum. This point is normally about 8–10 cm from the spectacle plane. If further away, the patient may have convergence insufficiency.
*See* **angle, metre; convergence insufficiency.**

**convergence, negative** *See* **divergence.**

**convergence, proximal** That component of convergence initiated by the awareness of a near object. For example, when looking into an instrument the image may be at optical infinity yet proximal convergence may be initiated. *Syn.* instrument convergence; psychic convergence; proximal vergence.
*See* **accommodative, proximal; convergence, accommodative; convergence, fusional; convergence, initial.**

**convergence, psychic** *See* **convergence, proximal.**

**convergence, relative** That amount of convergence which can be exerted while the accommodation remains unchanged. Clinically, it is measured by using prisms base-out (**positive relative convergence** or **positive fusional convergence**) (Fig. C14) and/or base-in (**negative relative convergence** or **negative fusional convergence**) to the limits of blur but single binocular vision. Beyond that limit accommodation changes. If the power of the base-out prism is increased the image, though blurred, will still appear single until the limit of fusional convergence is reached and the image appears double (break point). The prism before the eyes now represents the **positive fusional reserve convergence** (or **positive fusional reserve**). Similarly, increasing the base-in prism, one reaches the break point which represents the **negative fusional reserve convergence** (or **negative fusional reserve**). *Syn.* relative vergence.
*See* **criterion, Percival; criterion, Sheard; zone of clear, single, binocular vision.**

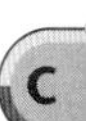

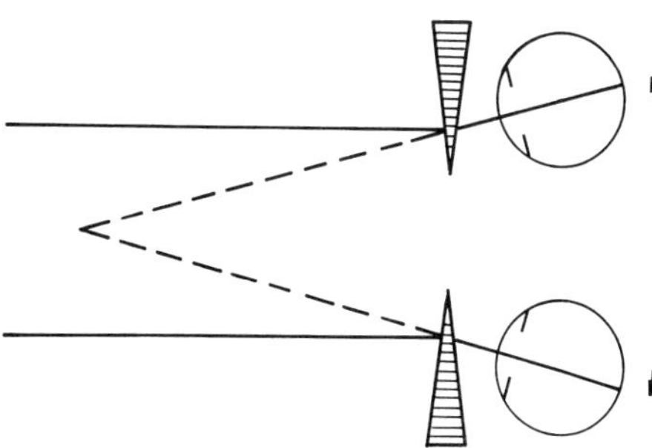

**Fig. C14** Base-out prisms cause positive relative convergence movements of the eyes

**convergence-retraction nystagmus** *See* **nystagmus, convergence-retraction.**

**convergence, tonic** *See* **vergence, tonic.**

**convergence, total** *See* **angle of convergence.**

**convergence, voluntary** Ability to converge the eyes without the aid of a fixation stimulus. Few people possess this ability but it can be trained in most people.

**convex** Having a surface curved like the exterior of a sphere.
*See* **lens, converging; mirror, convex.**

**copper deposits** *See* **chalcosis.**

**copper wire artery** *See* **arteriosclerosis.**

**coquille** An unsurfaced lens, approximately plano, made by allowing sheet material to sag onto a shaped former (British Standard). This lens is often employed for goggles.

**corectopia** A condition in which the pupil is not situated in the centre of the iris. It may occur

as a result of ocular surgery, trauma or from a congenital defect. *Syn.* ectopia pupillae.
*See* **luxation of the lens; pupil.**

**coreometer** *See* **pupillometer.**

**cornea** The transparent anterior portion of the fibrous coat of the globe of the eye. It has a curvature somewhat greater than the rest of the globe, so a slight furrow marks its junction with the sclera. Looked at from the front the cornea is about 12 mm horizontally and 11 mm vertically. It is the first and most important refracting surface of the eye, having a power of about 42 D. The anterior surface has a radius of curvature of about 7.8 m, the posterior surface 6.5 mm, and the central thickness is about 0.5 mm. It consists of five layers, starting from the outside: (1) the stratified squamous epithelium; (2) Bowman's membrane; (3) the stroma (or substantia propria); (4) Descemet's membrane; and (5) the endothelium. The cornea is avascular, receiving its nourishment by permeation through spaces between the lamellae. The sources of nourishment are the aqueous humour, the tears and the limbal capillaries. The cornea is innervated by the long ciliary and other nerves of the surrounding conjunctiva which are all branches of the ophthalmic division of the trigeminal nerve. Innervation is entirely sensory. Within the cornea there are only unmyelinated nerve endings. The density of nerves in the cornea is very high, making it the most sensitive structure in the body. The cornea owes its transparency to the regular arrangement of the collagen fibres, but any factor which affects this lattice structure (e.g. swelling, pressure) results in a loss of transparency. The cornea contains some 78% water, some 15% collagen and some 5% of other proteins (Fig. C15).
*See* **bedewing, endothelial; dellen; deturgescence; dyskeratosis; glycosaminoglycan; keratitis; keratometer; keratomycosis; limbus; line, Hudson–Stahli; membrane, Bowman's; membrane, Descemet's; microcornea; microscope, specular; optical zone of cornea; pachometer; theory, Maurice's.**

**cornea, conical** *See* **keratoconus.**

**cornea guttata** Dystrophy of the endothelial cells of the cornea which may result from corneal trauma, cataract surgery, keratic precipitates, tonography, ageing, continuous contact lens wear, or as part of the early stages of **Fuch's endothelial dystrophy** (a disease associated with ageing and with females more than males). It is seen clinically by slit-lamp examination as

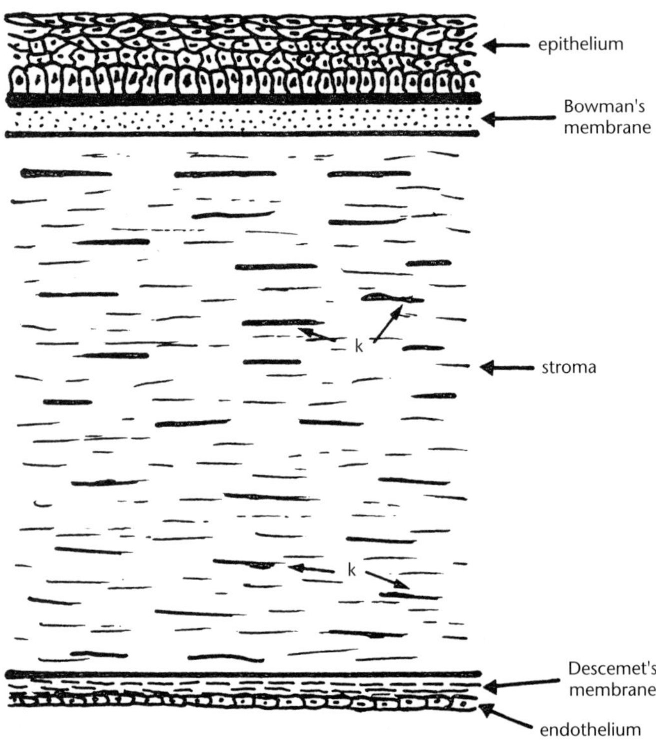


**Fig. C15** Diagram showing the various layers of the cornea (k, keratocytes)

black spherules in the endothelial pattern. The condition is bilateral, although one eye may be affected more than the other. As the condition progresses the cornea becomes oedematous with a consequent loss of vision and eventually turns into bullous keratopathy. If the degenerated cells are located at the periphery of the cornea they are called **Hassall–Henle bodies** and are of no clinical significance except as an indication of ageing. *Syn.* corneal guttae; endothelial corneal dystrophy.
*See* **clouding, central corneal; corneal endothelium; illumination, specular reflection; keratic precipitates; keratopathy, bullous.**

**cornea, optical zone of** *See* **optical zone of cornea.**

**corneal abrasion** An area of the cornea which has been removed by rubbing. The condition ranges from punctate staining with fluorescein to a total removal of the epithelium. Corneal abrasions may result from overwear of contact lenses, foreign bodies, fingernail scratches, etc. Symptoms may be pain, photophobia, tearing and blepharospasm. The condition usually heals quickly if not severe and if infection has not occurred. Treatment consists of removal of the foreign bodies, if any, usually by irrigation, tight patching of the eye, and antibiotic ointment; if due to contact lenses, discontinue wear until full recovery. Local anaesthetics should not be used in the treatment as they tend to delay the regeneration of the corneal epithelium.
*See* **fluorescein; irrigation; mitosis; syndrome, overwear; rose bengal.**

**corneal apex** *See* **apex, corneal; optical zone of cornea.**

**corneal arcus** *See* **arcus, corneal.**

**corneal cap** *See* **optical zone of cornea.**

**corneal clouding, central** *See* **clouding, central corneal.**

**corneal corpuscle** Main cellular element of the stroma. It is a flattened, dendritic cell located between the lamellae with a large flattened nucleus and lengthy processes which may communicate with neighbouring cells. These cells have fibroplastic and phagocytic functions. *Syn.* corneal fibrocyte; fixed cell; keratocyte.
*See* **corneal stroma.**

**corneal dellen** *See* **dellen.**

**corneal dystrophy; ectasia** *See* under the nouns.

**corneal endothelium** The posterior layer of the cornea consisting of a single layer of cells, about 5 μm thick, bound together and predominantly hexagonal in shape. The posterior border is in direct contact with the aqueous humour while the anterior border is in contact with Descemet's membrane. The endothelium is the structure responsible for the relative dehydration of the corneal stroma. The endothelium receives most of its energy from the oxidative breakdown of carbohydrates via the Krebs cycle. With age, disease or trauma the density of cells decreases but with disease or trauma this reduction may affect corneal transparency as some fluid then leaks into the cornea.
*See* **bedewing, endothelial; blebs, endothelial; cornea; cornea guttata; cycle, Krebs; illumination, specular reflection; microscope, specular; phacoemulsification; polymegethism, endothelial.**

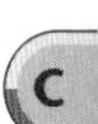

**corneal epithelium** The outermost layer of the cornea consisting of stratified epithelium mounted on a basement membrane. It is made up of various types of cells; next to the basement membrane are the **basal cells** (columnar in shape), then two or three rows of **wing cells** and near the surface are two or three layers of thin surface **squamous cells** (or **superficial cells**). The outer surfaces of the squamous cells have projections (called **microvilli** and **microplicae**) which extend into the mucin layer of the precorneal tear film and are presumed to help retain the tear film. The epithelium in humans has a thickness of about 51 μm. Some dendritic cells of mesodermal origin are also normally present. The corneal epithelium receives its innervation from the conjunctival and the stromal nerves. The life cycle of epithelial cells is about a week (Fig. C16 ).
*See* **epikeratoplasty; mitosis; pachometer; palisades of Vogt.**

**corneal erosion, recurrent** Periodic loss of some of the corneal epithelium, due to its detachment from the basement membrane. It may be the result of trauma (e.g. fingernail scratch) or of some corneal dystrophy. There is severe pain, redness, lacrimation and photophobia, typically upon awakening. Management usually begins with artificial tear drops and a lubricating ointment but the acute phase requires antibiotic ointment and pressure patching or a therapeutic soft contact lens or debridement.
*See* **desmosome; dystrophy, Cogan's microcystic epithelial; dystrophy, lattice; dystrophy, Reis–Buckler's.**

**corneal exhaustion syndrome** *See* **syndrome, corneal exhaustion.**

**corneal facet** *See* **facet, corneal.**

**corneal fibrocyte** *See* **corneal corpuscle.**

**corneal fold** *See* **oedema.**

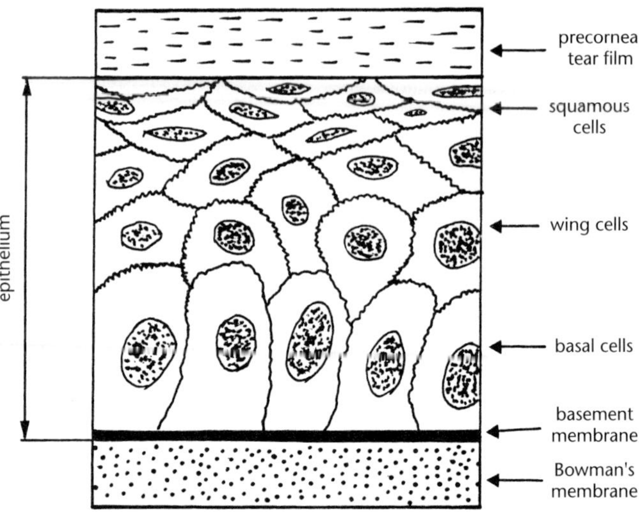


**Fig. C16** Diagram showing the various layers of the corneal epithelium

**corneal fragility** The ability of the cornea to withstand damage. It is quantified by measuring the corneal damage threshold (CDT) (or corneal epithelial fragility threshold (CFT)), that is the lowest pressure exerted on the cornea (using, e.g., a Cochet–Bonnet aesthesiometer) which produces some ruptured epithelial cells; they can be seen after fluorescein instillation with a slit-lamp and UV filter.
*See* **aesthesiometer; fluorescein.**

**corneal graft** *See* **graft, corneal; keratoplasty.**

**corneal granular dystrophy** *See* **dystrophy, granular.**

**corneal hydrops; hyperaesthesia; hypoxia; image** *See* under the nouns.

**corneal infiltrates** Small hazy greyish areas (local or diffuse) located in the cornea typically near the limbus. The adjacent conjunctiva is usually hyperaemic. They appear as a result of corneal inflammation, reaction to solution preservatives and some contact lens wear (especially extended wear) which causes prolonged hypoxia. Management depends on the cause; for example, if due to contact lenses, cessation of wear is usually indicated.
*See* **keratitis, acanthamoeba; keratoconjunctivitis, superior limbic; lens, extended wear.**

**corneal keratocyte** *See* **corneal corpuscle.**

**corneal lens** *See* **lens, contact.**

**corneal limbus** *See* **limbus, corneal.**

**corneal neovascularization** *See* **pannus.**

**corneal opacity** *See* **leukoma.**

**corneal parallelepiped** A section of the cornea illuminated by the thin slit of light of a slit-lamp, when viewed obliquely.
*See* **slit-lamp.**

**corneal reflex; sensitivity** *See* under the nouns.

**corneal stria** *See* **oedema; stria.**

**corneal stroma** The thickest layer of the cornea located behind Bowman's membrane and in front of Descemet's membrane. It represents approximately 90% of the total corneal thickness and gives the cornea its strength. The stroma consists of about 200 layers or lamellae of parallel collagen fibrils, but embedded in a hydrated matrix of proteoglycans. The orientation of the alternate layers differs with each other. Between the layers are found the corneal corpuscles (or keratocytes). When the cornea becomes oedematous due to trauma, disease or hypoxia, some of the fibrils lose their usual uniform calibre, become displaced and fluid accumulates between the lamellae, the stroma then loses its transparency. *Syn.* substantia propria.
*See* **cornea; corneal corpuscle; membrane, Bowman's; membrane, Descemet's.**

**corneal topography** *See* **photokeratoscopy.**

**corneal touch threshold (CTT)** The minimum pressure (in force per unit area, such as $mg/mm^2$) exerted against the cornea which can just be felt.
*See* **aesthesiometer; hyperaesthesia; sensitivity, corneal.**

**corneal transplant** *See* **keratoplasty.**

**corneal ulcer** *See* **ulcer, corneal.**

**corneal warpage** Irregular shape of the corneal surface produced by contact lenses, especially rigid lenses with low or no oxygen transmissibility. It affects vision. It is noted when measuring corneal topography.
*See* **videokeratoscope.**

**corneoscleral junction** *See* **limbus, corneal.**

**corneoscleral meshwork** *See* **meshwork, trabecular.**

**corona ciliaris** *See* **ciliary body.**

**corpora quadrigemina** *See* **colliculi, inferior; colliculi, superior.**

**corpus callosum** Transverse white fibres connecting the two cerebral hemispheres.
*See* **commissure; stereoblindness.**

**correction 1.** Term used to designate the prescription of spectacle or contact lenses to compensate for ametropia (Figs. C17 and C18). *Syn.* refractive correction. **2.** The process whereby the aberrations of an optical system are minimized.
*See* **doublet; lens, achromatic; lens, aplanatic; metamorphopsia; refractive error; triplet.**

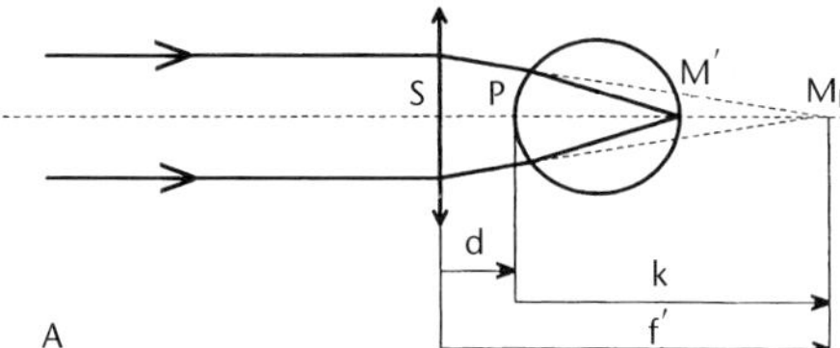


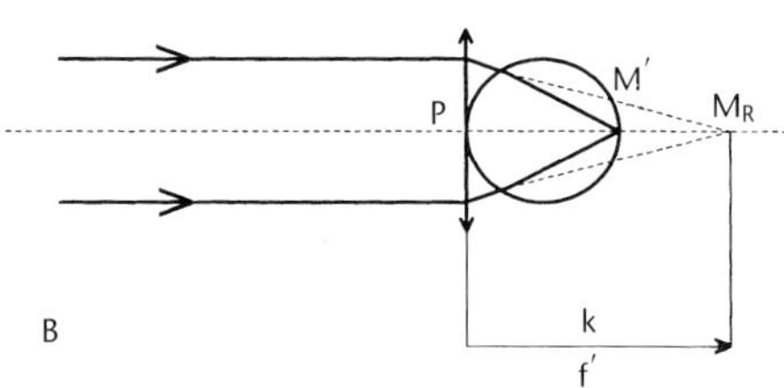


**Fig. C17** Optical principle of the correction of a hypermetropic eye with, A a spectacle lens, B a contact lens ($M_R$, far point of the eye)

**correspondence, abnormal retinal** *See* **retinal correspondence, abnormal.**

**corresponding points** *See* **retinal corresponding points.**

**cortex of the crystalline lens** *See* **lens, crystalline.**

**cortex, motor** Area of the frontal lobe of the brain just anterior to the central sulcus which is responsible for voluntary movements of the eyes (as well as other voluntary movements of other parts of the body). The motor cortex in each hemisphere controls mainly muscles on the opposite side of the body. It is laid out according to the parts of the body with the region controlling the feet at the top and the region controlling the legs, the trunk, the arms and the head in descending order.
*See* **movements, eye.**

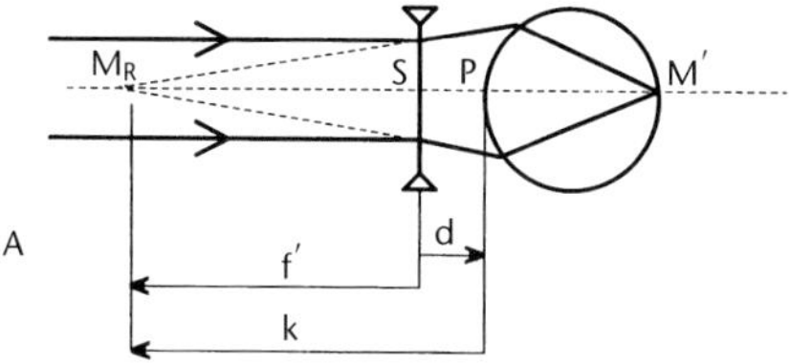


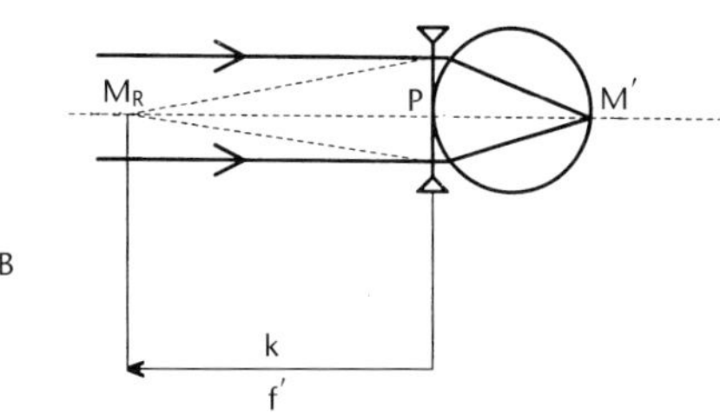


**Fig. C18** Optical principle of the correction of a myopic eye with, A a spectacle lens, B a contact lens ($M_R$, far point of the eye)

**cortex, occipital** The superficial grey matter on the posterior part of each hemisphere comprising Brodmann's areas 17, 18 and 19.
*See* **area, visual.**

**cortex, prestriate** *See* **areas, visual association.**

**cortex, striate; visual** *See* **area, visual.**

**cortical blindness** *See* **blindness, cortical.**

**cortical magnification** *See* **magnification, cortical.**

**corticosteroid** *See* **antiinflammatory drug.**

**cosine law** *See* **diffusion.**

**cotton thread test** *See* **test, phenol red cotton thread.**

**cotton-wool spots** *See* **bodies, cytoid; exudate.**

**counting fingers (CF)** A method of recording vision in patients who are unable to identify any optotype on an acuity chart. If a patient correctly counts the numbers of the examiner's fingers shown, this is recorded with the distance at which it is performed.

**cover test** *See* **test, cover.**

**CR-39 material** Allyl diglycol carbonate or Columbia Resin. CR-39 is a light transparent plastic material (refractive index 1.498, V = 57.8)

used in the manufacture of spectacle lenses and much harder than polymethyl methacrylate. It is not quite as hard as glass. *Syn.* hard resin.
*See* **constringence; lens, absorptive; lens, plastic, polymethyl methacrylate.**

**crescent, congenital scleral** A white semilunar patch of sclera seen adjacent to the optic disc due to the fact that the choroid and retinal pigment epithelium do not extend to the optic disc. This condition is present at birth, unlike myopic crescent, and is often associated with defective vision. *Syn.* Fuch's coloboma; tilted optic disc. It may also result from an ectasia, typically of the nasal or inferior part of the fundus. In this case there is usually **situs inversus of the disc** in which the retinal vessels course nasally from the disc instead of temporally and the eye has myopic astigmatism. This is called the **tilted disc syndrome.**
*See* **ectasia.**

**crescent, myopic** A white area of sclera seen adjacent to the temporal side of the optic disc mainly in pathological myopia, but also sometimes in nonpathological myopia. The choroid and retinal pigment epithelium have atrophied in the crescent area, allowing the sclera to be seen. *Syn.* myopic conus; myopic scleral crescent.
*See* **myopia, pathological.**

**crest, lacrimal** *See* **lacrimal crest, anterior; lacrimal crest, posterior.**

**cribriform plate** This is a part of the sclera which is situated at the site of attachment of the optic nerve, 3 mm to the inner side of and just above the posterior pole of the eye. There, the sclera is a thin sieve-like membrane through which pass fibres of the optic nerve. *Syn.* lamina cribrosa (although this term also refers to the striated portion of the bulbar optic nerve which includes the cribriform plate).
*See* **fibres, myelinated nerve; nerve, optic.**

**criterion, Percival** Rule proposed by Percival to establish whether a patient is going to experience discomfort in binocular vision. It states that if Donders' line (or demand line) lies within the **zone of comfort** which is the middle third of the total range of relative convergence (to the blur points), Percival's criterion of comfortable binocular vision is fulfilled. If it is not, appropriate prisms, spherical lenses or visual training can be used to shift the demand point within the zone of comfort. In this criterion, no reference is made to the actual phoria of the subject and for this reason it has been criticized by several authors. *Syn.* middle third technique.
*See* **convergence, relative; Donders' diagram; line, demand; phoria; zone of clear, single, binocular vision.**

**criterion, Rayleigh** Observation first made by Rayleigh that the images of two point objects will be resolved when the central maximum in the diffraction pattern of one image coincides with the first minimum of the diffraction pattern of the other image. For a perfect eye, with a 2 mm pupil, this criterion corresponds to a theoretical tolerance in focusing equal to about 0.075 D.
*See* **disc, Airy's; diffraction; resolution, limit of.**

**criterion, Sheard** Rule proposed by Sheard to establish whether a patient is going to experience discomfort in binocular vision. It states that the amount of heterophoria should not be less than half the opposing fusional convergence in reserve. If the criterion is not met, appropriate prisms, spherical lenses or visual training can be used. If a patient has 10 Δ of exophoria, the positive fusional vergence should be at least 20 Δ to satisfy this criterion.
*See* **convergence, relative; zone of clear, single, binocular vision.**

**critical angle** *See* **angle, critical.**

**critical fusion frequency** *See* **frequency, critical fusion.**

**critical oxygen requirement** *See* **oxygen requirement, critical.**

**critical period** *See* **period, critical.**

**crocodile shagreen; tears** *See* under the nouns.

**Crohn's disease** *See* **disease, Crohn's.**

**cromolyn sodium** *See* **mast cell stabilizers.**

**cross-cylinder lens** *See* **lens, cross-cylinder.**

**cross-cylinder test for astigmatism** *See* **test for astigmatism, cross-cylinder.**

**cross, Maddox** *See* **Maddox cross.**

**crossed disparity** *See* **disparity, crossed.**

**crossed eyes** *See* **strabismus, convergent.**

**crowding phenomenon** *See* **phenomenon, crowding.**

**crown glass** *See* **glass, crown.**

**crutch, ptosis** *See* **ptosis.**

**cryotherapy** Method of treating a disease by the use of cold as a destructive medium. It may be used to treat retinal detachment and tears, conjunctival melanomas, lid tumours, uveitis, distichiasis and trichiasis.

**cryptophthalmia** A very rare congenital defect in which the skin of the eyelids is continuous over the eyeball, resulting in an absence of palpebral fissure. Eyelashes may or may not be present.

The cornea is fused with the overlying skin into one structure. *Note*: also spelt cryptophthalmos or cryptophthalmus.

**crypts of Fuchs** *See* **Fuchs, crypts of.**

**crypts of Henle** See **glands of Henle.**

**crystal, anisotropic** A crystal that exhibits birefringence (or double refraction).
*See* **birefringence.**

**crystal, dichroic** A birefringent crystal which absorbs the ordinary and extraordinary rays unequally. Natural light passing through a plate of a dichroic material becomes partially or totally polarized.
*See* **birefringence; dichroism; index of refraction; light, polarized.**

**crystal, isotropic** A crystal which has the same optical properties in all directions.

**crystal, tourmaline** *See* **polarizer.**

**crystalline lens** *See* **lens, crystalline.**

**crystalline lens, equator of the** *See* **equator of the crystalline lens.**

**cues, monocular** *See* **perception, depth.**

**cul-de-sac** *See* **conjunctiva.**

**cuneiform cataract** *See* **cataract, cuneiform.**

**cup–disc ratio** *See* **ratio, cup–disc.**

**cup, glaucomatous** A large and deep excavation within the optic disc due to a raised intraocular pressure. It is characterized by overhanging walls over which the blood vessels bend sharply and reappear at the bottom of the depression.
*See* **disc, cupped; glaucoma; ratio, cup–disc.**

**cup, ocular; ophthalmic** *See* **cup, optic.**

**cup, optic 1.** A double layered cup-shaped structure attached to the forebrain of the embryo by means of a hollow stalk. It develops into the retina and inner layers of the ciliary body and iris. It is formed by the invagination of the outer wall of the optic vesicle. Subsequently, nerve cells develop in its invaginated layer and some of these send their axons back along the hollow stalk (or **optic stalk** or **lens stalk**) to form the optic nerve. *Syn.* ocular cup; ophthalmic cup; secondary optic vesicle. **2.** Synonym for physiological cup.
*See* **anophthalmia; fissure, optic; vesicle, optic.**

**cup, physiological** A funnel-shaped depression at or near the centre of the optic disc through which pass the central retinal vessels. *Syn.* optic cup (although it would be preferable not to use this synonym since this term has another meaning); physiological excavation.
*See* **cup, optic; disc, cupped; disc, optic; ratio, cup–disc.**

**cupped disc** *See* **disc, cupped.**

**cupulifom cataract** *See* **cataract, cuneiform.**

**curettage** *See* **chalazion.**

**curl side** *See* **side; side, curl.**

**curvature ametropia** *See* **ametropia, refractive.**

**curvature of field** Aberration of an optical system due to the obliquity of the incident rays of light relative to the optical axis. The image corresponding to a plane object lies on a curved surface. This aberration does not usually affect the eye as the retina is itself curved.
*See* **aberration; Petzval surface.**

**curvature of a surface** A measure of the shape of a curved surface. It is expressed in a unit called **reciprocal metre,** usually written as $m^{-1}$, which is equal to the reciprocal of the radius of curvature of a surface in metres. *Example*: if a surface has a radius of curvature $r$ of +0.5 m, its curvature $R$ will be $R = 1/r = 1/+0.5 = 2\,m^{-1}$.

**curve, base (BC) 1.** The shallower principal meridian of a toroidal surface of a toric lens. The other meridian of the toroidal surface which has the maximum power is called the **cross curve. 2.** In a meniscus lens, the shallower of the two surfaces. **3.** Of a range of lenses of different powers, a surface power common to all the lenses in that range.
*See* **lens, meniscus; lens, periscopic; optic zone radius, back.**

**cyanolabe** *See* **pigment, visual.**

**cyanophobia** An abnormal aversion to blue.
*See* chromatophobia.

**cyanopsia** *See* **chromatopsia.**

**cycle, citric acid** *See* **cycle, Krebs.**

**cycle per degree** Unit of spatial frequency. It is equal to the number of cycles of a grating (one dark and one light band) which subtends an angle of one degree at the eye. *Abbreviated*: c/deg; cpd. This unit was developed because there is no finite width in a bar of a sine grating.
*See* **acuity, visual; frequency, spatial; grating; sensitivity, contrast.**

**cycle, Krebs** A series of reactions in which the intermediate products of carbohydrate, fat and protein metabolism are converted to carbon dioxide and hydrogen atoms (electrons and hydrogen ions). This cycle can only operate in the presence of oxygen. Further oxidation yields carbon dioxide, water and ATP. This cycle occurs in the mitochondria which are found in

**Table C9** Relationship between the minimum angle of resolution, the Snellen fraction and the equivalent spatial frequency of a sine wave

| resolution (min of arc) | Snellen fraction (m) | (ft) | spatial frequency (cpd) |
|---|---|---|---|
| 0.5 | 6/3 | 20/10 | 60 |
| 0.6 | 6/3.6 | 20/12 | 50 |
| 0.75 | 6/4.5 | 20/15 | 40 |
| 1.0 | 6/6 | 20/20 | 30 |
| 1.25 | 6/7.5 | 20/25 | 24 |
| 1.5 | 6/9 | 20/30 | 20 |
| 2.0 | 6/12 | 20/40 | 15 |
| 2.5 | 6/15 | 20/50 | 12 |
| 4.0 | 6/24 | 20/80 | 7.5 |
| 5.0 | 6/30 | 20/100 | 6 |
| 8.0 | 6/48 | 20/160 | 3.8 |
| 10.0 | 6/60 | 20/200 | 3 |
| 20.0 | 6/120 | 20/400 | 1.5 |

the cytoplasm of cells of living organisms. It forms one of the processes in the metabolism of glucose providing energy (stored in ATP) to maintain the vital functions of the cells (e.g. mitosis). This cycle represents the principal energy pathway of the corneal endothelium. *Syn.* citric acid cycle; tricarboxylic acid cycle.
*See* **mitosis.**

**cycle, tricarboxylic acid** *See* **cycle, Krebs.**

**cyclic heterotropia; strabismus** *See* **heterotropia, cyclic.**

**cyclitis** Chronic or acute inflammation of the ciliary body frequently associated with iritis and choroiditis.
*See* **cataract, complicated; iritis; syndrome, Fuchs'; uveitis.**

**cyclodialysis** Disinsertion of the ciliary body from the scleral spur.
*See* **angle recession.**

**cycloduction** Rotation of an eye around its anteroposterior axis. *Syn.* cyclorotation; cyclotorsion; torsion.
*See* **torsion.**

**cyclofusion** Rotation of the eyes about their anteroposterior axes in an attempt to align the two views of the visual field so that the presentations to the two eyes match up, in response to an appropriate stimulus.

**cyclopean eye** *See* **eye, cyclopean.**

**cyclopentolate hydrochloride** An antimuscarinic (or parasympatholytic) drug used as a short duration mydriatic and cycloplegic. Common concentrations are 0.5% and 1.0% as cycloplegic and 0.1% as mydriatic.
*See* **acetylcholine; cycloplegia; mydriasis.**

**cyclophoria** When binocular vision is dissociated (i.e. when stimuli to fusion are eliminated) one eye or both rotate about its/their respective anteroposterior axes to take up the passive position. If the upper portion of the eye rotates inward it is called **incyclophoria** and if it rotates outward it is called **excyclophoria**. It is usually caused by an anomaly of the oblique muscles. *Syn.* periphoria.
*See* **test, double prism; test, Maddox rod.**

**cycloplegia** Paralysis of the ciliary muscle resulting in a loss of accommodation. It is usually accompanied by dilatation of the pupil. Cycloplegic drugs (i.e. antimuscarinic drugs) include atropine, cyclopentolate, homatropine, hyoscine hydrobromide (scopolamine hydrobromide) and tropicamide.
*See* **acetylcholine; anisocycloplegia; atropine; cyclopentolate; homatropine; hypermetropia, latent; muscle, ciliary; mydriatic.**

**cycloplegic 1.** A drug which produces cycloplegia. **2.** Pertaining to cycloplegia.

**cycloplegic refraction** *See* **refraction, cycloplegic.**

**cyclorotation** Rotation of an eye about an anteroposterior axis.

**cyclotonic** A state of constant accommodation.
*See* **tonus.**

**cyclotropia** Type of strabismus in which there is a deviation around the anteroposterior axis of one eye (or both eyes) relative to the vertical meridian.

**cycloversion** Rotation of both eyes in the same direction, around their respective anteroposterior axes.
*See* **dextrocycloversion; laevocycloversion.**

**cylinder axis** *See* **axis, cylinder.**

**cylinder lens, cross-** *See* **lens, cross-cylinder.**

**cylindrical error** *See* **prescription.**

**cylindrical lens** *See* **lens, astigmatic.**

**cyst, dermoid** A tumour containing keratin, sebum, fibrous tissue, hair or fat globules which may be found in the cornea, interior of the eye, or in the subcutaneous tissue of the superotemporal orbital rim. It presents as a round mass, about 1 to 2 cm in diameter, pink to yellow in colour. Limbal dermoids may be associated with Goldenhar's syndrome. There may be induced astigmatism. If vision is impaired or it is cosmetically disfiguring, treatment is by excision.

**cyst, macular** *See* **macular cyst.**

**cyst, meibomian** *See* **chalazion.**

**cytoid bodies** *See* **bodies, cytoid.**

**cystoid macular oedema** *See* **oedema, cystoid macular.**

**cytology** A study of cells to detect diseases. The usual procedure is to obtain a sample, to fix it on a glass slide, treat it with various dyes and inspect it under a microscope. Differential staining allows identification of the cells and their state of health.

**cytology, impression** A simple, noninvasive means of studying cells on the conjunctiva. It is carried out by pressing a small piece of special filter paper against the anaesthetized bulbar conjunctiva for a few seconds after which it is removed. The operation is usually repeated two or three times over the same area. The filter paper is then fixed to a glass slide, stained and examined under a microscope. Mucin, goblet cells and many epithelial cells which stain in different colours, depending on the dyes used, can be assessed and facilitate the diagnosis of many external eye diseases and especially keratitis sicca and xerophthalmia.
*See* **Gram stain.**

**cytomegalovirus retinitis** *See* **retinitis, cytomegalovirus; syndrome, acquired immunodeficiency.**

# D

**D-15 test** *See* **test, Farnsworth.**

**dacryoadenitis** Inflammation of the lacrimal gland. The acute type is characterized by localized pain, swelling and redness over the upper temporal area of the eye. The chronic type is painless and develops slowly. A frequent cause is an associated systemic infection such as mumps, infectious mononucleosis, influenza, or it can be due to a local condition such as trachoma, herpes zoster or staphylococcal infection. The chronic type may be due to any of the granulomatous diseases (tuberculosis, syphilis, sarcoidosis). Treatment consists mainly of warm compresses and antibiotics.
*See* **gland, lacrimal; syndrome, Mikulicz's.**

**dacryocystectomy** Surgical removal of the lacrimal sac.

**dacryocystitis** Inflammation of the lacrimal sac. It is a rare condition which may occur when there is a blockage of the nasolacrimal drainage system. The acute type gives rise to redness, tenderness and swelling below the lid margin while in the chronic type there is epiphora and with pressure on the lacrimal sac pus will come out of the punctum. Treatment includes broad-spectrum antibiotics and warm compresses but surgery may be needed in the chronic type.
*See* **epiphora; lacrimal apparatus.**

**dacryoliths** Concretions found in the lacrimal apparatus, in the puncta or canaliculi which it may occlude. The concretions are usually composed of epithelial cells, lipid, nonspecific debris as well as calcium.

**dacryoma 1.** A tumour or swelling anywhere within the lacrimal apparatus. **2.** A blockage of a lacrimal punctum.
*See* **lacrimal apparatus.**

**dacryops 1.** A chronic watery eye. **2.** A cyst in a tear duct of the lacrimal gland.
*See* **epiphora; gland, lacrimal.**

**Dalen–Fuchs nodules** *See* **nodules, Dalen-Fuchs.**

**Dalrymple's sign** *See* **sign, Dalrymple's.**

**daltonism** Term used formerly to designate colour blindness, usually deutan, so named because John Dalton (1766–1844) was the first to describe his own anomaly.
*See* **colour vision, defective.**

**dapiprazole** *See* **alpha-adrenergic antagonist.**

**dark adaptation** *See* **adaptation, dark.**

**dark filter test** *See* **test, neutral density filter.**

**dark focus** *See* **accommodation, resting state of.**

**dark room test** *See* **test, provocative.**

**dark vergence** *See* **vergence, tonic.**

**day blindness** *See* **hemeralopia.**

**daylight, artificial** Illumination produced by a source of artificial light having a spectral

distribution similar to that of daylight. CIE Illuminant C is considered to almost fulfil this criterion.
*See* **illuminants.**

**daylight, natural** Illumination dependent on the sun and the extent of clear sky.

d

**daylight vision** *See* **vision, photopic.**

**deaf-blind** A person who has a severe hearing impairment in addition to a visual defect. It is usually congenital but it may result from ageing or some systemic disease or as part of a syndrome (e.g. Usher's syndrome which accounts for about half of all cases of deaf-blind people).
*See* **syndrome, rubella; syndrome, Usher's.**

**debility** The state of being feeble or without strength.

**debridement** Removal of dead or infected tissue or foreign material until surrounding healthy tissue is exposed. This is done to facilitate healing. Corneal debridement is usually performed with a cotton-tipped applicator, a spatula or with a sharp instrument. *Example*: debridement of some of the corneal epithelium in dendritic keratitis or in corneal erosion.
*See* **corneal erosion; keratitis, dendritic.**

**decibel (dB)** **1.** Unit used for the measurement of the intensity of a sound. **2.** Light intensities are often presented on a logarithmic (rather than linear) scale. This is done, in particular, to abbreviate large numbers. Moreover, it has become common, especially in perimetry, to use decibels rather than log units. A decibel scale is a logarithmic scale where 10 decibels are equal to 1 log unit; 20 decibels, to 2 log units, etc. In perimetry, decibels are used to indicate the attenuation of brightness of the stimulus. Thus, a 20 dB stimulus is equal to one-tenth the brightness of a 10 dB stimulus.

**decompensation** Failure of an organ to fulfil its function adequately. *Examples*: corneal decompensation following years of extended contact lens wear; a failure of the eye movement system to overcome a heterophoria.
*See* **heterophoria, uncompensated.**

**decongestant, ocular** A pharmaceutical agent used to reduce hyperaemia in the eye, usually by vasoconstriction. *Examples*: adrenaline (epinephrine); naphazoline hydrochloride; tetrahydrozoline hydrochloride. A decongestant can also be used to differentiate between conjunctival and ciliary injection. If the instillation of a decongestant alleviates eye redness the injection is primarily conjunctival, otherwise the redness is of ciliary origin.
*See* **injection, ciliary; injection, conjunctival.**

**decussation** Crossing of nerve fibres passing through the mid-sagittal plane of the central nervous system and connecting with structures on the opposite side. Partial decussation occurs at the optic chiasma.
*See* **chiasma, optic; pathway, visual.**

**degeneration** Deterioration of tissue or organ resulting in reduced efficiency. *Examples*: degeneration of the cornea; degeneration of the retina.
*See* **dystrophy, corneal; vision, low.**

**degeneration, age-related macular** *See* **maculopathy, age-related.**

**degeneration, cobblestone** *See* **degeneration, paving-stone.**

**degeneration, cone** *See* **dystrophy, cone.**

**degeneration, Doyne's honeycombed** *See* **drusen, familial dominant.**

**degeneration, lipid droplet** *See* **keratopathy, actinic.**

**degeneration, paving-stone** Discrete, yellowish round areas of retinal thinning and depigmentation located near the ora serrata. The underlying choroid may be seen. It is a benign degeneration occurring with advancing age. *Syn.* cobblestone degeneration; peripheral chorioretinal degeneration.

**degeneration, pellucid marginal corneal** A rare condition characterized by bilateral, slowly progressive thinning and protrusion of the inferior peripheral cornea. The involved area is clear (hence the word pellucid), but the condition may be complicated by hydrops and the central cornea typically develops against the rule astigmatism. Treatment usually consists of gas permeable scleral lenses, but keratoplasty may be necessary.
*See* **hydrops; keratoconus.**

**degeneration, peripheral chorioretinal** *See* **degeneration, paving-stone.**

**degeneration, peripheral cystoid** A degenerative process in the peripheral retina which occurs almost universally in the elderly. It consists of numerous, discrete cystic spaces in the outer plexiform or inner nuclear layer presenting a frothy appearance. The degeneration starts at the ora serrata and slowly progresses to the peripheral retina. If the cysts should join together, degenerative retinoschisis develops. It is not usually associated with retinal tears. The condition does not require any treatment.

**degeneration of the retina, lattice** *See* **retina, lattice degeneration of the.**

**degeneration, senile macular** *See* **maculopathy, age-related.**

**degeneration, tapetoretinal** A hereditary degeneration affecting the photoreceptors of the retina or the pigment epithelium layer. Some authors also include the choroid. *Syn.* tapetoretinopathy. *See* **choroideraemia; retinitis pigmentosa.**

**degeneration, Terrien's marginal** *See* **ectasia, corneal.**

**degeneration, vitreoretinal** *See* **disease, Wagner's.**

**dellen** A transient shallow depression in the cornea near the limbus which is caused by a local dehydration of the corneal stroma leading to a compression of its lamellae. It can occur as a result of strabismus surgery, cataract surgery, swelling of the limbus (as in episcleritis or pterygium), rigid contact lens wear or senility.
*See* **keratitis sicca.**

**DEM test** *See* **test, developmental eye movement.**

**demand line** *See* **line, demand.**

**demecarium bromide** *See* **anticholinesterase.**

**dendritic keratitis** *See* **keratitis, dendritic.**

**densitometry, retinal** A technique used to study visual pigments *in vivo*. It consists of measuring the small fraction of light that is reflected by the pigment epithelium of the retina before and after bleaching with a bright source of light.
*See* **pigment, visual.**

**density** An indication of the compactness of a substance. It is expressed as the ratio of the mass of the substance to its unit volume. The common units are $g/cm^3$ and $kg/m^3$. This property is usually given by lens manufacturers, the greater the density of a material, the greater its weight, all other factors being equal.

**Table D1** Density of optical lens materials

| | *n* | density ($g/cm^3$) |
|---|---|---|
| **glass** | | |
| spectacle crown | 1.523 | 2.54 |
| dense barium crown | 1.620 | 3.71 |
| dense flint | 1.706 | 3.20 |
| dense barium flint | 1.700 | 4.10 |
| titanium oxide | 1.701 | 2.99 |
| **plastics** | | |
| PMMA | 1.490 | 1.19 |
| CR-39 | 1.498 | 1.32 |
| polycarbonate | 1.586 | 1.2 |

**density, optical** A term applied to optical filters. It is equal to the logarithm to the base 10 of the reciprocal of the transmission factor *T* thus,

$$D = \log_{10} \frac{1}{T}$$

where *D* is the symbol for optical density. *Syn.* absorbance (not strictly correct).
*See* **absorption; filter; spectrophotometer.**

**Table D2** Relationship between optical density *D* and light transmission *T* of optical filters

| *D* | *T* (%) |
|---|---|
| 0.0 | 100 |
| 0.1 | 79.4 |
| 0.2 | 63.1 |
| 0.3 | 50.1 |
| 0.4 | 39.8 |
| 0.5 | 31.6 |
| 0.6 | 25.1 |
| 0.7 | 20.0 |
| 0.8 | 15.8 |
| 0.9 | 12.6 |
| 1.0 | 10.0 |
| 1.5 | 3.16 |
| 2.0 | 1.0 |
| 2.5 | 0.32 |
| 3.0 | 0.1 |
| 4.0 | 0.01 |

**Denver Developmental Screening Test** *See* **test, developmental and perceptual screening.**

**deorsumduction** *See* **depression.**

**deorsumvergence** *See* **infravergence.**

**deorsumversion** *See* **version.**

**depolarization** A change in the value of the resting membrane potential towards zero. The inside of the cell becomes less negative compared to the outside. This is due to a change in permeability and migration of sodium ions into the interior of the cell.
*See* **hyperpolarization; potential, resting membrane.**

**depolished glass** *See* **glass, ground.**

**deposits, contact lens** Accumulation of materials on or into the matrix of contact lenses. They are mainly tear components (proteins, calcium, lipids, mucin) but other materials can be found (e.g. mercurial or iron deposits, nicotine, hand cream). Deposits reduce comfort, vision, patient tolerance and discolour and spoil the lenses. They may act as antigens for the development of giant papillary conjunctivitis. Most of these deposits can be removed with a surfactant, an enzymatic system and a calcium-preventing solution.
*See* **conjunctivitis, giant papillary; enzyme; surfactant.**

**depression** Downward rotation of an eye. It is accomplished by the inferior rectus and superior oblique muscles. It can be induced by using base-up prisms. *Syn.* infraduction; deorsumduction.

**depressors** Extraocular muscles that move the eye downward, such as the inferior rectus and the superior oblique.
*See* **muscles, extraocular.**

**deprivation amblyopia** *See* **amblyopia, deprivation.**

d

**deprivation, sensory** The condition produced by a loss of all or most of the stimulation from the visual, auditory, tactile and other sensory systems. Often, deprivation involves only one modality (e.g. vision). Methods used for deprivation include diffusing goggles, white noise, padded gloves, etc. Its effect has shown the necessity of continuous sensory activity to maintain the normal development and functioning of any sensory system.

**deprivation, visual** The condition produced by a loss of form vision. It may occur as a result of an anomaly within the eye (e.g. opacification of the cornea), or it can be artificially induced (e.g. by placing a transparent plastic occluder in front of the eye, as used in myopia research with animals).

**depth of field** For a given setting of an optical system (or a steady state of accommodation of the eye) it is the distance over which an object may be moved without causing a sharpness reduction beyond a certain tolerable amount. Depth of field increases when the diaphragm (or pupil) diameter diminishes as, for example, in old eyes (Fig. D1). *Examples*: viewing at infinity, the depth of field varies between infinity and about 3.6 m for a pupil of 4 mm in diameter; and between infinity and about 2.3 m for a 2 mm pupil. At a viewing distance of 1 m, the depth of field ranges from about 1.4 m to 80 cm with a 4 mm pupil; and from about 1.8 m to 70 cm with a 2 mm pupil.
*See* **distance, hyperfocal.**

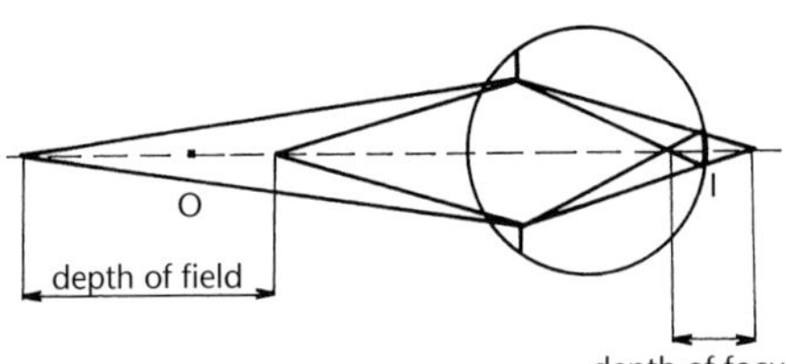


**Fig. D1** Schematic representation of the depth of field and the depth of focus of an eye fixating an object at O (I, retinal image size corresponding to the tolerable resolution)

**depth of focus** For a given setting of an optical system (or a steady state of accommodation of the eye) it is the distance in front and behind the focal point (or retina) over which the image may be focused without causing a sharpness reduction beyond a certain tolerable amount. (The criterion could be as much as a line of letters on a Snellen chart.) The depth of focus is represented by the total distance in front and behind (Fig. D1). As with depth of field, it is inversely proportional to the diameter of the diaphragm (or pupil).

**depth perception** *See* **perception, depth.**

**dermatitis** *See* **eczema.**

**dermatochalasis** A condition in which there is a redundancy of the skin of the upper eyelids. It is often associated with a protrusion of fat through a defective orbital septum. The condition occurs usually in old people. The excess skin may cause pseudoptosis. In severe cases it may obstruct vision. Treatment is surgical. *Syn.* ptosis adiposa; ptosis atrophica.
*See* **blepharochalasis; orbital septum; pseudoptosis.**

**dermoid cyst** *See* **cyst, dermoid.**

**desaturated D-15 test** *See* **test, Farnsworth.**

**Descartes' law** *See* **law of refraction.**

**Descemet's membrane** *See* **membrane, Descemet's.**

**descemetocele** A forward bulging of Descemet's membrane due to either trauma or a deep corneal ulcer which has eroded the overlying stroma. *Syn.* keratocele.
*See* **membrane, Descemet's.**

**desiccation** The process of becoming dry.
*See* **eye, dry.**

**desmosome** A site of adhesion between two adjacent cells, such as in the corneal epithelium. It consists of a small, dense body in which the two halves are separated by an intercellular gap filled with extracellular substance. The basal cells are attached at irregular intervals to the underlying basement membrane adjacent to Bowman's membrane by **hemidesmosomes** (one half of a desmosome). Thus, scraping off the epithelium usually leaves fragments of the basal cells attached to the basement membrane.
*See* **corneal epithelium.**

**deturgescence** State of relative dehydration maintained by the normal cornea which is necessary for transparency. It is maintained by the epithelium which, to a large extent, is impermeable to water, and also by a metabolic transport system in the endothelium.

**deutan** A person who has either deuteranomaly or deuteranopia.

**deuteranomal** Person who has deuteranomaly.

**deuteranomaly** A type of anomalous trichromatism in which an abnormally high proportion of green is needed when mixing red and green light to match a given yellow. This is the most common type of colour vision deficiency occurring in about 4.6% of males and 0.35% of the female population. *Syn.* deuteranomalous trichromatism; deuteranomalous vision; green-weakness.
*See* **anomaloscope; colour vision, defective; plates, pseudoisochromatic; trichromatism.**

**deuteranope** Person who has deuteranopia.

**deuteranopia** Type of dichromatism in which red and green are confused, although their relative spectral luminosities are practically the same as in normals. In the spectrum, the deuteranope only sees two primary colours, the long wavelength portion of the spectrum (yellow, orange or red) appears yellowish and the short wavelength portion (blue or violet) appears bluish. There is, in between, a neutral point which appears whitish or colourless, at about 498 nm. It occurs in slightly over 1% of the male population and only rarely in females. *Syn.* green blindness (although this term is incorrect as green lights appear to a deuteranope as bright as to a normal observer).
*See* **colour vision, defective; dichromatism; plates, pseudoisochromatic; point, neutral.**

**developmental and perceptual screening test** *See* **test, developmental and perceptual screening.**

**deviating eye** *See* **eye, deviating.**

**deviation 1.** In strabismus, the departure of the visual axis of one eye from the point of fixation. **2.** A change in direction of a light ray resulting from reflection or refraction at an optical surface.
*See* **angle of deviation; strabismus.**

**deviation, angle of** *See* **angle of deviation.**

**deviation, conjugate** The simultaneous and equal rotations of the eyes in any direction. It may be physiological such as versions, or pathological due to, either muscular spasm or paralysis.
*See* **movements, disjunctive; version.**

**deviation, dissociated vertical (DVD)** A form of strabismus in which one eye apparently moves vertically without any compensatory movement from the other eye. Although initially felt to disobey Hering's law, it is now felt that Hering's law is observed if the horizontal, vertical and rotational aspects of the condition are considered together. This form of strabismus often accompanies infantile esotropia and is almost always noted from the period of infancy. The misalignment can be either latent or manifest, and may require operative intervention if of a great degree.

**deviation, Hering–Hillebrand** The deviation of the apparent frontoparallel plane horopter from the Vieth–Müller circle (Fig. D2).
*See* **horopter; plane, apparent frontoparallel.**

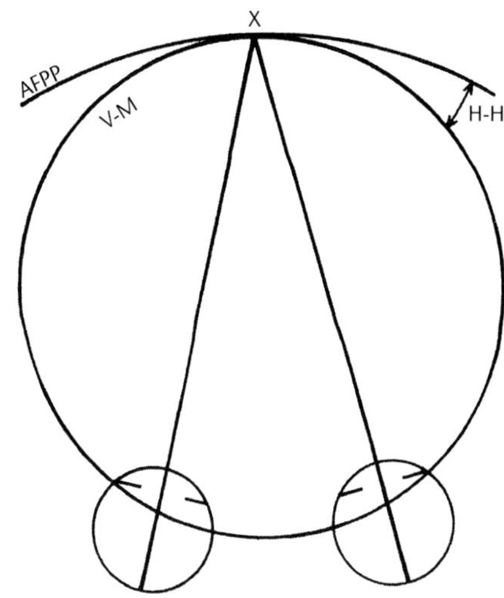


**Fig. D2** Hering–Hillebrand deviation H-H (AFPP, apparent frontoparallel plane horopter); V-M (Vieth–Müller circle; X, fixation point)

**deviation, minimum of a prism** *See* **prism, minimum deviation of a.**

**deviation, primary** The deviation found in paralysis of an extraocular muscle when the unaffected eye is fixating.

**deviation, secondary** The deviation found in paralysis of an extraocular muscle when the eye with the paralytic muscle is fixating.

**deviation, skew** A form of strabismus, typically vertical, that does not follow any standard or typical pattern and is usually difficult to quantify. It may be due to a midbrain disorder, multiple sclerosis or myasthenia gravis.

**deviation, vertical 1.** Type of ocular deviation found in strabismus in which the deviating eye is rotated upward with respect to the fixating eye. **2.** Upward ocular deviation of an occluded eye in the cover test, as found in hyperphoria or hypophoria.

**Devic's disease** *See* **disease, Devic's.**

**dexamethasone** *See* **antiinflammatory drug.**

**dextroclination** Rotation of the upper pole of the vertical meridian of an eye to the subject's right. *Syn.* dextrocycloduction; dextrotorsion.

**dextrocycloversion** Rotation of the upper poles of the vertical meridians of both eyes towards the subject's right.
*See* **laevocycloversion.**

**dextrodeorsumversion** Movement of the eyes down and to the right.

**dextroduction** Rotation of one eye to the right. *See* **duction.**

**dextrophoria** A tendency of the visual axes of both eyes to deviate to the right, in the absence of a stimulus to fusion.
*See* **heterophoria; laevophoria.**

**dextrotorsion** *See* **dextroclination.**

**dextroversion** Movement of both eyes to the right. *See* **version.**

**diabetes** A disease characterized by an excessive excretion of urine. The most common type is **diabetes mellitus** in which there is a disorder of glucose metabolism. There are two types of diabetes mellitus: type I (or juvenile form) in which the patient is dependent on insulin and type II (or adult form) in which the patient is not dependent on insulin, usually obese and treated with diet. The main complications in the eye are retinopathy, cataract, rubeosis iridis, xanthelasma and ptosis.
*See* **accommodative insufficiency; anisocoria; cataract, diabetic; glaucoma, neovascular; glaucoma, open-angle; hypoxia; myopia, lenticular; paralysis of the fourth nerve; paralysis of the sixth nerve; paralysis of the third nerve; ptosis; pupil, Adie's; retinopathy, diabetic; retinopathy, proliferative; rubeosis iridis; tritanopia; vitrectomy; vitreous detachment; xanthelasma.**

**diabetic retinopathy** *See* **retinopathy, diabetic.**

**diagnosis 1.** Term that indicates the disease (e.g. pulmonary tuberculosis) or the refractive error (e.g. compound myopic astigmatism) which a person has. **2.** The art of determining a disease or visual anomaly based on the signs, symptoms and tests.
*See* **aetiology; prognosis; sign.**

**diagnostic positions of gaze** *See* **positions of gaze, diagnostic.**

**dialysis, retinal** *See* **retinal dialysis.**

**diameter, total (TD)** The linear measurement (usually specified in millimetres) of the maximum external dimension of a contact lens. It is equal to the BOZD plus twice the width of each of the back peripheral optic zones (if any) or twice the width of the edge in a spherical lens. Formerly, it was called overall size (OS).
*See* **optic zone diameter; v gauge.**

**diaphragm 1.** In optics, an aperture generally round and of variable diameter placed in a screen and used to limit the field of view of a lens or optical system (**field stop**). It also limits stray light (**light stop**). *Syn.* stop; aperture-stop. **2.** In anatomy, a dividing membrane.

**diascope** A projector used to project transparent objects.

**dibropropamidine** *See* **antibiotic.**

**dichlorphenamide** *See* **carbonic anhydrase inhibitors.**

**diclofenac** *See* **antiinflammatory drug.**

**dichoptic** Viewing a separate and independent field by each eye, in binocular vision, as for example in a haploscope.
*See* **haploscope; masking, dichoptic.**

**dichroism** Property exhibited by certain transparent substances of producing two different colours depending upon the thickness of substance traversed, the directions of transmission of light and/or viewing, the concentration of the substance, etc. The most common example is that of crystals (e.g. tourmaline) which absorb unequally the ordinary and extraordinary rays.
*See* **anisotropic; crystal, dichroic; pleochroism.**

**dichromat** Person having dichromatism, i.e. a deuteranope, a protanope or a tritanope.
*See* **deuteranope; protanope; tritanope.**

**dichromatism** A form of colour vision deficiency in which all colours can be matched by a mixture of only two primary colours. The spectrum appears as consisting of two colours separated by an achromatic area (the neutral point). There are several types of dichromatism: deuteranopia, protanopia and tritanopia. *Syn.* daltonism; dichromatopsia; dichromatic vision.
*See* **colour vision, defective; deuteranopia; pigment, visual; protanopia; tritanopia.**

**dicoria** A condition in which there are two pupils in one iris. It may be congenital or the result of surgery or injury. *Syn.* diplocoria.
*See* **polycoria.**

**differential threshold** *See* **threshold, differential.**

**diffraction** Deviation of the direction of propagation of a beam of light which occurs when the light passes the edge of an obstacle such as a diaphragm, the pupil of the eye or a spectacle frame. There are two consequences of this phenomenon. First, the image of a point source cannot be a point image but a **diffraction pattern**. This pattern depends upon the shape and size of the diaphragm as well as the wavelength of light. Second, a system of close, parallel and equidistant grooves, slits or lines ruled on a polished surface can produce a light spectrum by diffraction. This is called a **diffraction grating.**

See **disc, Airy's; fringes, diffraction; theory, Maurice's.**

**diffractive contact lens** See **lens, contact.**

**diffuser** A device used to scatter light. It can be a reflecting surface (e.g. matt paint) or a transmitting medium (e.g. ground glass).

**diffusion** Scattering of light passing through a heterogeneous medium, or being reflected irregularly by a surface, such as a sand blasted opal glass surface. Diffusion by a perfectly diffusing surface occurs in accordance with **Lambert's cosine law**. In this case, the luminance will be the same, regardless of the viewing direction. *See* **light, diffuse; reflection, diffuse.**

**diffusion circle** See **blur circle.**

**diisopropyl fluorophosphate (DFP)** See **anticholinesterase.**

**dilator pupillae muscle** See **muscle, dilator pupillae.**

**dioptre 1.** A unit proposed by Monoyer to evaluate the **refractive power** of a lens or of an optical system. It is equal to the product of the refractive index in the image space and the reciprocal of the focal length in metres. (*Symbol*: D.) Thus a lens with a focal length (in air) of 1 m has a power of 1 D, one with a focal length of 1/2 m, has a power of 2 D, etc. **2.** It is also incorrectly used to represent a unit of curvature, being equal to the reciprocal of the radius of curvature expressed in metres. *See* **curvature of a surface; myodioptre; paraxial equation, fundamental; power, refractive; refractive error; vergence.**

**dioptre, prism 1.** A unit specifying the amount of light deviation by an ophthalmic prism. One prism dioptre (written 1 Δ) represents a deviation of 1 cm on a flat surface 1 m away from the prism. The surface is perpendicular to the direction of the original light ray (Fig. D3). Similarly, a 2 Δ prism deviates light 2 cm at a distance of 1 m and so on. For small angles, conversion between prism dioptres and degrees is given by the approximate formula

$7\ \Delta = 4° \text{or } 1\ \Delta = 0.57° \text{ or } 1° = 1.75\ \Delta$

The exact formula for any angle α less than 90° is

$\alpha \text{ in } \Delta = 100 \tan \alpha$

*Note*: the current British Standard regarding ophthalmic lenses specifies a deviation (in Δ) of a ray of light of wavelength 587.6 nm incident normally at one surface. **2.** A unit of convergence of the eyes.
*See* **law, Prentice's; power, prism; prism, ophthalmic.**

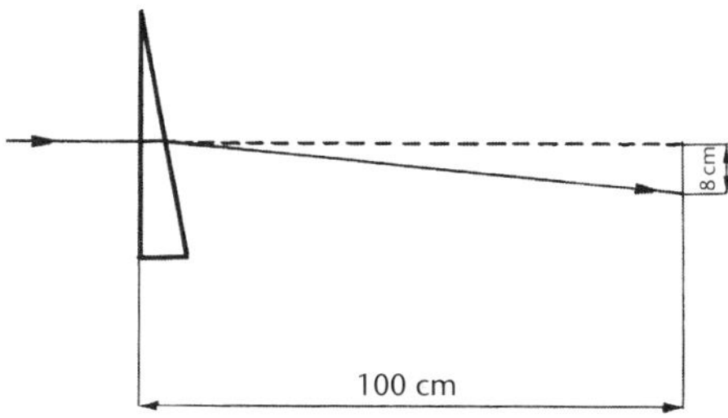


Fig. D3 Effect of an 8 Δ prism

**Table D3** Relationship between dioptres and focal length (in air)

| dioptre value | focal length (cm) | (in) |
|---|---|---|
| 0.25 | 400 | 157 |
| 0.50 | 200 | 79 |
| 1.00 | 100 | 39 |
| 1.50 | 67 | 26 |
| 2.00 | 50 | 20 |
| 2.50 | 40 | 16 |
| 3.00 | 33.3 | 13 |
| 4.00 | 25 | 10 |
| 5.00 | 20 | 7.9 |
| 6.00 | 16.7 | 6.6 |
| 7.00 | 14.3 | 5.6 |
| 8.00 | 12.5 | 4.9 |
| 9.00 | 11.1 | 4.4 |
| 10.00 | 10 | 3.9 |
| 12.00 | 8.3 | 3.3 |
| 14.00 | 7.1 | 2.8 |
| 16.00 | 6.2 | 2.4 |
| 20.00 | 5.0 | 2.0 |

**Table D4** Relationship between prism dioptres and degrees

| prism dioptres (Δ) | degrees (°) | minutes (′) |
|---|---|---|
| 1 | 0.573° | 0°34′ |
| 2 | 1.14° | 1°8′ |
| 3 | 1.71° | 1°43′ |
| 4 | 2.28° | 2°17′ |
| 5 | 2.85° | 2°51′ |
| 6 | 3.43° | 3°26′ |
| 7 | 4.0° | 4°0′ |
| 8 | 4.57° | 4°34′ |
| 9 | 5.14° | 5°8′ |
| 10 | 5.71° | 5°43′ |
| 15 | 8.57° | 8°34′ |

**dioptric power** See **power, refractive.**

**dioptrics** That branch of optics which deals with the refraction of light (as opposed to reflection). *Example*: the dioptrics of the eye.

**diplocoria** See **dicoria.**

d

**diplopia** The condition in which a single object is seen as two rather than one. This is usually due to images not stimulating corresponding retinal areas. Other causes are given below. *Syn.* double vision (colloquial).
*See* **cataract; diplopia, monocular; diplopia, pathological; effect, differential prismatic; haplopia; myasthenia gravis; retinal corresponding points; polyopia; sclerosis, multiple; strabismus; test, diplopia; triplopia.**

**diplopia, binocular** Diplopia in which one image is seen by one eye and the other image is seen by the other eye.

**diplopia, crossed** *See* **diplopia, heteronymous.**

**diplopia, heteronymous** Binocular diplopia in which the image received by the right eye appears to the left and that received by the left eye appears to the right. In this condition the images are formed on the temporal retina. *Syn.* crossed diplopia.

**diplopia, homonymous** Binocular diplopia in which the image received by the right eye appears to the right and that received by the left eye appears to the left. In this condition, the images are formed on the nasal retina. *Syn.* uncrossed diplopia.

**diplopia, incongruous** Diplopia present in individuals with abnormal retinal correspondence in which the relative positions of the two images differ from what would be expected on the basis of normal retinal correspondence. *Example*: an exotrope experiencing homonymous diplopia instead of heteronymous diplopia. *Syn.* paradoxical diplopia.
*See* **retinal correspondence, abnormal.**

**diplopia, monocular** Diplopia seen by one eye only. It is usually caused by irregular refraction in one eye (e.g. in early cataracts) or by dicoria or polycoria. It may be induced by placing a biprism in front of one eye.
*See* **cataract; dicoria; diplopia, pathological; image, ghost; luxation of the lens; polycoria.**

**diplopia, paradoxical** *See* **diplopia, incongruous.**

**diplopia, pathological** Any diplopia due to an eye disease (e.g. proptosis), an anomaly of binocular vision (e.g. strabismus), a variation in the refractive index of the media of the eye (e.g. cataract), a subluxation of the crystalline lens, or to a general disease (e.g. multiple sclerosis).
*See* **exophthalmos; luxation of the lens; myasthenia gravis; strabismus.**

**diplopia, physiological** Normal phenomenon which occurs in binocular vision for nonfixated objects whose images fall on disparate retinal points. It is easily demonstrated to persons with normal binocular vision: fixate binocularly a distant object and place a pencil vertically some 25 cm in front of your nose. You should see two rather blurred pencils. The observation of physiological diplopia has been found to be useful in the management of eso or exo deviations, suppression, ARC, etc. (Fig. D4).
*See* **Brock string; disparity, retinal.**

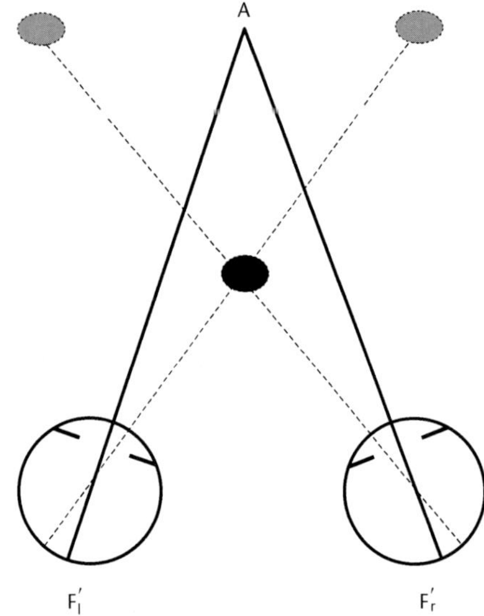


**Fig. D4** Physiological diplopia. The subject fixates a distant object A. The near object appears in crossed diplopia ($F_l'$, $F_r'$, foveas of the left and right eye, respectively)

**diplopia test** *See* **test, diplopia.**

**diplopia, uncrossed** *See* **diplopia, homonymous.**

**diploscope** Instrument used to evaluate binocular vision and which may be used for the treatment of anomalies of binocular vision.

**direct ophthalmoscopy** *See* **ophthalmoscopy, direct.**

**direction, oculocentric** Direction associated with a particular retinal point. It is always perceived in the same direction if the light is received by the same retinal receptor. The capacity of a receptor to distinguish its excitation from that of its neighbours is referred to as **local sign** (or **Lotze's local sign**). This characteristic means that each retinal receptor has a unique oculocentric direction.
*See* **line of direction; oculocentre.**

**disc, Airy's** Owing to the wave nature of light, the image of a point source consists of a diffraction pattern. If light passes through a circular aperture, the diffraction pattern will appear as a bright central disc, called Airy's disc, surrounded by concentric light and dark rings. Airy's disc receives about 90% of the luminous flux. The radius of Airy's disc equals

$$\frac{1.22\lambda f}{d}$$

where $d$ is the radius of the entrance pupil of the optical system of focal length $f$ and $\lambda$ the wavelength of the light used. In the eye, with a pupil of 4 mm diameter and $\lambda$ = 507 nm, the diameter of Airy's disc is about 5 µm which corresponds to a visual angle of about one minute of arc. *Syn.* diffraction disc.
*See* **criterion, Rayleigh; diffraction; function, point-spread; image, retinal; resolution, limit of.**

**disc, choked** *See* **papilloedema.**

**disc, cupped** An enlarged and deepened excavation of the physiological cup. It may be physiological, or due to glaucoma (**glaucomatous cup**), or following atrophy of the optic nerve (as in papilloedema).
*See* **cup, glaucomatous; cup, physiological; papilloedema.**

**disc, diffraction** *See* **disc, Airy's.**

**disc, Maxwell** A rotating disc onto which differently coloured discs which are radially slit can be fitted together to overlap and divide the surface into sectors of different colours. It may be used to investigate colour mixture.

**disc, morning glory** A congenital, usually unilateral, anomaly of the optic disc. It may be due to a failure of the embryonic fissure such that the optic disc and some peripapillary tissue prolapse posteriorly. The optic disc is abnormally large and a white-grey tuft of glial tissue covers its centre. The annular zone surrounding the disc has irregular areas of pigmentation and depigmentation. The optic disc thus resembles a morning glory flower. Patients present with reduced visual acuity and strabismus and, in about one-third of patients, retinal detachment.

**disc, optic** Region of the fundus of the eye corresponding to the optic nerve head. It can be seen with the ophthalmoscope as a pinkish-yellow area with usually a whitish depression called the physiological cup. The optic disc has an area of about 2.7 mm², a horizontal width of about 1.75 mm and a vertical height of about 1.9 mm. The optic disc is the anatomical correlate of the physiological blind spot. *Syn.* optic nerve head; optic papilla (this is not strictly correct because the disc is not elevated above the surrounding retina).
*See* **blind spot; cup, physiological; neural rim; papilloedema; retina; syndrome, Swann's.**

**disc, pinhole (ph)** A blank disc with a small aperture (2 mm diameter or less) mounted in a trial lens rim. It is used to reduce the size of the blur circle in an ametropic eye. In this condition vision will improve giving an indication of the final visual acuity which will be obtained with corrective lenses. If no improvement occurs, the eye is amblyopic. This procedure is called the **pinhole test.**
*See* **amblyopia.**

**disc, Scheiner's** An opaque disc in which there are two pinholes separated by a distance less than the pupil diameter. It is used to measure the dioptric changes during accommodation or to detect the type of ametropia (Fig. D5).
*See* **experiment, Scheiner's.**

**disc, stenopaeic 1.** A pinhole disc. **2.** A blank disc with a slit used in detecting and measuring the astigmatism of the eye (Fig. D6). *Syn.* stenopaeic slit. *Note*: also spelt stenopeic or stenopaic.
*See* **astigmatism; disc, pinhole; kinescope; spectacles, stenopaeic.**

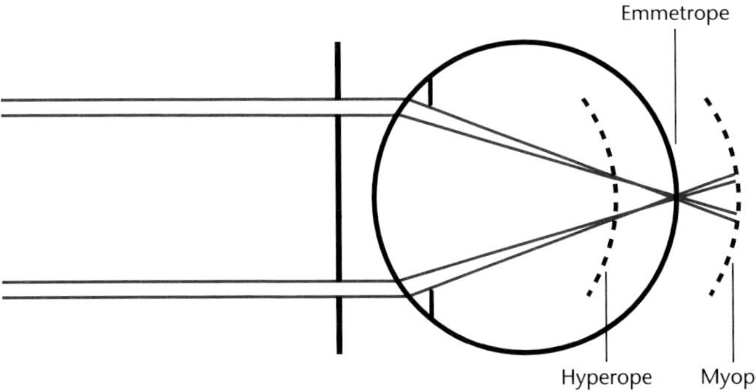


**Fig. D5** Images of a distant object formed on the retina of an unaccommodated emmetrope (clear, single image), a hyperope and a myope (blurred, double images) looking through a Scheiner's disc. To determine the type of ametropia, cover one of the pinholes; if the top hole is covered a hyperope will report that the lower image disappears (because the retinal image is inverted perceptually), whereas a myope will report that the upper image disappears

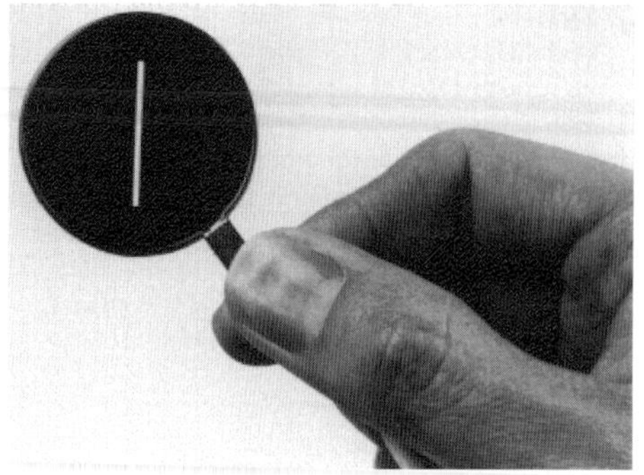

Fig. D6 Stenopaeic slit

**disciform keratitis** *See* **keratitis, disciform.**

**disciform scar** A subretinal scar, most often located in the macular area. It results from the haemorrhages that sometimes follow choroidal neovascularization (consisting of fibrovascular tissue) in the exudative type of age-related maculopathy. It causes irreparable damage to vision.
*See* **maculopathy, age-related.**

**discomfort glare** *See* **glare, discomfort.**

**disconjugate movements** *See* **movements, disjunctive eye.**

**disease, autoimmune** A disease produced when the immune response of an individual is directed against its own cells or tissues. It is not yet known exactly what causes the body to react to one's own antigens as if they were foreign. *Examples*: diabetes mellitus; rheumatoid arthritis; Graves' disease; Reiter's disease.

**disease, Basedow's** *See* **disease, Graves'.**

**disease, Batten–Mayou** Juvenile form of amaurotic family idiocy. It is characterized by progressive degeneration of the retina which eventually leads to blindness. *Syn.* Spielmeyer–Stock disease.

**disease, Behçet's** Disease consisting of ulceration of the mouth and genital region with anterior uveitis and hypopyon. This disease tends to recur at regular intervals. It usually affects individuals below the age of 40 and frequently results in blindness about 3 years after the onset of ocular symptoms.
*See* **hypopyon; uveitis.**

**disease, Benson's** *See* **asteroid hyalosis.**

**disease, Berlin's** A traumatic phenomenon in which the posterior pole of the retina develops oedema (and haemorrhages). *Syn.* commotio retinae.

**disease, Best's** Hereditary degeneration characterized by the appearance on the retina in the first and second decades of life of a bright orange deposit, resembling the yolk of a fried egg, with practically no effect on vision. It eventually absorbs, leaving scarring, pigmentary changes and impairment of central vision in most cases, although in some cases the retinal lesion may be eccentric, with very little effect on vision. The electro-oculogram is abnormal throughout the development of the disease. *Syn.* Best's vitelliform macular dystrophy; vitelliform degeneration; vitelliform macular dystrophy.
*See* **electro-oculogram.**

**disease, Bowen's** A disease characterized by a slow growing tumour of the epidermis of the skin which may involve the corneal or conjunctival epithelium.

**disease, Coats'** Chronic, progressive retinal abnormality occurring predominantly in young males. It is characterized by retinal exudates and usually associated with malformation of retinal blood vessels and appears as a whitish fundus reflex. Subretinal haemorrhages are frequent and eventually retinal detachment may occur. The main symptom is a decrease in central or peripheral vision. *Syn.* exudative retinitis; retinitis exudativa externa.
*See* **leukocoria.**

**disease, Crohn's** A type of inflammatory, chronic bowel disease characterized by granulomatous inflammation of the bowel wall causing fever, diarrhoea, abdominal pain and weight loss. The ocular manifestations include acute iridocyclitis, scleritis, conjunctivitis and corneal infiltrates.

**disease, Devic's** A demyelinative disease of the optic nerve, the optic chiasma and the spinal cord characterized by a bilateral acute optic neuritis with a transverse inflammation of the spinal cord. Loss of visual acuity occurs very rapidly and is accompanied by ascending paralysis. There is no treatment for this disease. *Syn.* neuromyelitis optica.
*See* **neuritis, optic.**

**disease, Eales'** A nonspecific peripheral periphlebitis that usually affects young males. It is characterized by recurrent haemorrhages in the retina and vitreous. This disease is a prime example of retinal vasculitis.

**disease, Graves'** Hyperthyroidism in which there are eye changes such as retraction of the eyelids (**Dalrymple's sign**), exophthalmos, lid lag in which the upper lid follows after a latent period when the eye looks downward (**von Graefe's sign**), raised IOP, especially on upgaze, and defective eye movements (**restrictive myopathy**) besides increased pulse rate, tremors, loss of weight and diarrhoea. It typically affects women between the ages of 20 and 50 years.

Most common signs associated with the disease are those of von Graefe and Moebius. *Syn.* Basedow's disease; exophthalmic goitre. If only the eye signs of the disease are present without clinical evidence of hyperthyroidism, the disease is called **euthyroid** or **ophthalmic Graves' disease**. Treatment begins with control of the hyperthyroidism (if present). Some cases may recover spontaneously with time. Mild cases of ocular deviations and restrictions may benefit from a prismatic correction. Corticosteroids and radiotherapy may be needed and surgery is a common form of management especially when there is diplopia in the primary position of gaze.
*See* **accommodative infacility; exophthalmos; ophthalmopathy, thyroid; ophthalmoplegia; positions of gaze, diagnostic; sign, Dalrymple's; sign, von Graefe's; sign, Moebius.**

**disease, Harada's** A disease characterized by bilateral exudative uveitis associated with alopecia, vitiligo and hearing defects. However, as many aspects of this entity overlap clinically and histopathologically with the Vogt–Koyanagi syndrome it is nowadays combined and called the Vogt–Koyanagi–Harada syndrome.
*See* **syndrome, Vogt–Koyanagi–Harada.**

**disease, von Hippel's** A rare disease, sometimes familial, in which haemangiomata occur in the retina where they appear ophthalmoscopically as one or more round elevated reddish nodules. The condition is progressive and takes years before there is a complete loss of vision. *Syn.* angiomatosis retinae.
*See* **disease, von Hippel–Lindau.**

**disease, von Hippel–Lindau** Retinal haemangioblastoma involving one or both eyes associated with similar tumours in the cerebellum and spinal cord and sometimes cysts of the kidney and pancreas. Ophthalmoscopic examination shows a reddish slightly elevated tumour.

**disease, Leber's** *See* **Leber's hereditary optic atrophy.**

**disease, Niemann–Pick** Inherited lipoid degeneration which produces a partial destruction of the retinal ganglion cells and a demyelination of many parts of the nervous system. The condition usually involves children of Jewish parentage. When the retina is involved there is a reddish central area (a cherry-red spot) surrounded by a white oedematous area. The disease usually leads to death by the age of two. This disease is differentiated from **Tay–Sachs disease** because of its widespread involvement and gross enlargement of the liver and the spleen. *Syn.* sphingomyelin lipidosis.
*See* **cherry-red spot; disease, Tay–Sachs.**

**disease, Oguchi's** Congenital and hereditary night blindness occurring mainly in Japan. All other visual capabilities are usually unimpaired. It is presumed to be due to an abnormality in the neural network of the retina.
*See* **hemeralopia.**

**disease, ophthalmic Graves'** *See* **disease, Graves'.**

**disease, Paget's** Hereditary systemic disorder of the skeletal system accompanied by visual disturbances, the most common being retinal arteriosclerosis.
*See* **angioid streaks; arteriosclerosis.**

**disease, von Recklinghausen's** Congenital benign tumours of the neural tissues characterized by pigmentation of the skin and a tumour growth in any of the structures of the eye or adnexa. *Syn.* neurofibromatosis.

**disease, Reiter's** A systemic syndrome characterized by a triad of three diseases: urethritis, arthritis and conjunctivitis. Keratitis and iridocyclitis may follow as complications. It occurs mainly in young men typically following urethritis and less commonly after an attack of dysentery or acute arthritis which usually affects the knees, ankles and Achilles tendon. *Syn.* Reiter's syndrome.

**disease, Sandhoff's** An autosomal recessive inherited disease similar to Tay–Sachs disease with the same signs, but differing in that both the enzymes hexosaminidase A and B are defective and it develops more rapidly and can be found among the general population. *Syn.* gangliosidosis type II.
*See* **disease, Tay–Sachs.**

**disease, sickle-cell** A hereditary anaemia encountered among Negro and other dark-skinned people due to a defect in the haemoglobin. It is characterized by retinal neovascularization, haemorrhages and exudates, cataract and subconjunctival haemorrhage. *Syn.* sickle-cell anaemia.

**disease, Spielmeyer–Stock** *See* **disease, Batten–Mayou.**

**disease, Stargardt's** An autosomal recessive inherited disorder of the retina occurring in the first or second decade of life and affecting the central region of the retina. With time a lesion develops at the macula which has a 'beaten-bronze' reflex. It is often surrounded by yellow-white flecks. There is a loss of central vision but peripheral vision is usually normal. Myopia is very common. Management usually consists of a high plus correction for near to magnify the retinal image. *Syn.* Stargardt's macular dystrophy.
*See* **fundus flavimaculatus.**

**disease, Still's** Juvenile rheumatoid arthritis; it occurs insidiously at about the time of second

dentition. In the eye it is associated with keratopathy (90%) usually accompanied by iridocyclitis. Secondary cataract may also develop. *Syn.* juvenile rheumatoid arthritis.
*See* **rheumatoid arthritis.**

**disease, Sturge–Weber** *See* **syndrome, Sturge–Weber.**

**disease, Tay–Sachs** Amaurotic family idiocy in which there is a widespread lipoid degeneration of the ganglion cells of both the retina and the brain. It has its onset in the first year of life, vision is affected and the central retina shows a whitish area with a reddish central area (cherry-red spot). Eventually the eye becomes blind and death occurs, usually at about the age of 30 months. It affects Jewish infants more than others by a factor of about ten to one.
*See* **cherry-red spot; disease, Niemann–Pick.**

**disease, Terrien's** *See* **ectasia, corneal.**

**disease Wagner's** An autosomal dominant inherited disease linked to an abnormality or mutation on chromosome 5q. It is characterized by an empty vitreous cavity or dense membranes within the vitreous, myopia, retinal perivascular pigmentation, retinal degeneration, cataract and less frequently retinal detachment. Vision is usually normal until adulthood. *Syn.* vitreoretinal degeneration.

**disease, Wernicke's** A disease characterized by disturbances in ocular motility, pupillary reactions, nystagmus and ataxia. It is mainly due to thiamin deficiency and is frequently encountered in chronic alcoholics. *Syn.* Wernicke's syndrome.

**disease, Wilson's** A systemic disease resulting from a deficiency of the alpha-2-globulin ceruloplasmin beginning in the first or second decade of life. It is characterized by widespread deposition of copper in the tissues, tremor, muscular rigidity, irregular involuntary movements, emotional instability and hepatic disorders. The ocular features are degenerative changes in the lenticular nucleus and most noticeably a Kayser–Fleischer ring. *Syn.* hepatolenticular degeneration; lenticular progressive degeneration; pseudosclerosis of Westphal.
*See* **ring, Kayser–Fleischer.**

**disinfectant** *See* **antiseptic.**

**disinfection by boiling** A method of killing all organisms (including acanthamoeba) in soft contact lenses, based on heating the lens to a temperature of at least 80° for 10 minutes. This is achieved in specially manufactured heating units in which the lenses are kept in physiological saline solution. However, repeated boiling of soft lenses may cause some degradation of the lens material and tear mucoproteins which have not been previously removed with a surface cleaning agent tend to become coagulated on the lens surface.
*See* **antiseptic; sterilization; surfactant.**

**disintersion, retinal** *See* **retinal dialysis.**

**disjunctive movements; nystagmus** *See* under the nouns.

**dislocation of the lens** *See* **luxation of the lens.**

**disparate retinal points** Non-corresponding retinal points.
*See* **disparity, retinal; retinal corresponding points.**

**disparity, binocular** *See* **acuity, stereoscopic visual; disparity, retinal; perception, depth.**

**disparity, crossed** Retinal disparity induced by an object nearer to the eyes than the point of fixation and focused on the temporal retina. Thus, the image received by the right eye appears to the left and that received by the left eye appears to the right. *Syn.* crossed retinal disparity.
*See* **disparate retinal points; horopter.**

**disparity, fixation** *See* **disparity, retinal.**

**disparity, retinal** Binocular vision in which the two retinal images of a single object do not fall on corresponding retinal points, i.e. when the object lies off the horopter. If, however, the two retinal images still fall within Panum's area the object will still be seen single. At the fixation point this may cause over or under convergence of the eyes. This particular case is called **fixation disparity** (or **retinal slip**). The presence of fixation disparity often indicates that binocular vision is under stress and the patient has an uncompensated heterophoria. Optical correction or orthoptic exercises usually eliminate the symptoms. Fixation disparity can be measured either (1) directly (e.g. Disparometer, Wesson Fixation Disparity Card, both consisting of targets with pairs of vernier lines of various angular separation, each line being seen by one eye through polarizing filters), or (2) indirectly as an associated phoria (e.g. Mallett fixation disparity unit). *Syn.* binocular disparity.
*See* **acuity, stereoscopic visual; anaglyph; area, Panum's; Disparometer; esodisparity; exodisparity; fusional movements; heterophoria, uncompensated; Mallett fixation disparity unit; perception, depth; retinal corresponding points; stereogram, random-dot; stereopsis; stereotest.**

**disparity, uncrossed** Retinal disparity induced by an object farther away from the eyes than the point of fixation and focused on the nasal retina. Thus, the image received by the right eye appears to the right and that received by the left eye appears to the left. *Syn.* uncrossed retinal disparity.
*See* **disparate retinal points; horopter.**

**disparity vergence** *See* **fusion, motor.**

**Disparometer** Tradename for a clinical instrument designed to measure fixation disparity at near. The target does not have a binocular fixation point and the fusion lock is parafoveal. The instrument fits on the near point rod of a standard phoropter. The Disparometer has two stimuli: one for vertical disparity measurement and the other for horizontal disparity measurement. The test consists of successive pairs of vernier lines of increasing angular separation within a structureless field, each line being viewed by one eye through polarizing filters. The edge of the field provides a peripheral fusion stimulus. Fixation disparity is measured when the vernier lines appear to be aligned and the amount is given by the angular separation (in minutes of arc) of the lines indicated on the back of the instrument. A fixation disparity curve can be obtained by determining the fixation disparity for various amounts of prism power placed in front of the eyes.
*See* **disparity, retinal; heterophoria, associated; Mallett fixation disparity unit.**

**dispensing, optical** The act of issuing an optical appliance which corrects, remedies or relieves defects of vision (definition of the World Council of Optometry). *Syn.* dispensing; ophthalmic dispensing.
*See* **appliance, optical; optician, dispensing; optics, ophthalmic.**

**dispersion** Phenomenon of the change in velocity of propagation of radiation in a medium, as a function of its frequency, which causes a separation of the monochromatic components of a complex radiation. All optical media cause dispersion by virtue of their variation of refractive index with wavelengths. Dispersion is specified by the difference in the refractive index of the medium for two wavelengths. The difference between the blue F (486.1 nm) and the red C (656.3 nm) spectral lines is called the **mean dispersion**, i.e. $n_F - n_C$. Dispersion is usually represented by its **dispersive power** ω or **relative dispersion** which is equal to the mean dispersion divided by the excess refractive index of the sodium D (589.3 nm) spectral line ($n_D-1$), often called the **refractivity** of the material,

$$\omega = \frac{n_F - n_C}{n_D - 1}$$

The reciprocal of the dispersive power is called the Abbé's number or constringence (Fig. D7).
*See* **aberration, lateral chromatic; aberration longitudinal chromatic; axis, achromatic; constringence; index of refraction; lines, Fraunhoffer's; prism, achromatic.**

**dispersion, mean; relative** *See* **dispersion.**

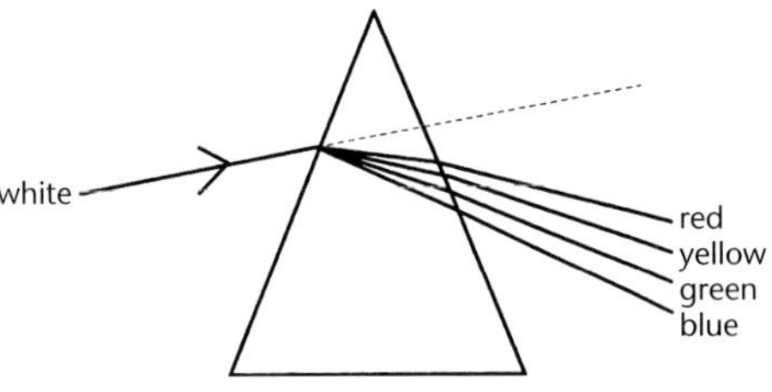


**Fig. D7** Dispersion of a white beam of light by a prism

**dispersive power** *See* **constringence.**

**disposable contact lens** *See* **lens, contact.**

**dissociated nystagmus** *See* **nystagmus.**

**dissociated vertical deviation** *See* **deviation, dissociated vertical.**

**dissociated vertical divergence** *See* **hypermetropia, alternating.**

**dissociating test** *See* **test, dissociating.**

**dissociation** Elimination of the stimulus to fusion. It is usually accomplished by occluding one eye, or by inducing gross distortion of the image seen by one eye (e.g. Maddox rod), or by placing a strong prism in front of one eye (e.g. von Graefe's test) with the result that the eyes will move to the passive position (or heterophoria position).
*See* **heterophoria, dissociated; position, passive; test, diplopia; test, dissociating.**

**distal** Farthest from a central point.
*See* **proximal.**

**distance, abathic** *See* **plane, apparent frontoparallel.**

**distance between lenses (DBL)** Horizontal distance between the nasal parts of the spectacle lenses in a frame, measured either along the datum line (datum system) or between the nasal peaks of the bevels of the two spectacle lenses (boxing system).
*See* **spectacle frame markings; system, boxing.**

**distance between rims (DBR)** Horizontal distance between the bearing surfaces of a regular bridge of a spectacle frame, usually measured along the datum line, or at a specified distance below the crest of the bridge.

**distance, centration** *See* **centration distance.**

**distance of distinct vision** A conventional distance used in calculating the magnifying power of a loupe or microscope. It is usually taken as 25 cm (or 10 inches) from the eye.
*See* **magnification, apparent; magnifier; microscope.**

**distance, focal** *See* **length, focal.**

**distance, hyperfocal** That distance from a lens or optical system at which the depth of field, on the far side of an object in focus, extends to infinity. On the near side of the object the depth of field then extends to half that distance. This is a useful distance in photography as it represents the shortest distance on which to focus in order to obtain a reasonable image definition of an object at infinity and the longest total depth of field. This distance depends on the focal length and the diameter of the entrance pupil of the system as well as the amount of the allowable blur.
*See* **depth of field.**

**distance, image** The distance along the optical axis of a lens or optical system between the image plane and the secondary principal plane. If the system consists of a single thin lens the image distance is measured from the optical surface and the reciprocal of this quantity is called the **reduced image vergence** or **image vergence** (in air).
*See* **plane, principal; power, back vertex; vergence.**

**distance, interocular** The distance between the centres of rotation of the eyes, i.e. the length of the base line.
*See* **line, base.**

**distance, interpupillary (IPD, PD)** The distance between the centres of the pupils of the eyes. It usually refers to the eyes fixating at distance, otherwise reference must be made to the fixation distance (e.g. near interpupillary distance). The average interpupillary distance for men is about 64 mm and for women about 62 mm (in Caucasians). *Syn.* pupillary distance. The interpupillary distance is often measured from the median plane to the centre of the pupil of each eye. This is referred to as the **monocular pupillary distance** (MPD): it is a useful measurement, especially in dispensing progressive lenses. The interpupillary distance for near vision can be calculated using the following formula:

near PD = ({$d/d'$}) distance PD

where $d$ is the distance between the target plane and the spectacle plane and $d'$ the distance between the target plane and the midpoint between the centres of rotation of the eyes.
*See* **angle of convergence; angle, metre; lens, progressive; pupillometer; rule, PD.**

**distance, object** The distance along the optical axis of a lens or optical system between the object plane and the primary principal plane. If the system consists of a single thin lens the object distance is measured from the optical surface and the reciprocal of this quantity is called the **reduced object vergence** or **object vergence** (in air).
*See* **plane, principal; power, front vertex; vergence.**

**distance, reading** The normal distance at which people read. It is about 33–44 cm for men and 29–40 cm for women. It is a useful measurement in determining the reading addition.
*See* **addition, near.**

**distance vision** *See* **vision, distance.**

**distance, working (WD) 1.** The distance at which a person reads or does close work. **2.** In retinoscopy, the distance between the plane of the sighthole and that of the patient's spectacles. **3.** In microscopy, the distance between an object and the front surface of the objective.
*See* **microscope, specular; retinoscope.**

**distances, conjugate** An optical system will form an image of an object. As the path of light is reversible, the position of object and image are interchangeable. These pairs of object and image points are called **conjugate points** (or **conjugate foci**) and the distances of the object and the image from the optical surface are called the **conjugate distances** (Fig. D8). When an eye is accurately focused for an object, object and retina are conjugate.
*See* **ametropia; emmetropia; experiment, Scheiner's.**

**distichiasis** Congenital anomaly in which there is a double row of eyelashes in the lid margin, one row being normal and the other row turning inward towards the eye. Distichiasis can also be acquired following scarring or chemical and physical injury. If there are symptoms treatment consists of removal of the aberrant eyelashes,

**Table D5** Calculated near PD (in mm) as a function of distance PD for three reading distances (target plane to spectacle plane). The distance between the spectacle plane and the midpoint of the base line is assumed to be 27 mm (vertex distance 12 mm)

| distance PD | 56 | 58 | 60 | 62 | 64 | 66 | 68 | 70 | 72 | 74 |
|---|---|---|---|---|---|---|---|---|---|---|
| near PD for 45 cm | 52.8 | 54.7 | 56.6 | 58.5 | 60.4 | 62.3 | 64.2 | 66.0 | 67.9 | 69.8 |
| difference | 3.2 | 3.3 | 3.4 | 3.5 | 3.6 | 3.7 | 3.8 | 4.0 | 4.1 | 4.2 |
| near PD for 40 cm | 52.5 | 54.3 | 56.2 | 58.1 | 59.9 | 61.8 | 63.7 | 65.6 | 67.4 | 69.3 |
| difference | 3.5 | 3.7 | 3.8 | 3.9 | 4.1 | 4.2 | 4.3 | 4.4 | 4.6 | 4.7 |
| near PD for 35 cm | 52.0 | 53.8 | 55.7 | 57.6 | 59.4 | 61.3 | 63.1 | 65.0 | 66.8 | 68.7 |
| difference | 4.0 | 4.2 | 4.3 | 4.4 | 4.6 | 4.7 | 4.9 | 5.0 | 5.2 | 5.3 |

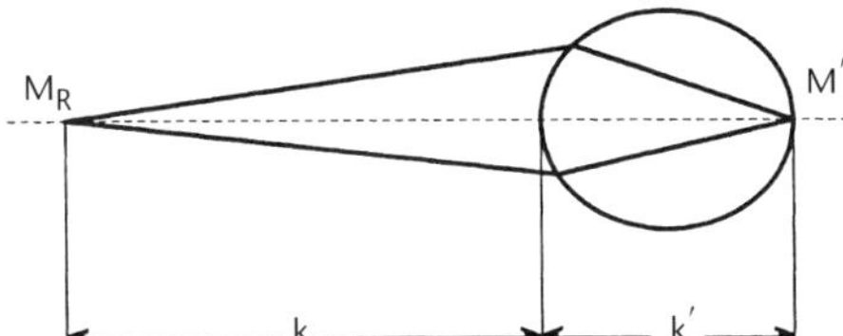


**Fig. D8** Conjugate distances k and k′ and conjugate points $M_R$ and M′ in the eye ($M_R$, far point of the eye; M′, foveola)

usually by cryotherapy (removal under cold or freezing conditions) or electrolysis.
*See* **epilation; eyelashes; polystichia; trichiasis.**

**distometer** An instrument for measuring the distance between the back surface of a spectacle lens and the apex of the cornea. It is usually carried out by having the patient close the eyes and one end of the instrument or caliper rests against the upper eyelid and the other presses against the back surface of the spectacle lens. The measurements are most commonly given to the nearest 0.5 mm. *Syn.* Lenscorometer (a tradename); vertexometer.

**distortion** Aberration of an optical system resulting in an image which does not conform to the shape of the object, somewhat resembling the image viewed through a cylindrical lens. This is due to an unequal magnification of the image. Distortion can be barrel-shaped (**barrel-shaped distortion**) in which the corners of the image of a square are closer to the centre than the middle part of the sides; or pincushion (**pincushion distortion**) in which the corners of the image of a square are farther from the centre than the middle part of the sides (Fig. D9). *Example* of barrel-shaped distortion: a square object seen through an uncorrected negative spectacle lens. *Example* of pincushion distortion: a square object seen through an uncorrected positive spectacle lens.
*See* **aberration; correction; lens, fisheye; sine condition.**

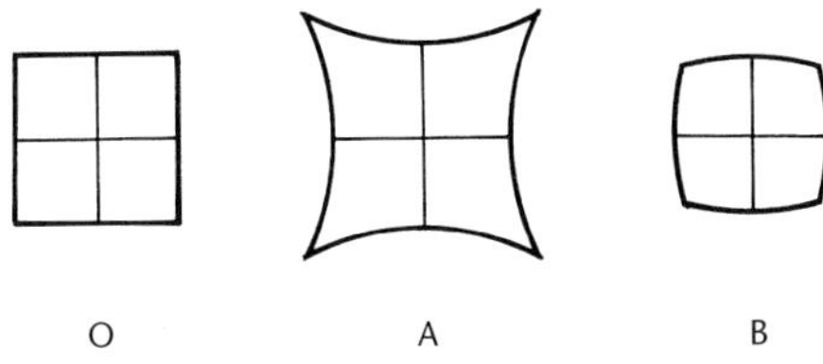


**Fig. D9** Distortion (O, object; A, pincushion distortion; B, barrel-shaped distortion)

**distortion test** *See* **test, distortion.**

**diurnal cycle** *See* **rhythm, circadian.**

**diurnal variations, in intraocular pressure** Normal intraocular pressure varies throughout the day within a range of about 4 mmHg, being higher in the morning than in the evening. In patients with primary open-angle glaucoma this range is greater. This variation must be taken into consideration when measuring intraocular pressure.
*See* **pressure, intraocular.**

**diurnal vision** *See* **vision, diurnal.**

**divergence** 1. Movement of the eyes turning away from each other. 2. Characteristic of a pencil of light rays, as when emanating from a point source. *Syn.* **negative convergence.**
*See* **vergence.**

**divergence excess** A high exophoria at distance associated with a much lower exophoria at near. It may occasionally give rise to diplopia in distance vision.
*See* **exophoria.**

**divergence, fusional** A movement of the eyes away from each other in response to retinal disparity, in order to restore single binocular vision. It occurs most commonly when induced by a base-in prism.

**divergence insufficiency** A high esophoria at distance associated with esophoria at near. It often gives rise to symptoms of asthenopia in both distance and near vision.
*See* **asthenopia; esophoria.**

**divergence paralysis** *See* **paralysis, divergence.**

**divergence, vertical** Relative vertical movement between the two eyes.

**diverging lens** *See* **lens, diverging.**

**doll's head phenomenon** *See* **phenomenon, doll's head.**

**Dolman's test** *See* **test, hole in the card.**

**dominance, ocular** The superiority of one eye whose visual function predominates over the other eye. It is that eye (called the **dominant eye**) which is relied upon more than the other in binocular vision. It is not necessarily the eye with the best acuity. The lack of ocular dominance is referred to as **ambiocularity** and such a person is **ambiocular.**
*See* **manoptoscope; occlusion treatment; test, hole in the card.**

**dominant eye** *See* **eye, dominant.**

**dominant wavelength (of a colour stimulus, not purple)** *See* **wavelength, dominant.**

**Donders' diagram** Graphical representation of total convergence as a function of accommodation for any fixation distance. The accommodation in dioptres is represented on the ordinate and the convergence in prism dioptres (or metre angles) on the abscissa. It is used to represent the binocular

status of the two eyes, as well as evaluating the patient's visual discomfort at any distance.
*See* **accommodation, relative amplitude of; angle, metre; convergence, relative; criterion, Percival; criterion, Sheard; line, demand; zone of clear, single, binocular vision.**

**Donders' law** *See* **law, Donders'.**

**Donders' line** *See* **line, demand.**

**Donders' method** *See* **method, push-up.**

**Donders' reduced eye** *See* **eye, reduced.**

**Doppler's ophthalmodynamometer** *See* **ophthalmodynanometer.**

**dorsal midbrain syndrome** *See* **syndrome, Parinaud's.**

**dorzolamide** *See* **carbonic anhydrase inhibitors.**

**dot haemorrhage** *See* **haemorrhage, blot.**

**double elevator palsy** *See* **palsy, double elevator.**

**double lid eversion** *See* **eversion, lid.**

**double refraction** *See* **birefringence.**

**double prism test** *See* **test, double prism.**

**double vision** *See* **diplopia.**

**doublet** A combination of two lenses usually cemented to each other used to correct chromatic aberration. Typically it consists of a positive crown lens and a negative flint lens.
*See* **glass, crown; glass, flint; lens, achromatizing; triplet.**

**Down's syndrome** *See* **syndrome, Down's.**

**downbeat nystagmus** *See* **nystagmus.**

**Doyne's honeycomb choroiditis** *See* **drusen, familial dominant.**

**Draper's law** *See* **law, Draper's.**

**drift** *See* **movements, fixation.**

**droopy eyelid** *See* **ptosis.**

**drusen** Small, circular, yellow or white dots located throughout the fundus but more so in the macular region, around the optic disc or the periphery. They consist of deposits lying between the basement membrane of the retinal pigment epithelium and Bruch's membrane. Although they may be found in young people, they almost universally occur with ageing but also with retinal and choroidal degeneration (e.g. age-related maculopathy, retinitis pigmentosa, angioid streaks) and primary dystrophy (e.g. fundus flavimaculatus). There are several main types of drusen: (1) **Hard** (or **nodular**) drusen are small, round and discrete. They are deposits of granular material as well as of abnormal collagen. They are the most common type and are usually innocuous. (2) **Soft** (or **diffuse** or **granular**) drusen are often large with indistinct edges and with time they may enlarge, coalesce and increase in number. They are due to either a focal thickening of the inner layer of Bruch's membrane or to amorphous material located between that thickened, detached part and the rest of Bruch's membrane. They represent an early feature of age-related maculopathy. (3) **Cuticular** (or **basal laminar**) drusen are small subretinal nodular thickening of the basement membrane of the pigment epithelium. They occur in younger patients more often than hard or soft drusen. (4) With time, the above drusen may calcify (**calcific** drusen) and take on a glistening appearance. Drusen rarely produce any symptoms and if there is a visual loss it is usually due to an accompanying macular haemorrhage. *Syn.* colloid bodies; hyaline bodies.
*See* **maculopathy age-related; naevus, choroidal.**

**drusen, familial dominant** An autosomal dominant hereditary degeneration of the choroid characterized by light-coloured patches of colloid material in the area around the macula and often the optic disc. There is no loss of vision unless it is followed by macular degeneration. *Syn.* Doyne's honeycomb choroiditis; Doyne's honeycombed degeneration; Tay's choroiditis (used more commonly for the elderly).

**dry eye** *See* **eye, dry; glands, meibomian; keratitis sicca.**

**Drysdale's method** *See* **method, Drysdale's.**

**Duane's syndrome** *See* **syndrome, Duane's.**

**duction 1.** Movement of one eye alone as in abduction, adduction, depression, elevation, etc. **2.** Disjunctive binocular movements (although it is more correct to call these movements vergences). **Binocular duction** refers to the maximum vergence powers that can be exerted while maintaining single binocular vision through prisms, either in the base-in or base-out direction. Binocular ductions are measured from the passive position (or phoria position) to the break point.
*See* **abduction; adduction; depression; dextroduction; elevation of the eye; laevoduction; movements, disjunctive eye; vergence.**

**duochrome test** *See* **test, duochrome.**

**duplicity theory** *See* **theory, duplicity.**

**Dutch telescope** *See* **telescope, galilean.**

**Dvorine's pseudoisochromatic plates** *See* **plates, pseudoisochromatic.**

**dye dilution test** *See* **test, dye dilution.**

**dynamic acuity; retinoscopy** *See* under the nouns.

**dyschromatopsia** General term given to deficiencies of colour vision, especially acquired defects. *See* **colour vision, defective.**

**dyscoria** Anomaly in the shape of the pupil. *See* **pupil.**

**dyskeratosis** Abnormal process which, in the eye, results in hornification of the epithelial layer of the conjunctiva or cornea. It may be hereditary or due to irritation (e.g. radiation) or to prolonged drug administration in the eye. It appears as a dry white plaque (called **leucoplakia** or **leucokeratosis**). It may be benign or malignant, in which case it must be surgically excised.
*See* **pterygium.**

**dyslexia** A condition characterized by difficulty with reading and spelling. Words may be read but not recognized or understood. It is independent of intelligence, motivation or visual correction. Its origin may be due to a disorder of the fast processing magnocellular visual system. The condition is commonly associated with the Meares–Irlen syndrome.
*See* **alexia; magnocellular visual system; syndrome, Meares–Irlen; test, developmental and perceptual screening.**

**dysmegalopsia** A condition in which the perceptual size of objects is abnormal. Objects may appear larger (**macropsia**) or smaller (**micropsia**). *See* **macropsia; micropsia.**

**dysmetria, ocular** Abnormality of eye movements in which the eyes overshoot when attempting to fixate an object. It is a sign of cerebellar disease. *See* **flutter; opsoclonus.**

**dystrophy** A non-inflammatory developmental, nutritional or metabolic disorder.

**dystrophy, anterior membrane** *See* **dystrophy, Cogan's microcystic epithelial.**

**dystrophy, band-shaped corneal** *See* **keratopathy, band.**

**dystrophy, Best's vitelliform macular** *See* **disease, Best's.**

**dystrophy, bleb-like** *See* **dystrophy, Cogan's microcystic epithelial.**

**dystrophy, central areolar choroidal** An autosomal dominant dystrophy of the macula with onset in the third to fifth decades of life. It causes a progressive decrease in visual acuity. It is characterized by bilateral, atrophic macular lesions, between one and three disc diameters in size and through which choroidal vessels can be seen. The prognosis of this condition is poor as it is progressive. *Syn.* central aerolar choroidal sclerosis. *See* **choroideraemia.**

**dystrophy, central crystalline** An autosomal dominant stromal corneal dystrophy. Yellow-white crystals are scattered throughout the central cornea. Since the lesions are usually found below Bowman's layer, the corneal epithelium remains unaffected. The crystals consist of cholesterol and fats. They do not affect vision.

**dystrophy, Cogan's microcystic epithelial** A bilateral corneal dystrophy located in the corneal epithelium and occurring most commonly in females. It is characterized by variously shaped greyish-white microcysts and debris which vary in shape and location over time, coalescing with other microcysts, forming lines, and resembling a fingerprint pattern. Symptoms are minimal and vision is unaffected unless the lesions are in the central zone of the cornea. The condition may be associated with **recurrent epithelial erosions** which cause pain, lacrimation, photophobia and blurred vision. Management normally includes artificial tears, patching and antibiotics and occasionally therapeutic soft contact lenses for frequent or more severe types. *Syn.* anterior membrane dystrophy; bleb-like dystrophy; epithelial basement membrane dystrophy; fingerprint dystrophy.
*See* **corneal erosion, recurrent; lens, therapeutic soft contact.**

**dystrophy, cone** A degeneration of the cone photoreceptors which, in most cases, is inherited in an autosomal dominant or X-linked recessive fashion, but some cases are sporadic. It appears in the first or second decades of life and is characterized by a progressive loss of visual acuity, colour vision impairment, photophobia and central scotoma. Ophthalmoscopic examination may show a demarcated circular atrophic area in the macular region (**bull's eye maculopathy**). There is no known treatment. *Syn.* cone degeneration.
*See* **achromatopsia; monochromat.**

**dystrophy, cone-rod** A bilateral degeneration of the photoreceptors affecting the cones first and the rods later. It may be inherited in an autosomal dominant or X-linked recessive fashion but many cases are sporadic. It appears in the first to third decades of life. It is characterized by poor visual acuity, colour vision impairment and photoaversion to bright sunlight. The ocular fundus may eventually show an atrophy of the retinal pigment epithelium which appears as a **bull's eye maculopathy**. Eventually as the rods degenerate there is progressive night blindness. There is no known treatment.

**dystrophy, corneal** Hereditary disorders affecting both corneas. It is occasionally present at birth but, more frequently, it develops during adolescence and progresses slowly throughout life. It varies in appearance and is often described on that basis (e.g. band-shaped corneal dystrophy), or on the basis of which layer is affected. Dystrophies affecting the anterior part of the cornea include **Cogan's microcystic epithelial dystrophy, Meesmann's dystrophy** and **Reis–Bucklers dystrophy.** Stromal dystrophies include **central crystalline dystrophy, granular dystrophy, lattice dystrophy, macular dystrophy,** and posterior corneal dystrophies include **Fuch's endothelial dystrophy** and **posterior polymorphous dystrophy.**
*See* **cornea guttata; keratopathy, band.**

**dystrophy, endothelial corneal** *See* **cornea guttata; dystrophy, Fuchs' endothelial.**

**dystrophy, epithelial basement membrane** *See* **dystrophy, Cogan's microcystic epithelial.**

**dystrophy, fingerprint** *See* **dystrophy, Cogan's microcystic epithelial.**

**dystrophy, Fuchs' endothelial** A progressive dystrophy of the corneal endothelium seen more commonly in women than in men, usually in the fifth decade of life. It may be transmitted in an autosomal dominant fashion. It is characterized by wart-like deposits on the endothelial surface. As the condition progresses there is oedema of the stroma and eventually of the epithelium and bullous keratopathy causing blurring of vision and pain. The stroma may also become vascularized. It is often associated with glaucoma and nuclear lens opacity. Treatment includes hypertonic agents (e.g. sodium chloride 5%), a bandage soft contact lens and in severe cases penetrating keratoplasty.
*See* **cornea guttata; keratopathy, bullous; keratoplasty.**

**dystrophy, granular** A hereditary condition characterized by the presence of irregularly shaped white granules of hyaline in the stroma of the cornea surrounded by clear areas. It usually develops during the first decade of life and progresses slowly throughout life. It rarely results in loss of vision although the granules are located in the centre of the cornea. If severe, though, a corneal graft is the main treatment. *Syn.* corneal granular dystrophy; Groenouw's nodular type I corneal dystrophy.
*See* **keratoplasty.**

**dystrophy, Grayson–Wilbrant** *See* **dystrophy, Reis–Buckler's.**

**dystrophy, lattice** An autosomal dominant, hereditary disorder characterized by the appearance in the corneal stroma of fine branching filaments interlacing and overlapping at different levels, as well as white spots and stellate opacities. These filaments are deposits of amyloid. The onset usually begins in the first decade of life and progresses in the following decades. Recurrent corneal erosions are common. When visual acuity becomes impaired, keratoplasty may be necessary. *Syn.* Biber–Haab–Dimmer corneal dystrophy; lattice corneal dystrophy type I.
*See* **corneal erosion, recurrent; keratoplasty.**

**dystrophy, macular** An autosomal recessive disorder characterized by bilateral, grey-white nodules which progressively develop into a generalized opacification of the corneal stroma. By about the fifth decade of life visual acuity is markedly diminished and penetrating keratoplasty may be necessary. Histological examination shows an accumulation of mucopolysaccharide in the stroma and degeneration of Bowman's membrane.

**dystrophy, Meesman's** A dominant, hereditary, bilateral disorder characterized by numerous small punctate opacities in the corneal epithelium. It appears in infancy. It is usually asymptomatic but in some cases there is discomfort and a slight decrease in visual acuity. In severe cases, keratoplasty may be necessary. *Syn.* juvenile epithelial corneal dystrophy; hereditary epithelial dystrophy.

**dystrophy, posterior polymorphous** An autosomal dominant, usually bilateral, dystrophy of the endothelium and Descemet's membrane appearing either at birth or in early childhood. It is characterized by polymorphous plaques of calcium crystals and vesicular lesions in the endothelium and on its surface. It is usually asymptomatic, but in some cases corneal oedema occurs and it may require penetrating keratoplasty.

**dystrophy, Reis–Buckler** An autosomal dominant disorder of the cornea characterized by ring-shaped opacities occurring at the level of Bowman's membrane and protruding into the epithelium. The opacities increase in density with time giving rise to a honeycomb appearance. The condition begins in childhood and progresses with frequent recurrent corneal erosions resulting in scarring, decreased visual acuity and reduced corneal sensitivity. In severe cases, keratoplasty may be necessary. A similar condition is **Grayson–Wilbrant dystrophy** in which visual acuity is less affected, corneal erosions are less frequent and corneal sensitivity is normal.
*See* corneal erosion, recurrent; keratoplasty.

**dystrophy, Stargardt's macular** *See* **disease, Stargardt's.**

**dystrophy, vitelliform macular** *See* **disease, Best's.**

# E



**'E' game** A technique used to evaluate visual acuity in young children. The letter 'E' is shown to the child who is instructed to either state or point his or her fingers in the direction of the open side of the letter. The 'E' is subsequently rotated left, right, up and down randomly as its size is decreased, and acuity is obtained when the smallest letter is just recognizable.
*See* **chart, illiterate E.**

**Eales' disease** *See* **disease, Eales'.**

**eccentric fixation; viewing** *See* under the nouns.

**eccentricity** Term referring to the angular distance from the centre of the visual field or from the foveola of the retina. *Example*: the maximum density of rods in the retina is at a retinal eccentricity of about 20°.
*See* **blind spot; cell, rod; field, visual; foveola.**

**ecchymosis** *See* **eye, black.**

**echo** *See* **ultrasonography.**

**echography** *See* **ultrasonography.**

**echothiophate iodide** *See* **acetylcholinesterase.**

**eclipse blindness** *See* **blindness, eclipse.**

**ectasia, corneal** A forward bulging and thinning of the cornea. It may result from a disease of the cornea (e.g. keratoconus), trauma, atrophy or raised intraocular pressure. If uveal tissue is included in the protrusion, the condition is called a **staphyloma**. If the ectasia is limited to a peripheral part of the cornea, it is called **Terrien's disease** or **Terrien's marginal degeneration**. It is due to degeneration of marginal corneal tissue. It affects adult males more commonly than females and the eye has progressive astigmatism. Therapy includes rigid contact lenses and occasionally keratoplasty. *Syn.* keratectasia; keratoectasia; kerectasis.
*See* **degeneration, pellucid marginal corneal; keratoconus; keratoglobus; staphyloma.**

**ectasia, scleral** A bulging and thinning of the sclera, due to disease, trauma, atrophy or raised intraocular pressure. It may be total as in buphthalmos, or partial as in staphyloma. *Syn.* sclerectasia.
*See* **glaucoma, congenital; staphyloma.**

**ectopia lentis** *See* **luxation of the lens.**

**ectopia of the macula** *See* **macula, ectopia of the.**

**ectopia pupillae** *See* **corectopia.**

**ectropion** Outward turning of the eyelid margin. The most common cause is a loss of tonus of the pretarsal orbicularis muscle combined with laxity of the medial and lateral canthal tendons, which occurs in old people and affects only the lower eyelid (**involutional ectropion**). Tears collect in the lacrimal lake and overflow onto the skin of the face. Other causes of ectropion are scarring, burns, trauma (called **cicatricial ectropion**), spasm of the orbicularis muscle which may affect either the upper or lower eyelid, or paralysis of the orbicularis muscle in which only the lower eyelid is affected. Ectropion may lead to exposure keratitis as the lower part of the cornea remains exposed. Management includes instilling an ocular lubricant and patching the eye during sleep as a temporary measure, but, if severe, the treatment is surgical.
*See* **entropion; eyelids; keratitis, exposure.**

**ectropion, cicatricial; involutional** *See* **ectropion.**

**ectropion uveae** An ectropion affecting the iris and characterized by a portion of the posterior pigment epithelium of the iris growing or being drawn around the pupillary margin onto the anterior iris surface. It may be acquired (e.g. following iris neovascularization, neovascular glaucoma) or congenital (e.g. neurofibromatosis).
*See* **disease, von Recklinghausen's; glaucoma, neovascular; neovascularization, iris.**

**eczema** An inflammatory disease of the skin characterized by a rash of red spots, rough scaling, dryness and soreness of the skin sometimes leading to the formation of blisters. It often gives rise to itching or to a burning sensation. It may occur on the skin of the face where parts of spectacles rest. Frames should be cleaned regularly to avoid causing skin irritation. *Syn.* contact dermatitis.

**edema** *See* **oedema.**

**edge clearance** A small, peripheral gap between the edge of a rigid contact lens and the cornea. It is important as it allows tear exchange and eases lens removal. The absence of edge clearance in rigid contact lenses may lead to superficial corneal damage.

**edge lift** Deviation of the posterior surface of a contact lens from a sphere at a given diameter. This is produced by either the peripheral curve(s) or the edging process. Edge lift provides **peripheral clearance** of a rigid contact lens, which is assessed by fluorescein pattern. If the edge lift is

specified axially (as an extension of the back central optic zone, measured parallel to the axis of symmetry) it is referred to as **axial edge lift**. If specified radially as an extension along the back optic zone radius it is referred to as **radial edge lift.**
*See* **optic zone diameter; optic zone radius, back.**

**edging** Grinding the edge of a lens to the finished shape and size required, at the same time imparting the desired edge form, e.g. flat, bevelled, etc. This is accomplished with a machine called an **edger**, either by hand with a grinding wheel or automatically operating from a lens pattern or former.
*See* **former; glazing.**

**Edinger–Westphal nucleus** *See* **nucleus, Edinger–Westphal.**

**Edridge-Green lantern** An occupational colour vision test which consists of small round and variable sized coloured lights produced by coloured and neutral density filters.
*See* **colour vision, defective; test, lantern.**

**edrophonium chloride** *See* **anticholinesterase.**

**effect, Aubert's** *See* **phenomenon, Aubert's.**

**effect, Bezold–Brücke** *See* **phenomenon, Bezold–Brücke.**

**effect, Broca–Sulzer** The brightness produced by a flash of a given luminance depends upon its duration. It is maximum for durations around 30–40 ms when the flash luminance is photopic.

**effect, Brücke–Bartley** An increased brightness produced by an intermittent light source (usually around 8–10 Hz) compared to the same light source viewed in steady illumination.

**effect, Cheshire cat** A form of binocular rivalry in which a moving object seen by one eye can cause the entire image, or parts of the image, of a stationary object seen by the other eye to disappear. The effect can be observed by dividing the field of vision with a mirror placed edge-on in front of the nose at a slight angle. One eye looks straight at a stationary object, such as a sleeping cat, while the other eye sees a reflection through the mirror of a white wall or background. If a hand is waved on the mirror side in the region of the field where the cat is seen, the whole cat or part of it may be seen to disappear.
*See* **retinal rivalry.**

**effect, crowding** *See* **phenomenon, crowding.**

**effect, differential prismatic** The difference in prism power induced by a pair of ophthalmic lenses of different power when the eyes look in various directions of gaze (except through the optical centres). Large amounts of differential prismatic effect can hinder fusion and give rise to diplopia. *Example*: A patient's right eye is corrected by +5 D, the left eye by +2 D. When the eye rotates upward so that the visual axes intersect the lenses 1 cm above the optical centres, the induced prism power becomes 5 Δ base down on the right and 2 Δ base down on the left. The differential prismatic effect is 3 Δ base down in front of the right eye, probably too large for fusion to be maintained. *Syn.* prismatic imbalance; relative prismatic effect.
*See* **anisophoria; law, Prentice's.**

**effect, Gelb** In a faintly illuminated room a piece of black paper (or a rotating black disc) is illuminated by a high intensity projector. The beam of the projector falls exactly on the area of the black surface. The paper or disc will then appear to be white. A reversal of the perception is accomplished by placing a small piece of white paper near the disc in front of the projected light, at which time the paper or disc reappears in its true colour, i.e. black.

**effect, kinetic depth** An impression of a three-dimensional structure of an object produced by a moving two-dimensional object. It is most easily demonstrated by casting a shadow of a moving two-dimensional object on a translucent screen.

**effect, Mandelbaum** A tendency for the accommodative response to be altered when interposing a conflicting visual stimulus to the one being viewed. If the eyes are viewing a distant object through a dirty window or a wire fence the actual accommodative response will tend to be raised. If the eyes are viewing a near object in front of a dirty window or wire fence the actual accommodative response will be less than if there were no conflicting stimulus.
*See* **accommodative response.**

**effect, McCollough** A visual after-effect of colour that is seen when viewing, for a minute at least, two differently oriented and differently coloured gratings, such as a vertical grating with blue and black stripes and a horizontal grating with orange and black stripes. After adapting to these the subject looks at a figure containing a grating of vertical black and white stripes and a grating of black and white horizontal stripes of the same size as the original coloured gratings. The white stripes will then appear to be of the complementary colour, that is the vertical stripes appear pinkish and the horizontal stripes appear bluish.

**effect, moiré** *See* **moiré effect.**

**effect, oblique** In central vision, contours with oblique orientations are perceived and discriminated less easily than those close to the horizontal or vertical.

**effect, Pulfrich** *See* **stereophenomenon, Pulfrich.**

**effect, Raman** In certain substances scattered light may be of a slightly different wavelength from that of the incident light.

**effect, Stiles–Crawford** Variation of the luminosity of a pencil of light stimulating a given receptor with the position of entry of the pencil through the pupil. The maximum luminosity occurs for pencils passing through the centre of the pupil and stimulating the receptor along its axis. This phenomenon is attributed to the particular shape of the cone cells of the retina and occurs only in photopic vision.
*See* **cell, cone.**

**effect, Tyndall** Diffusion of light by the particles present in a liquid or gas. It is because of this effect that heterogeneities (e.g. increased proteins) of the media of the eye can be seen, as occurs in iris and/or ciliary body inflammation. *Syn.* Tyndall scatter.
*See* **aqueous flare.**

**effective power** *See* **power, effective.**

**efferent** Carrying nervous impulses away from the central nervous system to the periphery.
*See* **afferent.**

**efficiency scale, Snell–Sterling** *See* **visual efficiency scale, Snell–Sterling.**

**efficiency, spectral luminous (of a monochromatic radiation of wavelength λ)** Ratio of the radiant flux at wavelength $\lambda_m$ to that at wavelength $\lambda$ such that both radiations produce equally intense luminous sensations under specified photometric conditions and $\lambda_m$ is chosen so that the maximum value of this ratio is equal to one. *Symbols*: $V(\lambda)$ for photopic vision. $V'(\lambda)$ for scotopic vision (Fig. E1). *Note*: unless otherwise indicated, the values used for the spectral luminous efficiency in **photopic vision** are the values agreed internationally in 1931 by the CIE and adopted in 1933 by the International Committee on Weights and Measures. For **scotopic vision** the CIE in 1951 provisionally adopted new values for young observers (CIE).
*See* **vision, photopic; vision, scotopic.**

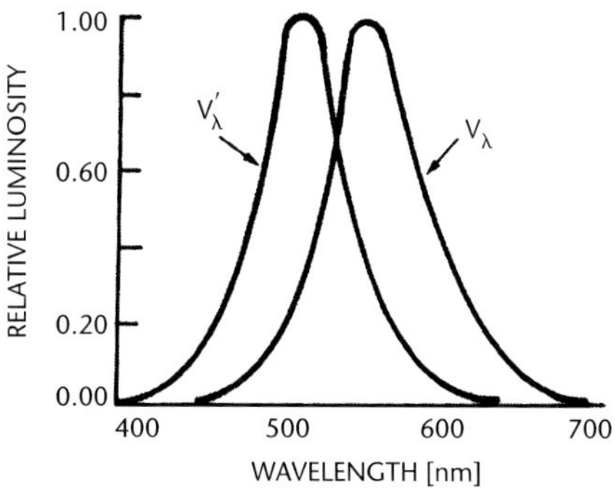


**Fig. E1** Relative luminous efficiency curves for photopic $V_\lambda$ and scotopic $V'_\lambda$ levels of adaptation for an equi-energy spectrum. These data represent the sensitivity (i.e. 1/threshold energy) typically obtained by flicker photometry

**Table E1** Photopic and scotopic relative luminous efficiency factors. The data are based on an average from a large number of individuals agreed by the CIE in 1931 for the photopic factor $V_\lambda$ and in 1951 for the scotopic factor $V'_\lambda$

| wavelength (in nm) | $V_\lambda$ | $V'_\lambda$ |
|---|---|---|
| 380 | 0.000 0 | 0.000 589 |
| 400 | 0.000 4 | 0.009 292 |
| 420 | 0.004 0 | 0.096 61 |
| 440 | 0.023 0 | 0.328 1 |
| 460 | 0.060 0 | 0.567 2 |
| 480 | 0.139 0 | 0.793 0 |
| 500 | 0.323 0 | 0.981 8 |
| 507 | – | 1.000 0 |
| 520 | 0.710 0 | 0.935 2 |
| 540 | 0.954 0 | 0.649 7 |
| 555 | 1.000 0 | – |
| 580 | 0.870 0 | 0.121 2 |
| 600 | 0.631 0 | 0.033 15 |
| 620 | 0.381 0 | 0.007 374 |
| 640 | 0.175 0 | 0.001 497 |
| 660 | 0.061 0 | 0.000 312 9 |
| 680 | 0.017 0 | 0.000 071 55 |
| 700 | 0.004 1 | 0.000 017 80 |
| 720 | 0.001 05 | 0.000 004 78 |
| 740 | 0.000 25 | 0.000 001 379 |
| 760 | 0.000 06 | 0.000 000 425 |
| 780 | 0.000 00 | 0.000 000 139 |

**Egger's line** *See* **ligament of Wieger.**

**egocentre** A point of reference in the self usually located between the eyes. Absolute judgement of distances and visual directions of objects fixated binocularly are referred to the egocentre.
*See* **localization; oculocentre.**

**egocentric localization** *See* **localization.**

**Ehlers–Danlos syndrome** *See* syndrome, Ehlers–Danlos.

**eidetic image** *See* **image, eidetic.**

**eikonometer** Instrument for measuring aniseikonia. The **direct comparison eikonometer** (or **standard eikonometer**) uses as a target a cross with a small white disc at the centre of a black square at its intersection (Fig. E2). Four pairs of opposing arrows are placed four degrees away from the centre of the cross with the even numbered arrows polarized in one direction and the odd numbered ones in the other direction. The subject wears polarizing lenses so that each set of

four arrows is seen by one eye. If the subject has aniseikonia, one set of arrows will not appear aligned with the other. Aniseikonia either in one or more meridians can be measured by means of an adjustable magnifying device before one eye. There is also a **space eikonometer** in which the parts of the target are seen three-dimensionally in space. An office model of this type has been manufactured. The space eikonometer is based on a modification of stereopsis. Aniseikonia will make the target appear tilted. The amount of aniseikonia is indicated by the power of the size lens that swings the target back into a frontoparallel plane. *Syn.* aniseikonometer.
*See* **aniseikonia; lens, aniseikonic; plane, frontoparallel.**

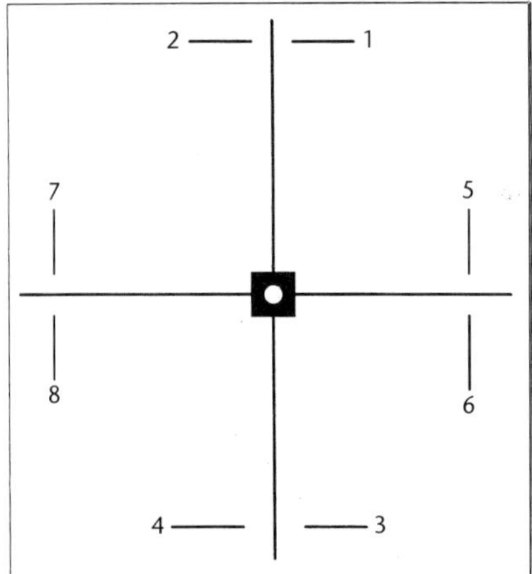


**Fig. E2** Target of the direct comparison eikonometer

**electrodiagnostic procedures** Methods such as the electroretinogram, the electro-oculogram and the visually evoked cortical potentials which are used to facilitate the diagnosis of some ocular diseases (e.g. retinitis pigmentosa) or the objective measurement of some visual functions (e.g. refractive error, visual acuity).
*See* **electro-oculogram; electroretinogram; potential, visual evoked cortical.**

**electroluminescence** *See* **luminescence.**

**electromagnetic spectrum** *See* **spectrum, electromagnetic.**

**electromyogram (EMG)** Recording of electrical activity of a muscle associated with contraction and relaxation. This is obtained by placing a microelectrode within a muscle. The recording process is called **electromyography.**
*See* **law of reciprocal innervation, Sherrington's.**

**electro-oculogram (EOG)** Recording of eye movements and eye position provided by the difference in electrical potential between two electrodes placed on the skin on either side of the eye. The EOG consists of two potentials: the **standing** or **resting potential** (or **dark phase**) which is evoked by moving the eyes in the dark and originates from the retinal pigment epithelium and the **light potential** (or **light rise**) which is evoked by moving the eyes in a lighted environment and originates from the photoreceptors. Clinically, the ratio between the light and dark potentials (sometimes also called the **Arden index** or **Arden ratio**) is assessed. If that ratio is less than 1.8 it indicates a malfunction of the structures from which the potential originates.

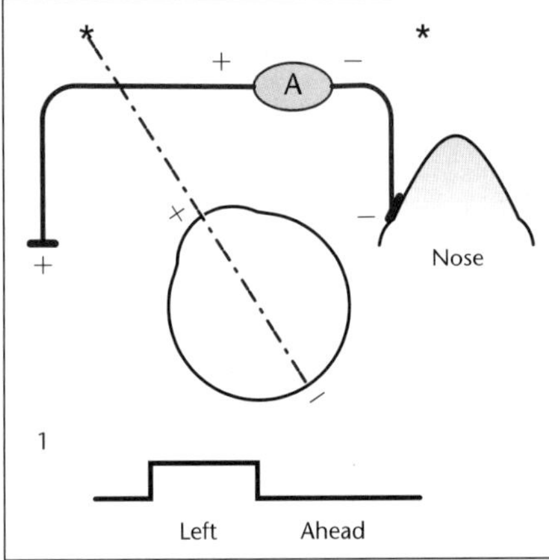


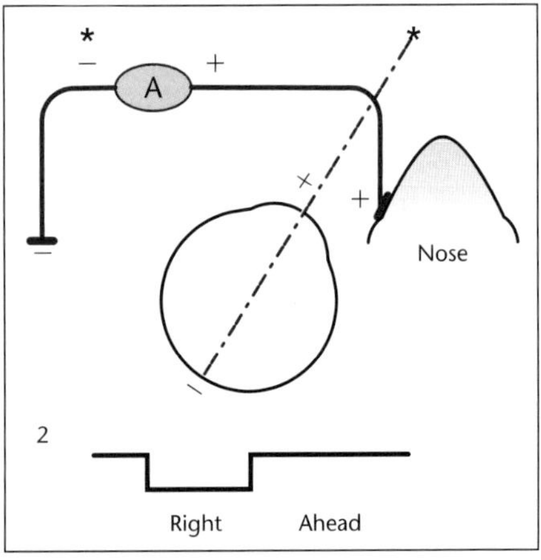


**Fig. E3** Principle of electro-oculography. The eye acts as a dipole in which the anterior pole is positive and the posterior pole is negative. 1. Left gaze; the cornea approaches the electrode near the outer canthus resulting in a positive-going change in the potential difference recorded from it. 2. Right gaze; the cornea approaches the electrode near the inner canthus resulting in a positive-going change in the potential difference recorded from it (A, an AC/DC amplifier). Below each diagram is a typical tracing displayed by a pen recorder

The EOG is also used to monitor eye movements (Fig. E3).
*See* **disease, Best's; fundus flavimaculatus; potential of the eye, resting.**

**electroretinogram (ERG)** Recording of mass electrical response of the retina when it is stimulated by light. It is recorded by placing an electrode in contact with the cornea (often with the aid of a contact lens) or around the eye under the eyelid. A second electrode is placed either on the forehead or the face. The response is complex as many cells of various types contribute to it and varies according to whether the eye is dark or light adapted, the colour of the stimulus, the health of the retina, etc. The curve consists of two major components: a negative a-wave and a positive b-wave. The a-wave originates in the photoreceptors while the b-wave originates in the bipolar and Mueller cells. Both waves also have a photopic and a scotopic component.
pERG indicates that this potential is pattern-elicited. The ERG and pERG are useful indicators of the health of all the layers of the retina and can differentiate between the functioning of the rods and cones.
*See* **alternating checkerboard stimulus; Leber's congenital amaurosis; potential, early receptor; potentials, oscillatory; retinitis pigmentosa.**

**electroretinography, multifocal (mfERG)** Simultaneous recording of the electroretinogram from small retinal areas (e.g. 103 hexagonal areas in the central 50 degrees of the retina) which are independently light stimulated according to a binary m-sequence (e.g. a random reversal at 75 Hz). This method enables evaluation of specific regions of the retina (e.g. macular degeneration) and mainly of the cone pathway.

**elephantiasis oculi** **1.** Enlargement of the eyelids due to lymphatic obstruction. *Syn.* elephantiasis palpebral. **2.** Extreme exophthalmos.
*See* **exophthalmos.**

**elephantiasis palpebral** *See* **elephantiasis oculi.**

**elevation of the eye** Upward rotation of an eye. It is accomplished by the superior rectus, inferior oblique, lateral rectus (very slightly) and medial rectus (very slightly) muscles. It can be produced voluntarily or by using base-down prisms. *Syn.* supraduction; sursumduction.
*See* **depression.**

**elevator** An extraocular muscle involved in rotating the eye upward such as the superior rectus and inferior oblique muscles.

**ellipse, Tscherning** A graphical representation of the front surface power as a function of total lens power in best-form lenses. There are two possible solutions: (1) Those lenses which are the least curved and represented by the lower portion of the Tscherning ellipse. This portion is called the **Oswalt branch** of the ellipse. (2) Those lenses which are most curved and represented by the upper portion of the ellipse. This latter portion is called the **Wollaston branch** of the ellipse.
*See* **lens, best-form.**

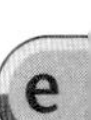

**ellipsoid** **1.** The refractile outer portion of the inner member of a rod or cone cell. It is located between the myoid and the outer member of the cell, and contains mitochondria. The **myoid** is in contact with the external limiting membrane of the retina while the outer member is next to the pigment epithelium. **2.** Surface of revolution generated by rotating an ellipse about a major or minor axis.
*See* **cell, cone; cell, rod.**

**Elschnig's spots** *See* **spots, Elschnig's.**

**embolism, retinal** Obstruction of a retinal artery or arteriole by a clot (embolus) which may result in atrophy or blindness in the area of the retina affected.
*See* **retinal arterial occlusion.**

**embryotoxon, anterior** *See* **arcus, corneal.**

**embryotoxon, posterior** A condition in which a thickened and anteriorly displaced Schwalbe's line is visible on external examination. The condition is inherited as an autosomal dominant trait and is usually not associated with any other ocular abnormality.
*See* **gonioscopy; ring of Schwalbe, anterior limiting.**

**emedastine** *See* **antihistamine.**

**Emmert's law** *See* **law, Emmert's.**

**emmetrope** One who has emmetropia.

**emmetropia** The refractive state of the eye in which, with accommodation relaxed, the conjugate focus of the retina is at infinity. Thus, the retina lies in the plane of the posterior principal focus of the eye and distant objects are sharply focused on the retina. This is the ideal refractive state of the eye. *Note*: the concept of emmetropia is not simple because accommodation is not inactive when fixating at distance (tonic accommodation). In fact, some authors consider hypermetropia of up to 1.00 D, in a pre-presbyope, as emmetropia.
*See* **accommodation, resting state of; ametropia; distances, conjugate.**

**emmetropization** A process that is presumed to operate to produce a greater frequency of emmetropic eyes than would otherwise occur on the basis of chance. This mechanism would coordinate the development of the various components of the optical system of the eye (e.g.

axial length, refracting power of the cornea, depth of the anterior chamber, etc.) to prevent ametropia.
*See* **ametropia.**

**emmetropization theory** *See* **theory, emmetropization.**

**empirical horopter** *See* **horopter, empirical.**

e

**empiricism** The belief that knowledge or behaviour stems from experience, learning or data acquired by observation or experimentation.
*See* **nativism; theory, empiricist.**

**empiricist theory** *See* **theory, empiricist.**

**Emsley's reduced eye** *See* **eye, reduced.**

**endophthalmitis** Inflammation of the intraocular structures. It can occur after a penetrating wound of the eye (either surgical or accidental), bacterial infection, or intraocular foreign bodies.
*See* **panophthalmitis; vitrectomy.**

**endoscope** Instrument designed to examine cavities which are not accessible for direct examination with the eye. It usually incorporates fibre optics to increase the flexibility of the instrument. *Examples*: a laryngoscope which is introduced through the mouth to examine the larynx; an ophthalmic endoscope to examine the intraocular structures by inserting a fibre optics system through the sclera, as may be used in ocular surgery.
*See* **optics, fibre.**

**endothelial bedewing; blebs** *See* under the nouns.

**endothelial corneal dystrophy** *See* **cornea guttata; dystrophy, Fuchs' endothelial; dystrophy, posterior polymorphous.**

**endothelial polymegethism; polymorphism** *See* under the nouns.

**enhancement, brightness** An increase in brightness resulting either from making a stimulus intermittent, or when a surface is surrounded by a dark area, as compared to when it is surrounded by a light area.
*See* **contrast; effect, Brücke–Bartley.**

**enophthalmos** Recession of the eyeball into the orbit. It is caused by a degeneration and shrinking of the orbital fat, a tumour, or an injury to the orbit or to shortening of the extraocular muscles following excessive resections.
*See* **entropion; exophthalmometer; exophthalmos; resection.**

**entoptic image** *See* **image, entoptic.**

**entoptoscope, blue field** An instrument enabling the visualization, especially by patients with a dense cataract, of the shadows of leucocytes flowing in the retinal capillaries and therefore providing a test of macular function. It consists of a very bright light source, an interference filter with a maximum transmission in the blue end of the spectrum, and a diffuser. The instrument is held close to the eye of the patient who is asked to describe his or her observations. The leucocytes appear as flying corpuscles and if many corpuscles (at least 15) are seen moving in the entire field the test is considered positive whereas if none or only a few corpuscles are seen the test is considered negative. Positive responses usually indicate that the patient has good macular function and negative responses usually indicate that the patient has poor macular function. This test is very useful in predicting central vision before cataract extraction.
*See* **angioscotoma; cataract extraction; image, entoptic; maxwellian view system, clinical.**

**entrance pupil** *See* **pupil, entrance.**

**entropion** Inward turning of the eyelid. It results in the eyelashes rubbing the cornea (as in trichiasis) and this usually causes discomfort. The most common cause of entropion which occurs in old people (called **involutional entropion**) and only affects the lower eyelid is due to a combination of atrophy and weakening of the tarsus, loss of tone of the subcutaneous tissues and loss of elasticity of the skin. Other causes are scarring (e.g. trachoma), or burns of the palpebral conjunctiva (called **cicatricial entropion**) which may affect either the upper or the lower eyelid, or spasm of the orbicularis muscle which may subside spontaneously once the original cause has been removed. Temporary relief of entropion may be provided by the taping of the lower eyelid to the cheek but the treatment is usually surgical.
*See* **ectropion; lens, therapeutic soft contact; spectacles, orthopaedic; tarsus; trichiasis.**

**entropion, cicatricial; involutional** *See* **entropion.**

**enucleation** Removal of an eye from its socket. It is usually performed to reduce pain in a blind eye, when there is a risk of sympathetic ophthalmia, or a malignant tumour in the eye.
*See* **epithelioma; evisceration; eye, artificial; melanoma, choroidal; ophthalmia, sympathetic.**

**enzyme** A protein substance which catalyses (i.e. enhances a chemical reaction in other bodies without undergoing a change in itself) and is formed by living cells but can act independently of their presence. *Example*: Enzyme preparations used to break down tear proteins which become attached to the surface of contact lenses.
*See* **conjunctivitis, giant papillary; deposits, contact lens; surfactant; wetting solution.**

**ephedrine hydrochloride** *See* **mydriatic.**

**epiblepharon** A congenital anomaly in which a fold of skin lies across the upper or lower lid margin. In the lower eyelid it causes a turning inward of the eyelashes without causing entropion. The condition commonly resolves itself with facial growth.
*See* **blepharochalasis; entropion.**

**epibulbar** Situated on the eyeball. *Syn.* epiocular.

**epicanthus** A condition in which a fold of skin that stretches from the upper to the lower eyelid partially covers the inner canthus. It is normal in the fetus, in Down's syndrome and in many infants, especially of oriental origin, where it may give the impression of a convergent strabismus (**pseudoesotropia**). The condition is normally bilateral. As the bridge of the nose develops, the folds eventually disappear. *Syn.* epicanthal fold.
*See* **ptosis; strabismus, apparent.**

**epicanthus inversus** A condition in which a fold of skin that stretches from the lower eyelid upward and toward the nose partially covers the inner canthus. It is often associated with ptosis.

**epichoroid** Synonym of suprachoroid.
*See* **sclera.**

**epidemiology** A branch of health science that deals with the incidence, distribution and aetiology of disease in a population.
*See* **aetiology.**

**epidiascope** A projector used to project by reflection opaque pictures (such as the page of a book) onto a screen.

**epikeratophakia** *See* **epikeratoplasty.**

**epikeratoplasty** A surgical procedure on the cornea aimed at curing ametropia. The patient's corneal epithelium is removed and a donor's corneal disc (or lenticule) which was previously frozen and reshaped to produce a new anterior curvature is rehydrated and sutured to Bowman's membrane. The lenticule can be removed and exchanged to provide a different power. There are many problems associated with this procedure, in particular the surface re-epithelialization. *Syn.* epikeratophakia; refractive keratoplasty and keratorefractive surgery (both terms also include keratomileusis, keratophakia and radial keratotomy).
*See* **Intacs; keratomileusis; keratophakia; keratotomy, radial; LASIK; lenticule.**

**epilation** The removal of hair by the roots as in the case of ingrowing eyelashes. The eyelashes are removed with forceps but, unfortunately, they tend to regrow.
*See* **distichiasis; eyelashes; trichiasis.**

**epinephrine** *See* **adrenaline (epinephrine).**

**epiocular** *See* **epibulbar.**

**epiphora** Overflow of tears due to faulty apposition of the lacrimal puncta in the lacrimal lake, scarring of the puncta, paresis of the orbicularis muscle, obstruction of the lacrimal passage or ectropion. This impairment of the outflow of tears is often unilateral. The main symptoms are discomfort and blurring of vision and sometimes embarrassment. Management depends on the cause. *Syn.* watery eye (colloquial).
*See* **dacryocystitis; dacryops; ectropion; hyperlacrimation; lacrimal apparatus; lacrimal lake; lacrimation.**

**epiretinal membrane** *See* **fibrosis, preretinal macular.**

**episclera** A loose connective and elastic tissue which covers the sclera and anteriorly connects the conjunctiva to it. It is a vascularized tissue whose deeper layers merge with the scleral stroma. It sends connective tissue bundles into Tenon's capsule. The episclera becomes progressively thinner towards the back of the eye.
*See* **episcleritis; sclera; Tenon's capsule.**

**episcleritis** Inflammation of the episclera. It is a benign, self-limiting, frequently recurring condition that typically affects adults. The disease is characterized by redness (usually in one quadrant of the globe) and varying degrees of discomfort. There are two types of episcleritis: **simple** which is the most common and **nodular** which is localized to one area of the globe forming a nodule. Simple episcleritis usually subsides spontaneously within 1–2 weeks while the nodular type usually takes longer. If the discomfort is intense topical corticosteroids may be used.
*See* **dellen; episclera; scleritis.**

**epithelial arcuate lesion; plug; splitting** *See* **staining, fluorescein.**

**epithelial downgrowth** Abnormal growth of epithelium into the interior of the eye, as a complication of a penetrating corneal injury and much more rarely following cataract extraction.

**epithelial keratitis** *See* **keratitis, punctate epithelial; keratitis, Thygeson's superficial punctate.**

**epithelial microcysts** *See* **microcysts, epithelial.**

**epithelioma** A tumour of epithelial cells, ranging from benign to malignant (e.g. carcinoma). *Example*: epithelioma of the conjunctival epithelium which begins near the limbus and spreads to the fornices and cornea. Treatment usually consists of excision, cryotherapy or both, or even enucleation if the tumour is very advanced.
*See* **carcinoma; enucleation.**

**equation, paraxial** *See* **paraxial equation, fundamental.**

**equator of the crystalline lens** The circle formed by the outer margin of the lens. The equator is not smooth, but shows a number of indentations corresponding to the zonular fibres. The indentations tend to disappear during accommodation, when the zonular fibres are loose.
*See* **lens, crystalline; Zinn, zonule of.**

e

**equatorial plane of the eye** *See* **plane, equatorial.**

**equivalent oxygen pressure** *See* **oxygen pressure, equivalent.**

**equivalent points** *See* **points, nodal.**

**equivalent power** *See* **power, equivalent.**

**equivalent, spherical** A spherical power whose focal point coincides with the circle of least confusion of a spherocylindrical lens. Hence, the spherical equivalent of a prescription is equal to the algebraic sum of the value of the sphere and half the cylindrical value, i.e. sphere + cylinder/2. *Example*: the spherical equivalent of the prescription –3 D sphere –2 D cylinder axis 180° is equal to –4 D.

**erector** A lens (for example an erecting eyepiece) or prism system (erecting prism such as a **Dove** or a **Porro prism**) placed in an optical system for the purpose of forming an erect image. *Syn.* erecting prism.
*See* **binoculars; image, erect; telescope, terrestrial.**

**error, cylindrical; spherical** *See* **prescription.**

**error of refraction of the eye** *See* **ametropia; refractive error.**

**erythema multiforme** A mucocutaneous disease that occurs as a hypersensitivity to drugs (e.g. sulfonamides) or as a consequence of infection. The condition which principally affects young people is characterized by the sudden appearance of various erosions of the mucous membranes and epidermis. A common complication is conjunctivitis which may become severe with cicatrization, abnormal lid margin function, symblepharon, corneal ulceration and vascularization and keratoconjunctivitis sicca. The patient complains of pain, discharge, photophobia and reduced vision if the cornea is involved. Treatment includes cleansing of the eyelids with antibiotic ointment and, if severe, topical steroids. *Syn.* Stevens–Johnson syndrome (although this term applies to the severe form of the disease).
*See* **conjunctivitis; keratitis sicca; symblepharon; syndrome, Stevens–Johnson.**

**erythrolabe** *See* **pigment, visual.**

**erythromycin** *See* **antibiotic.**

**erythrophobia** *See* **chromatophobia.**

**erythropsia** *See* **chromatopsia.**

**erythropsin** *See* **rhodopsin.**

**eserine** *See* **physostigmine.**

**eso deviation** Term referring to either esophoria or esotropia.
*See* **esophoria; strabismus, convergent.**

**esodisparity** Fixation disparity characterized by a slight overconvergence of the eyes, while still retaining single binocular vision.
*See* **disparity, retinal.**

**esophoria (E, ESOP, SOP, eso)** Turning of the eye inward from the active position when fusion is suspended. If symptomatic, treatment may be by means of base-out prisms, plus spherical lenses or visual training.
*See* **convergence excess; criterion, Percival; criterion, Sheard; divergence insufficiency; heterophoria; position, active.**

**esotropia** *See* **strabismus, convergent.**

**esotropia, blind spot** *See* **syndrome, Swann's.**

**esotropia, consecutive** *See* **strabismus, consecutive.**

**esotropia, infantile** *See* **strabismus, infantile.**

**esotropia, non-accommodative acquired** A form of ocular misalignment, in which the visual axes are convergent. This form of strabismus differs from other types in so much that it presents after normal ocular alignment has been established and is not related to a subject's accommodative effort. Although this technically includes nerve paresis, and other forms of acquired strabismus, the term is usually reserved for types of strabismus not due to an identifiable systemic cause. Examples of non-accommodative acquired esotropia include cyclic esotropia and stress-induced esotropia.

**esthesiometer** *See* **aesthesiometer.**

**ethmoid bone** *See* **orbit; sinus, ethomoidal.**

**ethylenediamine tetraacetic acid (EDTA)** A chelating agent used in ophthalmic preparations to remove metals which are essential for the metabolism of bacteria and viruses, and therefore inactivate them. It enhances the bactericidal effect of preservatives and is commonly combined with benzalkonium chloride, chlorhexidine and thiomersalate.
*See* **antiseptic.**

**etiology** *See* **aetiology.**

**euchromatopsia** Normal perception of colours. *Syn.* euchromatopsy
*See* **chromatopsia.**

**euryopia** Abnormally wide palpebral aperture.

**euthyroid** *See* **disease, Graves'.**

**Euthyscope** *See* **Visuscope.**

**eversion, lid** Turning of the eyelid inside out so as to expose the palpebral conjunctiva. For the upper lid this is accomplished by grasping the lid by the central eyelashes, pulling it downward and forward and then folding it back over a cotton applicator (or thin plastic rod) placed at the upper margin of the tarsus, while the patient continually maintains downward fixation. Return to the normal lid position is obtained by asking the patient to look up and gently pushing the eyelashes in an outward and downward direction. Foreign bodies and even contact lenses are often lodged under the upper eyelid or in the conjunctival fornix of the upper eyelid. To inspect the superior conjunctival fornix **double lid eversion** is necessary. Following lid eversion (and usually with local anaesthesia of the conjunctiva), a retractor is placed between the two skin surfaces of the lid with the retractor engaging the tarsus and, after gently pulling outward and upward, the fornix will become visible. Eversion of the lower lid is performed easily by drawing the margin downward while the patient looks upward.
*See* **eyelids; irrigation; sulcus, subtarsal.**

**evisceration** Removal of the inner contents of the eye with the exception of the sclera. It is usually performed when there is intraocular suppuration.
*See* **enucleation.**

**evoked potential** *See* **potential, visual evoked cortical.**

**excavation, physiological** *See* **cup, physiological.**

**excimer laser** *See* **laser, excimer.**

**excyclophoria** *See* **cyclophoria.**

**excyclovergence** Rotary movements about their respective anteroposterior axes of one eye relative to the other. If the upper pole of the cornea of one eye moves away from that of the other eye, it is called **excyclovergence**. If, however, the upper pole of the cornea of one eye moves towards that of the other eye, it is called **incyclovergence.**
*See* **vergence.**

**exenteration** Removal of the entire contents of the orbit, including the eyeball, the extraocular muscles, the optic nerve, nerves and blood vessels, the orbital fat and connective tissues. It is performed in cases of malignant tumours.
*See* **enucleation; evisceration.**

**exfoliation of the lens** Shedding of the layers of the lens capsule. It often occurs as a result of exposure to prolonged and intense heat.
*See* **cataract, heat-ray; pseudoexfoliation.**

**exit pupil** *See* **pupil, exit.**

**exo deviation** Term referring to either exophoria or exotropia.
*See* **exophoria; strabismus, divergent.**

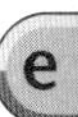

**exodisparity** Fixation disparity characterized by a slight underconvergence of the eyes, while still retaining single binocular vision.
*See* **disparity, retinal.**

**exophoria (X, XOP, exo)** Turning of the eye outward from the active position when fusion is suspended. If symptomatic, treatment may be by means of base-in prisms, minus spherical lenses or visual training.
*See* **convergence insufficiency; criterion, Percival; criterion, Sheard; divergence excess; heterophoria; position, active.**

**exophoria, physiological** The relative exophoria at near, when the heterophoria in near vision is compared to the heterophoria in distance vision. It is, on average, of the order of 3–4 Δ at a fixation distance of 40 cm. *Example*: if distance heterophoria is 6 Δ eso and near heterophoria is 2 Δ eso, the physiological exophoria is 4 Δ exo.

**exophthalmic goitre** *See* **disease, Graves'.**

**exophthalmometer** Instrument for measuring the amount of exophthalmos (or enophthalmos). There are several types, the most common being the **Hertel exophthalmometer**: it measures the distance between the corneal apex and the apex of the deepest angle of the lateral orbital margin of both eyes simultaneously, using either mirrors or prisms and a superimposed millimetre scale. The average distance for normal eyes is about 16 mm.
*See* **enophthalmos; exophthalmos.**

**exophthalmos** Abnormal protrusion of the eyeball(s) from the orbit, caused by exophthalmic goitre, endocrine malfunction, paralysis of the extraocular muscles, injury of the orbit, cavernous sinus thrombosis or a tumour behind the eye. The palpebral fissure is usually wider and a rim of sclera may be visible above and below the cornea. Unilateral displacement is usually referred to as **proptosis.**
*See* **aperture, palpebral; diplopia, pathological; disease, Graves'; elephantiasis oculi; enophthalmos; exophthalmometer.**

**exotropia** *See* **strabismus, divergent.**

**exotropia, consecutive** *See* **strabismus, consecutive.**

**exotropia, paralytic pontine** *See* **syndrome, 'one and one half'.**

**experiment, Bidwell's** Experiment aimed at producing the complement of a colour stimulus by viewing it through a rotating disc which presents the sequence: black, colour stimulus and white. *See* **colour, complementary.**

**experiment, Scheiner's** A demonstration of the refractive changes occurring in the eye when accommodating. The subject observes a target monocularly (such as a simple point of light) through a **Scheiner disc** (an opaque disc with two pinholes separated by a distance less than the pupil diameter). It will be seen singly at only one distance where the eye is focused, because target and retina are then conjugate. If the eye accommodates, two points of light are seen. The principle of this experiment is incorporated in several refractometers.
*See* **disc, Scheiner's; distances, conjugate; optometer, infrared; optometer, Young's.**

**experiment, Young's** Method of producing interference of light which was shown by Young in 1801. He used two coherent beams of light that were produced by passing light through a very small circular aperture in one screen, then through two small circular apertures very close together in a second screen. On a third screen, behind the second screen, there will be two overlapping sets of waves and, if the original source is emitting monochromatic light, interference fringes will appear on the third screen (Fig. E4).
*See* **coherent sources; interference fringes.**

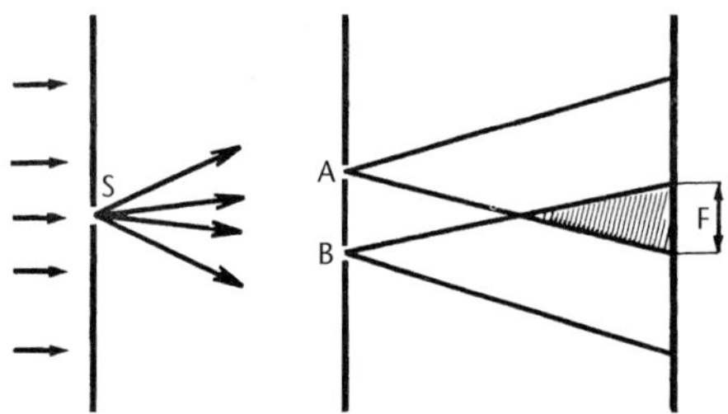


Fig. E4 Young's experiment (S, source of light (illuminated pinhole); A and B, pinholes; F, circular interference fringes)

**exposure keratitis** *See* **keratitis, exposure.**

**exposure meter** Light measuring instrument for ascertaining the setting (lens aperture, shutter speed, etc.) of a camera for correct light exposure of the photographic material (CIE).

**extended object; source; wear lens** *See* under the nouns.

**external hordeolum; limiting membrane; ophthalmoplegia** *See* under the nouns.

**extinction phenomenon** *See* **phenomenon, extinction.**

**extorsion** *See* **torsion.**

**extraction, cataract** *See* **cataract extraction; phacoemulsification.**

**extraocular muscles** *See* **muscles, extraocular.**

**extrinsic muscles** *See* **muscles, extraocular.**

**exudate** A liquid or semisolid which has been discharged through the tissues to the surface or into a cavity. Exudates in the retina are opacities which result from the escape of plasma and white blood cells from defective blood vessels. They usually look greyish white or yellowish and are circular or ovoid in shape. They are sometimes classified into three groups according to size: (1) **punctate hard** exudates which often tend to coalesce; (2) exudates of moderate size, such as '**cotton-wool** or **soft** exudates' as, for example, in hypertension or in diabetic retinopathy. These 'exudates' have ill-defined margins and are actually areas of ischaemia containing cytoid bodies, unlike hard exudates which are generally lipid deposits; (3) larger exudates, as found in the severe forms of retinopathy.
*See* **retinopathy, diabetic; retinopathy, hypertensive.**

**exudative retinitis** *See* **disease, Coats'.**

**eye** The peripheral organ of vision, in which an optical image of the external world is produced and transformed into nerve impulses. It is a spheroidal body approximately 24 mm in diameter with the segment of a smaller sphere (of about 8 mm radius), the cornea, in front. It consists of an external coat of fibrous tissue, the sclera and transparent cornea; a middle vascular coat, comprising the iris, the ciliary body and the choroid; and an internal coat, the retina, which includes the cones and rods photoreceptors. Within the eye, there are the aqueous humour located between the cornea and the crystalline lens, the crystalline lens held by the zonule of Zinn and the vitreous body located between the crystalline lens and the retina. The movements of the eye are directed by six extraocular muscles (Fig. E5). *Syn.* organ of sight; visual organ.

**eye, amaurotic** *See* **amaurosis.**

**eye, amblyopic** An eye which has amblyopia. *Syn.* lazy eye (colloquial).
*See* **amblyopia.**

**eye, aphakic** An eye without the crystalline lens.
*See* **aphakia.**

**eye, artificial** A prosthesis made of glass or plastic which resembles the eye and which is placed in the socket after enucleation.
*See* **ocularist; prosthesis, ocular.**

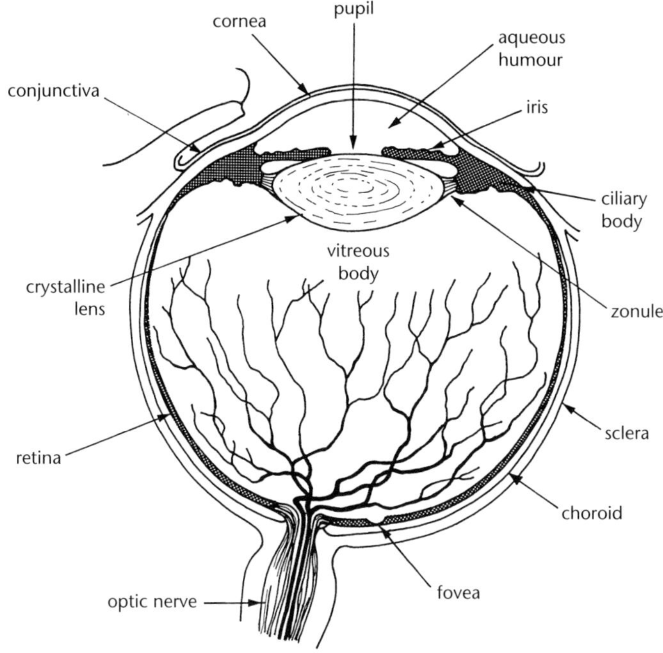


**Fig. E5** Cross-section of the eye

**eye, axial length of the** *See* **length of the eye, axial.**

**eye bank** An organization that collects, evaluates, stores and distributes eyes from donors. The eyes are used for corneal transplants and research.
*See* **keratoplasty.**

**eye, black** A colloquial term for a swollen or blue-black spot on the skin of the eyelid caused by effusion of blood as a result of a superficial injury in which the skin is not broken. The correct term is **ecchymosis** of the eyelid. The condition recovers by itself within 2–3 weeks while changing in colour to yellow. Immediately after the injury, application of ice helps minimize the haemorrhage and swelling.
*See* **haematoma.**

**eye, bleary** A red and watery eye, with a lacklustre appearance. Lack of sleep is a common cause. *Syn.* blear eye.

**eye blink** *See* **blink.**

**eye, compound** The eye of arthropods composed of a variable number of ommatidia.
*See* **facet, corneal; ommatidium.**

**eyes, crossed** *See* **strabismus, convergent.**

**eye, cyclopean** Imaginary eye located at a point midway between the two eyes. When the two visual fields overlap and the impressions from the two eyes are combined into a single impression, the apparent direction of a fixated object appears in a direction which emanates from the cyclopean eye.

**eye, dark-adapted** An eye that has been in darkness and is sensitive to low illumination. *Syn.* scotopic eye.
*See* **adaptation, dark; theory, duplicity.**

**eye, deviating** The non-fixating eye in strabismus or under heterophoria testing. *Syn.* squinting eye.
*See* **eye, fixating; heterophoria; strabismus.**

**eye, dominant** The eye that is dominant when ocular dominance exists.
*See* **dominance, ocular; manoptoscope; monovision; test, hole in the card.**

**eye, dry** An eye in which there is a minimum of moisture which causes damage to the interpalpebral ocular surface. It may result from tear deficiency, excessive tear evaporation, meibomian gland dysfunction, abnormal blink reflex, damage to the conjunctival or corneal surface or lacrimal apparatus, soft contact lens wear, Sjögren's syndrome, menopause, etc. Symptoms are irritation, foreign body sensation and sometimes transient blurring of vision. It often leads to keratitis sicca. Management consists mainly of artificial tears and frequent blinking exercises.

*See* **glands, meibomian; keratitis sicca; mucin; syndrome, Sjögren's; syndrome, Stevens–Johnson; tear meniscus; tears; tears, artificial; test, break-up time; test, Norn's; test, phenol red cotton thread; test, Schirmer's; xerophthalmia.**

**eye, equatorial plane of the** *See* **plane, equatorial.**

**eye, exciting** *See* **ophthalmia, sympathetic.**

**eye, fixating** The eye which is directed towards the object of regard in strabismus.
*See* **eye, deviating; strabismus.**

**eye, glass** An artificial eye made of glass.
*See* **eye, artificial; ocularist; prosthesis, ocular.**

**eye impression** *See* **impression, eye.**

**eye, lazy** *See* **eye, amblyopic.**

**eye lens** *See* **eyepiece.**

**eye, light-adapted** An eye which has been exposed to light and is insensitive to low illumination. *Syn.* photopic eye.
*See* **adaptation, light; theory, duplicity.**

**eye movements** *See* **movements, eye.**

**eye patch** A piece of material or plastic which is worn over the eye when it has been injured or over the socket when it is missing.

**eye, phakic** An eye which contains the crystalline lens.
*See* **phakic.**

**eye, photopic** *See* **eye, light-adapted.**

**eye, pink** *See* **conjunctivitis, contagious.**

**eye, pseudophakic** An eye fitted with an intraocular lens implant.
*See* **implant, intraocular lens.**

**eye, red** A colloquial term often used for any condition in which the blood vessels of the conjunctiva or ciliary body are congested. Many conditions result in a red eye (e.g. subconjunctival haemorrhage, pterygium, conjunctivitis, episcleritis, ulcerative keratitis, corneal dendritic ulcer, acute iritis, angle-closure glaucoma, orbital cellulitis, and possibly contact lens wear).
*See* **injection, ciliary; injection, conjunctival.**

**eye, reduced** A mathematical model of the optical system of the eye. It consists of a single refracting surface with one nodal point, one principal point and one index of refraction. In the first such model, proposed by **Listing** in 1853, the refracting surface had a power of 68.3 D and was situated 2.34 mm behind the schematic eye's cornea. It had an index of refraction of 1.35, a radius of curvature of 5.124 mm and a length of 20 mm. **Donders'** reduced eye was even more simplified. It has a power of 66.7 D, a radius of curvature of 5 mm, an index of refraction of 4/3 and anterior and posterior focal lengths of – 15 and 20 mm, respectively, with a refracting surface situated 2 mm behind the schematic eye's cornea. **Gullstrand's** reduced eye has a radius of curvature of 5.7 mm, an index of refraction of 1.33, a power of 61 D with the refracting surface situated 1.35 mm behind the schematic eye's cornea. **Emsley's** reduced eye has a power of 60 D, an index of refraction of 4/3 and is situated 1.66 mm behind the schematic eye's cornea, with anterior and posterior focal lengths of – 16.67 and 22.22 mm, respectively.
*See* **ultrasonography.**

**eye, schematic** A model consisting of various spherical surfaces representing the optical system of a normal eye based on the average dimensions (called the **constants of the eye**) of the human eye. There are many schematic eyes, although the most commonly used is that of Gullstrand. A great deal of variation among authors stemmed from the difficulty in giving an index of refraction which would represent the heterogeneous character of the crystalline lens. Gullstrand in fact proposed two schematic eyes, one which he called the **exact schematic eye** and the other which he called the **simplified schematic eye** in which the divergent effect of the posterior corneal surface is ignored and the cornea replaced by an equivalent surface; the crystalline lens is homogeneous and the optical system is free from aberrations.
*See* **constants of the eye; ultrasonography.**

**eye, scotopic** *See* **eye, dark-adapted.**

**eye shield** **1.** *See* **occluder**. **2.** A protective device to cover the eye against injury, glare or in radiotherapy of the face.

**eye, sighting-dominant** The eye which is preferred in monocular tasks, such as looking through a telescope or aiming a firearm.

**eye socket** The bony orbit which contains the eyeball, the muscles, the nerves, the vessels, the orbital fat and the orbital portion of the lacrimal gland.

**eye speculum** An instrument designed to hold the eyelids apart during surgery. *Syn.* blepharostat.

**eye, squinting** *See* **eye, deviating.**

**eye stone** A small, smooth shell or other object that can be inserted beneath the eyelid to facilitate the removal of a foreign body from the eye.

**eye, sympathetic** The uninjured eye in sympathetic ophthalmia which becomes secondarily affected. *Syn.* sympathizing eye.
*See* **ophthalmia, sympathetic.**

**eye, wall** A colloquial term referring to (1) a white opaque cornea or (2) a divergent strabismus.

**eye, watery** *See* **epiphora.**

**eyeball** The globe of the eye without its appendages. *See* **appendages of the eye; eye.**

**eyebrow** A transverse elevation covered with hairs and situated at the junction of the forehead and upper lid. *Syn.* supercilium.
*See* **ophryosis.**

**eyecup** A small vessel made of glass, plastic or porcelain, used to bathe the eye.

**eyeglass 1.** Synonym for monocle. In the plural (**eyeglasses**) it refers to pince-nez or a similar type of eyewear without sides, or to spectacles. **2.** The eyepiece of an optical instrument.
*See* **eyepiece; spectacles.**

**eyelashes** Rows of stiff hairs (cilia) growing on the margin of the upper and lower eyelids. The upper eyelashes are longer and more numerous and curl upward, while the lower ones turn downward. *Syn.* cilia; lashes.
*See* **distichiasis; epilation; madarosis; polystichia; trichiasis.**

**eyelid eversion** *See* **eversion, lid.**

**eyelid twitch** *See* **ciliosis; myasthenia gravis; myokymia.**

**eyelids** A pair of movable folds of skin which act as protective coverings of the eye. The upper eyelid extends downward from the eyebrow. It is the more moveable of the two, due to the action of a levator palpebrae muscle. When the eye is open and looking staight ahead, it just covers the upper part of the cornea; when it is closed, it covers the whole cornea. The lower eyelid reaches just below the cornea when the eye is open and rises only slightly when it shuts. Each eyelid consists of the following layers, starting anteriorly: (1) the skin, (2) a layer of subcutaneous connective tissue, (3) a layer of striated muscle, (4) the submuscular connective tissue, (5) the fibrous layer, including the tarsal plates, (6) a layer of smooth muscle, (7) the palpebral conjunctiva. *Syn.* blephara; lids; palpebrae.
*See* **ablephary; blepharitis; ciliosis; ectropion; entropion; epicanthus; eversion, lid; eye, black; hordeolum; lagophthalmos; ligament, palpebral; muscle, orbicularis; myokymia; phthiriasis; sign, Cogan's lid twitch; sulcus, inferior palpebral; sulcus, superior palpebral; tarsorrhaphy; tarsus; xanthelasma.**

**eyepiece** The lens or combination of lenses in an optical instrument (microscope, telescope, etc.) through which the observer views the image formed by the objective. The most common eyepieces are composed of two single lenses or two doublets: the lens or doublet nearer the eye is called the **eye lens** and the one nearer the objective is called the **field lens**. The role of the eyepiece is to magnify the image and to reduce the aberrations of the image formed by the objective. *Syn.* eye lens; eyeglass; ocular.
*See* **doublet; microscope; objective; telescope.**

**eyepiece, Huygens'** Negative eyepiece used commonly in microscopes. It consists of two planoconvex lenses mounted with their plane surfaces facing the eye. In the most common type the eye lens has a focal length half that of the field lens and the separation is equal to half the sum of the two focal lengths.

**eyepiece, negative** Eyepiece made up of two lenses, in which the first principal focus of the eyepiece lies between the two lenses, such as in a Huygens' eyepiece.

**eyepiece, orthoscopic** An eyepiece corrected for distortion, and which provides a wide field of view and high magnification. It consists of a triplet field lens and a single eye lens. It is used in high-power telescopes and range finders.
*See* **triplet.**

**eyepiece, positive** Eyepiece made up of two lenses in which the first principal focus of the eyepiece lies in front of the field lens such as in a Ramsden eyepiece.

**eyepiece, Ramsden** Positive eyepiece consisting of two planoconvex lenses mounted with their convex side facing each other and having equal focal lengths. The lenses are usually separated by two-thirds the focal length of either.

**eyesight** Vision.

**eyesize** The horizontal dimension of the lens opening of a frame which is bounded by two vertical lines at a tangent to the left and right sides of the opening.
*See* **spectacle frame markings; spectacles.**

**eyestrain** *See* **asthenopia.**

**eyewash** Any liquid which is used for bathing the eye. *Example*: physiological saline.
*See* **saline, physiological.**

**eyewear** *See* **spectacles.**

**eyewire** The rim which surrounds the lens of a spectacle frame.

# F

**f number** Designation for a photographic lens which gives the ratio of the focal length to the diameter of the effective aperture or entrance pupil. *Example*: f/8 means that the lens has a focal length eight times the diameter of the entrance pupil. *Syn.* f/stop; f-value; focal ratio; lens speed. *See* **aperture, relative.**

**facet, corneal 1.** Small flattened depression on the outer surface of the cornea, due to a healed ulcer which has failed to fill with tissue. **2.** The corneal element in the ommatidium of the compound eye.
*See* **eye, compound; ulcer, corneal.**

**factor, absorption** Ratio of the absorbed luminous flux to the incident flux. *Syn.* absorbance.
*See* **absorption; density, optical.**

**factor, reflection** Ratio of the reflected luminous flux to the incident flux. There are the regular reflection factor and the diffuse reflection factor. The reflection factor is given by Fresnel's formula. *Symbol*: ρ. *Syn.* reflectance.
*See* **diffusion; Fresnel's formula; reflection.**

**factor, spectral transmission** *See* **spectrophotometer.**

**factor, transmission** *See* **transmittance.**

**facultative hypermetropia** *See* **hypermetropia, facultative.**

**Falant** *See* **test, lantern.**

**fallen eye syndrome** *See* **syndrome, fallen eye.**

**false macula** *See* **macula, false.**

**false negative** *See* **sensitivity.**

**false positive** *See* **specificity.**

**familial autonomic dysfunction** *See* **syndrome, Riley–Day.**

**fan and block test** *See* **test, fan and block.**

**fan chart** *See* **chart, astigmatic fan.**

**far point of accommodation** *See* **accommodation, far point of.**

**far point of convergence** *See* **convergence, far point of.**

**far point of the eye** *See* **accommodation, far point of.**

**far point sphere** *See* **sphere, far point.**

**far sight** *See* **hypermetropia.**

**Farnsworth–Munsell 100 Hue test** *See* **test, Farnsworth.**

**Farnsworth test** *See* **test, Farnsworth; test, lantern.**

**fascia** A sheet of connective tissue covering, partitioning or binding together muscles and certain other organs, such as the lacrimal sac, the orbital septum and other organs within the orbit, the sclera (e.g. Tenon's capsule), etc.
*See* **Tenon's capsule.**

**Table F1** Sequence of f numbers used in photography with the corresponding relative image brightness and exposure time to maintain constant film exposure. The relative image brightness is equal to the square of the f number fraction

| f number | focal length/ pupil diameter | exact f number | relative image brightness | relative exposure time |
|---|---|---|---|---|
| f/0.5 | 0.5 | f/0.500 | 1/0.25 | 0.12 |
| f/0.7 | 0.7 | f/0.707 | 1/0.5 | 0.25 |
| f/1 | 1 | f/1.000 | 1/1 | 0.5 |
| f/1.4 | 1.4 | f/1.414 | 1/2 | 1 |
| f/2 | 2 | f/2.000 | 1/4 | 2 |
| f/2.8 | 2.8 | f/2.828 | 1/8 | 4 |
| f/4 | 4 | f/4.000 | 1/16 | 8 |
| f/5.6 | 5.6 | f/5.657 | 1/32 | 16 |
| f/8 | 8 | f/8.000 | 1/64 | 32 |
| f/11 | 11 | f/11.314 | 1/128 | 64 |
| f/16 | 16 | f/16.000 | 1/256 | 128 |
| f/22 | 22 | f/22.627 | 1/512 | 256 |
| f/32 | 32 | f/32.000 | 1/1024 | 512 |

**fascia bulbi** *See* **Tenon's capsule.**

**fascia, palpebral** *See* **orbital septum.**

**fasciculus, medial longitudinal** One of a pair of nerve fibres, one on each side of the midline and extending from the upper midbrain to the cervical spinal cord. It is composed largely of ascending fibres from the vestibular nuclei ascending to the motor nuclei (third, fourth and sixth) and innervating the extraocular muscles; and to a lesser extent of descending fibres from the medial vestibular nuclei, the reticular formation, the superior colliculi and nucleus of Cajal innervating the musculature of the neck. *Syn.* medial longitudinal bundle; posterior longitudinal bundle.

**fast eye movements** *See* **movements, saccadic eye.**

**fat, orbital** Fat (e.g. adipose tissue) which fills all the space not occupied by the other structures of the orbit (eyeball, optic nerve, muscles, vessels, etc.). It extends from the optic nerve to the orbital wall and from the apex of the orbit to the septum orbitale.

**fatigue, visual** A feeling of weariness resulting from a visual task. It can be of ocular, muscular or psychic origin. However, there does not seem to be objective proof of a reduction in visual aptitude (e.g. visual acuity) accompanying visual fatigue.
*See* **asthenopia.**

**Fechner's law** *See* **law, Fechner's.**

**Fechner's paradox** Subjective impression of a decrease in the brightness of a field when viewing it binocularly, after one eye which was closed looks through a dark filter (about 5% transmission). This is paradoxical since more light is received by the eyes when the field is viewed binocularly, as compared to monocularly.

**felderstruktur muscle fibres** *See* **fibres, felderstruktur muscle.**

**fenestration** *See* **lens, fenestrated; lens, scleral contact.**

**Fermat's law** *See* **law, Fermat's.**

**Ferry–Porter law** *See* **law, Ferry–Porter.**

**fibre, Henle's** *See* **layer of Henle, fibre.**

**fibre optics** *See* **optics, fibre.**

**fibres, arcuate** Axons of the ganglion cells of the retina which are temporal to the optic disc and pass above and below the papillomacular bundle in an arcuate course. *Syn.* arcuate nerve fibres bundle.
*See* **fibres, papillomacular; raphe, retinal; scotoma, arcuate; scotoma, Bjerrum's.**

**fibres, cilio-equatorial; cilio-posterior capsular** *See* **Zinn, zonule of.**

**fibres, circular** *See* **muscle, ciliary.**

**fibres, felderstruktur muscle** A type of extraocular muscle fibre whose effect is to produce slow, and tonic contraction. They are mainly responsible for maintaining smooth pursuit movements. The fibres are located in the superficial portions of the extraocular muscle and are unique to this type of muscle.
*See* **muscles, extraocular.**

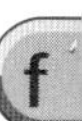

**fibres, fibrillenstruktur muscle** A type of extraocular muscle fibre whose effect is to produce fast and twitch type of contractions. They are mainly responsible for saccadic eye movements. The fibres are located deep within the extraocular muscle and are the type usually found in skeletal muscle.
*See* **muscles, extraocular.**

**fibres, lens** Long, six-sided bands containing few organelles and mostly lacking a nucleus, derived from epithelial cells just within the capsule of the crystalline lens and attached to an anterior and to a posterior suture.
*See* **capsule; suture, lens.**

**fibres, longitudinal** *See* **muscle, ciliary.**

**fibres, macular** *See* **fibres, papillomacular.**

**fibres, medullated nerve** *See* **fibres, myelinated nerve.**

**fibres, meridional** *See* **muscle, ciliary.**

**fibres of Mueller** *See* **cell, Mueller's.**

**fibres, myelinated nerve** Anomalous congenital extension onto the retina of the myelin sheaths covering the optic nerve fibres. This myelination beyond the lamina cribrosa normally disappears soon after birth. Ophthalmoscopically, it appears as whitish, striated feather-shaped patches which may or may not obscure retinal vessels. Vision in these areas may be reduced, although visual acuity is not affected as the patches are most frequently located adjacent to the optic disc and sometimes in the periphery. The most characteristic sign may be an enlargement of the blind spot. *Syn.* medullated nerve fibres; opaque nerve fibres.
*See* **blind spot; cribriform plate.**

**fibres, orbiculo-anterior capsular; orbiculo-posterior capsular** *See* **Zinn, zonule of.**

**fibres, papillomacular** Axons of the ganglion cells of the macular region of the retina which

enter the temporal portion of the optic disc and travel in the central region of the optic nerve. In the chiasma, the temporal macular fibres remain on the same side, while the nasal ones cross to the other side. These fibres make up the **papillomacular bundle** (Fig. F1).
*See* **chiasma, optic; retina.**

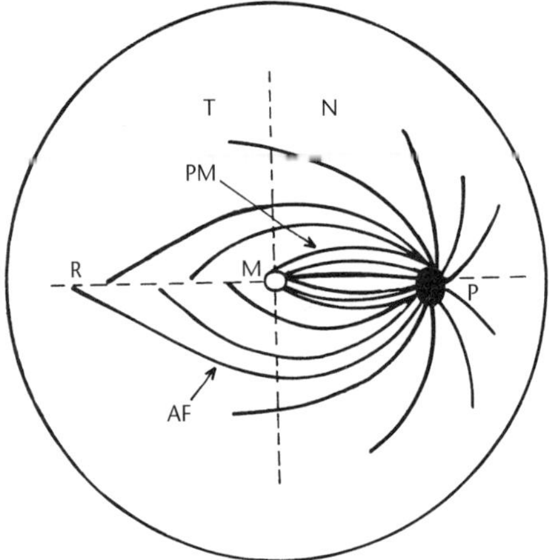


**Fig. F1** Diagram of the optic nerve fibres of the right eye seen from the front (M, macula; P, optic disc; R, retinal raphe; PM, papillomacular fibres; AF, arcuate fibres; T, temporal side; N, nasal side)

**fibres, pupillary** Axons of the optic nerve which branch off from the visual portion of the optic tract, before the lateral geniculate body, to run in the superior brachium towards the pretectal region anterior to the superior colliculus. They mediate the pupillary reflexes.
*See* **colliculi, superior; nerve, optic; reflex, pupil light; tectum of the mesencephalon; tracts, optic.**

**fibres, radial** *See* **muscle, ciliary.**

**fibres, visual** Axons from the ganglion cells of the retina, making up the optic nerves and optic tracts. They synapse in the lateral geniculate body and then project to the region of the calcarine fissure of the cortex conveying the nervous impulses associated with vision.
*See* **geniculate bodies, lateral; nerve, optic; tracts, optic.**

**fibres, zonular** *See* **Zinn, zonule of.**

**fibrillenstruktur muscle fibres** *See* **fibres, fibrillenstruktur muscle.**

**fibrinoplatelet** *See* **plaques, Hollenhorst's.**

**fibrocyte, corneal** *See* **corneal corpuscle.**

**fibroplasia, retrolental** *See* **retinopathy of prematurity.**

**fibrosis, preretinal macular** Proliferation of glial cells over the surface of the internal limiting membrane of the macular region of the retina. Ophthalmoscopically the retina presents a glinting reflex. The condition may occur after trauma, eye surgery, retinal vascular disease and inflammation and with any of the causes of retinitis proliferans and most commonly in elderly patients. Initially the patient is asymptomatic or reports some distortion of vision (metamorphopsia). This stage is often called **cellophane maculopathy**. As the condition develops, visual acuity diminishes, there is retinal wrinkling and the preretinal membrane becomes denser obscuring some retinal vessels in ophthalmoscopy. Some patients may also develop a macular hole and posterior vitreous detachment. If vision is significantly reduced the main treatment is by vitreous surgery with removal of the layer of preretinal proliferative tissue. *Syn.* epiretinal membrane; macular epiretinal membrane; macular pucker; premacular fibrosis; preretinal membrane; preretinal vitreous membrane; surface wrinkling retinopathy.
*See* **retinopathy, proliferative.**

**Fick, axes of** *See* **axes of Fick.**

**field, binocular visual** An approximately circular zone of radius about 60° centred on the point of fixation (slightly larger in the lower part of the field) in which an object stimulates both retinas simultaneously. Beyond that area on each side, the visual field is monocular.
*See* **field, visual.**

**field of excursion** *See* **field of fixation.**

**field of fixation** The area in space over which an eye can fixate when the head remains stationary. The field of fixation is smaller than the field of vision. It extends to approximately 47° temporally, 45° nasally, 43° upward and 50° downward. *Syn.* field of excursion; motor field.
*See* **field of view, apparent; field of view, real; field, visual.**

**field glasses** *See* **binoculars.**

**field, keyhole visual** A term used to describe a visual field defect in which there is a bilateral homonymous hemianopsia with macular sparing. An occipital lobe lesion sparing the posterior tips of the occipital lobe usually causes this lesion.
*See* **hemianopia, homonymous.**

**field lens** *See* **eyepiece.**

**field, motor** *See* **field of fixation.**

**field, receptive** The retinal area within which a light stimulus can produce a potential difference in a single ganglion cell. Retinal receptive

fields are circular, often with a response different in the centre than in the periphery (also referred to as on-centre/off-centre or centre/surround organization). Receptive fields also exist at other levels of the visual pathway all the way to the visual cortex where they have various shapes and sizes and may only respond to either a vertical bar or a black dot moving in a given direction and at a given speed, etc. Receptive fields reflect the interaction between excitation and inhibition between neighbouring neurons. The term can also describe the region of space that induces these neural responses.
*See* **cell, complex; cell, hypercomplex; cell, simple; inhibition, lateral; summation.**

**field stop** *See* **diaphragm.**

**field, surrounding** That area of the field of view surrounding any object.

**field of view** The extent of an object plane seen through an optical instrument.

**field of view, apparent** Angle subtended by the exit port of a sighting instrument or an empty frame aperture at the centre of the entrance pupil of the eye. *Syn.* apparent peripheral field of view. *Note*: when referring to the apparent field of fixation, the reference point is the centre of rotation of the eye. *Syn.* apparent macular field of view (Fig. F2).
*See* **field of fixation.**

**field of view, real** Angle subtended by the effective diameter of a lens at the point conjugate with the centre of the entrance pupil of the eye. *Syn.* real peripheral field of view; true field of view. *Note*: when referring to the real field of fixation, the reference point is the centre of rotation of the eye. *Syn.* real macular field of view (Fig. F2).
*See* **distances, conjugate; phenomenon, jack-in-the-box.**

**field of vision** *See* **field, visual.**

**field, visual (VF)** The extent of space in which objects are visible to an eye in a given position. The extent of the visual field tends to diminish with age. The visual field can be measured either monocularly or binocularly. In the latter case its extent is much larger, especially in the horizontal plane. *Syn.* field of vision.
*See* **eccentricity; field, binocular visual; hemianopsia; perimetry, kinetic; perimetry, static; test, confrontation; vision, low.**

**fifth cranial nerve** *See* **nerve, trigeminal.**

**figure** A part or pattern in the visual field which has the perceptual attribute of completeness and is perceived as distinct from the rest of the field which forms the ground. *Example*: a printed word against a background page.

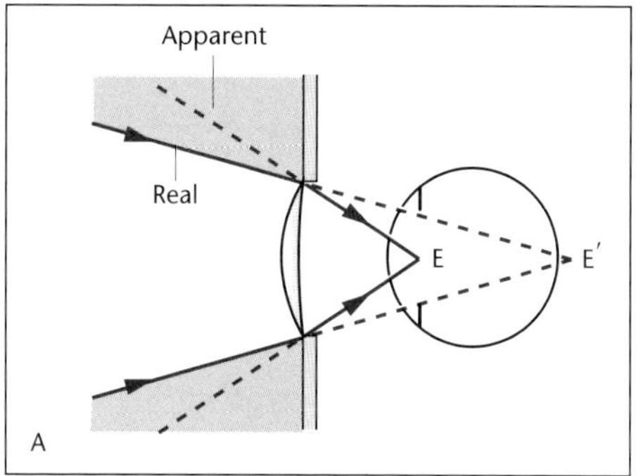


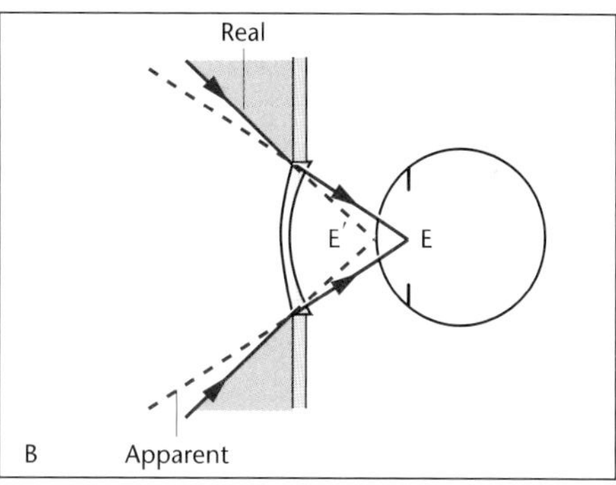


**Fig. F2** Apparent and real field of view seen through A, a converging lens, and B, a diverging lens, placed in a diaphragm. The apparent field of view is decreased by the converging lens and increased by the diverging lens (E, centre of the entrance pupil; E′, its image formed by the lens). The hatched area is not seen

**Table F2** Average extent of the normal visual field (in degrees) of one eye of a young adult looking in the straight ahead position, and measured with a white target subtending 1.0° under normal room illumination

| | |
|---|---|
| temporally | 94° |
| down and temporally | 88° |
| down | 70° |
| down and nasally | 54° |
| nasally | 60° |
| up and nasally | 56° |
| up | 54° |
| up and temporally | 64° |

**figure, ambiguous** *See* **cube, Necker; figure, Blivet; Schroeder's staircase; vase, Rubin's.**

**figure, Blivet** An 'impossible' figure in which three apparently solid tubes are attached at one end of a rectangular base which projects only two bars (Fig. F3).
*See* **Necker cube; Schroeder's staircase; vase, Rubin's.**

Fig. F3 Blivet figure

**figure, fortification** *See* **scotoma, scintillating.**

**figure, Kanisza** An ambiguous figure in which the illusory contour of a square (or triangle) appears in the middle of four (or three) truncated solid squares (or circles). It is an illustration of the perceptual ability to make sense of an incomplete figure. Some people cannot perceive the contour. *Syn.* Kanisza square (Fig. F4).

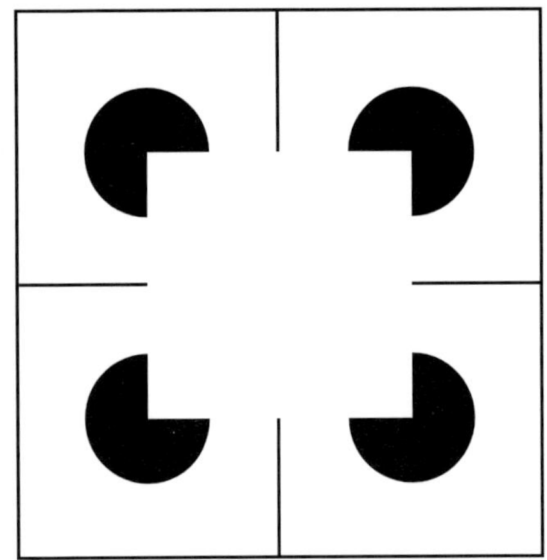

Fig. F4 Kanisza figure

**filamentary keratitis** *See* **keratitis, filamentary.**

**film, anti-reflection** *See* **anti-reflection coating.**

**film, precorneal** The field covering the anterior surface of the cornea which consists of lacrimal fluid and of the secretion of the meibomian and conjunctival glands. Its total thickness was thought to be about 9 μm but recent investigations have questioned that value and point to a much larger figure. It is composed of three layers: (1) The deepest and densest is the **mucin layer** (or **mucous layer**) which derives from the conjunctival goblet cells, as well as some secretion from the lacrimal gland. (2) The watery lacrimal fluid is the middle layer, called the **lacrimal** (or **aqueous layer**). It is secreted by the lacrimal gland and the accessory glands of Krause and Wolfring. It forms the bulk of the film and contains most of the bactericidal lysosyme and other proteins, inorganic salts, sugars, amino acids, urea, etc. (3) The **oily layer** (or **lipid layer**) is the most superficial and is derived principally from the meibomian glands in the lids as well as some secretion from the glands of Zeis. It greatly slows the evaporation of the watery layer and may provide a lubrication effect between lid and cornea (Fig. F5). *Note*: Recent research is pointing to a precorneal film made up of only two layers; an innermost aqueous and mucin gel layer and an outer lipid layer. *Syn.* lacrimal layer; preocular tear film; tear film; tear layer.
*See* **cell, goblet; gland, conjunctival; glands of Krause; gland, lacrimal; glands, meibomian; glands of Wolfring; hyperlacrimation; mucin; tear meniscus; tears; Tearscope; test, break-up time.**

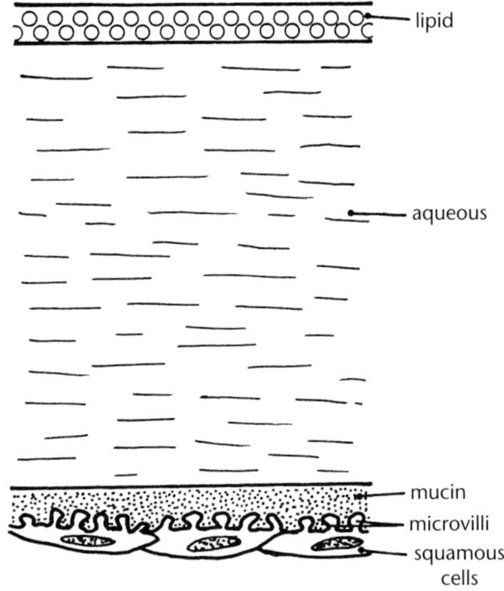


Fig. F5 Diagram of the three layers of the precorneal film attached to the squamous epithelial cells

**filter** Material or device used to absorb or transmit light of all wavelengths equally (**neutral density filter** which is abbreviated **ND filter**) or selectively, such as the **coloured filters** (blue filter transmits only blue light, green filter transmits only green light, etc.).
*See* **density, optical; filter, interference; lens, absorptive; light; test, neutral density filter; wavelength; wedge, optical.**

**filter, bandpass** A filter which allows the passage of radiations only within a narrow band of wavelengths around a central wavelength. This is done by multilayer coating which produces destructive interference.
*See* **coating; lens, coated.**

**filter, green** A filter which transmits only green light. It may be used in ophthalmoscopy to increase the contrast of the blood vessels to the background facilitating the visibility of retinal circulation defects, haemorrhages and

microaneurysms and the distinction between retinal and choroidal lesions. However, ophthalmoscopes actually use a filter which transmits a certain amount of red light as otherwise the observation would be so dark as to make it extremely difficult. *Syn.* red-free filter.
*See* **ophthalmoscope.**

**filter, interference** A coloured filter consisting of five layers, two outside glass, two intermediate evaporated metal films and one central evaporated layer of transparent material. These filters act not by absorption of light, but by destructive interference for all but a very narrow band of wavelengths which is transmitted. *Syn.* coloured filter.

**filter, neutral density** *See* **filter.**

**filter, red** A filter which transmits only red light. It may be used in ophthalmoscopy to facilitate viewing the yellow macular pigment, but other structures are seen with less contrast. It also produces a larger pupil allowing observation of a larger fundus area.
*See* **pigment, macular.**

**filter, red-free** *See* **filter, green.**

**filter, Wood's** *See* **light, Wood's.**

**Fincham, coincidence optometer of** *See* **optometer of Fincham, coincidence.**

**Fincham's theory** *See* **theory, Fincham's.**

**finished lens** *See* **lens, finished.**

**first-degree fusion** *See* **vision, Worth's classification of binocular.**

**first-order optics** *See* **optics, paraxial.**

**fisheye lens** *See* **lens, fisheye.**

**fissure, calcarine** Fissure on the medial aspect of the occipital lobe. Its anterior portion is in front of the parieto-occipital fissure and the posterior portion extends round the occipital pole and even appears on the lateral surface. *Syn.* calcarine sulcus.
*See* **area, visual.**

**fissure, embryonic** *See* **fissure, optic.**

**fissure, inferior orbital** An elongated opening lying between the lateral wall and the floor of the orbit. It is bounded anteriorly by the maxilla and the orbital process of the palate bone and posteriorly by the great wing of the sphenoid bone. *Syn.* sphenomaxillary fissure.
*See* **artery, infraorbital; nerve, zygomatic.**

**fissure, interpalpebral** *See* **aperture, palpebral.**

**fissure, optic** An invagination of the inferior portion of the optic stalk of the embryo. The hyaloid vessels pass through that fissure to supply the developing crystalline lens. In cases in which the invagination (or fissure) fails to fully close, colobomas will be formed. *Syn.* embryonic fissure; choroidal fissure.
*See* **artery, hyaloid; cup, optic.**

**fissure, palpebral** *See* **aperture, palpebral.**

**fissure, sphenoidal** *See* **fissure, superior orbital.**

**fissure, sphenomaxillary** *See* **fissure, inferior orbital.**

**fissure, superior orbital** An elongated opening lying between the roof and the lateral walls of the orbit, that is, between the two wings of the sphenoid bone. *Syn.* sphenoidal fissure.
*See* **nerve, abducens; nerve, oculomotor; nerve, ophthalmic; nerve, trochlear; orbit; vein, superior ophthalmic.**

**fit-over** *See* **clipover.**

**fitted on K** Refers to a contact lens in which the back optic zone radius is the same as that of the flattest meridian (or the mean of the two principal meridians) of the cornea. K is a symbol referring to the keratometer reading of the principal meridians of the cornea. *Syn.* alignment fit.
*See* **keratometer; lens, flat; lens, steep; optic zone radius, back.**

**fitting** Technique and art of selecting and adjusting spectacles or contact lenses following a visual examination.
*See* **dispensing, optical.**

**fixation** The act of directing the eye to a given object so that its image is formed on the foveola.
*See* **foveola.**

**fixation, anomalous** *See* **fixation, eccentric.**

**fixation axis** *See* **axis, fixation.**

**fixation, bifoveal** *See* **bifixation.**

**fixation, binocular** Fixation on an object with both eyes simultaneously.

**fixation disparity** *See* **disparity, retinal; fusional movements.**

**fixation disparity unit, Mallett** *See* **Mallett fixation disparity unit.**

**fixation, eccentric** Monocular condition in which the image of the point of fixation is not formed on the foveola. In this condition, the patients feel that they are looking straight at the object stimulating the non-foveolar retinal area and the visual acuity of that eye is reduced. The condition occurs most commonly in strabismic amblyopia but can also occur when the fovea has been destroyed by some pathological process. *Syn.* anomalous fixation.

*See* **acuity, central visual; amblyopia; Haidinger's brushes; Maxwell's spot; occlusion treatment; penalization; pleoptics; test, after-image transfer; viewing, eccentric; Visuscope.**

**fixation, foveal** Normal fixation in which the image of an object falls on the foveola.

**fixation, line of** *See* **axis, fixation.**

**fixation movements** *See* **movements, fixation.**

**fixation, parafoveal** Fixation by a retinal area located outside the fovea but within the macula (or fovea centralis ), i.e. within 5 degrees of the central visual field. It may occur in amblyopia.

**fixation, plane of** *See* **plane of regard.**

**fixation, point of** Point in space upon which the eye is directed, either monocularly or binocularly. If there is no eccentric fixation, the image of that point is formed on the foveola. *Syn.* object of regard.
*See* **point of regard.**

**fixation reflex** *See* **reflex, fixation.**

**fixation response** Eye movement aimed at placing the image of a point of fixation on the foveola.
*See* **foveola.**

**fixation, voluntary** Conscious fixation of an object as distinguished from the fixation reflex.
*See* **reflex, fixation.**

**flame haemorrhage** *See* **haemorrhage, preretinal.**

**flash** An intense light of short duration.

**flash blindness** *See* **keratoconjunctivitis, actinic.**

**flat lens** *See* **lens, flat.**

**flavimaculatus fundus** *See* **fundus, flavimaculatus.**

**Fleischer's ring** *See* **ring, Fleischer's.**

**flicker** Perception produced when the retina is stimulated by an intermittent light stimulus which fluctuates between a frequency of a few hertz and the critical fusion frequency.
*See* **frequency, critical fusion.**

**flicker photometer** *See* **photometer, flicker.**

**flint glass** *See* **glass, flint.**

**flippers** *See* **lens flippers.**

**floaters** Heterogeneities in the vitreous humour which may be of embryonic origin or pathological (e.g. in retinal detachment, vitreous detachment). The patient sees spots which float as the eye moves. Floaters are common in normal old eyes. *Syn.* vitreous floaters.
*See* **image, entoptic; iritis; muscae volitantes; photopsia; retina, lattice degeneration of the; retinal detachment; retinitis, cytomegalovirus; uveitis; vitreous detachment.**

**floccules of Busacca** *See* **Koeppe's nodules.**

**fluid, lacrimal** *See* **film, precorneal; tears.**

**fluorescein** A fluorescent, weak dibasic acid with a molecular weight of 376 whose sodium salt is used in dilute solution as a dye in the fitting of contact lenses, in the detection of corneal abrasions, etc. It is a yellowish-red compound which fluoresces a brilliant yellow-green under ultraviolet or blue illumination (Fig. F6). *Syn.* sodium fluorescein.
*See* **angiography, fluorescein; corneal abrasion; corneal fragility; edge lift; fluorescence; fluorexon; lamp, Burton; light, Wood's; rose bengal; staining; test, break up time; test, fluorescein.**

**fluorescein angiography** *See* **angiography, fluorescein.**

**fluorescence** Property of a substance that, when illuminated absorbs light of a given wavelength and re-emits it as radiations of a longer wavelength. *Example*: fluorescein.
*See* **lamp, fluorescent; law, Draper's; light, Wood's; luminescence; wavelength.**

**fluorescent lamp** *See* **lamp, fluorescent.**

**fluorexon** A staining agent similar to fluorescein but with a much higher molecular weight (710) and which is less readily absorbed by soft contact lens material. It is used in the fitting of soft or hybrid lenses (e.g. a piggyback lens). It stains a pale yellow-brown. However, it is not recommended for use with high water contact lenses (above 65%).

**fluorometholone** *See* **antiinflammatory drug.**

**flush bridge** *See* **bridge, flush.**

**flush, choroidal** This is the first evidence of fluorescein dye reaching the eye during the method of fluorescein angiography. It occurs approximately 1 second before reaching the retinal circulation because the route from the ophthalmic artery to the choroidal circulation is shorter.

**flutter, ocular** An involuntary, rapid, horizontal saccadic oscillation of both eyes while attempting to fixate an object. It is a sign of cerebellar disease.
*See* **myoclonus, ocular; opsoclonus.**

**flux, luminous** Flow of light which produces a visual sensation. It is measured in lumens.
*See* **lumen.**

**flux, radiant** Power emitted in the form of radiation. It is measured in watts or ergs per second.

**FM 100 Hue test** *See* **test, Farnsworth.**

**focal interval** *See* **Sturm, interval of.**

**focal length** *See* **length, focal.**

**focal length, equivalent** *See* **length, equivalent focal.**

**focal length, vertex** *See* **vertex focal length.**

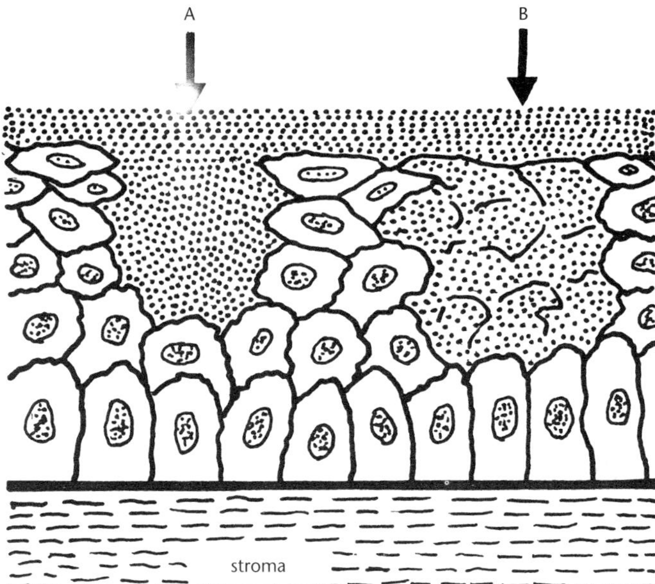


Fig. F6 Fluorescein on the corneal surface staining A, an abraded area, and B, some damaged epithelial cells

**focal line; plane** *See* under the nouns.

**focal point** *See* **focus, principal.**

**focal power** *See* **paraxial equation, fundamental; power, refractive.**

**focal ratio** *See* **f number.**

**foci, conjugate** *See* **distances, conjugate.**

**focimeter** An optical instrument for determining the vertex power, axis direction and optical centre of an ophthalmic lens (Fig. F7). *Syn.* Lensometer (a tradename); vertexometer; Vertometer (a tradename).
*See* **lens measure; neutralization; power, back vertex; transposition.**

**focus 1.** The point at which rays of light converge after passing through a convex lens to form a real image (**real focus**), or diverge from (**virtual focus**) after passing through a concave lens. **2.** The centre or starting point of a disease process. **3.** To adjust an optical system (e.g. camera or projector) in order to obtain a sharp image. *Plural*: foci. *Syn.* focusing.
*See* **confocal; focus, principal; line, focal.**

**focus, dark** *See* **accommodation, resting state of.**

**focus, depth of** *See* **depth of focus.**

**focus, principal** The axial image point produced by an optical system of an infinitely distant object (the **second principal focus** or **posterior principal focus**), or that axial object point for which the image will be formed at infinity (the **first principal focus** or **anterior principal focus**). A converging

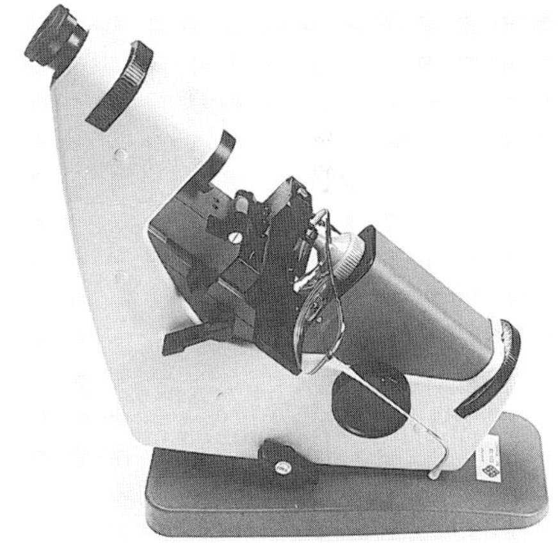

Fig. F7 Focimeter (Shin Nippon)

optical system or lens has two principal foci which are real. A diverging optical system or lens has a second principal focus which is virtual. In curved mirrors the two principal foci coincide. Depending upon whether the object is at infinity or at the principal focus, this same focal point becomes either the second principal focus or the first principal focus, respectively. *Syn.* focal point.
*See* **focus; length, focal; points, cardinal; power, equivalent; sign convention.**

**focus, real** *See* **focus.**

**focus, sagittal; tangential** *See* **astigmatism, oblique.**

**focus, virtual** *See* **focus.**

**focusing** *See* **focus.**

**fogging method** *See* **method, fogging.**

**fold, conjunctival** *See* **conjunctiva.**

**fold, corneal** *See* **oedema.**

**fold, semilunar** *See* **plica semilunaris.**

**follicle** **1.** A small gland. **2.** A small cavity or deep narrow depression with excretory or secretory function. **3.** A small nodule of lymphocytes and other cells occurring as a result of chronic inflammation.
*See* **follicle, conjunctival; papilla.**

**follicle, conjunctival** Small localized aggregation of lymphocytes, plasma and other cells appearing as white or grey elevations on the palpebral conjunctiva (tarsal area) as a result of chronic irritation (allergic, viral or mechanical such as contact lenses).
*See* **conjunctivitis, adult inclusion; conjunctivitis, follicular.**

**follicles, palpebral** *See* **glands, meibomian.**

**follicular conjunctivitis** *See* **conjunctivitis, follicular.**

**footcandle** Non-metric unit of illuminance. It is equal to a flux of 1 lumen per $ft^2$. *Symbol*: fc. 1 fc = 10.764 lux.
*See* **illuminance; lux.**

**footlambert** Non-metric unit of luminance. It is equal to the average luminance of a surface emitting or reflecting 1 lumen per $ft^2$. *Symbol*: fL. 1 fL = 3.426 cd/$m^2$.
*See* **luminance.**

**foramen, optic** *See* **canal, optic.**

**forced duction test** *See* **test, forced duction.**

**former** A pattern, usually made of plastic, used to guide the automatic machines which cut and edge lenses. *Syn.* lens pattern.
*See* **edging.**

**fornix** *See* **conjunctiva.**

**Forster–Fuchs spot** *See* **Fuchs' spot.**

**fortification spectrum** *See* **scotoma, scintillating.**

**fossa, hyaloid** A cup-shaped depression in the anterior vitreous body which accommodates the posterior part of the crystalline lens. It is actually separated from the lens itself by the postlenticular space of Berger. *Syn.* lenticular fossa; patellar fossa.
*See* **ligament of Wieger; postlenticular space, Berger's.**

**fossa for the lacrimal gland** A depression in the frontal bone in which rests the orbital portion of the lacrimal gland, as well as some orbital fat which itself lies in the posterior part of the fossa called the **accessory fossa of Rochon–Duvigneaud**. The fossa is located behind the zygomatic process of the frontal bone in the anterior and lateral part of the orbital roof.

**fossa for the lacrimal sac** A vertical groove, some 5 mm deep and about 14 mm high, formed by the frontal process of the maxilla and lacrimal bones and which contains the lacrimal sac. The fossa is bounded by the anterior and posterior lacrimal crests coming from the maxilla (frontal process) and lacrimal bone respectively, with no definite boundary above. It leads downward to the nasolacrimal canal which contains the nasolacrimal duct.
*See* **lacrimal apparatus; orbit.**

**fossa, trochlear** A small depression in the frontal bone which contains the pulley (or **trochlea**), a cartilagenous structure surrounded by a thick fibrous sheath 1 mm thick and through which passes the superior oblique muscle. The fossa is located about 4 mm behind the medial upper margin of the orbit.

**Foster Kennedy syndrome** *See* **syndrome, Foster Kennedy.**

**Foucault grating** *See* **grating.**

**four prism dioptre base out test** *See* **test, four prism base out.**

**Fourier analysis** The mathematical breakdown of waveforms into simple sine wave constituents. Any complex waveform consists of sine waves of different frequencies: the slowest (fundamental) frequency and harmonics thereof (these are frequencies which are odd multiples of the fundamental frequency). It is used in analysis and reconstruction of waveforms as, for example, analysing the spatial frequency components of a visual image. *Syn.* Fourier transform.
*See* **sensitivity, contrast.**

**fourth cranial nerve** *See* **nerve, trochlear.**

**fourth nerve paralysis** *See* **paralysis of the fourth nerve.**

**fovea** *See* **foveola.**

**fovea centralis** A small area of the retina of approximately 1.5 mm in diameter situated within the macula lutea. At the fovea centralis, the retina is the thinnest as there are no supporting fibres of Mueller, no ganglion cells and no bipolar cells. These cells are shifted to the edge of the depression. The fovea centralis contains mainly cone cells, each one being connected to only one ganglion cell and thus contributing to the highest visual acuity of the retina. The visual field represented by the fovea centralis is equal to about 5° (Fig. F8). *Syn.* foveal pit; macula (term often used by clinicians).
*See* **acuity, central visual; foveola; image, retinal; macula lutea.**

**foveal avascular zone** *See* **foveola.**

**foveal fixation** *See* **fixation, foveal.**

**foveal pit** *See* **fovea centralis.**

**foveola** It is the base of the fovea centralis with a diameter of about 0.4 mm (or about 1° of the visual field). The image of the point of fixation is formed on the foveola in the normal eye. The foveola contains cone cells only (**rod-free area**). The **foveal avascular zone** is slightly larger (about 0.5 mm in diameter) (Fig. F8). *Syn.* fovea (term often used by clinicians).
*See* **eccentricity; fixation.**

**Foville's syndrome** *See* **syndrome, Foville's.**

**fragile X syndrome** *See* **syndrome, fragile X.**

**frame** A structure in metal, plastic, tortoiseshell, wood, leather, etc. for enclosing or supporting ophthalmic lenses but usually considered without the lenses.
*See* **spectacles.**

**frame, eyeglass 1.** Synonym for spectacles. **2.** Synonym for rimless spectacles.
*See* **spectacles.**

**frame heater** A device used to warm plastic spectacle frames in order to soften its material sufficiently to allow insertion of lenses and/or adjustment. Some frame heaters warm air which is directed to the area of the frame which is to be altered. Others heat salt or glass beads to a given temperature and the part of the frame which is to be altered is placed into the heated material. *Syn.* frame warmer.
*See* **plastic; spectacle frame, plastic.**

**frame markings, spectacle** *See* **spectacle frame markings.**

**framycetin** *See* **antibiotic.**

**Fraunhofer's lines** *See* **lines, Fraunhofer's.**

**frequency, critical fusion (CFF)** Frequency of a light stimulation at which it becomes perceived as a stable and continuous sensation. That frequency depends upon various factors: luminance, colour, contrast, retinal eccentricity, etc. *Syn.* critical flicker frequency.
*See* **flicker; law, Ferry–Porter; law, Granit–Harper; law, Talbot–Plateau; photometer, flicker.**

**frequency, cut-off** *See* **sensitivity, contrast.**

**frequency of light** *See* **hertz; spectrum, electromagnetic; wavelength.**

**frequency, spatial** The rate of alternation of the luminance in a visual stimulus as a function of length, usually expressed in cycles per degree.
*See* **contrast; cycle per degree; Fourier analysis; function, modulation transfer.**

**Fresnel lens** *See* **lens, Fresnel.**

**Fresnel Press-On prism** *See* **prism, Fresnel Press-On.**

**Fresnel's bi-prism** *See* **bi-prism, Fresnel's.**

**Fresnel's formula** Formula used to determine the proportion of light lost by reflection at the interface between two transparent media. The reflection is

$$\rho = \left(\frac{n_2 - n_1}{n_2 + n_1}\right)^2$$

where $n_1$ is the index of refraction of the first medium and $n_2$ that of the second medium. For a lens surface in air, the percentage of light reflected is given by

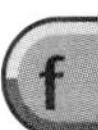

$$\rho = \left(\frac{n - 1}{n + 1}\right)^2 \times 100\%$$

*Example*: the reflection from the two surfaces of a glass lens made of crown ($n = 1.523$) is equal to 8.6%.
*See* **factor, reflection; image, ghost; index of refraction; lens, high index; reflection, surface.**

**Table F3** Percentage of light reflected in normal incidence ρ at the surface of several transparent substances of varying refractive indices, in air

| Refractive index | ρ (%) |
|---|---|
| 1.333 | 2.04 |
| 1.4 | 2.78 |
| 1.45 | 3.35 |
| 1.5 | 4.0 |
| 1.523 | 4.3 |
| 1.55 | 4.65 |
| 1.6 | 5.32 |
| 1.65 | 6.02 |
| 1.7 | 6.72 |
| 1.75 | 7.44 |
| 1.8 | 8.16 |

**Friedmann visual field analyser** *See* **analyser, Friedmann visual field.**

**Friedreich's ataxia** *See* **ataxia, hereditary spinal.**

**FRIEND test** *See* **test, FRIEND.**

**fringes, diffraction** A pattern of alternate dark and light bands produced by diffracted light passing the edge of an opening.
*See* **diffraction.**

**fringes, interference** *See* **interference fringes.**

**Frisby stereotest** *See* **stereotest, Frisby.**

**front** The part of a spectacle frame without the sides.
*See* **side; spectacles.**

**front silvered mirror** *See* **mirror, front surface.**

**front vertex focal length** *See* **vertex focal length.**

**front vertex power** *See* **power, front vertex.**

**frontal plane** *See* **plane, frontal.**

**frontoparallel plane** *See* **plane, frontoparallel.**

**frosted lens** *See* **lens, frosted.**

**Fuchs' coloboma** *See* **crescent, congenital scleral.**

**Fuchs, crypts of** Pit-like depressions found near the collarette of the iris.
*See* **collarette.**

**Fuchs' endothelial dystrophy** *See* **dystrophy, Fuchs' endothelial.**

**Fuchs' heterochromic iridocyclitis** *See* **iridocyclitis, Fuchs' heterochromic.**

**Fuchs' spot** A round or elliptical, pigmented spot, usually located in the macular or paramacular area. It occurs in patients who have pathological myopia. It is due to breaks in Bruch's membrane (called **lacquer cracks**) and to the development of a choroidal neovascular membrane followed by subretinal haemorrhage which has changed colour and has become pigmented. The patient may notice photopsia when the membrane breaks but eventually it causes a loss of vision with a central scotoma. *Syn.* **Forster–Fuchs spot.**
*See* **photopsia.**

**Fuchs' spur** A few fibres located about midway along the length of the sphincter muscle which join with a few fibres of the dilator muscle of the iris.

**Fuchs' syndrome** *See* **syndrome, Fuchs'.**

**function, line-spread** A mathematical description of the distribution of light across the image of a very thin bright line object. On the retina the image of a thin bright slit spreads over a distance subtending about six minutes of arc at which point the intensity is less than two log units below the maximum.

**function, modulation transfer (MTF)** A relationship between the spatial frequency of an image (e.g. in number of cycles per degree or lines per inch) and the modulation amplitude (i.e. the difference between the luminance at the peaks and troughs of a grating). This gives an indication of the ability of a lens to resolve a grating. The greater the quality of a lens, the higher the spatial frequency at which the modulation amplitude falls to zero. At this point the lens can no longer transfer spatial modulation of intensity from the object to the image and the image appears as a uniform intensity distribution. This technique has been applied to assess the quality of the retinal image. One way of doing so is by measuring contrast thresholds for detecting a grating of a given spatial frequency and varying the modulation amplitude until the presence of the grating is just detected. This procedure is repeated for a number of different spatial frequencies and the results form a function which is more commonly referred to as a **contrast sensitivity function** (CSF).
*See* **frequency, spatial; sensitivity, contrast.**

**function, point-spread (PSF)** The mathematical description of the light distribution across the image of a point source. The shape and width of the function depends upon the amount of diffraction, aberrations and scatter and in the eye, the shape of the pupil. Its shape, which resembles a normal distribution, is conventionally defined by its 'half-width', being the width of the curve at half the peak luminance. If only diffraction is considered the point-spread function is known as Airy's disc.
*See* **disc, Airy's.**

**functional visual loss** Reduced vision experienced by an individual, but which is not based on objective measurements that could explain the symptom.
*See* **amblyopia, hysterical; malingering.**

**fundoscopy** The act of examining the fundus of the eye, as with an ophthalmoscope or a slit-lamp.

**fundus albipunctatus** A recessively inherited, nonprogressive tapetoretinal degeneration. It is characterized by a multitude of small, grey or whitish dots scattered throughout the fundus at the level of the pigment epithelium and accompanied by night blindness. The macula is spared and the retinal blood vessels, optic disc, visual field, colour vision and visual acuity are normal.

**fundus camera** *See* **camera, fundus.**

**fundus flavimaculatus** A retinal degeneration characterized by prominent, irregular-shaped whitish or yellow flecks scattered throughout the posterior fundi of both eyes. There is usually no loss of vision unless one of the flecks involves the fovea. It is a variant of Stargardt's disease. The electro-oculogram is useful in diagnosing this condition.
*See* **disease, Stargardt's; electro-oculogram.**

**fundus, leopard** An ocular fundus marked with dark blotches on its surface as a result of a tapetoretinal degeneration, such as retinitis pigmentosa. *Syn.* leopard retina.
*See* **retinitis pigmentosa.**

**fundus, ocular** The interior of the eye (as may be seen with the aid of an ophthalmoscope) consisting of the retina, the retinal blood vessels and even sometimes the choroidal vessels when there is little pigment in the pigment epithelium

(e.g. albinos), the foveal depression, and the optic disc. The fundus appears red, owing mainly to the choroidal blood supply. The colour is lighter in fair people than in darker races and is dependent upon the amount of pigment in the pigment epithelium and in the choroid. In dark races the fundus is almost dark grey (Fig. F8). *Plural*: fundi.
*See* **camera, fundus; fuscin; melanin; ophthalmoscope; plaques, Hollenhorst's; retina; tapetum lucidum.**

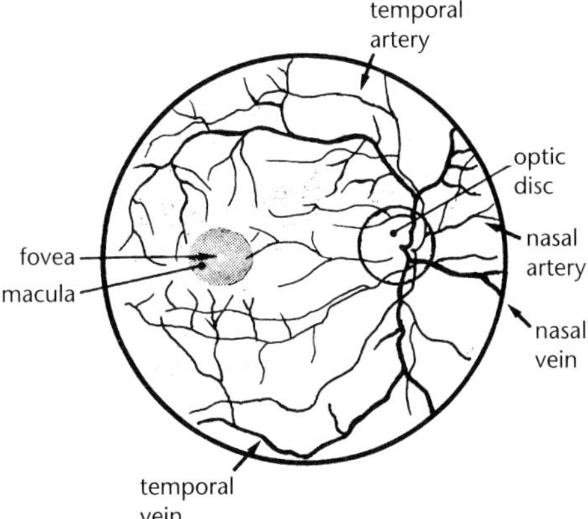


**Fig. F8** Diagram of the fundus of the right eye

**fundus reflex** *See* **reflex, fundus.**

**fundus, salt and pepper** The appearance of the ocular fundus characterized by a stippling of dark pigmented spots and yellowish-red spots of atrophy, as is found in congenital syphilis, choroideraemia, Leber's congenital amaurosis, rubeola, poliomyelitis, etc.
*See* **choroideraemia; Leber's congenital amaurosis.**

**fundus, tessellated** A normal ocular fundus in which the choroidal pattern appears as roughly polygonal dark areas in between choroidal vessels because the retinal pigment epithelium layer is thin and the choroid heavily pigmented. *Syn.* tessellated retina; tigroid fundus; tigroid retina.

**fundus, tigroid** *See* **fundus, tessellated.**

**fungal keratitis** *See* **keratitis, fungal.**

**fuscin** A pigment present in granules in the pigment epithelium of the retina consisting of residual bodies ingested by lysosomes and sometimes fused with melanin granules. The residual bodies are thought to be mainly the undigested elements of disc membrane phagocytosis. In albinos the pigment granules are immature and colourless.
*See* **albinism; cell, cone; cell, rod; melanin; retinal pigment epithelium.**

**fused bifocal** *See* **lens, bifocal.**

**fusidic acid** A product used as an antibiotic agent in solution 1%. It is synthesized as sodium fusidate from the microorganism *Fusidium coccineum*. It is effective against gram-positive bacteria. It is used in the treatment of bacterial blepharoconjunctivitis, especially staphylococcal infection.

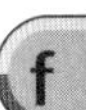


**fusion, binocular** *See* **fusion, sensory.**

**fusion, central** *See* **fusion, sensory.**

**fusion, chiastopic** Fusion obtained by voluntary convergence on two targets separated in space and such that the right eye fixates the left target and the left eye the right target. This is often facilitated by fixating a small mark above a single aperture placed in front of the two targets and then slowly shifting one's gaze to the targets. The procedure is aimed at improving positive fusional convergence.
*See* **convergence, fusional; fusion, orthopic.**

**fusion, first-degree; flat** *See* **vision, Worth's classification of binocular.**

**fusion field** An area around the fovea of each eye within which the fusion reflex is initiated. If the disparate images fall within this area motor fusion will occur, but if the disparity is too great there will be no fusional movement. This field is much larger horizontally than vertically.

**fusion frequency, critical** *See* **frequency, critical fusion.**

**fusion lock** *See* **heterophoria, associated.**

**fusion, motor** One of the components of convergence in which the eyes move until the object of regard falls on corresponding retinal areas (e.g. the foveas) in response to disparate retinal stimuli. *Syn.* disparity vergence; fusion reflex.
*See* **convergence, fusional; disparate retinal points; fusion field; fusion, sensory; retinal corresponding points; vergence facility.**

**fusion, orthopic** Fusion obtained by voluntary convergence on two targets separated in space and such that the right eye fixates the right target and the left eye the left target. This is often facilitated by looking beyond the targets and then slowly shifting one's gaze to the targets through double apertures placed in front of them. This procedure is aimed at improving negative fusional convergence.
*See* **convergence, fusional; fusion, chiastopic.**

**fusion, peripheral** *See* **fusion, sensory.**

**fusion reflex** *See* **fusion, motor.**

**fusion, second-degree** *See* **vision, Worth's classification of binocular.**

**fusion, sensory** The neural process by which the images in each retina are synthesized or integrated into a single percept. In normal binocular vision, this process occurs when corresponding (or nearly corresponding) regions of the retina are stimulated. This process can occur when the images are either in the central part of the retinae (**central fusion**) or in the peripheral part of the retinae (**peripheral fusion**). *Syn.* **binocular fusion.**
*See* **amblyoscope; anaglyph; convergence, fusional; convergence insufficiency; haploscope; response, SILO; retinal corresponding points; stereogram, random-dot; test, bar reading; test, diplopia; test, Worth's four dot; vision, binocular; vision, central; vision, peripheral; vision, Worth's classification of binocular.**

**fusion, third-degree** *See* **vision, Worth's classification of binocular.**

**fusional convergence** *See* **convergence, fusional; convergence, relative.**

**fusional divergence** *See* **divergence, fusional.**

**fusional movements** Reflex movements of the eyes occurring in response to retinal disparity (even though it may be below the threshold for diplopia to be seen) in order to produce a single image. If the fusional movements are such that although diplopia is eliminated there is still some disparity, this is **fixation disparity.**
*See* **disparity, retinal.**

**fusional reserve, convergence; vergence** *See* **convergence, relative.**

**f-value** *See* **f number.**

# G

**GABA** *See* **neurotransmitter.**

**galilean telescope** *See* **telescope, galilean.**

**galvanic nystagmus** *See* **nystagmus.**

**ganciclovir** *See* **antiviral agents.**

**ganglion** An aggregation of nerve cell bodies found in numerous locations in the peripheral nervous system.

**ganglion cell** *See* **cell, ganglion.**

**ganglion, ciliary** A small reddish-grey body about the size of a pinhead situated at the posterior part of the orbit about 1 cm from the optic foramen between the optic nerve and the lateral rectus muscle. It receives posteriorly three roots: (1) the long, nasociliary or sensory root (or ramus communicans), which contains sensory fibres from the cornea, iris and ciliary body and some sympathetic postganglionic axons going to the dilator muscle; (2) the short (or motor root or oculomotor root) which comes from the Edinger–Westphal nucleus through the third nerve. It carries fibres supplying the sphincter pupillae and ciliary muscles; (3) the sympathetic root which comes from the cavernous and the internal carotid plexuses. It carries fibres mediating constriction of the blood vessels of the eye and possibly mediating dilatation of the pupil. The ciliary ganglion gives rise to 6–10 short ciliary nerves. *Syn.* lenticular ganglion; ophthalmic ganglion.
*See* **nerve, oculomotor; nerve, short ciliary; nucleus, Edinger–Westphal; reflex, pupil light.**

**ganglion, gasserian** Sensory ganglion of the fifth nerve located in a bony fossa on the front of the apex of the petrous temporal bone. It receives the sensory portion of the fifth nerve in the posterior part of the ganglion. From its anterior part the three divisions of the fifth nerve are given off: the ophthalmic (which contains the sensory fibres from the cornea and the eye in general), the maxillary and the mandibular nerves. *Syn.* semilunar ganglion; trigeminal ganglion.
*See* **herpes zoster ophthalmicus; nerve, trigeminal.**

**ganglion, lenticular; ophthalmic** *See* **ganglion, ciliary.**

**ganglion, semilunar** *See* **ganglion, gasserian.**

**ganglion, superior cervical** One of the uppermost and largest ganglion in the two chains of

sympathetic ganglia lying alongside the vertebral column. It is located just below the base of the skull between the internal carotid artery and the internal jugular vein. It gives rise to the internal carotid nerve, which forms the internal carotid plexus.
*See* **plexus, internal carotid.**

**ganglion, trigeminal** *See* **ganglion, gasserian.**

**ganzfeld** A visual stimulus which consists of completely homogeneous and colourless luminance conditions throughout. It is used especially when recording the standard electroretinogram.
*See* **electroretinogram.**

**Gardner Reversal-Frequency Test** *See* **test, developmental and perceptual screening.**

**gasserian ganglion** *See* **ganglion, gasserian.**

**gaussian approximation** *See* **ray, paraxial.**

**gaussian optics** *See* **optics, paraxial.**

**gaussian points** *See* **points, cardinal.**

**gaussian space** *See* **paraxial region.**

**gaussian theory** *See* **theory, gaussian.**

**gaze** To fixate steadily or continuously.

**gaze palsy** *See* **palsy, gaze.**

**Gelb effect** *See* **effect, Gelb.**

**gene therapy** A therapeutic method in which a defective gene is replaced by a normal copy of itself, thus restoring its function. There are several ways in which a new gene is carried into a diseased cell. Common methods include the use of a retrovirus, an adenovirus or an adeno-associated virus. This therapy has been used in the treatment of several eye diseases, especially retinoblastoma and retinitis pigmentosa, but so far with limited success.

**geniculate bodies, lateral (LGB, LGN)** Ovoid protuberances lateral to the pulvinar of the thalamus in the diencephalon of the forebrain and into which the fibres of the optic tract synapse on their way to the visual cortex. However, because of the semidecussation of the optic nerve fibres in the chiasma, the lateral geniculate body in the right thalamus receives the fibres originating on the temporal retina of the right eye and the nasal fibres of the left. Each body appears, in cross-section, to consist of alternating white and grey areas. The white areas are formed by the medullated nerve fibres of the optic tract while the grey areas consist largely of the cell bodies of the optic radiations which synapse with the fibres of the optic tract. There are six grey areas or layers of cells, with layer 1 being the most ventral and layer 6 the most dorsal (or posterior). Layers 1, 4 and 6 receive the crossed or nasal fibres from the contralateral retina, while layers 2, 3 and 5 receive the uncrossed or temporal fibres of the ipsilateral retina. There are two main types of cells in the lateral geniculate bodies: in layers 1 and 2 (those most ventral) the cells are substantially larger than in the other four layers and are called **magno cells** and the layers, **magnocellular layers**. The main input to these cells are the retinal rods and the magno ganglion cells. In the other four layers (those most dorsal) the cells are smaller and are called **parvo cells** and the layers, **parvocellular layers**. The main input to these cells are the retinal cones and the parvo ganglion cells. The cells of the parvocellular layers seem to be mainly responsible for transmitting information about visual acuity, form vision, colour perception and low contrast targets. The cells in the magnocellular layers seem to be mainly responsible for transmitting information about motion and flicker perception, stereopsis and high contrast targets. The magnocellular and parvocellular cells project to different cells in the primary visual cortex (V1), where they retain the same segregation as in the lateral geniculate bodies. The receptive field of the cells in the lateral geniculate body is circular with either an 'on' or 'off' centre with the opposite behaviour in the surround, but they are more sensitive to contrast than the retinal ganglion cells (Fig. G1).
*Syn.* lateral geniculate nucleus (although this is not strictly correct as this term refers only to the grey matter of the body).
*See* **cell, ganglion; cell, X; cell, Y; chiasma, optic; fibres, visual; field, receptive; radiations, optic; tracts, optic.**

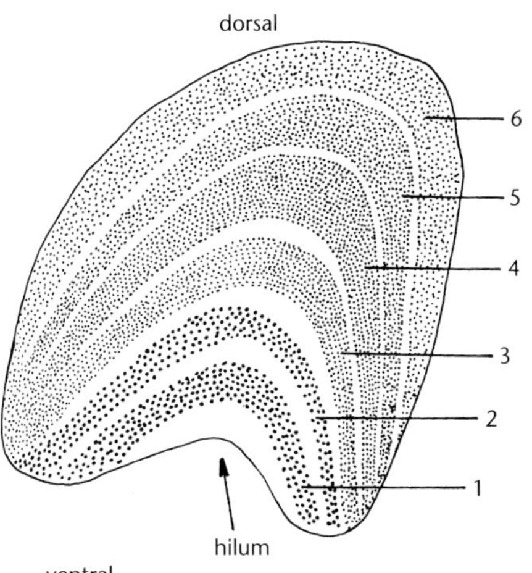


**Fig. G1** Section through the lateral geniculate body

**general refraction formula** *See* **paraxial equation, fundamental.**

**geniculocalcarine tract** *See* **radiations, optic.**

**Gennari, line of** *See* **area, visual.**

**gentamicin** *See* **antibiotic.**

**geometrical axis; optics** *See* under the nouns.

**gerontopia** *See* **sight, second.**

**gerontoxon** *See* **arcus, corneal.**

**Gerstmann syndrome** *See* **syndrome, Gerstmann.**

**ghost image** *See* **image, ghost.**

**giant cell arteritis** *See* **arteritis, temporal.**

**giant papillary conjunctivitis** *See* **conjunctivitis, giant papillary.**

**giantophthalmos** Megalocornea associated with an enlargement of the anterior segment of the eye.
*See* **keratoglobus.**

**Giles–Archer lantern** *See* **test, lantern.**

**glabella 1.** A prominent area of the frontal bone situated above the root of the nose. **2.** The skin between the eyebrows, which is usually hairless. *Syn.* intercilium.

**glands, accessory lacrimal** They are the glands of Krause and Wolfring. These glands are histologically identical to the main lacrimal gland, but are located within the eyelids. These glands are responsible for basal (not reflex) tear secretion and appear to be under sympathetic neural control.
*See* **tear secretion.**

**gland, conjunctival** Any gland which secretes a substance into the conjunctiva such as the lacrimal, meibomian, Krause and Wolfring glands or a goblet cell.
*See* **cell, goblet; conjunctiva; tears.**

**gland, lacrimal** A compound gland situated above and to the outer side of the globe of the eye. It consists of two portions: (1) a large orbital or superior portion; and (2) a small palpebral or inferior portion. It secretes the middle aqueous layer of the tears through about a dozen fine ducts into the conjunctival sac at the upper fornix although one or two may also open into the outer part of the lower fornix (Fig. G2).
*See* **cell, goblet; dacryoadenitis; dacryops; film, precorneal; glands, meibomian; mucin; nerve, zygomatic; tear duct; tears.**

**glands of Ciaccio** *See* **glands of Wolfring.**

**glands, ciliary sebaceous** *See* **glands of Zeis.**

**glands, ciliary sweat** *See* **glands of Moll.**

**glands of Henle** These are not really glands. They are folds in the mucous membrane of the palpebral conjunctiva, situated between the tarsal plates and the fornices, in which there are goblet cells (Fig. G2). *Syn.* crypts of Henle (strictly speaking this term refers only to the pit-like depressions).
*See* **cell, goblet; film, precorneal.**

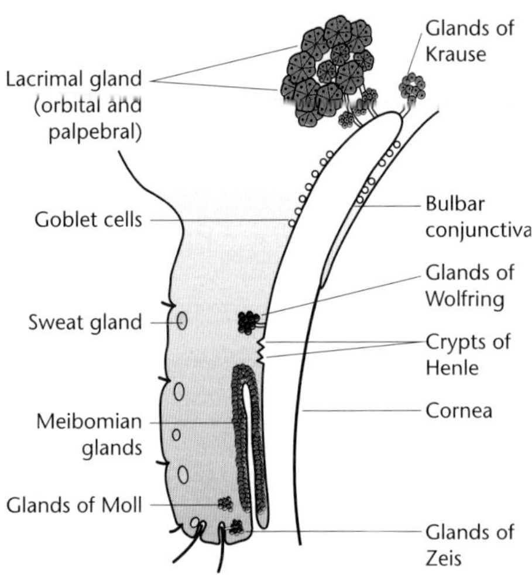


**Fig. G2** Section diagram of the upper eyelid showing the various glands

**glands of Krause** Accessory lacrimal glands of the conjunctiva having the same structure as the main lacrimal gland. They are located in the subconjunctival connective tissue of the fornix, especially the superior fornix (Fig. G2).
*See* **film, precorneal; gland, lacrimal; glands of Wolfring.**

**glands of Manz** Tiny glands located near the limbus. They secrete mucin. The existence of these glands in man is not established.

**glands, meibomian** Sebaceous glands located in the tarsal plates of the eyelids whose ducts empty into the eyelid margin. They are arranged parallel with each other, perpendicular to the lid margin, about 25 for the upper lid and 20 for the lower. They secrete **sebum**. This sebaceous material provides the outermost oily (or lipid) layer of the precorneal tear film. It prevents the lacrimal fluid from overflowing onto the outer surface of the eyelid. It also makes for an airtight closure of the lids and prevents the tears from macerating the skin. The meibomian glands can be seen showing through the conjunctiva of fair-skinned people as yellow streaks (Fig. G2). **Meibomian gland dysfunction** (MGD) may be induced by blepharitis, chalazion, contact lens wear (particularly soft lenses) and ageing. The most common sign is a cloudy or absent secretion upon expression with symptoms of a mild dry eye. Hot compresses and lid massage will cure more than half of the patients; oral tetracycline will help in many of the others. *Syn.* palpebral follicles; tarsal glands. *See* **blepharitis, marginal; chalazion; film, precorneal; gland, lacrimal; hordeolum, internal; meibomianitis; tarsus; tears; Tearscope plus.**

**glands of Moll** Sweat glands of the eyelids. They are situated in the region of the eyelashes (Fig. G2). *Syn.* ciliary sweat glands.
*See* **eyelids; hordeolum.**

**glands, tarsal** *See* **glands, meibomian.**

**glands of Wolfring** Accessory lacrimal glands of the upper eyelid situated in the region of the upper border of the tarsus (Fig. G2). *Syn.* glands of Ciaccio.
*See* **film, precorneal; gland, lacrimal; glands of Krause.**

**glands of Zeis** Sebaceous glands of the eyelids which are attached directly to the follicles of the eyelashes. Their secretion contributes to the oily layer of the precorneal film (Fig. G2). *Syn.* ciliary sebaceous glands.
*See* **blepharitis, marginal; film, precorneal; hordeolum.**

**glare** A visual condition in which the observer feels either discomfort and/or exhibits a lower performance in visual tests (e.g. visual acuity or contrast sensitivity). This is produced by a relatively bright source of light (called the **glare source**) within the visual field. A given bright light may or may not produce glare depending upon the location and intensity of the light source, the background luminance, the state of adaptation of the eye or the clarity of the media of the eye.

**glare, direct** Glare produced by a source of light situated in the same or nearly the same direction as the object of fixation.

**glare, disability** Glare which reduces visual performance without necessarily causing discomfort.

**glare, discomfort** Glare which produces discomfort without necessarily interfering with visual performance.

**glare, eccentric** *See* **glare, indirect.**

**glare, indirect** Glare produced by an intense light source situated in a direction other than that of the object of fixation. *Syn.* eccentric glare.

**glare source** *See* **glare.**

**glare tester** An instrument for measuring the effect of glare on visual performance. There exist several (e.g. Brightness Acuity Tester (BAT), Miller–Nadler Glare Tester, Optec 1500 Glare Tester). The Miller–Nadler Glare Tester consists of a glare source surrounding a Landolt C. The instrument contains 19 black Landolt C, all of the same size, 6/120 (or 20/400). Each Landolt C is presented in one of four orientations and from the highest to the lowest contrast at which the subject can no longer judge in which direction the letter appears. The contrast threshold is expressed in percentage disability glare. Glare testing is valuable in patients with corneal and lenticular opacities before and after surgery and in elderly patients in whom adaptation to glare is usually more difficult.
*See* **adaptation, dark.**

**glare, veiling** Glare caused by scattered light and producing a loss of contrast.

**glass 1.** Material from which lenses and optical elements may be made. It is hard, brittle and lustrous and usually transparent. It is produced by fusing sand (silica) at about 1400°C with various oxides (potassium, sodium, etc.) and other ingredients such as lead oxide, lime, etc. Glass may be produced in various colours by the addition of different substances (e.g. metal oxides). **2.** A lens.
*See* **index of refraction; lens blank; stria; surfacing.**

**glass, absorption** Glass which transmits only a certain portion of the incident light, the rest being absorbed.

**glass, Bagolini's** A lens on which fine parallel striations have been grooved. It produces a slight reduction in acuity but a light source observed through this lens appears as a streak of light orientated at 90° from the striations. Such a lens is used in the analysis of anomalous correspondence, suppression, etc. For example, in testing suppression the lenses can be placed in a trial frame with the striations at an angle of 135° for one eye and 45° for the other eye. A spotlight stimulus at distance or near is used, and if there is no suppression, the patient will see two diagonal lines crossing at, above or below the light source. If there is suppression, all or part of one line will not be seen. If the two diagonal lines cross at the source when the cover test indicated an ocular deviation, the patient has harmonious, abnormal retinal correspondence. *Syn.* Bagolini's lens.
*See* **retinal correspondence, abnormal.**

**glass, cobalt-blue** *See* **lens, cobalt.**

**glass, crown** Glass characterized by low dispersion. The most commonly used crown glass in ophthalmic lenses, called **ophthalmic crown** or **spectacle crown**, has a refractive index $n = 1.523$ and a constringence or V-value of 59. There are

other types of crown glass (e.g. dense barium crown $n = 1.623$, V-value 56; fluor crown $n = 1.485$, V-value 70).
*See* **constringence; dispersion; doublet; Fresnel's formula; triplet.**

**glass, depolished** *See* **glass, ground.**

**glass eye** *See* **eye, glass.**

**glass, flint** Glass containing lead or titanium besides the usual ingredients and having a high dispersion (*example*: Tital, V-value 31) compared to crown glass and a high refractive index ($n = 1.701$). It is, however, a softer and heavier material than crown. It is used in ophthalmic lenses of high power as it can be made much thinner than a crown glass lens of the same power.
*See* **constringence; dispersion; doublet; Fresnel's formula; index of refraction; lens, high index; triplet.**

**glass, ground** Glass which has been ground with emery, sandblasted or etched with fluoric acid to give it a matt surface. Such glass is usually translucent but not transparent. *Syn.* depolished glass.
*See* **lens, frosted; translucent; transparent.**

**glass, magnifying** *See* **lens, magnifying.**

**glass, opal** A white or milky translucent glass used to diffuse light.

**glass, photochromic** *See* **lens, photochromic.**

**glass, safety 1.** Glass which has been ground and polished and then heated just below its softening point and rapidly cooled. Such treatment renders the glass highly resistant to fracture, and breakage causes it to crumble rather than shatter. Safety glass can also be produced chemically. In this process the lens is immersed in a molten salt bath (e.g. 99.5% potassium nitrate and 0.5% silicic acid at a temperature of 470°C for some 16 hours). The lens surface thus becomes compressed as larger potassium ions replace the smaller sodium ions which are in the glass. Chemically strengthened lenses have greater impact resistance and can be made thinner than air-tempered glass lenses. However, when broken the fragments of the chemically strengthened lenses are not as blunt as those of air-tempered glass lenses. *Syn.* toughened glass. **2.** Non-shatterable laminated glass used in automobiles and goggles.
*See* **goggles; lens, laminated; lens, plastic; lens, safety; lens, toughened; polariscope; spectacles, industrial.**

**glass, toughened** *See* **glass, safety.**

**glass, Wood's** *See* **light, Wood's.**

**glasses** *See* **spectacles.**

**glasses, field** *See* **binoculars.**

**glaucoma** Eye disease characterized by an elevated or unstable intraocular pressure which cannot be sustained without damage to the eye's structure or impairment to its function. The increased pressure may cause optic atrophy with excavation of the optic disc as well as characteristic loss of visual field. Glaucoma is usually divided into **open-angle** and **angle-closure** types. If the cause of the glaucoma is a recognized ocular disease or injury (e.g. corneal laceration), it is called **secondary**, whereas if the cause is unknown it is called **primary.**
*See* **atrophy, optic; campimetry; cup, glaucomatous; disease, Sturge–Weber; hyphaemia; iridectomy; neuroprotection; perimeter; perimetry, frequency doubling; perimetry, short wavelength automated; pressure, intraocular; ratio, cup–disc; scotoma, Bjerrum's; syndrome, Marfan's; tonography; tonometry; tritanopia.**

**glaucoma, absolute** Final stage of the disease which has been either untreated or unsuccessfully treated. The eye is blind and hard, the optic disc is white and the pupil dilated.

**glaucoma, acute angle-closure (AACG)** A form of raised intraocular pressure in which the pressure within the eye increases rapidly due to blockage of the trabecular meshwork. Symptoms include: intense pain, redness, blurred vision, haloes around lights, as well as nausea. Findings on examination include: reduced visual acuity, greatly elevated intraocular pressure (in the range of 40–50 mmHg), corneal epithelial oedema, semi-dilated and fixed pupil, shallow anterior chamber and mild aqueous cell and flare. Elevated intraocular pressure often causes glaucomatous optic nerve damage, as well as iris atrophy and damage to the anterior epithelial cells of the lens (**glaukomflecken**). Treatment should be commenced as soon as possible and be directed at lowering the intraocular pressure. Therapeutic agents include: topical beta-adrenergic agents, oral or topical carbonic anhydrase inhibitors, and oral hyperosmotic agents. Surgery is often necessary. *Syn.* acute glaucoma; congestive glaucoma.

**glaucoma, angle-closure (ACG)** Glaucoma in which the angle of the anterior chamber is blocked by the root of the iris which is in apposition to the trabecular meshwork and thus the aqueous humour cannot reach the drainage apparatus to leave the eye. (As the blockage persists, anterior synechia may result.) This condition occurs usually in anatomically shallow anterior chambers, as is often the case in hypermetropes. **Angle-closure** glaucoma can either be primary (PACG) or secondary following iritis, iridocyclitis, postoperative complications,

traumatic cataract, tumours, etc. Moreover, angle-closure glaucoma is divided into **acute** and **chronic**. In **chronic angle-closure glaucoma** (CACG) there may never be an attack but intermittent periods of increased intraocular pressure caused by progressively extensive peripheral anterior synechia. Symptoms may be absent or there may be periodic episodes of mild congestion and blurred vision. Gonioscopy is essential to differentiate this condition from open-angle glaucoma. Treatment of angle-closure glaucoma is essentially surgical. However, initially therapeutic agents are used. They include: miotics (e.g. pilocarpine, carbachol, dapiprazole), the hyperosmotic agents which cause a rapid reduction of the IOP (e.g. glycerin, isosorbide), beta-blockers (e.g. timolol) and carbonic anhydrase inhibitors (e.g. acetazolamide). *Syn.* closed-angle glaucoma; narrow-angle glaucoma.
*See* **anisocoria; gonioscope; iridectomy; iridoschisis; iris bombé; iris, plateau; iritis; method, van Herick, Shaffer and Schwartz; pupillary block; synechia; test, provocative; test, shadow; trabeculectomy.**

**glaucoma, capsular** *See* **pseudoexfoliation.**

**glaucoma, chronic** *See* **glaucoma, open-angle.**

**glaucoma, chronic angle-closure** *See* **glaucoma, angle-closure.**

**glaucoma, ciliary block** A secondary glaucoma which occurs when aqueous fluid becomes misdirected into the vitreous cavity. The accumulating fluid then produces a displacement of the lens and iris, causing a narrowing of the anterior chamber angle with resultant raised intraocular pressure. This condition occurs most commonly following intraocular surgery, especially glaucoma surgery after the cessation of cycloplegic medications. Treatment consists of medical intervention (cycloplegics, beta-adrenergic agents, carbonic anhydrase inhibitors and hyperosmotic agents) or puncture of the vitreous face with the Nd-YAG laser if medical treatment is unsuccessful. In phakic eyes, vitrectomy is sometimes required to open the anterior vitreous face. *Syn.* malignant glaucoma.

**glaucoma, closed-angle** *See* **glaucoma, angle-closure.**

**glaucoma, compensated** *See* **glaucoma, open-angle.**

**glaucoma, congenital** Glaucoma occurring with developmental anomalies that are manifest at birth and interfere with the drainage of the aqueous humour causing an increase in intraocular pressure. This in turn causes stretching of the elastic coats of the eye, enlargement of the globe as the sclera and cornea stretch, optic atrophy, marked cupping of the optic disc and loss of vision. Most noticeable is the enlargement of the cornea. Congenital glaucoma is inherited as an autosomal recessive condition with incomplete penetrance. *Syn.* buphthalmos; hydrophthalmos; infantile glaucoma.
Glaucoma occuring after the age of about 3 years is more often referred to as **juvenile glaucoma** as it follows a course similar to adult glaucoma without enlargement of the globe.
*See* **luxation of the lens.**

**glaucoma, congestive** *See* **glaucoma, angle-closure.**

**glaucoma, infantile; juvenile** *See* **glaucoma, congenital.**

**glaucoma, low tension (LTG)** Ocular condition in which there is a glaucomatous cupping and visual field defects with an intraocular pressure of 22 mmHg or less. This glaucoma is usually associated with a cardiovascular disease or migraine.

**glaucoma, narrow-angle** *See* **glaucoma, angle-closure.**

**glaucoma, neovascular** A secondary glaucoma due to new vessel formation on the anterior surface of the iris blocking the exit of the aqueous humour through the angle of filtration. It may occur as a result of central retinal vein occlusion (this type typically develops within 3 months and is sometimes called '**ninety-day glaucoma**'), or diabetes mellitus. Other causes include carotid artery occlusion, central retinal artery occlusion, retinal and choroidal tumours. The condition may initially be open-angle but eventually becomes angle-closure with severe loss of visual acuity, pain, congestion, high intraocular pressure, corneal oedema, aqueous flare, synechia and severe rubeosis iridis. The presence of new blood vessels on the iris and drainage angle distinguishes this condition from primary angle-closure glaucoma. Treatment includes topical steroids to decrease the inflammation, beta-blockers and carbonic anhydrase inhibitors to lower the intraocular pressure and laser treatment of the iris neovascularization and sometimes cilio-destructive procedures.
*See* **ectropion uvea; glaucoma, angle-closure; neovascularization, iris; rubeosis iridis.**

**glaucoma, ninety-day** *See* **glaucoma, neovascular.**

**glaucoma, open-angle** Glaucoma in which the angle of the anterior chamber is open and provides the aqueous humour free access to the drainage apparatus. It can occur: (1) As a **primary open-angle glaucoma** (POAG) (also called **simple glaucoma, compensated glaucoma,**

chronic glaucoma). The increased intraocular pressure leads to atrophy and excavation of the optic disc and typical defects of the visual field. It is the most common type of glaucoma (opinions of incidence vary between 0.5% and 3% of the Caucasian population over 40) and because of its insidious nature is difficult to detect. It tends to occur more often in people after the age of 35, in people who have a family history of the disease, who have high myopia and who have diabetes mellitus. It is characterized by an almost complete absence of symptoms. Haloes around lights and blurring of vision occur in some patients when there has been a sudden increase in intraocular pressure or when the disease is very advanced. The diagnosis of this disease is made by demonstrating that the eye has a characteristic visual field loss (Fig. G3). There may also be a raised intraocular pressure, although this is not always the case. (2) The other form is **secondary open-angle glaucoma** in which the intraocular pressure is elevated as a result of ocular trauma or iridocyclitis, crystalline lens abnormalities, etc. Management of open-angle glaucoma is usually by medication, unless this proves ineffective and surgery may be necessary. Formerly, pilocarpine (or carbachol) or adrenaline (epinephrine) drops were the most commonly used drugs. Nowadays, β-adrenergic blocking agents such as timolol maleate or betaxolol which act by reducing aqueous humour formation and do not affect pupil size or accommodation, are employed as the initial treatment. Also used are the carbonic anhydrase inhibitors (e.g. acetazolamide) the alpha-adrenergic agonist (e.g. brimonidine), and the prostaglandin derivatives (e.g. latanoprost) which enhance the uveoscleral outflow.
*See* **adrenergic receptors; alpha-adrenergic agonists; atrophy, optic; blind spot, baring of the; carbonic anhydrase inhibitors; cup, glaucomatous; gonioscope; hypertension, ocular; iris, plateau; miotics; perimetry, frequency doubling; pseudoexfoliation; scotoma, Bjerrum's; test, provocative; test, shadow; trabeculoplasty, laser; vision, tunnel.**

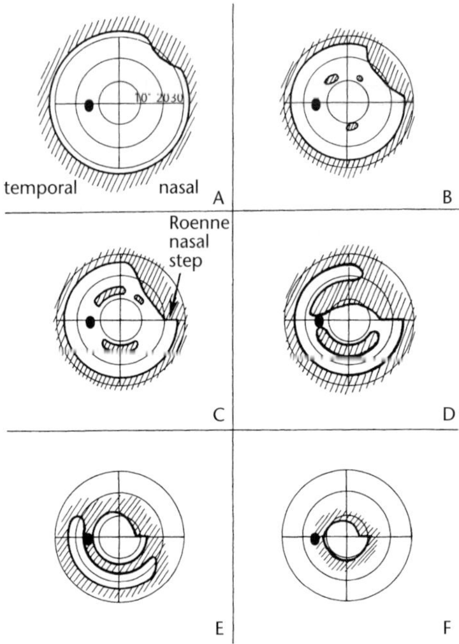

**Fig. G3** Typical evolution of field defects in primary open-angle glaucoma of the left eye (A and B, early field defects; C, more field defects with Roenne nasal step; D, Bjerrum scotoma; E and F, advanced field defects)

**glaucoma, phacolytic** An open-angle glaucoma secondary to a hypermature or mature cataract. It is due to a leakage of lens proteins into the anterior chamber which blocks the outflow of aqueous humour through the trabecular meshwork. It is characterized by an acute onset of pain and redness with high intraocular pressure.
*See* **cataract, hypermature; cataract, mature; glaucoma, open-angle; meshwork, trabecular.**

**glaucoma, phacomorphic** A form of secondary angle-closure glaucoma in which the angle of the anterior chamber is closed due to swelling of the lens. Angle closure may be due to pupillary block or in some cases due to anterior pressure on the iris.
*See* **pupillary block.**

**glaucoma, pigmentary** *See* **syndrome, pigment dispersion.**

**glaucoma, primary** *See* **glaucoma, angle-closure; glaucoma, open-angle.**

**glaucoma, pseudoexfoliation** *See* **pseudoexfoliation.**

**glaucoma, secondary** Glaucoma occurring as a result of intraocular tumour, iritis, iridocyclitis, uveitis, rubeosis iridis, traumatic cataract, tumours, etc.
*See* **disease, Graves'; glaucoma, angle-closure; glaucoma, neovascular; glaucoma, open-angle; hyphaemia; iritis; luxation of the lens; rubeosis iridis; syndrome, Rieger's; syndrome, ICE; uveitis.**

**glaucoma, simple** *See* **glaucoma, open-angle.**

**glaucomatocyclitic crisis** *See* **syndrome, Posner–Shlossman.**

**glaukomfleken** *See* **glaucoma, acute angle-closure.**

**glazing** Strictly, the fitting of lenses to a frame or mount, but often to include the cutting and edging processes (British Standard).
*See* **edging.**

**glial cell of the retina** *See* **astrocyte; cell, Mueller's.**

**glial veil** An irregular greyish membrane just anterior to the optic disc and obscuring its full view or usually only part of it. It is actually a cone-shaped mass of glial cells which enclosed the hyaloid vessels during embryonic development but has remained after birth. It may sometimes suggest a tumour of the disc but it is in fact benign, stable and does not interfere with vision. *Syn.* Bergmeister's papilla.
*See* **hyaloid remnant.**

**glioma, retinal** *See* **retinoblastoma.**

**globe of the eye** *See* **eyeball.**

**gloss** Shiny appearance of a surface.
*See* **matt surface.**

**glossmeter** Instrument for measuring the ratio of the amount of light specularly reflected from a surface to that diffusely reflected.
*See* **reflection, diffuse; reflection, regular.**

**glycerin** *See* **hyperosmotic agent.**

**glycocalyx** *See* **mucin.**

**glycosaminoglycan** A complex macromolecule considered to be the 'glue' of the cornea. It is responsible for providing the plasticity and structural support needed for successful corneal function. Along with other molecules, it comprises the solid portion of the cornea (~22%, the remainder being water). The distribution and arrangement of glycosaminoglycans are responsible for corneal transparency and thickness.

**goblet cell** *See* **cell, goblet.**

**goggles** Type of spectacles, usually large with shields and perhaps padding, used as eye protectors from flying particles, dust, wind, chemical fumes or other external hazards.
*See* **glass, safety; shield, eye; spectacles, industrial.**

**goitre, exophthalmic** *See* **disease, Graves'.**

**gold deposits** *See* **chrysiasis.**

**Goldmann lens** *See* **gonioscope.**

**Goldmann perimeter** *See* **perimeter, Goldmann.**

**Goldmann tonometer** *See* **tonometer, applanation.**

**Goldmann–Weekers adaptometer** *See* **adaptometer.**

**goniolens** *See* **lens, gonioscopic.**

**gonioprism, Allen–Thorpe** A prism in which the base has been curved so that it can rest on the cornea in gonioscopic examination.
*See* **gonioscope; prism.**

**gonioscope** Instrument used to observe the angle of the anterior chamber of the eye usually consisting of a biomicroscope in conjunction with a prismatic contact lens (e.g. Allen–Thorpe gonioprism) or a contact lens and mirror (e.g. Goldmann lens). It is an instrument which facilitates the diagnosis of angle-closure and open-angle glaucoma, as well as the diagnosis of secondary glaucoma (Fig. G4).
*See* **angle of the anterior chamber; glaucoma; lens, gonioscopic; lens, Koeppe; method, van Herick, Shaffer and Schwartz; slit-lamp.**

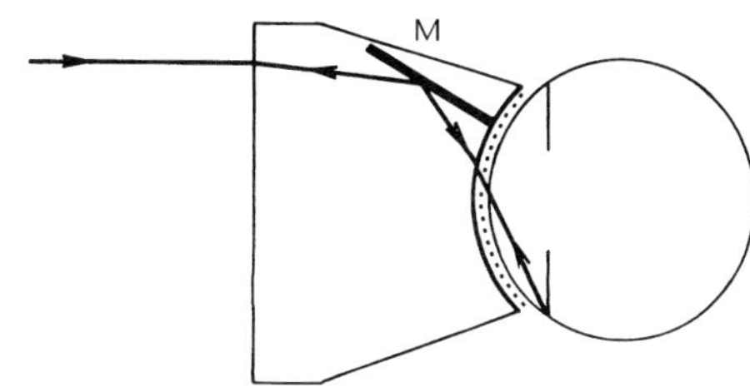


**Fig. G4** Optical principle of the Goldmann gonioscopic lens (M, mirror)

**gonioscopy** Observation of the angle of the anterior chamber of the eye with a gonioscope.

**gonioscopy, direct** Observation of the virtual, erect image of the angle of the anterior chamber as formed by a gonioscopic lens (e.g. Koeppe lens). The image can be viewed with a hand-held magnification system with the patient in a supine position.

**gonioscopy, indentation** Gonioscopy performed when the angle of the anterior chamber is closed in order to determine whether the closure is appositional or synechial. It is usually done with the four-mirror Zeiss lens by pressing the lens against the cornea forcing the aqueous into the peripheral part of the angle and pushing the iris posteriorly. If the angle is closed by apposition between the iris and cornea (appositional closure) the angle will open. If the angle is closed by adhesion between the iris and cornea (synechial closure) it will remain closed.
*See* **lens, Zeiss; synechia, anterior.**

**gonioscopy, indirect** Observation of the real, inverted image of the angle of the anterior chamber as formed by a gonioscopic lens. The image is viewed through a biomicroscope. This is the most commonly used gonioscopic method.

**gonococcal infection** *See* **conjunctivitis, acute; ophthalmia neonatorum.**

**Gradenigo's syndrome** *See* **syndrome, Gradenigo's.**

**gradient method; test** *See* **AC/A ratio.**

**Table G1** Structures of the angle of the anterior chamber as seen by gonioscopy in an individual in whom the angle is open and none of the structures is obscured by the iris

| structure (anterior to posterior) | anatomy/physiology | normal appearance |
|---|---|---|
| Schwalbe's ring | posterior termination of Descemet's membrane | not always discernible off-white ridge; pigment may collect on it |
| trabecular meshwork | site of aqueous flow; covers internal part of Schlemm's canal | variable degree of pigmentation |
| scleral spur | strip of scleral tissue | thin white line |
| ciliary body band | anterior face of ciliary body in the angle recess | pigmented seen more easily if iris is moved backward |



**gradient-index lens** *See* **lens, gradient-index.**

**von Graefe's test** *See* **test, diplopia.**

**graft, corneal** Corneal tissue of a donor used to replace a diseased or opaque cornea.
*See* **keratoplasty.**

**Gram stain** A procedure for detecting and identifying bacteria and certain other microbes. Microorganisms, such as those found in corneal or conjunctival samples, are stained with crystal violet, rinsed in water, treated with iodine solution, decolorized with ethyl alcohol or acetone and counterstained with a contrasting dye, usually safranin, a pink dye. The preparation is then rinsed with water, dried and examined. Microorganisms that retain the crystal violet stain are said to be **gram-positive**, while those that retain the counterstain are said to be **gram-negative**. Common **gram-negative** bacteria include *Acinetobacter, Chlamydia trachomatis, Enterobacter, Escherichia coli, Haemophilus influenzae, Moraxella lacunata, Neisseria gonorrhoeae, Proteus vulgaris, Pseudomonas aeruginosa.* Common **gram-positive** bacteria include *Mycobacterium chelonae, Mycobacterium fortuitum, Staphylococcus aureus, Staphylococcus epidermidis, Streptococcus pneumoniae, Streptococcus pyogenes.*

**Granit–Harper law** *See* **law, Granit–Harper.**

**granular dystrophy** *See* **dystrophy, granular.**

**granuloma** Growth appearing like a nodule consisting essentially of granulation tissue and occurring as a result of localized inflammation. It can appear on the conjunctiva, the iris, the lacrimal gland, the orbit.

**graticule** Graduated transparent scale engraved or photographed, placed in the front focal plane of the eyepiece of an optical instrument for direct observation of the apparent image size or position in the field of view. *Example*: the focusing screen of a focimeter. *Syn.* reticule.

**grating** A series of black and white parallel bars of equal width used to measure visual acuity, contrast sensitivity, and resolution of optical systems. The grating can be either square-wave (also called **Foucault grating** or **Foucault pattern**), in which the luminance across a bar is constant, or sine-wave, in which the luminance varies sinusoidally (Fig. G5).
*See* **cycle per degree; function, modulation transfer; sensitivity, contrast; test type.**

**Fig. G5** Square-wave grating

**grating, diffraction** *See* **diffraction.**

**Gratiolet, optic radiations of** *See* **radiations, optic.**

**Graves' disease** *See* **disease, Graves'.**

**Grayson–Wilbrant dystrophy** *See* **dystrophy, Reis–Buckler's.**

**green** The hue sensation evoked by stimulating the retina with rays of wavelength 490–560 nm and situated between blue and yellow. The

complementary colour of green is a **nonspectral colour** situated in the red-purple region.
*See* **colour, complementary; purple.**

**green blindness** *See* **deuteranopia.**

**gregorian telescope** *See* **telescope.**

**grey** A colour said to be achromatic or without hue. It varies in magnitude from white to black. *Note*: also spelt gray.
*See* **colour, achromatic.**

**grid, Amsler** *See* **chart, Amsler.**

**grid, Hering–Hermann** *See* **Hering–Hermann grid.**

**grid, Javal's** A test for simultaneous binocular vision and for detecting ocular suppression. It consists of five equally spaced opaque, parallel bars crossed by two perpendicular bars. It is held between the reader's eyes and a page of print. The bars being perpendicular to the lines of the text occlude some letters (along vertical strips) to one eye but these letters are seen by the other eye. If binocular vision is present no difficulty is experienced in reading the page. This instrument represents the most common type of **bar reader**.
*See* **suppression; vision, binocular.**

**Groenouw's nodular type 1 corneal dystrophy** *See* **dystrophy, granular.**

**Grotthus' law** *See* **law, Draper's.**

**ground** *See* **figure.**

**Gullstrand's reduced eye** *See* **eye, reduced.**

**Gullstrand's schematic eye** *See* **eye, schematic.**

**guttata, cornea** *See* **cornea guttata.**

**gyrus** One of the prominent rounded elevations between the sulci or grooves on the surface of the hemispheres of the brain. There are numerous gyri. Those associated with the visual association areas are the angular and lingual gyri. *Plural*: gyri.



# H

**Haab's pupillometer** *See* **pupillometer.**

**haemangioma, retinal** A benign tumour affecting the retinal capillaries and sometimes the optic nerve. It is often associated with systemic lesions, such as von Hippel–Lindau disease. The retinal lesion grows from a small red nodule to a larger yellowish mass accompanied by dilatation and tortuosity of the supplying artery and draining vein, and perhaps hard exudates, macular oedema, epiretinal membrane and retinal detachment. Treatment includes laser photocoagulation, cryotherapy and radiotherapy.

**haematoma** A swelling containing blood. It may result from injury (e.g. black eye) or from some blood disease, such as leukaemia. *Note*: also spelt hematoma.
*See* **eye, black.**

**haemotoma, ocular** A swelling due to a large haemorrhage into the tissues of the eye.

**haemophthalmia** An effusion of blood into the eye.

**haemorrhage** The escape of blood from any part of the vascular system. *Note*: also spelt hemorrhage.

**haemorrhage, blot** A form of intraretinal haemorrhage often noted in background (nonproliferative) diabetic retinopathy, branch retinal vein occlusion, carotid occlusive disease and child abuse. The haemorrhage is located within the inner retina and is limited by the orientation of the inner nuclear and plexiform layers. A small blot haemorrhage is often referred to as a '**dot**' haemorrhage.

**haemorrhage, flame** *See* **haemorrhage, preretinal.**

**haemorrhage, preretinal** Haemorrhage occurring between the retina and the vitreous body. It is usually large and often shaped like a D with the straight edge at the top. *Syn.* subhyaloid haemorrhage. Others are flame shaped and occur at the level of the nerve fibre layer and tend to parallel the course of the nerve fibres (**flame haemorrhage**). Retinal haemorrhages are usually round and originate in the deep capillaries of the retina. Retinal and preretinal haemorrhages usually absorb after a period of time (except those that break into the vitreous), but **subarachnoid haemorrhage** (which is usually due to a rupture of an aneurysm in an

artery of the circle of Willis) must be suspected as they often accompany it.
*See* **circle of Willis; retinopathy, diabetic.**

**haemorrhage, subconjunctival** A red patch of blood on the conjunctiva of the eye due to the rupture of a small blood vessel beneath. The condition is nearly always unilateral and the haemorrhage absorbs spontaneously although it frequently alarms the subject.
*See* **disease, sickle-cell.**

**haemorrhage, subarachnoid; subhyaloid** *See* **haemorrhage, preretinal.**

**Haidinger's brushes** An entoptic phenomenon observed when viewing a large diffusely illuminated blue field through a polarizer. It appears as a pair of yellow, brush-like shapes which seem to radiate from the point of fixation. The brushes are believed to be due to double refraction by the radially oriented fibres of Henle around the fovea. This phenomenon is used in detecting and treating eccentric fixation.
*See* **fixation, eccentric; image, entoptic; layer of Henle, fibre.**

**Halberg clip** *See* **clip, Halberg.**

**half-eyes** *See* **spectacles, half-eye.**

**Haller's layer** *See* **choroid.**

**hallucination, visual** Visual perception not evoked by a light stimulus.

**halo** A coloured ring of light seen around a light source as a result of aberrations, internal reflections, diffraction or scattering. It also appears when the eye is diseased and the cornea is oedematous, as in glaucoma.
*See* **glaucoma, open-angle; Sattler's veil.**

**haplopia** Single normal vision, as distinguished from diplopia.
*See* **diplopia.**

**haploscope** Instrument used mainly in the laboratory to study various aspects of binocular vision. It presents separate fields of view to the two eyes while allowing changes in convergence or accommodation of one or both eyes, as well as providing for controls of colour, intensity or size of target and field.
*See* **amblyoscope, Worth; dichoptic; masking, dichoptic; vision, binocular.**

**haptic 1.** *See* **scleral zone. 2.** Pertaining to the sense of touch.
*See* **lens, scleral contact.**

**Harada's disease** *See* **disease, Harada's.**

**hard resin** *See* **CR-39 material.**

**harmonious ARC** *See* **retinal correspondence, abnormal.**

**Harrington–Flocks visual field screener** *See* **screener, Harrington–Flocks visual field.**

**Hasner's valve** *See* **valve of Hasner.**

**Hassall–Henle bodies** *See* **cornea guttata.**

**head posture, abnormal** A deviation in position of the head, aimed at mitigating the effects of diplopia. It may be due to a field restriction or shyness, but the most frequent reason is an incomitant strabismus. Patients usually adjust their heads to permit fusion. If the deviation is too large to achieve fusion, patients may adjust their heads so as to increase the separation between the diplopic images and thereby making the diplopia less troublesome. *Examples*: if the right medial rectus or the left lateral rectus is affected, the face may be turned to the left, and vice versa if the other horizontal muscles are affected; if the left superior oblique is affected, the face may be turned to the right, the chin may be depressed and the head may be tilted to the right. If the cause of abnormal head posture remains untreated it may produce torticollis.
*See* **paralysis of the fourth nerve; paralysis of the sixth nerve; strabismus, incomitant; strabismus, paralytic; torticollis.**

**head tilt test** *See* **test, Bielschowsky's head tilt.**

**headache, ocular (HA)** A headache believed to result from excessive use of the eyes, uncorrected refractive error, especially hypermetropia and low grades of astigmatism, binocular vision anomaly or eye diseases. This headache typically occurs in the brow region but also in the occipital or neck regions.
*See* **accommodative insufficiency; asthenopia; astigmatism; hypermetropia.**

**headlamp 1.** Lighting device fitted to a vehicle and used to provide illumination on the road. **2.** A lamp strapped to the forehead of a surgeon or miner enabling light to be directed where required leaving both hands free.

**heliophobia** Neurotic fear of exposure to sunlight.

**Helmholtz's law of magnification** *See* **law, Lagrange's.**

**Helmholtz's theory of accommodation** *See* **theory, Helmholtz's of accommodation.**

**Helmholtz's theory of colour vision** *See* **theory, Young–Helmholtz.**

**HEMA** Transparent hydrophilic plastic used in the manufacture of soft contact lenses. It stands for 2-hydroxyethyl methacrylate.
*See* **index of refraction; lens, contact.**

**hematoma** *See* **haematoma.**

**hemeralopia** Term used to mean either **night blindness** in which there is a partial or total inability to see in the dark associated with a loss of rod function or vitamin A deficiency; or **day blindness** in which there is reduced vision in daylight while vision is normal in the dark. *Syn.* nyctalopia (this term is only synonymous with night blindness); night sight (this term is only synonymous with day blindness).
*See* **adaptation, dark; disease, Oguchi's; retinitis pigmentosa.**

**hemianopia** *See* **hemianopsia.**

**hemianopsia** Loss of vision in one half of the visual field of one eye (**unilateral hemianopsia**) or of both eyes (**bilateral hemianopsia**). *Syn.* hemianopia.
*See* **quadrantanopsia; perimeter; reflex, hemianopic pupillary; scotoma; screen, tangent; screener.**

**hemianopsia, absolute** Hemianopsia in which the affected part of the retina is totally blind to light, form and colour.

**hemianopsia, altitudinal** Hemianopsia in either the upper or lower half of the visual field.

**hemianopsia, binasal** Hemianopsia in the nasal halves of the visual fields of both eyes.

**hemianopsia, bitemporal** Hemianopsia in the temporal halves of the visual fields of both eyes.

**hemianopsia, congruous** Hemianopsia in which the defects in the two visual fields are identical.

**hemianopsia, heteronymous** Hemianopsia involving either both nasal halves (binasal hemianopsia) or both temporal halves of the visual field (bitemporal hemianopsia). A common cause of the latter is a lesion in the optic chiasma.
*See* **circle of Willis.**

**hemianopsia, homonymous** Hemianopsia involving the nasal half of the visual field of one eye and the temporal half of the visual field of the other eye. Common causes are occlusion of the posterior cerebral artery (stroke), trauma and tumours.
*See* **macula, sparing of the.**

**hemianopsia, incongruous** Hemianopsia in which the defects in the two affected visual fields differ in one or more ways. A common cause of incongruous homonymous hemianopsia is a lesion of the optic tract.

**hemianopsia, quadrantic** *See* **quadrantanopsia.**

**hemianopsia, relative** Hemianopsia involving a loss of form and colour but not of light.

**hemianopsia spectacles** *See* **spectacles, hemianopsia.**

**hemidecussation** The re-arrangement of the fibres of the optic nerves occurring in the optic chiasma in which about half of them from each optic nerve pass on to the contralateral optic tract. Thus each optic tract contains one half of the fibres of the ipsilateral optic nerve (representing the ipsilateral half visual field) and one half from the contralateral optic nerve (representing the contralateral half visual field). *Syn.* semidecussation.
*See* **chiasma, optic; decussation.**

**hemidesmosome** *See* **desmosome.**

**hemifield** One half of the visual field, usually divided vertically through the fovea into the left or the right visual field. It occurs following transection of the optic chiasma. Hemifield neglect sometimes occurs following trauma to the posterior lobe of one hemisphere.
*See* **visual neglect.**

**hemorrhage** *See* **haemorrhage.**

**Henle, crypts; glands of** *See* **glands of Henle.**

**Henle, fibre layer of** *See* **layer of Henle, fibre.**

**hepatolenticular degeneration** *See* **disease, Wilson's.**

**Herbert's pits** *See* **trachoma.**

**van Herick, Shaffer and Schwartz method** *See* **method, van Herick, Shaffer and Schwartz.**

**Hering's after-image; after-image test** *See* under the nouns.

**Hering's law** *See* **law of equal innervation, Hering's.**

**Hering's theory of colour vision; visual illusion** *See* under the nouns.

**Hering–Hermann grid** A grid consisting of perpendicularly crossed white stripes on a black background. The observer sees a dark shadow at the intersections of the white stripes. This phenomenon is due to lateral inhibition and does not occur for the fixated point (Fig. H1). *Syn.* Hermann's grid; Hermann's visual illusion.
*See* **inhibition, lateral.**

**Hering–Hillebrand deviation** *See* **deviation, Hering–Hillebrand.**

**herpes simplex of the cornea** *See* **keratitis, dendritic; keratitis, punctate epithelial.**

**herpes zoster** A viral infection of the posterior root ganglia of the spinal cord due to a reactivation of the chickenpox virus which has remained latent. It is characterized by a circumscribed vesicular eruption of the skin and neuralgic pain in the areas supplied by the sensory nerves.

h

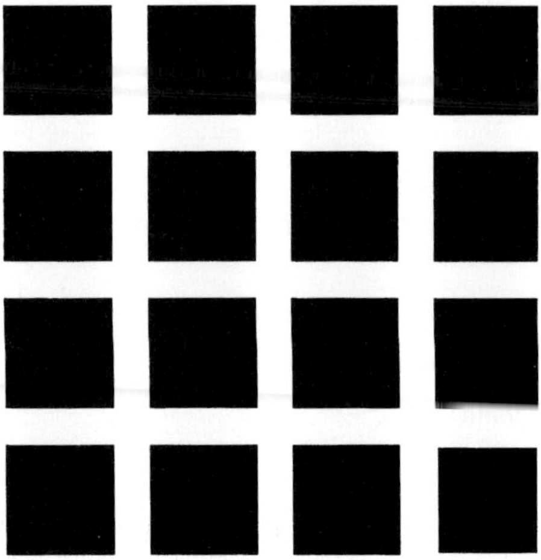

Fig. H1 Hering–Hermann grid

This is due to the migration of the virus from the affected ganglia to the sensory nerves. *Syn.* shingles; varicella zoster. (The term varicella is a synonym for chickenpox. The herpes zoster virus is identical to that of varicella.)
*See* **herpes zoster ophthalmicus; syndrome, acquired immunodeficiency.**

**herpes zoster ophthalmicus** An inflammation of that portion of the gasserian ganglion receiving fibres from the ophthalmic division of the trigeminal nerve, due to an infection by a latent virus identical to that causing chickenpox. The disease that occurs most commonly in people over 50 years of age begins with a severe, unilateral, disabling neuralgia in the region of distribution of the nerve. It is followed by a vesicular eruption of the epithelium of the forehead, the nose, eyelids and sometimes the cornea. The vesicles rupture leaving haemorrhagic areas that heal in several weeks. Pain usually disappears in about 2 weeks but in a few cases neuralgia persists for a long time. Ocular complications occur in approximately 50% of all cases of herpes zoster ophthalmicus. Corneal involvement appears as **acute epithelial keratitis** which is characterized by small fine dendritic or stellate lesions in the peripheral cornea in association with a conjunctivitis. This keratitis usually resolves within a week. As the disease progresses it may give rise to **mucous plaque keratitis** which occurs usually between the third and the sixth month after the onset of the rash. It is characterized by the plaque lines on the surface of the cornea which can be easily lifted and stromal haze. Iritis also accompanies this keratitis in approximately 50% of cases.
*See* **antiviral agents; ganglion, gasserian; herpes zoster; iritis; keratitis; scleritis.**

**herpetic keratitis** *See* **keratitis, herpetic.**

**Hess after-image** *See* **after-image.**

**Hertel exophthalmometer** *See* **exophthalmometer.**

**hertz** A unit of frequency equal to one cycle per second. *Symbol*: Hz.

**Hess screen** *See* **screen, Hess.**

**Hess–Lancaster test** *See* **test, Hess–Lancaster.**

**heterochromatic iridocyclitis** *See* **iridocyclitis, Fuchs' heterochromic.**

**heterochromatic stimuli** Visual stimuli which give rise to different colour sensations.

**heterochromia** Difference in colour of the two irides or of different parts of the same iris. It is usually congenital but some cases are associated with some eye diseases such as cataract, corneal precipitates, glaucoma, iridocyclitis or as a result of siderosis. *Syn.* anisochromia.
*See* **siderosis bulbi; syndrome, Fuchs'; syndrome, Horner's; syndrome, Marfan's.**

**heterodeviation** A form of ocular alignment that differs from the normal orthophoria. These include the general groups of **heterophoria** (e.g. esophoria, hyperphoria, etc.) and **heterotropia** (e.g. esotropia, exotropia, etc.).

**heterometropia** *See* **anisometropia.**

**heteronymous diplopia; hemianopsia** *See* under the nouns.

**heterophoria** The tendency for the two visual axes of the eyes not to be directed towards the point of fixation, in the absence of an adequate stimulus to fusion. Thus, the active and passive positions do not coincide for that particular fixation distance. This tendency is characterized by a deviation which can take various forms according to its relative direction such as **esophoria, exophoria, excyclophoria, incyclophoria, hyperphoria, hypophoria**. *Syn.* phoria.
*See* **anisophoria; cataphoria; dextrophoria; dissociation; laevophoria; Maddox rod; Maddox wing; position, active; position, passive; prism, relieving; test, cover; test, Thorington.**

**heterophoria, associated** A term sometimes used to denote the prism power necessary to align the nonius markers of a fixation disparity test. It is not strictly speaking a heterophoria because only part of the visual field is dissociated while the rest of the field is fused (that fused area is often referred to as **fusion lock** or **binocular lock**). The dissociation of only part of the field is achieved by using either a method of cross-polarization (e.g. Mallet fixation disparity unit)

or a septum (e.g. Turville infinity balance test). *Syn.* aligning prism; compensating prism.
*See* **disparity, retinal; Disparometer; dissociation; heterophoria, dissociated; heterophoria, uncompensated; Mallett fixation disparity unit; test, Turville infinity balance.**

**heterophoria, compensated** Any heterophoria which does not give rise to symptoms or to suppression.
*See* **heterophoria, uncompensated.**

**heterophoria, decompensated** *See* **heterophoria, uncompensated.**

**heterophoria, dissociated** Any heterophoria which is revealed by methods which produce complete dissociation such as the cover test, the Maddox rod test, the Thorington test, the von Graefe's test, etc.
*See* **dissociation; heterophoria, associated; Maddox rod; test, diplopia; test, Thorington.**

**heterophoria, uncompensated** Any heterophoria which gives rise to symptoms or to suppression. The symptoms are associated with visual tasks, especially close work, but also occasionally, inadequate illumination. Resting the eyes will usually lessen the symptoms. Unbalanced spectacle correction, a deterioration in the patient's general health, worry and anxiety can also sometimes give rise to an uncompensated heterophoria. This type of heterophoria is presumed to manifest itself as fixation disparity. *Syn.* decompensated heterophoria.
*See* **disparity, retinal; Disparometer; heterophoria, compensated; Mallett fixation disparity unit; prism, relieving.**

**heterophthalmia** A difference in the appearance of the two eyes as in heterochromia.
*See* **heterochromia.**

**heteropsia** *See* **anisometropia.**

**heterotopia maculae** *See* **macula, ectopia of the.**

**heterotropia** *See* **strabismus.**

**heterotropia, cyclic** A very rare and unusual form of strabismus occurring on a 48-hour rhythm in which a 24-hour period of normal binocular vision is followed by 24 hours of manifest heterotropia. The condition, which may have started in early infancy, only becomes apparent during early childhood. With time, cyclic heterotropia tends to become constant. *Syn.* cyclic strabismus.
*See* **strabismus.**

**von Hippel's disease** *See* **disease, von Hippel's.**

**von Hippel–Lindau disease** *See* **disease, von Hippel–Lindau.**

**hippus** Small rhythmic variations in the size of the pupils. They are present in everybody and increase slightly at high luminances. The frequency of these oscillations is about 1.4 Hz.
*See* **pupil.**

**Hirschberg's method** *See* **method, Hirschberg's.**

**history, case** A record of a patient's chief complaint, ocular and general health and that of close relatives, and visual requirements. It is a very important part of the examination which facilitates the diagnosis and treatment of the patient's complaint.

**hole in the card test** *See* **test, hole in the card.**

**hole in the hand test** *See* **test, hole in the hand.**

**Hollenhorst's plaques** *See* **plaques, Hollenhorst's.**

**Holmes–Adie syndrome** *See* **syndrome, Adie's.**

**Holmes–Wright lantern** *See* **test, lantern.**

**Holmgren's test** *See* **test, wool.**

**hologram** *See* **holography.**

**holography** A technique for obtaining a stereoscopic image of an object without the use of lenses. It consists of recording on a photographic plate the pattern of interference between coherent light reflected from the object and light that comes directly from the same source (or is reflected from a mirror). The coherent light is usually provided by a laser. The photographic recording on the plate (called a **hologram**) when illuminated with coherent light yields an image which is identical in amplitude and phase distribution with the original wave from the object. It thus provides a three-dimensional image of the object in the sense that the observer's eyes must refocus to examine foreground and background and indeed 'look around' objects by simply moving the head laterally.
*See* **coherent sources; interference.**

**homatropine** Alkaloid derived from atropine. It is an antimuscarinic drug used as a mydriatic and as a weak cycloplegic.
*See* **acetylcholine; cycloplegia; mydriasis.**

**homocentric pencil of rays 1.** One in which all rays converge or diverge from a single point. **2.** One in which more than one beam of light share the same pathway. *Example*: in an ophthalmoscope the illumination and observation paths are shared.

**homochromatic after-image** *See* **after-image, homochromatic.**

**homonymous diplopia; hemianopsia** *See* under the nouns.

**hordeolum, external** An acute suppurative infection (usually caused by staphylococci) of an eyelash follicle or of the sebaceous gland of Zeis or of the sweat gland of Moll (located in the region of an eyelash). The condition occurs most commonly in people who have a lower resistance to staphylococci as in debility, or who have a blepharitis. It has the appearance of a hyperaemic elevated area, indurated on the eyelid margin where it may rupture and discharge yellowish pus. The symptom is tenderness of the eyelid that may become marked as the suppuration progresses and the eyelid near the margin is red and swollen. Treatment usually consists of hot compresses and application of an antibiotic ointment and perhaps removal of the affected eyelash. Surgical incision is rare. *Syn.* stye.
*See* **eyelashes; glands of Moll; glands of Zeis.**

h

**hordeolum, internal** An acute purulent infection (usually caused by staphylococci) of the meibomian glands. It usually causes more discomfort than an external hordeolum as it is located on the conjunctival side of the eyelid. Treatment is similar to that of external hordeolum but surgical incision is required more frequently. *Syn.* meibomian stye.
*See* **chalazion; glands, meibomian; hordeolum, external; meibomianitis.**

**horizontal cell** *See* **cell, horizontal.**

**Horner's muscle; syndrome** *See* under the nouns.

**Horner–Trantas' dots** *See* **conjunctivitis, vernal.**

**horopter** The locus of object points in space that stimulate corresponding retinal points of the two eyes when the eyes are fixating binocularly one of these object points. The horopter is a curve that passes through the fixation point and changes shape with fixation distance. Objects closer to the eyes than the horopter are seen double (crossed disparity) and objects further than the horopter are seen double (uncrossed disparity). There are various types of horopters depending upon the method of determination.
*See* **area, Panum's; disparity, crossed; disparity, uncrossed; retinal corresponding points.**

**horopter, apparent frontoparallel plane** The locus of object points in space which appear to the observer to lie on a plane through the fixation point, parallel to the plane of the face. *Syn.* frontal plane horopter.
*See* **plane, apparent frontoparallel.**

**horopter, empirical** A horopter determined experimentally by having an observer judge a series of targets to be neither 'nearer than' nor 'farther than' the fixation point. *Examples*: the frontoparallel plane horopter; the nonius horopter.
*See* **horopter, theoretical.**

**horopter, longitudinal** Horopter that is plotted by only considering the longitudinal section where the rods meet the plane of fixation. Thus this horopter is a curve located in that plane and not a surface.

**horopter, nonius** Horopter plotted by fixating binocularly a central vertical rod while the other rods located in the periphery have their upper halves seen by one eye only and their lower halves seen by the other eye only. Each rod is moved individually until the two halves are seen aligned. *Syn.* vernier horopter.

**horopter, rectilinear** The assemblage of all lines in space that stimulate corresponding retinal lines. It is a pencil of quadric surfaces with the space horopter as their common curve of intersection.

**horopter, space** The horopter consisting of all object points in space which stimulate corresponding retinal points as distinguished from the two-dimensional cases such as the apparent frontoparallel plane, longitudinal or nonius horopters.

**horopter, vernier** *See* **horopter, nonius.**

**horopter, Vieth–Müller** A theoretical horopter formed by a circle passing through the point of fixation and the anterior nodal points of the two eyes. Thus any point on this horopter forms an image in the two retinas which is at equal distances from their respective foveas. *Syn.* Vieth–Müller circle.
*See* **deviation, Hering–Hillebrand.**

**horopter, theoretical** A horopter based on theoretical concepts. *Example*: the Vieth–Müller horopter.
*See* **horopter, empirical; horopter, Vieth–Müller.**

**horror fusionis** Avoidance of fusion resulting from two retinal images which are so different that they are impossible to fuse. This is often the case in strabismus. *Syn.* fusion aversion.

**horseshoe tear** A type of retinal tear in which a strip of tissue is torn from the retina. The tear commonly follows a vitreous detachment in which the vitreous adheres to the retina and pulls it from the point of adherence during or just after an abrupt eye movement. This type of retinal tear is particularly dangerous since it is often a precursor to a retinal detachment.
*See* **retinal tear; retinal detachment.**

**Howard–Dolman test** *See* **test, Howard–Dolman.**

**HRR test** *See* **plates, pseudoisochromatic.**

**Hruby lens** *See* **lens, Hruby.**

**Hudson–Stahli** *See* **line, Hudson–Stahli.**

**hue** Attribute of colour sensation, such as blue, red, green, etc., which is ordinarily associated with a given wavelength of the light stimulating the retina, as distinguished from the attributes of brightness and saturation.
*See* **brightness; phenomenon, Bezold–Brücke; saturation; threshold, differential.**

**humour, aqueous** Clear, colourless fluid that fills the anterior and posterior chambers of the eye. It is a carrier of nutrients for the lens and for part of the cornea. It contributes to the maintenance of the intraocular pressure. It is formed in the ciliary processes, flows into the posterior chamber, then through the pupil into the anterior chamber and leaves the eye through the trabecular meshwork passing to the canal of Schlemm and then to veins in the deep scleral plexus (Fig. H2). The aqueous in the anterior chamber is a component of the optical system of the eye. It has an index of refraction of 1.336, slightly lower than that of the cornea so that the cornea/aqueous surface acts as a diverging lens of low power.
*See* **adrenergic receptors; aqueous flare; canal, Schlemm's; ciliary processes; cornea; glaucoma, open-angle; meshwork, trabecular; tonography; transport, active; ultrafiltration; vein, aqueous.**

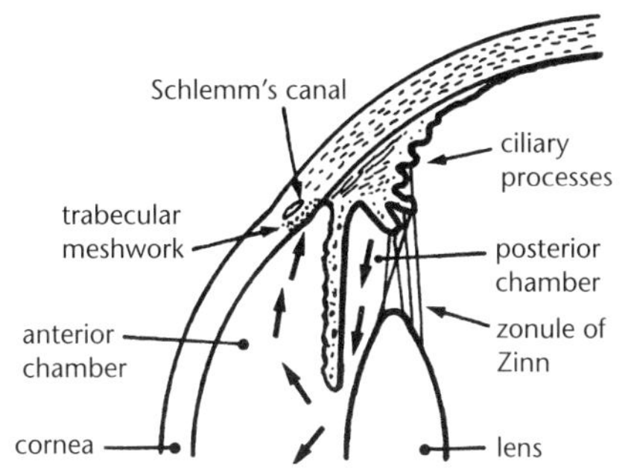


**Fig. H2** Outflow of aqueous humour

**humour, vitreous** A transparent, colourless, gelatinous mass of a consistency somewhat firmer than egg white which fills the space between the crystalline lens, the ciliary body and the retina. It is firmly attached to the pars plana of the ciliary body near the ora serrata in an area known as the **vitreous base** and around the optic disc. In older people and in pathological conditions the vitreous is no longer in a gel state tending to become fluid. It has a chemical composition similar to that of the aqueous humour, except for a greater content of collagen and hyaluronic acid. *Syn.* vitreous body.
*See* **artery, hyaloid; asteroid hyalosis; canal, hyaloid; chamber, vitreous; floaters; hyaloid remnant; synchisis scintillans; vitrectomy; vitreous base; vitreous detachment.**

**Humphrey Vision Analyser** *See* **Analyser, Humphrey Vision.**

**Humphriss immediate contrast test; method** *See* **method, Humphriss.**

**Hutchinson's pupil** *See* **pupil, Hutchinson's.**

**Huygens' eyepiece** *See* **eyepiece, Huygens'.**

**hyaline bodies** *See* **drusen.**

**hyaloid artery; canal; fossa** *See* under the nouns.

**hyaloid membrane** *See* **membrane, hyaloid.**

**hyaloid remnant** A rare condition in which there remain some parts of the hyaloid artery. Posteriorly there may be a vascular loop or the thread of an obliterated vessel running forward from the optic disc and floating freely in the vitreous. Anteriorly there may be some fibrous remnants attached to the posterior lens capsule and others sometimes floating in the vitreous. The anterior attachment of the hyaloid artery to the lens may also remain throughout life as a black dot, called **Mittendorf's dot**, and can be seen within the pupil by direct ophthalmoscopy (it appears as a white dot with the biomicroscope). There is rarely any visual interference although patients may sometimes report seeing muscae volitantes. *Syn.* persistent hyaloid artery.
*See* **glial veil; image, entoptic; vitreous, persistent hyperplastic primary.**

**hydrocortisone** *See* **antiinflammatory drug.**

**hydrogel** Type of plastic material which contains water, and is commonly used in the manufacture of soft contact lenses, e.g. HEMA.

**hydrogen peroxide** *See* **antiseptic.**

**hydrophilic lens** *See* **lens, contact.**

**hydrophthalmos** *See* **glaucoma, congenital.**

**hydrops, corneal** Excessive accumulation of watery fluid in the stroma of the cornea as a result of rupture of the posterior layers of the cornea (Descemet's membrane and the endothelium). It is often found in advanced keratoconus.
*See* **cornea; keratoconus.**

**hydroxyethylcellulose; hydroxymethylcellulose, hydroxypropylcellulose** *See* **tears, artificial.**

**hydroxypropylmethylcellulose** *See* **hypromellose.**

**hyoscine hydrobromide** An antimuscarinic (or parasympatholytic) drug with actions, similar to those of atropine, but of shorter duration. It is used in the measurement of refraction of children and in the treatment of keratitis, anterior uveitis and in cases of burns to the anterior segment of the eye to prevent posterior synechia, as well as to reduce the pain secondary to iridociliary spasm. *Syn.* scopolamine hydrobromide.

See **acetylcholine; atropine; cycloplegia; mydriatic.**

**hyperaccommodation** See **accommodative excess.**

**hyperacuity** The ability of the eye to detect the differences in the spatial locations of two or more stimuli. Hyperacuity thresholds are not based on resolution and are usually below about 15 seconds of arc. Hyperacuity tests include vernier acuity, stereoscopic acuity, orientation discrimination in which differences in the tilts of lines must be detected, the movement displacement threshold, the vertical alignment of a cluster of dots, or the ability to bisect two parallel lines. Hyperacuity is less affected by optical defocus or light scattering (as occurs for example in corneal leukoma, cataract, vitreous haemorrhage) than is Snellen acuity and can therefore be helpful in assessing macular function behind a cataract or other media opacity before surgery (Fig. H3).
See **acuity, stereoscopic visual; acuity, vernier visual; cataract; leukoma; maxwellian view system, clinical; threshold, movement.**

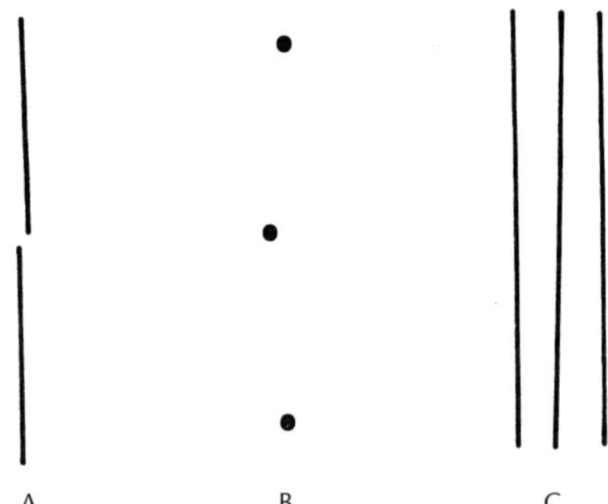


**Fig. H3** Examples of hyperacuity tests (A, detection of lack of alignment of two lines; B, of three dots; C, of the tilt of one line)

**hyperaemia** Excessive accumulation of blood in a part of the body. *Note*: also spelt hyperemia. *Syn.* injection.
See **injection, ciliary; injection, conjunctival.**

**hyperaesthesia, corneal** Abnormally high corneal sensitivity (threshold less than 15 mg/0.013 mm$^2$ near the limbus in the adult eye) as distinguished from **hypoaesthesia** (beyond 70 mg/0.013 mm$^2$ near the limbus in the adult eye) which is abnormally low corneal sensitivity.
See **aesthesiometer; corneal touch threshold; sensitivity, corneal.**

**hypercapnia** The presence of a raised carbon dioxide content or tension in a milieu (e.g. blood, tears). Contact lens wear tends to give rise to this condition, especially lenses of low gas transmissibility.

**hypercolumn** A complete set of orientation columns over a cycle of 180° and of right and left dominance columns in the visual cortex. A hypercolumn may be about 1 mm wide. A hypercolumn of orientation columns is perpendicular to a hypercolumn of ocular dominance columns (Fig. H4).
See **column, cortical.**

**hypercomplex cell** See **cell, hypercomplex.**

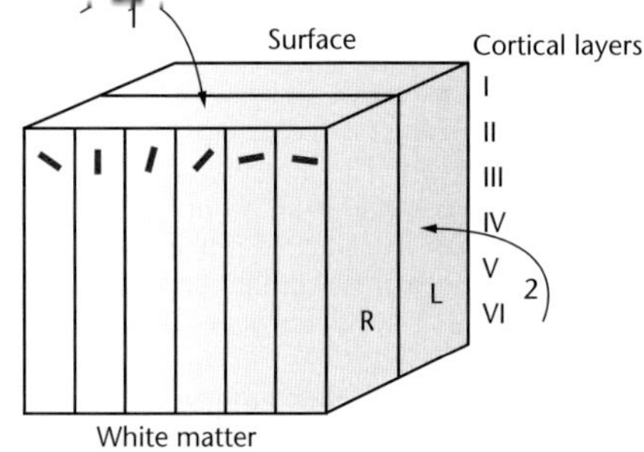


**Fig. H4** A hypercolumn consisting of one set of orientation columns and one set of ocular dominance columns in the visual cortex. Electrode 1 penetrating at right angle to the surface encounters neurons responding to the same orientation and the same (right) ocular dominance. Electrode 2 penetrating parallel to the surface encounters neurons responding to the left ocular dominance and to different orientations

**hyperfocal distance** See **distance, hyperfocal.**

**hyperlacrimation** Overflow of tears due to excessive secretion by the lacrimal gland. It may be caused by drugs (e.g. pilocarpine), strong emotion; or as a reflex from trigeminal stimulation by an inflamed eye; or irritation of the cornea or conjunctiva by a chemical irritant in the air; cold wind; or a foreign body in the eye. The main symptoms are discomfort and blurring of vision and sometimes embarrassment. Management depends on the cause. *Syn.* hypersecretion.
See **epiphora; gland, lacrimal; tears.**

**hypermature cataract** See **cataract, hypermature.**

**hypermetria** An abnormally large movement. *Example*: a saccade which overshoots its target.
See **movement, saccadic eye.**

**hypermetrope** A person who has hypermetropia.

**hypermetropia (H)** Refractive condition of the eye in which distant objects are focused behind the retina when the accommodation is relaxed. Thus, vision is blurred. In hypermetropia, the point conjugate with the retina, that is the far point of the eye, is located behind the eye (Fig. H5).

The percentage of people with hypermetropia increases beyond the age of 40. *Syn.* far sight; long sight; hyperopia.
*See* **glaucoma, angle-closure; headache, ocular; luxation of the lens; retinoschisis; test, plus 1.00 D blur.**

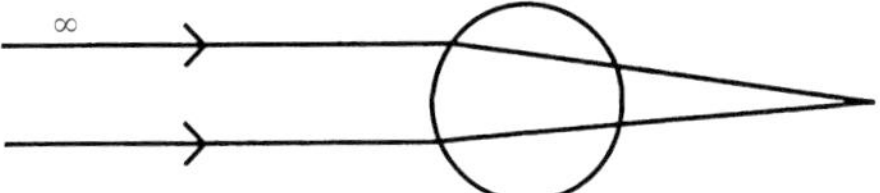


**Fig. H5** A hypermetropic eye looking at a distant axial point

**hypermetropia, absolute** That hypermetropia which cannot be compensated for by accommodation.

**Table H1** Approximate relationship between uncorrected absolute hypermetropia and visual acuity

| | Snellen visual acuity | |
|---|---|---|
| **hypermetropia** | **(m)** | **(ft)** |
| +4.5 D | 6/120 | 20/400 |
| +3.5 D | 6/90 | 20/300 |
| +2.5 D | 6/60 | 20/200 |
| +2.0 D | 6/36 | 20/120 |
| +1.5 D | 6/24 | 20/80 |
| +1.0 D | 6/18 | 20/60 |
| +0.75 D | 6/12 | 20/40 |
| +0.50 D | 6/9 | 20/30 |

**hypermetropia, acquired** Hypermetropia resulting from changes in the refractive indices of the media due to either age or disease, or to surgery.
*See* **hypermetropia, simple.**

**hypermetropia, facultative** That portion of hypermetropia which can be compensated for by accommodation.

**hypermetropia, latent** That portion of total hypermetropia which is compensated for by the tonus of the ciliary muscle. It can be revealed wholly or partially by the use of a cycloplegic.
*See* **hypermetropia, total.**

**hypermetropia, manifest** That portion of total hypermetropia which can be determined by the strongest convex lens in a subjective routine examination while retaining the best visual acuity.
*See* **hypermetropia, total.**

**hypermetropia, simple** Hypermetropia uncomplicated by disease, trauma or astigmatism.

**hypermetropia, total** The sum of the latent and manifest hypermetropia.

**hyperopia** *See* **hypermetropia.**

**hyperosmotic agent** A drug which makes blood plasma hypertonic thus drawing fluid out of the eye and leading to a reduction in intraocular pressure. It is used in solution in the treatment of angle-closure glaucoma and sometimes before surgery to decrease the intraocular pressure. Common agents include glycerine, isosorbide, mannitol and urea.
*See* **glaucoma, angle-closure; solution, hypertonic.**

**hyperphoria** The tendency for the line of sight of one eye to deviate upward relative to that of the other eye, in the absence of an adequate stimulus to fusion. If the deviation tends to be downward relative to the other eye or if the other eye in hyperphoria is used as a reference, the condition is called **hypophoria**.
*See* **kataphoria.**

**hyperphoria, left (L/R)** Hyperphoria in which the line of sight of the left eye deviates upward relative to the other eye.

**hyperphoria, paretic** Hyperphoria due to a paresis of one or several of the extraocular muscles.

**hyperphoria, right (R/L)** Hyperphoria in which the line of sight of the right eye deviates upward relative to the other eye.

**hyperplasia** Any condition in which there is an increase in the number of cells in an organ or a tissue. It usually excludes tumour formation. *Example*: choroidal naevus.
*See* **naevus, choroidal.**

**hyperpolarization** A change in the value of the resting membrane potential towards a more negative value. The inside of the cell becomes more negative than the outside. *Example*: the retinal photoreceptor potentials when stimulated by light.
*See* **depolarization; potential, receptor; potential, resting membrane.**

**hypersecretion** *See* **hyperlacrimation.**

**hypertelorism, ocular** A developmental, congenital anomaly in which the distance between the orbits is abnormally large resulting in a large distance between the eyes. This can be associated with mental deficiency, divergent strabismus, exophthalmos or optic atrophy.

**hypertension** Abnormally high blood pressure beyond 140–150 mmHg for systolic blood pressure or beyond 90–95 mmHg for diastolic blood pressure. These figures are higher for older people. Elevated blood pressure can give rise to hypertensive retinopathy.
*See* **paralysis of the fourth nerve; paralysis of the sixth nerve; paralysis of the third**

**nerve; retinopathy, hypertensive; sphygmomanometer.**

**hypertension, ocular** A condition in which the intraocular pressure is above normal but in which there are neither visual field defects nor optic disc changes. Open-angle glaucoma may or may not develop later.
*See* **glaucoma, open-angle; pressure, intraocular.**

**hypertensive retinopathy** *See* **retinopathy, hypertensive.**

**hyperthyroidism** *See* **disease, Graves'; ophthalmopathy, thyroid.**

**hypertonic solution** *See* **solution, hypertonic.**

h

**hypertropia** Strabismus in which one eye is directed to the fixation point while the other is directed upward (right or left hypertropia). If one eye fixates while the other is directed downward the condition is called **hypotropia** (right or left hypotropia). *Syn.* for hypertropia is sursumvergens strabismus; for hypotropia is deorsumvergens strabismus.
*See* **strabismus; test, three-step.**

**hypertropia, alternating** A condition in which, on dissociation (e.g. by occlusion) of either eye, the eye behind the cover deviates upward but reverts to its fixating position when dissociation ceases. The condition can either occur as an isolated phenomenon or be associated with strabismus or latent strabismus. *Syn.* anaphoria; anatropia; dissociated vertical divergence; double hyperphoria.
*See* **dissociation; phenomenon, Bielschowsky's; strabismus.**

**hyphaemia** Haemorrhage into the anterior chamber of the eye. It usually occurs as a result of trauma to the eye, especially in sports. It is usually advisable to have the patient admitted to hospital because of the possibility of recurrent haemorrhage and secondary glaucoma. *Note*: also spelt hyphema.
*See* **glaucoma.**

**hypoaesthesia** *See* **hyperaesthesia, corneal.**

**hypoexophoria** Combined hypophoria and exophoria.

**hypolacrima** *See* **alacrima.**

**hypophoria** *See* **hyperphoria.**

**hypoplasia** Any condition in which there is a decrease in the number of cells in an organ or tissue. *Example*: optic nerve hypoplasia in which there is a reduction of axons which, in severe cases, leads to visual impairment.
*See* **hyperplasia.**

**hypopyon** The presence of pus in the anterior chamber of the eye associated with infectious diseases of the cornea (e.g. corneal ulcer), the iris or the ciliary body. The pus usually accumulates at the bottom of the chamber and may be seen through the cornea.
*See* **disease, Behçet's; iritis; keratitis, hypopyon; keratomycosis; ulcer, corneal; uveitis.**

**hypothalamus** A group of nuclei at the base of the brain located in the floor of the third ventricle. It consists of the optic chiasma, the paired mammillary bodies, the tuber cinereum, the infundibulum and the pars posterior of the pituitary gland.

**hypotonia, ocular** Abnormally low intraocular pressure. *Syn.* ocular hypotonus; ocular hypotony.

**hypotonic solution** *See* **solution, hypotonic.**

**hypotropia** *See* **hypertropia.**

**hypoxia** An inadequate supply of oxygen to tissues. It may occur in some pathological conditions. *Examples*: in long-standing cases of diabetes there is corneal hypoxia (with consequent high epithelial fragility and some neovascularization) and retinal hypoxia (with consequent neovascularization). Corneal hypoxia (with consequent oedema, loss of sensitivity, etc.) may also occur in contact lens wear.
*See* **anoxia; hypercapnia; microcysts, epithelial; mitosis; oedema; oxygen requirement, critical; retinopathy, proliferative; syndrome, corneal exhaustion; syndrome, overwear; tear pumping.**

**hypoxic stress** *See* **strain.**

**hypromellose** A highly viscous, water-soluble, non-irritating compound used as a thickening, lubricating and clinging agent. It is used principally as artificial tears (as for example in the management of keratoconjunctivitis sicca) and sometimes as a wetting agent. *Syn.* hydroxypropylmethylcellulose.
*See* **alacrima; keratitis sicca; methylcellulose; staining, 3 and 9 o'clock; tears, artificial; wetting solution.**

**hysteresis, accommodative** A term used to indicate an incomplete and temporary relaxation of the accommodation of the eye after a period of fixation. The amount of relaxation varies according to the position of the fixation point relative to the position of the tonic accommodation, and to the ametropia of the eye. In general, a sustained near visual task leads to an increase in accommodation, while a sustained distant visual task leads to a decrease in accommodation.
*See* **accommodation, resting state of.**

**hysterical amblyopia** *See* **amblyopia, hysterical.**

**hysteropia** Visual disorder due to hysteria.
*See* **amblyopia, hysterical.**

# I

**iatrogenic** Relating to a disorder induced by the treatment itself. *Example*: the development of amblyopia in the good eye following occlusion treatment.

**idiopathic** Relating to any primary pathological condition of unknown origin.

**idoxuridine** *See* **antiviral agents.**

**illiterate chart** *See* **chart, illiterate.**

**illuminance** Quotient of the luminous flux, F, incident on an element of surface divided by the area, A, of that element of surface. *Symbol*: E. Thus,

$$E = \frac{F}{A}$$

The units are in lux or footcandles. *Syn.* illumination.
*See* **footcandle; law of illumination, inverse square; lux; photometer.**

**illuminance, retinal** *See* **retinal illuminance.**

**illuminants, CIE standard** The colorimetric illuminants A, B, C and D defined by the CIE in terms of relative spectral energy (power distribution): **standard illuminant A** representing the full radiator at T = 2854 K; **standard illuminant B** representing direct sunlight with a correlated colour temperature of T = 4874 K; **standard illuminant C** representing daylight with a correlated colour temperature of T = 6774 K; **standard illuminant D** representing daylight with a correlated colour temperature of T = 6504 K (CIE).
*See* **chromaticity diagram; lamp, Macbeth; light, white.**

**illumination** **1.** The action of brightening an object with light. **2.** The science of the application of lighting. **3.** Synonym for illuminance.
*See* **illuminance.**

**illumination, diffuse** In slit-lamp examination, it is the illumination obtained with a wide slit and an out of focus beam or with a diffuser, thus providing an overall view of the structures of the eye.

**illumination, direct** In slit-lamp examination, the slit beam and the microscope are both focused sharply on the structure to be observed. *Syn.* focal illumination.

**illumination, focal** *See* **illumination, direct.**

**illumination, indirect** In slit-lamp examination, the slit beam is focused on a structure located adjacent to the structure to be observed.

**illumination, inverse square law of** *See* **law of illumination, inverse square.**

**illumination, oscillation** In slit-lamp examination, it is a technique in which the beam of light is oscillated to provide alternative direct and indirect illumination. It sometimes allows one to see slight changes more easily which otherwise would remain unnoticed under sustained illumination of either kind.

**illumination, retinal** *See* **retinal illuminance.**

**illumination, retro-** In slit-lamp examination, it is a method of illuminating a structure by using the light that is reflected by the iris or an opaque or senescent lens. This method is closely related to indirect illumination and often in corneal examination, part of the cornea will simultaneously be under retro- and indirect illumination. *Syn.* transillumination.
*See* **clouding, central corneal; oedema.**

**illumination, sclerotic scatter** In slit-lamp examination, it is a method in which the beam of light is focused on the sclera near the limbus and the cornea remains uniformly dark in the absence of an opacity. However, an opacity in the cornea becomes easily visible as it scatters light.
*See* **clouding, central corneal; oedema.**

**illumination, specular reflection** In slit-lamp examination, it is a method in which the beam of light and the microscope are placed at equal angles from the normal to the corneal or lens surface to be viewed. This is a method for examining the quality of a surface. This method is particularly useful to observe the corneal endothelium.
*See* **blebs, endothelial; cornea guttata; corneal endothelium; shagreen.**

**illuminometer** *See* **photometer.**

**illusion, autokinetic visual** The apparent motion of a luminous object fixated in the dark, or in a large blank field. It is not due to eye movements and the illusion disappears as soon as the ambient luminance increases so that other objects become visible. *Syn.* visual autokinesis.

**illusion Baldwin's** **1.** Illusion in which a line connecting two large squares appears shorter than a line connecting two smaller squares (Fig. I1). **2.** Illusion in which a dot placed halfway between a large disc and a smaller disc appears to be nearer the large one.

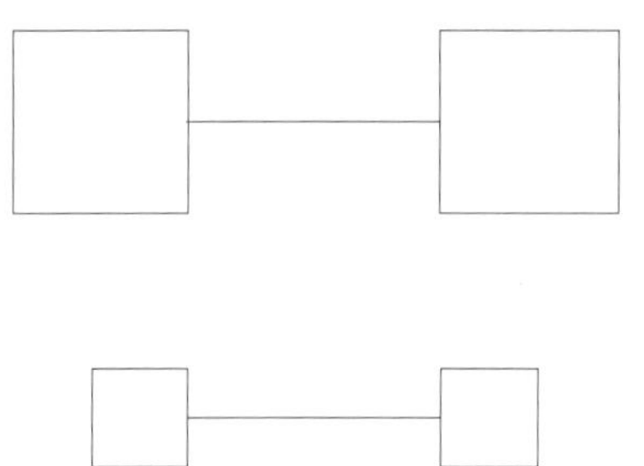

**Fig. I1** Baldwin's illusion

**illusion, café wall** An illusion induced by a pattern of alternating columns of black and white rectangles (or squares) placed in such a way that the lines that they compose do not appear to be parallel. *Syn.* Munsterberg illusion. A variant of this illusion consists of hollow squares without alternating colour and is called a 'hollow square illusion'.

**illusion, corridor** Illusion in which images of equal size in a perspective figure of a corridor, appear to be of different sizes. The figure that seems further away appears larger than the one in the foreground (Fig. I2).

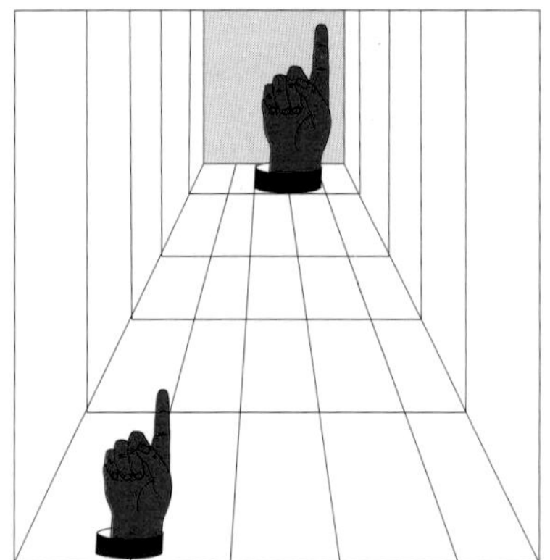

**Fig. I2** Corridor illusion

**illusion, Craik–Cornsweet** An illusion produced by separating two identical black (or grey) areas of equal average luminance separated by a border consisting of a narrow dark strip merging into a narrow light strip (or double cusp). It results in the whole area adjacent to the narrow light strip appearing much lighter than the other area adjacent to the narrow dark strip. It is often demonstrated by using a rotating disc. *Syn.* Craik–O'Brien effect; O'Brien edge illusion.

**illusion Delboeuf** Illusion in which a circle surrounded by a slightly larger concentric circle appears larger than another circle of the same size surrounded by a much larger concentric circle (Fig. I3).

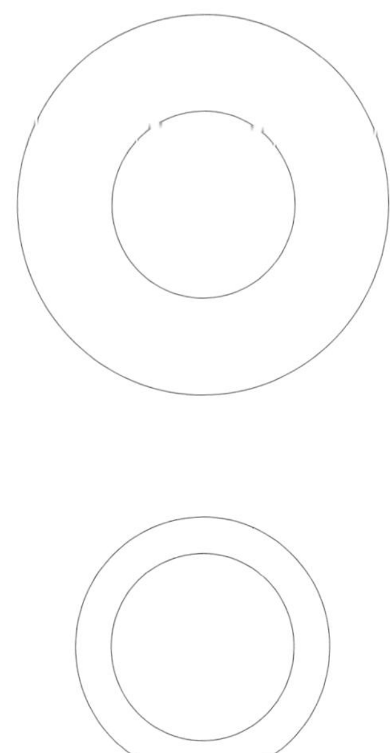

**Fig. I3** Delboeuf illusion

**illusion, Ebbinghaus** Illusion in which a circle usually appears larger when surrounded by smaller circles than by larger circles.

**illusion, Ehrenstein' brightness** Illusion in which the erased area at the intersection of radial (or horizontal and vertical) lines appears to be brighter than the background and with an illusory contour (Fig. I4).

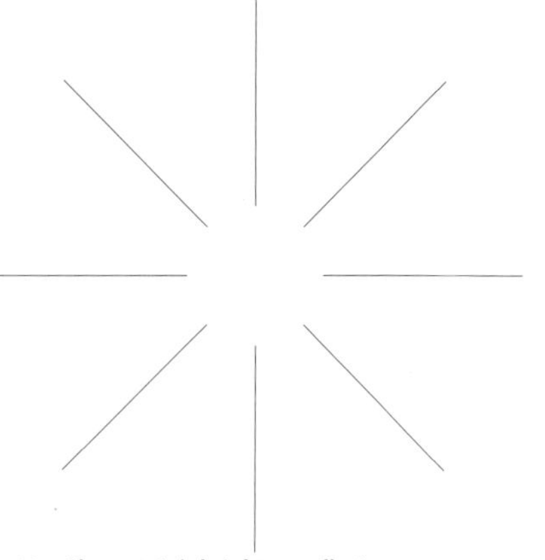

**Fig. I4** Ehrenstein's brightness illusion

**illusion, floating-finger** Illusion noted when fixating a point in the distance while the forefingers of each hand are held horizontally about 30 centimetres in front of the eyes, with the fingertips nearly touching. A small, disembodied finger

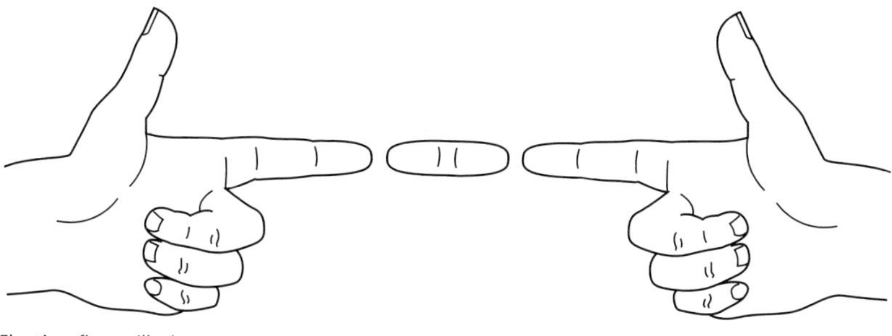

Fig. I5 Floating-finger illusion

with two tips appears floating in between and can be shortened or lengthened by varying the distance between the fingertips. It is a peculiar illustration of physiological diplopia (Fig. I5).
*See* **diplopia, physiological.**

**illusion, frequency doubling** Illusion in which a grating pattern appears to have twice as many black and white bars as it actually has. This happens when a sinusoidal grating with a low spatial frequency (less than 4 c/deg) flickers in a counterphase fashion (i.e. light bars become dark and vice versa) at a high temporal frequency (more than 15 Hz). This type of stimulation is assumed to stimulate the non-linear mechanism within the magnocellular visual system.
*See* **magnocellular visual system; perimetry, frequency doubling.**

**illusion, Hering's** Illusion in which a pair of parallel lines appear bent when placing diagonal lines across them. This illusion is most noticeable when radiating lines are crossing two parallel lines on opposite sides of the point of radiation. In this case, the two parallel lines appear to bend away from each other (Fig. I6).
*See* **illusion, Wundt's.**

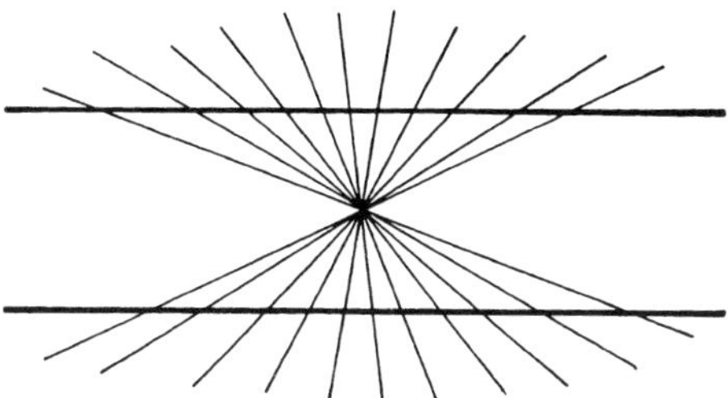

Fig. I6 Hering's illusion

**illusion, Helmholtz** *See* **irradiation.**

**illusion, Hermann's** *See* **Hering–Hermann's grid.**

**illusion, hole in the hand** *See* **test, hole in the hand.**

**illusion, hollow square** *See* **illusion, café wall.**

**illusion, horizontal–vertical visual** Illusion in which the vertical line appears longer than the horizontal line when two lines of equal length are placed with the vertical line at the midpoint of the horizontal.
*See* **illusion, top hat.**

**illusion, Jastrow** Illusion in which two identical curved and tapering ring segments placed one above the other appear unequal in size, the band nearer the centres of curvature appearing to be the longest (Fig. I7).

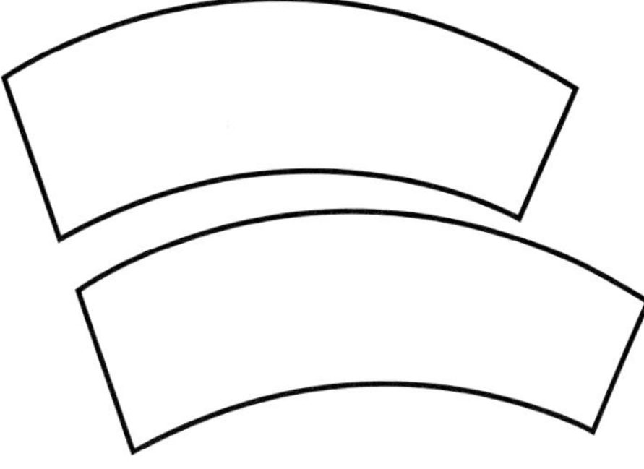

Fig. I7 Jastrow illusion

**illusion, Kundt's** Illusion occurring when one attempts to bisect a horizontal line with only one eye and the segment on the temporal side of the visual field is then larger than the other.

**illusion, moon** Illusion in which the moon appears much larger at the horizon than when viewed high in the sky. In fact, the actual size of the moon remains constant as does its distance from the earth. One possible explanation is that at the horizon there are many other cues in the field of view (e.g. houses, mountains) which make the moon appear to be much closer than when it is high in the sky and thus should be larger.
*See* **room, Ames.**

**illusion, Müller–Lyer** Illusion in which a line with outgoing fins on both ends appears longer than another of equal length but with arrowheads on both ends (Fig. I8).

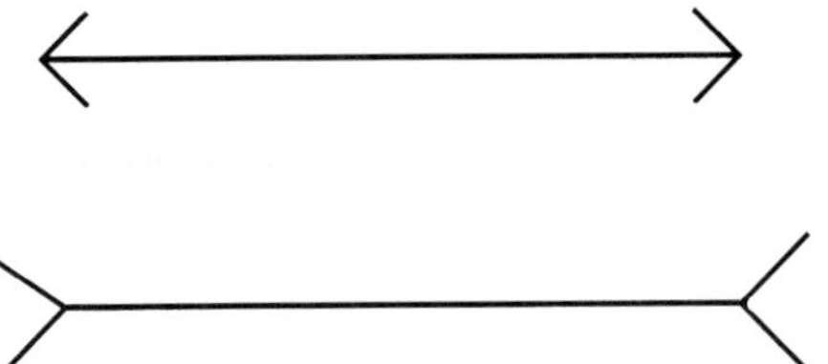

Fig. I8 Müller–Lyer illusion

**illusion, Munsterberg** *See* **illusion, café wall.**

**illusion, oculogyral** Illusion of apparent movement of viewed objects when the body is subjected to rotary acceleration. The initial apparent movement is opposite to that of the direction of rotation of the body and is followed by an apparent movement in the same direction.

**illusion, Oppel–Kundt** Illusion in which a divided, interrupted or filled area appears to be larger than an empty area of equal size.

**illusion, optical** *See* **illusion, visual.**

**illusion, Orbison** Illusion of a distorted geometric figure such as a square or a circle drawn on a background of radiating lines or concentric lines.

**illusion, Poggendorff's** Illusion in which two visible portions of a diagonal line overlayed by a rectangle do not appear to be continuous (Fig. I9).

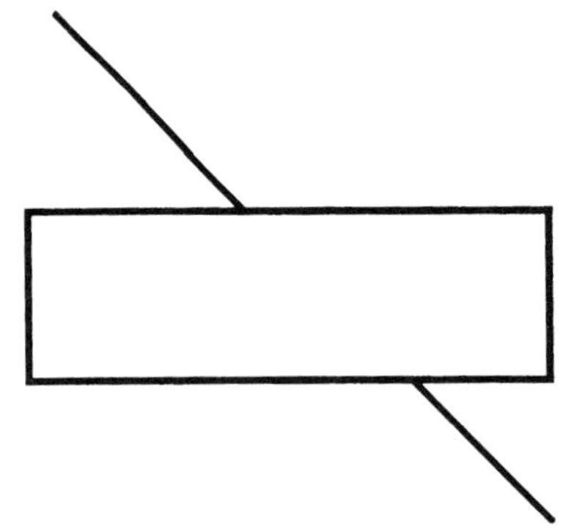

Fig. I9 Poggendorff's illusion

**illusion, Ponzo** Illusion in which two parallel lines of equal length do not appear equal when they are surrounded by two radiating straight lines, one on each side. The parallel line nearer the point of radiation appears to be longer (Fig. I10).

**illusion, Schroeder's staircase visual** *See* **Schroeder's staircase.**

**illusion, top hat** Illusion in which a top hat drawn with equal vertical and horizontal dimensions appears to be much greater vertically than

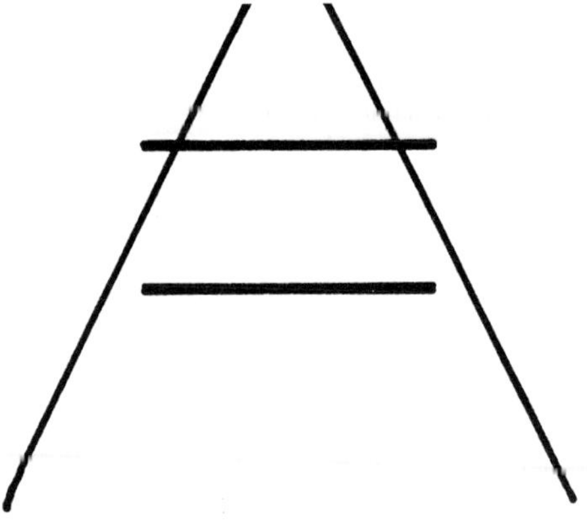

Fig. I10 Ponzo illusion

horizontally. It is closely related to the horizontal–vertical illusion (Fig. I11).
*See* **illusion, horizontal–vertical visual.**

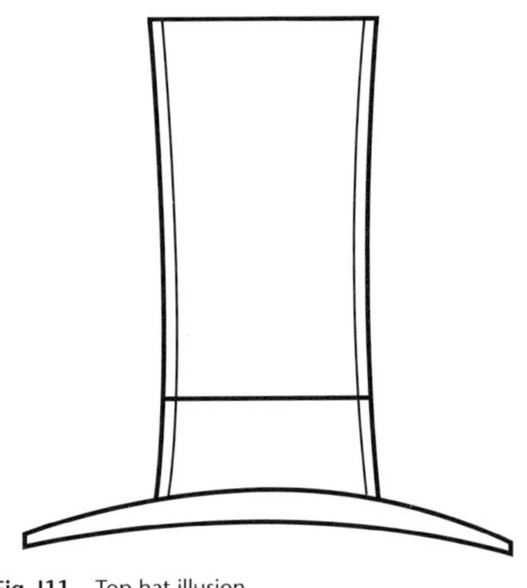

Fig. I11 Top hat illusion

**illusion, visual** Perception of an object or a figure which does not correspond to the actual physical characteristics of the stimulus.
*See* **optical illusion; geometrical optical illusion.**

**illusion, waterfall** *See* **after-effect, waterfall.**

**illusion, Wundt's** Illusion in which a pair of parallel lines appear bent towards each other when crossed by lines radiating from two points, one on each side of the parallel lines.
*See* **illusion, Hering's.**

**illusion, Zollner's** Illusion in which a series of parallel lines appear to converge or diverge from each other when crossed by short diagonal lines.

**image** A picture of an object formed by a lens, a mirror or other optical system.
*See* **object; plane, image.**

**image, aerial** An image found in space and not on a screen such as the image viewed in indirect ophthalmoscopy.
*See* **ophthalmoscopy, indirect.**

**image, after-** *See* **after-image.**

**image, axial point** The point of intersection of an image with the optical axis.

**image, catadioptric** Image formed by both reflecting and refracting surfaces.
*See* **catadioptric system.**

**image, catoptric** Image formed by regular reflection, either from a mirror or by reflection at refracting surfaces such as the optical surfaces of the eye which form the Purkinje–Sanson images.
*See* **images, Purkinje–Sanson.**

**image, corneal** Catoptric image formed by either the anterior or posterior surface of the cornea. They are also called the first and second Purkinje–Sanson images.
*See* **images, Purkinje–Sanson.**

**image, dioptric** An image formed by a refracting surface as distinguished from a catoptric image.

**image, direct** A virtual image such as the erect image seen in direct ophthalmoscopy.
*See* **ophthalmoscopy, direct.**

**image, double** A pair of images obtained either optically through a doubling system or due to diplopia.
*See* **diplopia.**

**image, eidetic** Visual perception arising from the imagination of the subject or what has previously been seen, and not from immediate retinal stimulation. That image may last from a few seconds to several minutes and appears to be located in front of the eyes.

**image, entoptic** Visual sensation arising from stimuli within the eye and perceived as in the external world. *Examples*: muscae volitantes; phosphene. *Syn.* entoptic phenomenon.
*See* **angioscotoma; arcs, blue; entoptoscope, blue field; floaters; Haidinger's brushes; Maxwell's spot; muscae volitantes; phosphene.**

**image, erect** Image which is not inverted with respect to the object such as a virtual image produced by a concave lens.
*See* **images, Purkinje–Sanson.**

**image, extraordinary** *See* **birefringence.**

**image, false** **1.** The retinal image in the deviating eye in strabismus. It is less well defined than the true image. **2.** *See* **image, ghost.**
*See* **image, true.**

**image, ghost** **1.** Unwanted image as may be formed by internal reflection in a lens or an optical system. These images are sometimes annoying to spectacle wearers, and even to observers as they detract from the appearance of the spectacle lens or hide the wearer's eyes behind a veil. The intensity of ghost images is diminished by antireflection coatings. **2.** The faint image seen in monocular diplopia. *Syn.* false image.
*See* **antireflection coating; diplopia, monocular; Fresnel's formula; lens flare; light, stray; mirror, front surface.**

**image, indirect** A real image such as the inverted image seen in indirect ophthalmoscopy.
*See* **ophthalmoscopy, indirect.**

**image, inverted** Image which is upside down and right for left with respect to its object. *Syn.* reversed image.
*See* **images, Purkinje–Sanson.**

**image jump** *See* **jump.**

**image line** *See* **line, focal.**

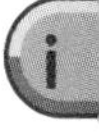

**image, ocular** **1.** The retinal image. **2.** The image formed by the refracting system of the eye, disregarding the presence or the position of the retina.
*See* **image, retinal.**

**image, perceptual; psychic** *See* **image, visual.**

**image, real** An image which can be formed on a screen.
*See* **focus; focus, principal; object, real.**

**image, retinal** Image formed on the retina by the optical system of the eye. The size of the retinal image $h'$ of a distant object subtending angle $u$ in an emmetropic eye is equal to

$$h' = \frac{u}{F}$$

where $h'$ is in metres, $u$ in radians and the power of the eye $F$ in dioptres. The formula is only valid for small angles. *Example*: a distant object subtends an angle of 5° viewed by an emmetropic eye of power 60 D ($\pi$ is equal to 3.1416)

$$u = 5 \times \frac{\pi}{180} = 0.0873\,\text{rad}$$

$$h' = \frac{0.0873}{60} = 0.00145\,\text{m or } 1.45\,\text{mm}$$

**image, reversed** *See* **image, inverted.**

**image shell** The curved surface containing either all the sagittal or all the tangential foci corresponding to a given object plane.
*See* **astigmatism, oblique.**

**image space** Region on one side of an optical system in which the image is formed.
*See* **object space.**

**image, stabilized retinal** *See* **stabilized retinal image.**

**image, true** The retinal image in the normally fixating eye in strabismus.
*See* **image, false.**

**Table I1** Approximate relationship between the retinal image size of an emmetropic eye with a power of 60 D and the angular subtense of a distant object

| angle (deg) | size (mm) |
|---|---|
| 0.017° (or 1′) | 0.0048 |
| 0.07° (or 4′) | 0.0194 |
| 0.013° (or 8′) | 0.039 |
| 0.2° (or 12′) | 0.058 |
| 0.4° (or 24′) | 0.12 |
| 0.6° (or 36′) | 0.17 |
| 0.8° (or 48′) | 0.23 |
| 1° | 0.29 |
| 2° | 0.58 |
| 3° | 0.87 |
| 4° | 1.16 |
| 5° | 1.45 |
| 6° | 1.75 |
| 8° | 2.33 |
| 10° | 2.91 |
| 12° | 3.49 |
| 15° | 4.36 |

**image, virtual** One from which refracted or reflected rays appear to have come. This image can be seen but it is not an actual image and cannot be formed on a screen. *Examples*: the image seen in a plane mirror; the image seen in the cornea.
*See* **focus; focus, principal; object, virtual.**

**image, visual 1.** Perceived image formed by the whole visual system. It includes the physiological and psychological processing. *Syn.* perceptual image; psychic image. **2.** A mental picture based on the recollection of a previous visual experience.
*See* **aniseikonia.**

**images, Purkinje–Sanson** Catoptric images produced by reflection from the optical surfaces of the eye. The **first image** is reflected by the anterior surface of the cornea, the **second image** by the posterior surface of the cornea, the **third image** by the anterior surface of the crystalline lens and the **fourth image** by the posterior surface of the crystalline lens. Only the fourth image is inverted. The third is the largest but the first is by far the brightest (Fig. I12). During accommodation, the third image becomes smaller while the size of the fourth diminishes only a little. Purkinje–Sanson images are used to measure or calculate various optical dimensions of the eye, to establish angle alpha or lambda and to contribute to some diagnostic tests of strabismus (e.g. Hirschberg's method; Krimsky's method). *Syn.* Purkinje images.
*See* **angle lambda; axis, optical; method, Hirschberg's; method, Krimsky's; ophthalmophakometer; phacoscope.**

**imagery 1.** Process of recalling past visual experiences. **2.** Synonym for visualization.
*See* **image, visual; visualization.**

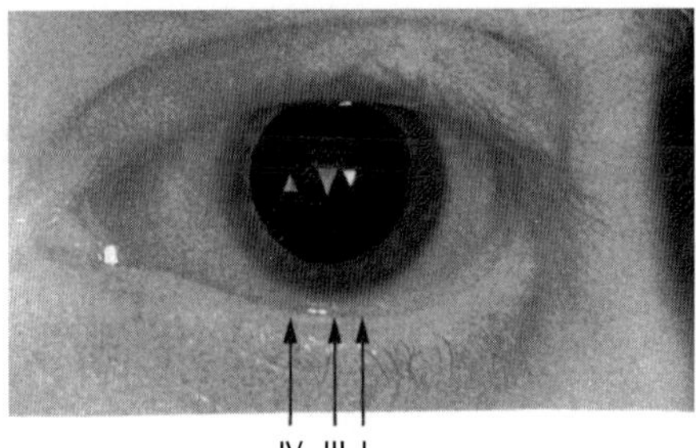


**Fig. I12** Purkinje–Sanson images I, III and IV. Image I is authentic, III and IV have been retouched for emphasis

**Table I2** Purkinje–Sanson images (all figures are calculated and rounded off and all distances are referred to the anterior corneal pole)

| source of reflection | type of image (object is at infinity) | relative brightness |
|---|---|---|
| I anterior corneal surface | – virtual<br>– erect<br>– smaller than object<br>– situated near plane of pupil (about 3.9 mm) | 1.0 |
| II posterior corneal surface | – virtual<br>– erect<br>– smaller than I (about × 0.8)<br>– situated near I (about 3.6 mm) | 0.01 |
| III anterior lens surface | – virtual<br>– erect<br>– larger than I (about × 2.0)<br>– situated in vitreous (about 10.7 mm) | 0.08 |
| IV posterior lens surface | – real<br>– inverted<br>– smaller than I (about × 0.8)<br>– situated in the lens (about 4.6 mm) | 0.08 |

**imbalance, muscular** Generic term referring to a defect in the oculomotor system, as in heterophoria or strabismus.
*See* **heterophoria; strabismus; test, motility.**

**Imbert–Fick law** *See* **law, Imbert–Fick.**

**immersion lens** *See* **lens, immersion.**

**implant, intraocular lens (IOL)** A lens inserted in the eye to replace the crystalline lens after cataract surgery. There are many types including multifocal ones.
*See* **eye, pseudophakic; phacoemulsification; SRK formula.**

**impression cytology** *See* **cytology, impression.**

**impression, eye** A negative form or replica of the anterior part of the eye. A substance with rapid gelling properties is held in contact with the eye until gelled. This **impression** (or **mould**) is then used in the preparation of a positive model called a **cast** (or casting) of the anterior part of the eye: it is made by filling the impression with a material containing a plaster of Paris base which hardens to artificial stone. Using this cast a **shell** of a scleral contact lens is produced with optimum shape of the back surface. *Syn.* impression; impression moulding; mould; ocular impression.

**impression tonometer** *See* **tonometer, impression.**

**in vitro** Term referring to a measurement or a process taking place in a test tube. *Example*: the measurement of the cholesterol content of the crystalline lens done in a test tube.

**in vivo** Term referring to a measurement or a process taking place in the living body. *Example*: the effect of a contact lens on the cornea.

**inadequate stimulus** *See* **stimulus, adequate.**

**incandescence** Emission of visible radiation by thermal excitation (CIE).
*See* **lamp, incandescent electric; luminescence.**

**incidence** **1.** The intersection of a ray of light with an optical surface. **2.** The number of new cases of a specific disease or condition occurring during a specific period of time (e.g. 1 year) divided by the population at risk during that period. *Example*: the incidence of keratoconus in Olmsted County, Minnesota was found to be 2 cases per 100 000 population a year.
*See* **prevalence.**

**incidence, angle of** *See* **angle of incidence.**

**incidence, plane of** *See* **plane of incidence.**

**incident ray** *See* **ray, incident.**

**incipient cataract** *See* **cataract, incipient.**

**inclusion conjunctivitis** *See* **conjunctivitis, adult inclusion.**

**incoherent** *See* **coherent sources.**

**incomitance** Condition in which the manifest or latent angle of deviation of the lines of sight of the two eyes differs according to which eye is fixating or in which direction the eyes are looking. This condition is usually attributed to a paresis or paralysis of one or more of the extraocular muscles. *Syn.* nonconcomitance.
*See* **angle of deviation; anisophoria; concomitance; strabismus, incomitant; strabismus, paralytic.**

**incongruity, retinal** *See* **retinal correspondence, abnormal.**

**incongruous diplopia; scotoma** *See* under the nouns.

**incyclophoria** *See* **cyclophoria.**

**incyclovergence** *See* **excyclovergence.**

**indentation, scleral** A clinical procedure used in conjunction with indirect ophthalmoscopy in which some slight pressure is applied to the sclera to bring the peripheral retina into view. Pressure is usually applied with an instrument called an **indentor**. The technique is contraindicated in patients with elevated intraocular pressure.
*See* **ophthalmoscope, indirect.**

**indentation tonometer** *See* **tonometer, impression.**

**indentor** *See* **indentation, scleral.**

**index myopia** *See* **myopia, lenticular.**

**index of refraction** The ratio of the speed of light in a vacuum or in air, $c$, to the speed of light in a given medium, $v$. *Symbol*: $n$. Hence,

$$n = \frac{c}{v}$$

The speed of light in a given medium depends upon its wavelength. Consequently, the index of refraction varies accordingly, being greater for short wavelengths (blue) than for longer wavelengths (red). The index of refraction forms the basis of Snell's law which quantitatively determines the deviation of light rays traversing a surface separating two media of different refractive indices. *Syn.* refractive index. *Plural*: indices.
*See* **dispersion; index of refraction, absolute; index of refraction, relative; law of refraction; lens, gradient-index; lens, high index; light, speed of; refract; refractometer; wavelength.**

**index of refraction, absolute** The ratio of the speed of light in a **vacuum** to the speed of light in a given medium.

**Table 13** Refractive indices of some transparent media at selected wavelengths

| **spectral line** | G | F | D | C | A |
|---|---|---|---|---|---|
| **origin** | calcium | hydrogen | sodium | hydrogen | oxygen |
| **wavelength (nm)** | 430.8 | 486.1 | 589.3 | 656.3 | 759.4 |
| **aqueous or vitreous humour** | 1.3440 | 1.3404 | 1.3360 | 1.3341 | 1.3317 |
| **crystalline lens** | 1.4307 | 1.4259 | 1.4200 | 1.4175 | 1.4144 |
| **spectacle crown** | 1.5348 | 1.5293 | 1.5230 | 1.5204 | 1.5163 |
| **dense flint** | 1.6397 | 1.6290 | 1.6170 | 1.6122 | 1.6062 |

**Table I4** Index of refraction *n* of various media for sodium light (λ = 589.3)

| | |
|---|---|
| air | 1.00 |
| water (at 20°C) | 1.333 |
| spectacle crown glass | 1.523 |
| flint glass (dense) | 1.62 |
| flint glass (extra dense) | 1.65–1.70 |
| titanium oxide glass | 1.701 |
| **calcite crystal** | |
| ordinary ray | 1.658 |
| extraordinary ray | 1.486 |
| **quartz crystal** | |
| ordinary ray | 1.544 |
| extraordinary ray | 1.553 |
| diamond | 2.42 |
| Canada balsam | 1.53–1.54 |
| CR-39 | 1.498 |
| polycarbonate | 1.586 |
| silicone rubber | 1.44 |
| CAB | 1.47 |
| PMMA | 1.49 |
| HEMA | 1.43 |
| **hydrogel polymer** | |
| 20% water content | 1.46–1.48 |
| 75% water content | 1.37–1.38 |
| **eye** | |
| tears | 1.336 |
| cornea | 1.376 |
| aqueous humour | 1.336 |
| crystalline lens (average effect) | 1.42 |
| vitreous humour | 1.336 |

**index of refraction, relative** The ratio of the speed of light in air (or other medium of reference) to the speed of light in a given medium.

**indirect ophthalmoscope** *See* **ophthalmoscope, indirect.**

**indirect vision** *See* **vision, peripheral.**

**indomethacin** *See* **antiinflammatory drug.**

**induced astigmatism** *See* **astigmatism, induced.**

**induced prism** *See* **prism, induced.**

**induction, colour** Modification of colour perception due either to another light stimulus nearby or to a previous light stimulus.

**induction, spatial** Modification of perception as a result of a simultaneous stimulation in another part of the visual field.
*See* **summation.**

**induction, temporal** Modification of perception as a result of a previous stimulus and in some cases a later stimulus, as in metacontrast.
*See* **metacontrast; summation.**

**industrial vision** *See* **vision, industrial.**

**infantile esotropia syndrome** *See* **strabismus, infantile.**

**infantile glaucoma** *See* **glaucoma, congenital.**

**infection** An invasion of the body by disease-producing microorganisms (e.g. bacteria, virus, fungus, parasite). Treatment typically includes anti-infective drugs, such as antibiotic, antifungal or antiviral agents.
*See* **antibiotic; antifungal agent; antiviral agents; inflammation.**

**inferior oblique muscle; orbital fissure; rectus muscle** *See* under the nouns.

**inferior tarsal muscle** *See* **muscles, Muller's palpebral.**

**infinity, optical** In optics, it is the region from which a point on an object sends rays of light which are considered to be parallel onto an optical system. Consequently it forms a clear image in the focal plane of that system. In clinical optometry, 6 metres is usually regarded as infinity.

**inflammation** A complex reaction that occurs in response to injury, infection, irritation, toxicity or hypersensitivity. The reaction is characterized by redness, heat, pain and swelling to different degrees. Treatment depends on the cause.
*See* **antiinflammatory drug; infection.**

**infraduction** *See* **depression.**

**infraorbital canal** *See* **canal, infraorbital.**

**infrared (IR)** Radiant energy of wavelengths between the extreme red wavelengths of the visible spectrum and a wavelength of a few millimetres. The wave band comprising radiations between 780 and 1400 nm is referred to as **IR-A**. Excessive exposure to these radiations can cause visual loss (e.g. eclipse blindness) and cataract. The waveband comprising radiations between 1400 and 3000 nm is referred to as **IR-B**. Excessive exposure to these radiations can cause cataract and corneal opacity. The wave band comprising radiations between 3000 and $1 \times 10^6$ nm (or 1 mm) is referred to as **IR-C**. Excessive exposure to these radiations can cause cataract.
*See* **blindness, eclipse; cataract, heat-ray; lens, absorptive; optometer, infrared; wavelength.**

**Table I5** Divisions of the infrared spectrum

| | |
|---|---|
| IR-A (near) | 780–1400 nm |
| IR-B (middle) | 1400–3000 nm |
| IR-C (far) | 3000–1 000 000 nm |

**infravergence** Movement of one eye downward relative to the other. *Syn.* deorsumvergence.
*See* **supravergence; vergence.**

**infraversion** *See* **version.**

**inheritance** The acquisition of traits, characteristics and disorders from parents to their children by transmission of genetic information. The genes controlling most characteristics come in pairs, one originating from the father, the other from the mother. If an individual presents only the hereditary characteristics determined by one gene of the pair on the autosomal chromosome, that gene is called **dominant**. The inheritance of diseases in which one parent has an abnormal dominant gene, even though its paired gene is normal, will produce the specific abnormality in about 50% of offspring of either sex. This is called **autosomal dominant inheritance**. *Examples*: Marfan's syndrome, congenital stationary night blindness, neurofibromatosis 1 and 2, von Hippel–Lindau disease. If the individual does not present the hereditary characteristics of the other gene (not dominant) in a pair of genes on the autosomal chromosome, that gene is called **recessive**. The inheritance of diseases from abnormal recessive genes must lie in pairs, that is each normal parent must contribute one recessive abnormal gene and about 25% of the offspring of either sex will be affected. This is called **autosomal recessive inheritance**. *Examples*: Laurence–Moon–Biedl syndrome, Tay–Sachs disease, oculocutaneous albinism, galactokinase deficiency. Thirdly, inheritance may be controlled by genes on the sex chromosomes. Abnormalities of these genes cause a disease in the male, whereas in the female an abnormal recessive gene of the sex chromosome is neutralized by the other gene of the pair. Therefore the disease is transmitted by the females and appears in about half of the male offspring. This is called **X-linked recessive inheritance** (or **sex-linked recessive inheritance**). *Examples*: colour blindness, ocular albinism.

**inhibition, lateral** Action of one neuron (e.g. in the retina) on the neighbouring neuron, the effect of which is to depress or prevent activity in the latter. This mechanism accounts for the increased contrast perception observed at the border of a black and white pattern. In the retina this is produced by the lateral connections of the amacrine and horizontal cells that interconnect the various retinal cells. *Syn.* lateral antagonism.
*See* **field, receptive; Hering–Hermann's grid; Mach's bands.**

**injection, ciliary** Redness (almost lilac) around the limbus of the eye caused by dilatation of the deeper small blood vessels located around the cornea. It occurs in inflammation of the cornea, iris and ciliary body, and in angle-closure glaucoma. Each of these conditions is associated with loss of vision and usually pain. *Syn.* ciliary flush.
*See* **decongestant, ocular; glaucoma, angle-closure; iritis; keratitis; keratomycosis; plexus, pericorneal; uveitis.**

**injection, conjunctival** Redness (bright red or pink) of the conjunctiva fading towards the limbus due to dilatation of the superficial conjunctival blood vessels occurring in conjunctival inflammations. There is no loss of vision but ocular discomfort and no pain.
*See* **conjunctivitis; decongestant, ocular; keratomycosis; ophthalmopathy, thyroid; plexus, pericorneal.**

**injury** *See* **irrigation.**

**inner nuclear layer; plexiform layer** *See* **retina.**

**innervation, reciprocal** *See* **law of reciprocal innervation, Sherrington's.**

**insertion** *See* **muscles, extraocular.**

**Intacs** Tradename of an intracorneal implant consisting of two tiny half ring segments which are inserted into the cornea to reshape its curvature and correct ametropia. The method is presently used to flatten the cornea by a given amount (the thicker the ring segments the flatter the cornea) in order to correct low myopia. It is an outpatient procedure carried out under local anaesthesia, takes less than half an hour and is reversible. The ring segments are made of clear biocompatible plastic inserted into the stroma and around the optical zone of the cornea.
*See* **LASIK.**

**intensity, luminous** Quotient of the luminous flux leaving the source, propagated in an element of solid angle containing the given direction, divided by the element of solid angle. *Symbol*: I. *Unit*: candela (CIE).

**intercilium** *See* **glabella.**

**interference** Modification of light intensity arising from the joint effects of two or more coherent trains of light waves superimposed at the same point in space and arriving at the same instant.
*See* **coherent sources; experiment, Young's; holography.**

**interference filter** *See* **filter, interference.**

**interference fringes** The alternate light and dark bands produced when two or more coherent rays of light are superimposed on a surface.
*See* **bi-prism, Fresnel's; coherent sources; experiment, Young's.**

**interferometer 1.** Instrument designed to measure the wavelength of light, the refractive index of a medium, as well as the flatness, thickness, the quality of optical surfaces, etc. The interferometer is based on the phenomenon of interference between two coherent beams of light. **2.** Name given to several types of clinical maxwellian view system used to measure visual acuity.
*See* **maxwellian view system, clinical; wavelength.**

**intermittent strabismus** *See* **strabismus, intermittent.**

**intermuscular membrane** *See* **membrane, intermuscular.**

**internal hordeolum; ophthalmoplegia** *See* under the nouns.

**internal limiting membrane** *See* **membrane of the retina, internal limiting.**

**internal rectus muscle** *See* **muscle, medial rectus; muscles, extraocular.**

**internuclear ophthalmoplegia** *See* **ophthalmoplegia, internuclear.**

**interocular** Situated between the eyes.

**interocular distance** *See* **distance, interocular.**

**interocular transfer (IOT)** Refers to a change in threshold in one eye which had been occluded, similar to, but of lower magnitude than that in the fixating eye, in response to a visual stimulation. *Example*: an elevation of contrast threshold with both eyes following adaptation to high contrast gratings of a given spatial frequency in one eye. The presence of interocular transfer indicates the existence of binocular cortical neurons.

**interpalpebral fissure** *See* **aperture, palpebral.**

**interposition** *See* **perception, depth.**

**interpupillary distance** *See* **distance, interpupillary.**

**interpupillometer** *See* **pupillometer.**

**interstitial keratitis** *See* **keratitis, interstitial.**

**intertrabecular spaces** *See* **meshwork, trabecular.**

**interval, achromatic** *See* **interval, photochromatic.**

**interval, astigmatic; focal** *See* **Sturm, interval of.**

**interval, photochromatic** Range of low luminances between the absolute threshold of light perception and the threshold of hue. The length of this interval varies with wavelength, being nearly nil around 650 nm (Fig. I13). *Syn.* achromatic interval.
*See* **Purkinje shift; theory, duplicity; threshold, absolute.**

**interval of Sturm** *See* **Sturm, interval of.**

**intorsion** *See* **torsion.**

**intracapsular cataract extraction** *See* **cataract extraction, intracapsular.**

**intraocular** Within the eye.

**intraocular lens implant** *See* **implant, intraocular lens.**

**intraocular muscles; pressure** *See* under the nouns.

**intrinsic light** *See* **light, idioretinal.**

**intrinsic muscles** *See* **muscles, intraocular.**

**inverse square law of illumination** *See* **law of illumination, inverse square.**

**inverted retina** *See* **retina, inverted.**

**invisible spectrum** *See* **spectrum, invisible.**

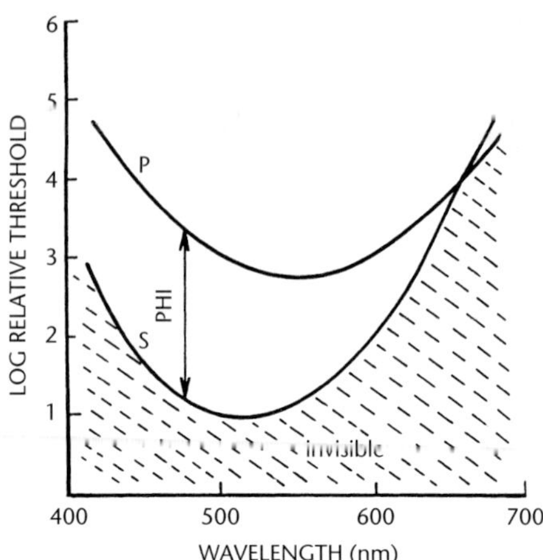


**Fig. I13** Photochromatic interval, PHI (P, curve of the threshold of hue; S, curve of the absolute threshold of light)

**involuntary eye movements** *See* **movements, fixation.**

**involutional ectropion; entropion** *See* under the nouns.

**iodine** *See* **antiseptic.**

**iodopsin** A photosensitive pigment found in the retinal cones of the chicken. Its maximum absorption is around 562 nm.
*See* **pigment, visual; rhodopsin.**

**ipsilateral** A term relating to the same side.
*See* **contralateral; geniculate bodies, lateral.**

**iridaemia** Haemorrhage from the iris. *Note*: also spelt iridemia.

**iridectomy** The surgical removal of part of the iris. The main reasons for iridectomy are to reduce the intraocular pressure, to enlarge an abnormally small pupil and, in cataract extraction, to prevent possible blockage of the angle of the anterior chamber. Nowadays, **laser iridotomy** is preferred in the treatment of angle-closure glaucoma because the incision obtained by this technique can be carried out as an outpatient procedure with only topical anaesthesia, although the cornea must not be hazy.
*See* **glaucoma, angle-closure; iridotomy; iris; iris, plateau; laser; phacoemulsification; pressure, intraocular.**

**irideremia** Absence of all or part of the iris. Strictly speaking a total absence of the iris is called aniridia.
*See* **aniridia.**

**iridescent** Presenting a rainbowlike play of colours as in soap bubbles.

**iridiagnosis** *See* **iridodiagnosis.**

**iridis rubeosis** *See* **rubeosis iridis.**

**iridocorneal angle** *See* **angle of the anterior chamber.**

**iridocorneal endothelial syndrome** *See* **syndrome, ICE.**

**iridocyclitis** Inflammation of both iris and ciliary body. The ciliary body is almost always involved with an inflammation of the iris. The clinical picture of iridocyclitis is practically the same as iritis. The condition is often associated with ankylosing spondylitis or sarcoidosis.
*See* **anisocoria; iritis; heterochromia; rheumatoid arthritis; syndrome, Behçet's; uveitis.**

**iridocyclitis, Fuchs' heterochromic** A chronic, idiopathic, non-granulomatous anterior uveitis characterized by heterochromia, often complicated by cataract which then leads to blurred vision, the main complaint. It is occasionally bilateral; in this case there is no heterochromia. The condition occurs in about 4% of all cases of uveitis. Keratic precipitates are usually present, being small, round or stellate, grey-white in colour and scattered throughout the posterior surface of the cornea. They do not conglomerate or become pigmented and filaments may be seen in between. Glaucoma may develop. Treatment may involve topical steroids as well as cataract or glaucoma therapy. *Syn.* Fuchs' uveitis syndrome; Fuchs' heterochromic cyclitis; heterochromatic iridocyclitis.
*See* **keratic precipitates.**

**iridodiagnosis** Diagnosis of systemic diseases through observation of changes in form and colour of the iris. The validity of this method is questionable. *Syn.* iridiagnosis.
*See* **iridology.**

**iridodialysis** A tearing away of the iris from its attachment to the ciliary body. It usually occurs as a result of blunt trauma to the eye.
*See* **ciliary body; iris.**

**iridology** The study of the iris (colour, shape, etc.), normal and abnormal.
*See* **iridodiagnosis.**

**iridodonesis** A tremulous condition of the iris. It usually occurs in aphakic eyes or when the lens is subluxated. *Syn.* tremulous iris.
*See* **aphakia; luxation of the lens; phacodonesis.**

**iridoplegia** Paralysis of the sphincter muscle of the iris resulting in a dilated pupil. The iridoplegia can be partial as in Argyll Robertson pupil, or complete in which case the pupil does not react to light or to a near object. It may be due to trauma, drugs (e.g. cocaine instilled in the eye) or a systemic disease (e.g. neurosyphilis).
*See* **pupil, Argyll Robertson.**

**iridoschisis** A condition in which the anterior stroma of the iris atrophies and separates from the posterior layer. It mostly affects the inferior iris in elderly patients. In advanced cases the ruptured anterior fibres float in the aqueous humour. It often accompanies angle-closure glaucoma.

**iridotomy** Creation of an opening in the iris to allow aqueous humour to flow from the posterior to the anterior chamber. It is commonly performed with a neodymium-yag or argon laser in angle-closure glaucoma, especially that caused by pupillary block.
*See* **glaucoma, angle-closure; iridectomy; pupillary block.**

**iris** The anterior part of the vascular tunic of the eye, which is situated in front of the crystalline lens and behind the cornea. It has the shape of a circular membrane with a perforation in the centre (the pupil) and is attached peripherally to the ciliary body. The iris forms a curtain dividing the space between the cornea and the lens into the **anterior** and **posterior chambers** of the eye. The anterior surface of the iris is divided into two portions: the largest peripheral **ciliary zone** and the inner **pupillary zone**. The two zones are separated by a zigzag line, the **collarette**. The iris consists of four layers which are, starting in the front: (1) the layer of fibrocytes and melanocytes; (2) the stroma in which are embedded the following structures: (a) the sphincter pupillae muscle which constricts the pupil and is supplied mainly by parasympathetic fibres via the third cranial nerve, (b) the vessels which form the bulk of the iris, and (c) the pigment cells; (3) the posterior membrane consisting of plain muscle fibres which constitute the dilator muscle which is supplied mainly by sympathetic motor fibres, via the long ciliary nerves; (4) the posterior epithelium which is highly pigmented. Sensory fibres from the iris are contained in the nasociliary branch of the ophthalmic nerve. The blood supply is provided by the ciliary arteries. The colour of the iris is blue in babies belonging to the white races and changes colour after a few months of life as pigment is deposited in the anterior limiting layer and the stroma. Iris colour is inherited; brown as a dominant trait and blue as a recessive trait.
*See* **arteries, ciliary; cell, clump; chamber, anterior; chamber, posterior; collarette; corectopia; Fuchs, crypts of; Fuchs' spur; heterochromia; inheritance; iridectomy; iridodialysis; iridology; iritis; melanin; membrane, pupillary; muscle, dilator pupillae; muscle, sphincter pupillae; polycoria; pupil.**

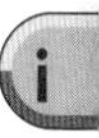


**iris bombé** A condition occurring in posterior annular **synechia** in which an increase of aqueous humour contained in the posterior chamber causes a forward bulging of the iris. It may provoke an attack of angle-closure glaucoma as the iris may block the drainage angle (Fig. I14). *See* **chamber, posterior; glaucoma, angle-closure; humour, aqueous; synechia, annular.**

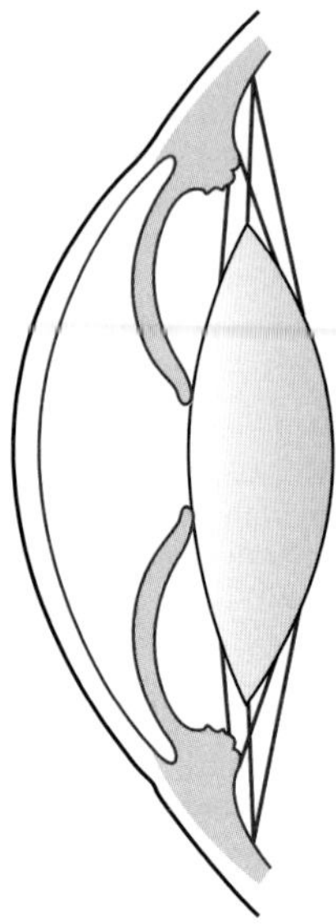

**Fig. I14** Iris bombé and posterior synechia

**iris coloboma; naevus; nodules** *See* under the nouns.

**iris naevus syndrome** *See* **syndrome, Cogan– Reese.**

**iris neovascularization** *See* **neovascularization, iris.**

**iris, plateau** An anatomical anomaly in which the iris lies in a plane rather than bulging anteriorly. This is due to the fact that the **root** (or **ciliary margin**) of the iris is inserted more anteriorly into the ciliary body than usual in apposition to the trabecular meshwork. It can predispose the eye to angle-closure glaucoma.
*See* **glaucoma, angle-closure; meshwork, trabecular.**

**iris processes** Fine bands of tissue extending from the anterior surface of the iris, bridging the angle of the anterior chamber from the root of the iris to the scleral spur or more often to the trabecular meshwork into which they usually merge. The processes are found in only about half of the population.
*See* **meshwork, trabecular; scleral spur.**

**iris, prolapse of the** Protrusion of a portion of the iris into a corneal wound. It results from either trauma, a severe corneal ulcer or an operation. In some cases an anterior synechia may develop as the iris remains fixed in the wound by scar tissue.
*See* **synechia, anterior; ulcer, corneal.**

**iris root** *See* **iris, plateau.**

**iris, tremulous** *See* **iridodonesis.**

**iritis** Inflammation of the iris. The condition is usually characterized by ciliary injection, exudates in the anterior chamber (aqueous flare), keratic precipitates, oedema, constricted and sluggish pupil, discoloration of the iris, posterior synechia, photophobia, lacrimation, loss of vision and pain. The chronic form exhibits most of the above signs and symptoms. In some cases the eye is not injected, in other cases there may be floaters and hypopyon and occasionally rubeosis iridis and an increase in intraocular pressure due to blocking of the angle of the anterior chamber. Iritis is most often associated with choroiditis and cyclitis. Treatment includes mydriatics (to prevent synechia) and topical corticosteroid drops. It is essential to differentiate acute iritis from angle-closure glaucoma because of the possible harm of using a mydriatic in the latter.
*See* **aqueous flare; choroiditis; cyclitis; floaters; hypopyon; injection, ciliary; iridocyclitis; iridodialysis; photophobia; syndrome, Fuchs'; synechia.**

**Irlen lens** *See* **syndrome, Meares–Irlen.**

**Irlen's syndrome** *See* **syndrome, Meares–Irlen.**

**iron deposits** *See* **line, iron; siderosis.**

**irradiation 1.** Application of electromagnetic radiations to an object. **2.** A phenomenon in which a bright area against a black background appears larger than a darker area of equal size against the same background. *Syn.* Helmholtz illusion.

**irregular astigmatism** *See* **astigmatism, irregular.**

**irrigation** The act of washing or cleansing a cavity or a surface with a stream of water or other solution (e.g. saline water) as in chemical or thermal burns or other superficial injuries to the eye, or to dislodge small foreign bodies on the cornea or in the conjunctival sac.
*See* **corneal abrasion; eversion, lid; saline, physiological.**

**Irvine–Gass syndrome** *See* **oedema, cystoid macular.**

**ischaemia** Insufficient blood supply for the need of a part of the body, usually as a result of a disease of the blood vessels supplying that part. *Note*: also spelt ischemia.

**ischaemia of the retina** Lack of blood in the retina due either to arterial narrowing or profuse haemorrhage from any part of the body.
*See* **arteritis, temporal.**

**ischaemic optic neuropathy; ocular syndrome** *See* under the nouns.

Table 16 Differential diagnosis* between acute conjunctivitis, acute iritis and angle-closure glaucoma

| | acute conjunctivitis | acute iritis | angle-closure glaucoma |
|---|---|---|---|
| **Signs** | | | |
| injection | conjunctival | ciliary | conjunctival and ciliary |
| pupil | normal | contracted | semi-dilated and fixed |
| intraocular pressure | normal | normal or low, occasionally increased | high |
| cornea | normal | KP | oedematous |
| anterior chamber | normal depth | normal depth, aqueous flare | shallow |
| iris | normal | faded | faded |
| view of fundus | clear | misty | almost invisible |
| **Symptoms** | | | |
| pain | irritation | moderate | very severe and radiating |
| photophobia | slight | marked | slight |
| lacrimation | watery, purulent or mucopurulent | watery | watery |
| vision | normal | slightly reduced | much reduced, haloes |
| onset | gradual | gradual | sudden |
| systemic complications | none | malaise or fever | nausea and vomiting |

*This is a guide, as individual cases vary according to the cause and severity of the disease.

**iseikonia** Condition in which the size and shape of the ocular images of the two eyes are equal, as distinguished from aniseikonia.
*See* **aniseikonia; image, ocular.**

**iseikonic lens** *See* **lens, aniseikonic.**

**Ishihara test** *See* **plates, pseudoisochromatic.**

**isoacuity area** **1.** An area surrounding the fixation point in which visual acuity is approximately constant. The width of this area varies with the test target, being smallest with resolution of two dots and largest with Landolt rings or gratings. **2.** An area of the visual field in which visual acuity is more or less constant.

**isoametropia** Condition in which the ametropia is similar in the two eyes. *Syn.* isometropia.

**isoametropic amblyopia** *See* **amblyopia.**

**isochromatic** Possessing the same colour.

**isocoria** Having two pupils of equal size.
*See* **anisocoria.**

**isoluminant** Possessing the same luminance. *Example*: red and green bars of a grating which have the same luminance. If such a grating is moving sideways, many observers will barely perceive its motion or fail to notice it altogether. *Syn.* equiluminant.

**isometropia** *See* **isoametropia.**

**isophoria** Constancy of the heterophoria in various directions of gaze.
*See* **heterophoria.**

**isopia** Identical vision in the two eyes.

**isopter** In the determination of visual fields, it is the contour line representing the limits of equal retinal sensitivity to a given test target.
*See* **field, visual; perimeter.**

**isotonic solution** *See* **solution, isotonic.**

**isotropic** Having the same properties of refraction in all directions.
*See* **anisotropic; birefringence.**

**ivermectin** *See* **onchocerciasis.**

# J

**J** *See* **Jaeger test types.**

**jack-in-the-box phenomenon** *See* **phenomenon, jack-in-the-box.**

**Jackson's crossed cylinder test** *See* **test for astigmatism, cross-cylinder.**

**Jaeger test types** Test types for measuring visual acuity at near. They consist of ordinary printers' types of various sizes and are arranged as words and phrases. Depending on the size of test types read, acuity is recorded as J.1, J.2 in ascending size up to J.20. The smallest Jaeger (J.1) subtends an angle of 5′ at 450 mm from the eye.
*See* **acuity, near visual.**

**Table J1** Approximate relationship between the Jaeger system, the point system (or N notation) and the Snellen equivalent

| | | Snellen equivalent at 40 cm | |
|---|---|---|---|
| Jaeger | point | (m) | (ft) |
| 1 | 3.5 | 6/7 | 20/23 |
| 2 | 4.5 | 6/8 | 20/27 |
| 3 | 5.5 | 6/11 | 20/37 |
| 4 | 6.5 | 6/13 | 20/43 |
| 5 | 7.5 | 6/14 | 20/47 |
| 6 | 8 | 6/15 | 20/50 |
| 7 | 9.5 | 6/17 | 20/57 |
| 8 | 11 | 6/20 | 20/67 |
| 9 | 12 | 6/24 | 20/80 |
| 10 | 13 | 6/26 | 20/87 |
| 11 | 14 | 6/28 | 20/93 |
| 12 | 16 | 6/30 | 20/100 |
| 13 | 18 | 6/36 | 20/120 |
| 14 | 22 | 6/45 | 20/150 |

**Jannelli clip** *See* **clipover.**

**Javal's grid** *See* **grid, Javal's.**

**Javal's method** *See* **method, Javal's.**

**Javal's rule** A relationship that relates corneal astigmatism to the total astigmatism of the eye. It states that

$$A_t = 1.25A_c - 0.50 \text{ axis } 90°,$$

where $A_t$ and $A_c$ are the total and corneal astigmatism, respectively. This relationship is relatively accurate in predicting the total astigmatism of the eye when corneal astigmatism is greater than 2 D. For smaller amounts of corneal astigmatism, a more appropriate version of Javal's rule is

$$A_t = 1.0A_c - 0.50 \text{ axis } 90°.$$

*See* **astigmatism, total; keratometer.**

**jaw-winking phenomenon** *See* **phenomenon, jaw-winking.**

**jerk nystagmus** *See* **nystagmus.**

**jnd** *See* **threshold, differential.**

**Jones I test** *See* **test, Jones I.**

**Jones II test** *See* **test, Jones II.**

**Julesz random-dot stereogram** *See* **stereogram, random-dot.**

**jump** The displacement of the image of an object occurring when viewing across the borderline between two portions of different power in a bifocal or trifocal lens. The jump is eliminated by placing the optical centres on the dividing line; the lens is then called a **no jump** bifocal (e.g. a monocentric bifocal with a straight dividing line) (Fig. J1). *Syn.* image jump; prismatic jump.
*See* **lens, bifocal; monocentric.**

**just noticeable difference** *See* **threshold, differential.**

**juvenile epithelial corneal dystrophy** *See* **dystrophy, Meesmann's.**

**juvenile glaucoma** *See* **glaucoma, congenital.**

**juvenile retinoschisis** *See* **retinoschisis.**

**juvenile rheumatoid arthritis** *See* **disease, Still's.**

**juvenile xanthogranuloma** *See* **xanthogranuloma, juvenile.**

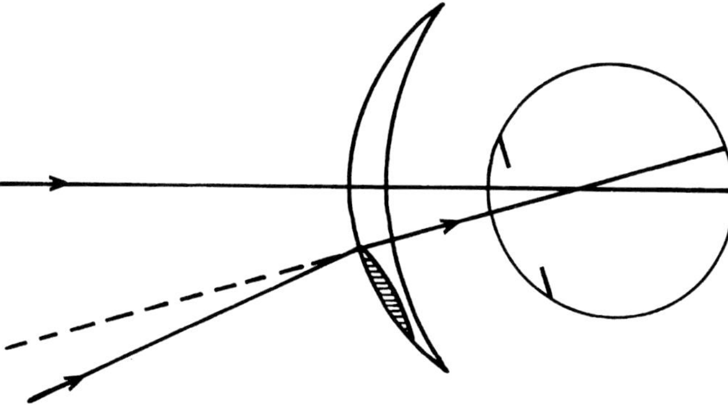

**Fig. J1** Image jump upward caused by the segment of a bifocal lens, as the direction of gaze is lowered across the dividing line

# K

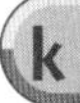

**Kanisza figure** *See* **figure, Kanisza.**

**kataphoria** **1.** A tendency of the visual axes of both eyes to deviate below the horizontal plane, in the absence of a stimulus to fusion. **2.** Synonym of alternating deorsumduction. *Note*: also spelt cataphoria.
*See* **depression; hyperphoria.**

**Kayser–Fleischer ring** *See* **ring, Kayser–Fleischer.**

**Kennedy syndrome** *See* **syndrome, Foster Kennedy.**

**Kepler telescope** *See* **telescope.**

**keratectasia** *See* **ectasia.**

**keratectomy, photorefractive** *See* **keratotomy, radial.**

**keratic precipitates (KP)** Cells (e.g. leukocytes) deposited on the endothelium of the cornea which occur as a result of inflammation of the iris or the ciliary body.
*See* **cornea guttata; iritis; uveitis.**

**keratitis** Inflammation of the cornea. It can arise from various sources, the most common being: infection by bacteria, fungi or viruses, hypersensitivity to staphylococcal exotoxins, nutritional deficiencies, failure of the eyelids to cover the cornea, deficiencies in the precorneal tear film, contact lens wear (especially extended wear), mechanical, radiation or chemical trauma or interruption of the ophthalmic branch of the trigeminal nerve. It is usually characterized by a dullness and loss of transparency of the cornea due to infiltrates, neovascularization, oedema and is accompanied by ciliary injection. The discomfort varies from a foreign body sensation to severe pain, with lacrimation, photophobia, blepharospasm and an impairment of vision. If the condition is severe, ulcers and pus (hypopyon) will appear and the iris and ciliary body may become involved. It is important to identify the cause and the organism in order to treat the condition. Keratitis of bacterial origin is treated with antibiotic drugs. Keratitis of viral origin (e.g. herpes) is treated with antiviral agents and that of fungal origin with antifungal agents.
*See* **corneal infiltrates; hypopyon; injection, ciliary; keratomalacia; keratomycosis; keratopathy; oedema; ulcer, corneal.**

**keratitis, acanthamoeba** A rare type of keratitis caused by the microorganism acanthamoeba which invades the cornea. The symptoms begin with a foreign body sensation which turns into pain, photophobia, tearing, blepharospasm and blurred vision. The signs are infiltrates that develop into a ring and eventually, in most cases, the cornea becomes opaque and the eye is blind. In a few cases, the disease develops into an

acute meningoencephalitis that is usually fatal. Diagnosis of the disease is made by laboratory analysis of a corneal scraping. Contact lens wear has been found to be associated with this disease in about three-quarters of the cases, especially when the patient has used homemade or unpreserved saline. The other cases were due to contact with stagnant water or following an abraded cornea. There is no therapy for this disease, as yet. However, strict compliance with contact lens regimens and avoidance of exposure to dirty, stagnant water diminishes the risks of contracting the disease.
*See* **corneal infiltrates; disinfection by boiling, propamidine isethionate.**

**keratitis, actinic** *See* **keratoconjunctivitis, actinic.**

**keratitis, acute epithelial** *See* **herpes zoster ophthalmicus.**

**keratitis, acute stromal** A complication of scleritis in which there are superficial and midstromal infiltrates in the limbal region. Lesions can also be noted in the central cornea and may develop vascularization and permanent opacification. In cases of scleritis that are limited (i.e. not diffuse), corneal changes are noted only in the bordering corneal region.
*See* **scleritis.**

**keratitis, dendritic** An acute and chronic corneal inflammation that occurs in a person who has had a primary infection with herpes simplex type 1. (Some cases occur with type 2 or 3.) It is characterized by the formation of small vesicles that break down and coalesce to form dendritic ulcers.
*See* **keratitis, ulcerative; ulcer, corneal.**

**keratitis, disciform** A deep localized keratitis involving the stroma usually characterized by a disc-shaped grey area (Wessley ring) that may spread to the whole thickness of the cornea. It is due to a viral infection or to an immune reaction, or it may also occur as a sequel to trauma. It may heal without residue or may cause scarring and vascularization of the cornea.
*See* **clouding, central corneal; ring, Wessley.**

**keratitis, exposure** Keratitis caused by the failure of the eyelids to cover the globe characterized by a haziness and desiccation of the corneal epithelium which may result in exfoliation. This condition is commonly associated with facial nerve disorders in which the orbicularis oculi muscle is paralysed. It may also occur as a result of hard contact lens wear, or sleep lagophthalmos. *Syn.* keratitis e lagophthalmos; lagophthalmic keratitis.
*See* **ectropion; lagophthalmos; staining, 3 and 9 o'clock; tears, artificial.**

**keratitis, filamentary** Keratitis characterized by the presence of fine epithelial filaments. It can occur as a result of herpes, thyroid dysfunction, corneal abrasions, keratitis sicca, etc.

**keratitis, fungal** A keratitis caused by a fungus, such as *Fusarium, Aspergillus*, or *Candida*. The condition may develop after eye injury (e.g. fingernail or contact lens scratch, tree branch), especially in agricultural areas. However, it has become more common since the use of corticosteroids. It may also occur in eyes suffering from corneal disease, after keratoplasty, diabetes or extended-wear contact lenses. It is characterized by greyish-white, rough ulcers with indistinct and feathery edges with filaments infiltrating into the stroma (filamentary keratitis). There is ciliary and conjunctival injection and it may be accompanied by ring abscesses and, in severe cases, hypopyon. The ulcers have oval or round outlines with a plaque-like surface and the cornea is fully oedematous. Differential diagnosis is facilitated by corneal scraping or biopsy of the ulcer. Management consists mainly of antifungal agents. *Syn.* mycotic keratitis.
*See* **antifungal agent; keratomycosis.**

**keratitis, herpetic** Keratitis caused by either herpes simplex (**dendritic keratitis**) or herpes zoster viruses.
*See* **herpes zoster ophthalmicus; keratitis, dendritic; keratitis, disciform; keratitis, interstitial; keratitis, punctate epithelial.**

**keratitis, hypopyon** Purulent keratitis with ulcer resulting in the presence of pus in the anterior chamber which gravitates to the bottom. The ulcer is a dirty grey colour and the conjunctiva is also inflamed. The usual cause of the infection is the pneumococcus which gives rise to a corneal ulcer (often called **serpiginous ulcer** because of its tendency to creep forward in the cornea).
*See* **hypopyon; keratitis, ulcerative; ulcer, corneal.**

**keratitis, interstitial** Keratitis involving the stroma. It is characterized by deep vascularization of the cornea and is often associated with iridocyclitis. Formerly, the most common cause was congenital syphilis (**syphilitic keratitis**). However, nowadays it is usually the result of a herpes simplex infection, or it may be part of a syndrome (Cogan's) or other systemic diseases (e.g. leprosy, tuberculosis). Management involves cycloplegics, topical antiviral agents and in severe cases corticosteroids. *Syn.* stromal interstitial keratitis.
*See* **sign, Hutchinson's; uveitis.**

**keratitis, lagophthalmic** *See* **keratitis, exposure.**

**keratitis, mucous plaque** *See* **herpes zoster ophthalmicus.**

**keratitis, mycotic** *See* **keratitis, fungal.**

**keratitis, non-ulcerative** *See* **contact lens acute red eye.**

**keratitis, neuroparalytic** Keratitis caused by a failure of blinking or infrequent or incomplete blinking causing inadequate spread of tears.
*See* **keratopathy, neurotrophic; keratitis sicca; tears, artificial.**

**keratitis, neurotrophic** *See* **keratopathy, neurotrophic.**

**keratitis, phlyctenular** Inflammation of the cornea characterized by the formation of small grey nodules (**phlyctens**) near the limbus. As the number of phlyctens in the cornea increases a neovascularization occurs which is called **phlyctenular pannus**. Phlyctenular keratitis is usually associated with an inflammation of the conjunctiva and raised nodules are also present there.
*See* **conjunctivitis, phlyctenular.**

**keratitis, punctate epithelial (PEK)** An inflammation of the cornea characterized by either multiple, small, superficial, punctate lesions or minute, flat, epithelial dots resulting from bacterial infection (e.g. chlamydial, staphylococcal), vitamin $B_2$ deficiency, virus infection (e.g. herpes) and also from exposure to ultraviolet light, injury to the eye with aerosol products or contact lens solutions. The condition is usually associated with a conjunctivitis. Treatment depends on the causative agent (e.g. antiviral agents will be used to suppress symptoms in viral infection). *Syn.* superficial punctate keratitis (SPK), although this term is more often used to describe a PEK of viral origin.
*See* **conjunctivitis, adult inclusion; keratitis, herpetic.**

**keratitis, rosacea** Keratitis associated with acne rosacea of the face. It is characterized by marginal vascularization at the limbus. The vessels extend into the cornea surrounded by a zone of grey infiltration. The infiltrate and vascularization are in the cornea proper and not raised above the surface (unlike phlyctens). There is little tendency to ulcerate. It is usually associated with an inflammation of the conjunctiva (**keratoconjunctivitis**). Treatment involves topical steroid drops as well as systemic antibiotic therapy.
*See* **acne rosacea; keratitis, phlyctenular; ulcer, corneal.**

**keratitis sicca** Keratitis due to an absence or deficiency of the lacrimal secretion. It is characterized by ciliary injection, loss of the usual glossy appearance of the cornea, mucous threads and filaments in the tear film and filamentary strands of epithelium which adhere to the cornea. The patient complains of burning, itching and foreign body sensations and transient blurring of vision which are worsened by hot, dry environments. The condition is usually associated with conjunctivitis (**keratoconjunctivitis sicca** KCS) and general dryness of the skin and of the membranes of the mouth and blepharitis. Tests with fluorescein or rose bengal show tissue stains and Schirmer's test is subnormal. Keratoconjunctivitis sicca may result from: (1) A fluid deficiency of the tear film. This deficiency is also encountered in **Sjögren's syndrome**, for example. (2) Mucin deficiency. In this case the condition is usually referred to as **xerophthalmia**. (3) Abnormal blinking as in **neuroparalytic keratitis**. (4) Lack of congruity between the cornea and the eyelids as occurs when there is a limbal lesion and dellen, for example. (5) It follows, in some cases, juvenile rheumatoid arthritis or sarcoidosis, certain medications such as antihistamines, oral contraceptives and antidepressants and living in a dry climate. Management consists mainly of artificial tears and frequent blinking. Occasionally, soft contact lenses may help although infection may be a problem. Treatment may also include moist goggles, and in severe cases, closure of the lacrimal puncta or tarsorrhaphy. *Syn.* dry eye.
*See* **alacrima; cytology, impression; eye, dry; fluorescein; glands, meibomian; keratitis, filamentary; keratitis, neuroparalytic; lacrimal apparatus; mucin; myasthenia gravis; occlusion, punctal; rose bengal; syndrome, Mikulicz's; syndrome, Sjögren's; syndrome, Stevens–Johnson; tarsorrhaphy; tears, artificial; test, Norn's; test, phenol red cotton; test, Schirmer's; xerophthalmia.**

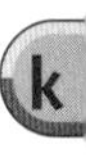


**keratitis, superficial punctate** *See* **keratitis, punctate epithelial.**

**keratitis, stromal; syphilitic** *See* **keratitis, interstitial.**

**keratitis, Thygeson's superficial punctate** A rare type of punctate epithelial keratitis. It is characterized by circular or oval, greyish-white epithelial lesions commonly located centrally and slightly elevated with a cluster of granular dots. The lesions show punctate staining with fluorescein. The cause is unknown, although a virus is suspected. It gives rise to mild irritation, photophobia and slight blurring of vision. Treatment includes artificial tears, corticosteroids (but this may induce recurrence) and therapeutic soft contact lenses. Untreated, it may subside within a few years.
*See* **keratitis, punctate epithelial.**

**keratitis, ulcerative** Any keratitis in which there is an ulcer of the cornea. The cause may be bacterial or viral infection, trauma or contact lens wear (particularly extended wear). The ulcer is a dirty grey coloured area on the cornea, the eye is red, the pain can be severe, there is photophobia, lacrimation and vision may be affected.

Immediate treatment is necessary: if due to contact lenses, cessation of wear and topical antibiotics will be used.
*See* **keratitis, dendritic; keratitis, hypopyon; ulcer, corneal.**

**keratitis, ultraviolet** *See* **keratoconjunctivitis, actinic.**

**keratocele** Hernia of Descemet's membrane through a hole in the cornea caused by a perforating corneal ulcer or wound.
*See* **ulcer, corneal.**

**keratoconjunctivitis** Inflammation of the conjunctiva and the cornea.
*See* **conjunctivitis; keratitis, punctate epithelial; keratitis, rosacea; keratitis sicca.**

**keratoconjunctivitis, actinic** Inflammation of the cornea and conjunctiva caused by exposure to ultraviolet light as, for example, from sun lamps, welder's arc or reflection from the snow. Both cornea and conjunctiva are usually involved although one tissue may be more affected than the other, hence the terms '**actinic conjunctivitis**' or '**actinic keratitis**'. Some time after exposure (4–8 hours) to the ultraviolet radiations, the patient experiences a marked sandy feeling in the eye, lacrimation, photophobia, blepharospasm, with congestion of the conjunctiva and swelling of the eyelids. The condition is usually self-limited and heals within 48 hours. Symptoms are relieved with cold compresses, firm patching and an analgesic. A local anaesthetic may sometimes be used but this delays the regeneration of the corneal epithelium and is not usually recommended. A topical antibiotic may also be used to prevent secondary infection. Sunglasses or suitable protection may prevent the condition. *Syn.* arc eye; flash blindness; photokeratitis; photokeratoconjunctivitis; photophthalmia; snow blindness (although this is not a strictly correct synonym it is often used as such); sun lamp conjunctivitis; ultraviolet keratitis.
*See* **actinic; blepharospasm; ultraviolet.**

**keratoconjunctivitis, phlyctenular** *See* **keratitis, phlyctenular.**

**keratoconjunctivitis sicca** *See* **keratitis sicca.**

**keratoconjunctivitis, superior limbic (SLK)** Chronic inflammation of the superior cornea and conjunctiva. It is characterized by hyperaemia, hazy epithelium and often corneal filaments near the upper limbus and the adjacent conjunctiva, and with the sensations of burning, itching, photophobia and hazy vision. The condition is bilateral in 50% of cases. Detection of the disease in its mild form is difficult as it requires lifting the upper eyelid. The condition typically affects middle-aged women with thyroid dysfunction. It may be induced by soft contact lens wear. Smaller hard lenses, especially gas permeable, rarely cause this disease. Management involves several options: application of silver nitrate, topical medication (e.g. sodium cromoglycate), thermal cauterization of the superior bulbar conjunctiva, or occlusion of the lacrimal puncta/um to increase tear volume over the conjunctiva.
*See* **ophthalmopathy, thyroid.**

**keratoconjunctivitis, vernal** *See* **conjunctivitis, vernal.**

**keratoconus (KC)** A developmental anomaly in which the central portion of the cornea becomes thinner and bulges forward in a cone-shaped fashion. Two types of cones are commonly described: a round cone and an oval (or sagging) cone. It usually appears around puberty, is bilateral, although one eye may be involved long before the other. Other corneal signs may be Vogt's striae, Fleischer's ring, scarring and corneal hydrops, as well as myopia and irregular astigmatism. The condition may be associated with osteogenesis imperfecta, ectopia lentis, aniridia, retinitis pigmentosa, Down's syndrome, Ehlers–Danlos syndrome, Marfan's syndrome. The main symptom is a loss of visual acuity due to irregular astigmatism and myopia. Correction is usually best achieved with contact lenses, especially rigid gas permeable, but if these cannot be worn or the condition is very severe, a corneal transplant is carried out (Fig. K1). *Syn.* conical cornea.
*See* **clouding, central corneal; ectasia, corneal; hydrops, corneal; keratoplasty; keratoscope; lens, combination; lens, piggyback; lenticonus; ring, Fleischer's; sclera, blue; sign, Munson's; sign, Rizzuti's; stria; striae, Vogt's; syndrome, Ehlers–Danlos; syndrome, Marfan's.**

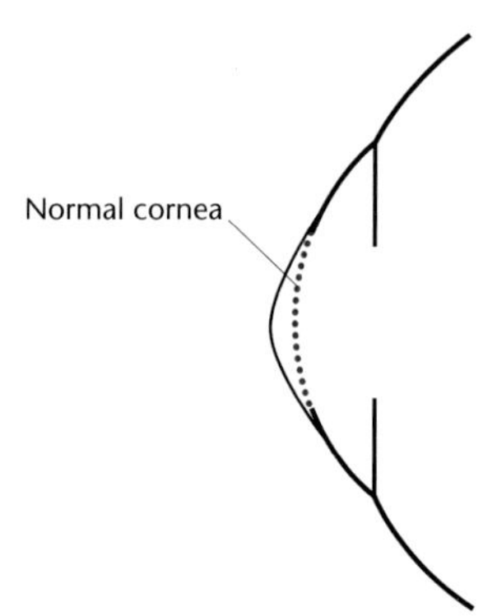


**Fig. K1** Schematic diagram of a keratoconus cornea

**keratoconus fruste** Term referring to subtle irregular astigmatism or moderate to high regular astigmatism usually measured by automated corneal topography and simulating keratoconus. However, the condition is usually stationary, corneal thickness is normal and there are none of the biomicroscopic signs of keratoconus (e.g. Vogt's striae, Fleischer's ring).

**keratoconus, posterior** A steep and irregular curvature of the posterior surface of the cornea, usually forming a depression in the central or paracentral area. The anterior surface is normal and vision is rarely affected. The condition is typically congenital, non-progressive and unilateral, but some cases are associated with some ocular abnormalities, such as anterior polar cataract, lenticonus, ectopia lentis, iris atrophy, etc. As the cornea is much thinner it represents a contraindication to LASIK procedure. The majority of cases do not require treatment.
*See* **LASIK; videokeratoscope.**

**keratocyte** *See* **corneal corpuscle.**

**keratoglobus** A rare, bilateral corneal ectasia, especially near the limbus. The condition is usually present at birth and generally does not progress. The diameter of the cornea is normal or slightly increased and the intraocular pressure is normal as the condition is not associated with congenital glaucoma. Complications include perforation after minor trauma and corneal hydrops. It is sometimes associated with Leber's congenital amaurosis, Ehlers–Danlos syndrome and blue sclera. *Syn.* macrocornea; megalocornea.
*See* **Leber's congenital amaurosis; megalophthalmos.**

**keratomalacia** Vitamin A deficiency in which the cornea becomes desiccated at first and then softens, at which stage it is associated with infiltration, pannus, necrosis, opacification and the eye becomes blind. There is also a lack of reaction to inflammation leading to a destruction of the eye if infection occurs. It is part of a general systemic condition due to malnutrition. Associated with this condition are night blindness, faulty growth of bone, xerophthalmia, etc.
*See* **hemeralopia; xerophthalmia.**

**keratome** A surgical instrument with a sharp edge for incising the cornea.
*See* **keratomileusis; LASIK.**

**keratometer** Optical instrument for measuring the radius of curvature of the cornea in any meridian. By measuring along the two principal meridians, corneal astigmatism can be deduced. The principle is based on the reflection by the anterior surface of a luminous pattern of **mires** in the centre of the cornea in an area of about 3.6 mm in diameter. Knowing the size of the pattern $h$ and measuring that of the reflected image $h'$ and the distance $d$ between the two, the radius of curvature $r$ of the cornea can be determined using the approximate formula

$$r = 2d \times \frac{h}{h'}$$

In addition, a doubling system (e.g. a bi-prism) is also integrated into the instrument in order to mitigate the effect of eye movements, as well as a microscope in order to magnify the small image reflected by the cornea. This instrument is used in the fitting of contact lenses and the monitoring of corneal changes occurring as a result of contact lens wear. The range of the instrument can be extended approximately 9 D by placing a +1.25 D lens in front of the objective to measure steeper corneas. The range in the other direction can be extended by approximately 6 D using a −1.00 D lens to measure flatter corneas (Fig. K2). *Syn.* ophthalmometer.
*See* **fitted on K; Javal's rule; keratoscope; lens, liquid; photokeratoscopy; prism, Wollaston; Topogometer; videokeratoscope.**

**Table K1** Extended keratometer range

| with 2 1.00 D | | with 1 1.25 D | |
|---|---|---|---|
| actual drum reading (D) | extended value (D) | actual drum reading (D) | extended value (D) |
| 36.00 | 30.87 | 45.00 | 52.46 |
| 36.50 | 31.30 | 45.50 | 53.05 |
| 37.00 | 31.73 | 46.00 | 53.63 |
| 37.50 | 32.16 | 46.50 | 54.21 |
| 38.00 | 32.59 | 47.00 | 54.80 |
| 38.50 | 33.02 | 47.50 | 55.38 |
| 39.00 | 33.45 | 48.00 | 55.96 |
| 39.50 | 33.88 | 48.50 | 56.55 |
| 40.00 | 34.30 | 49.00 | 57.13 |
| 40.50 | 34.73 | 49.50 | 57.71 |
| 41.00 | 35.16 | 50.00 | 58.30 |
| 41.50 | 35.59 | 50.50 | 58.88 |
| | | 51.00 | 59.46 |
| | | 51.50 | 60.04 |
| | | 52.00 | 60.63 |

**keratometer, auto** A keratometer using a microprocessor computer to facilitate the rapid measurement of the corneal curvature. Such instruments usually provide measurements of the peripheral and central corneal curvatures at different points providing a contour of the cornea in several meridians, as well as of the corneal apex.

**keratomileusis** A surgical procedure on the cornea aimed at curing ametropia. An anterior layer of the cornea is sliced off with a microkeratome, frozen, ground to a new curvature and sutured back in the same location. There are many complications and technical difficulties associated

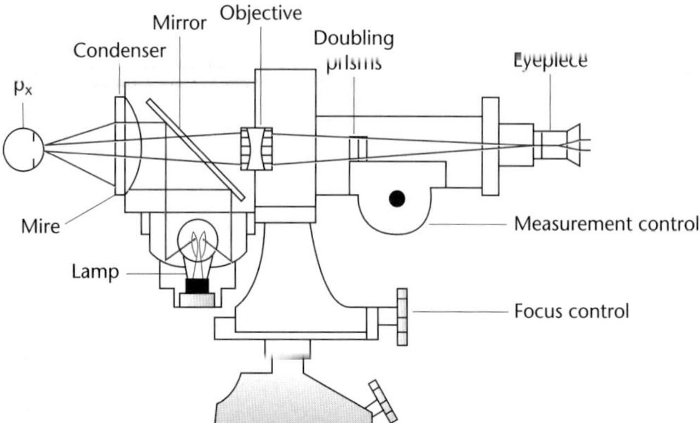


**Fig. K2** Schematic diagram of the Reichert keratometer

with this procedure. *Syn.* refractive keratoplasty and keratorefractive surgery (both terms also include epikeratoplasty, keratophakia and radial keratotomy).
*See* **epikeratoplasty; keratome; keratophakia; keratotomy, radial; LASIK.**

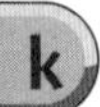

**keratomycosis** A fungus infection of the cornea which may result in keratitis and ulceration. It is usually introduced by injury and is characterized by an ulcer which appears as a fluffy white elevated protuberance surrounded by a shallow crater on the edge of which is a sharply demarcated halo. There is ciliary and conjunctival injection. Diagnosis is best provided by laboratory analysis of a specimen of these fungal organisms which are obtained by scraping the base of the ulcer.
*See* **hypopyon; injection, ciliary; injection, conjunctival; keratitis, fungal; ulcer, corneal.**

**keratopathy** A non-inflammatory disease of the cornea. *Examples*: band keratopathy; bullous keratopathy.
*See* **dystrophy, corneal.**

**keratopathy, actinic** A form of corneal degeneration characterized by white or yellowish stromal deposits consisting of cholesterol, fats and phospholipids, and in some cases corneal vascularization. The condition may be caused by exposure to sunlight (especially ultraviolet radiations) or trauma. The deposits are usually present within the pupillary area, often as elevated nodules distributed in a band-shaped configuration and can have a dramatic effect on visual function. The damage is similar to that found in pterygium and pinguecula. Treatment consists of resorbing the lipid infiltrates and, in severe cases, keratoplasty. *Syn.* Bietti's band-shaped nodular dystrophy; climatic droplet keratopathy; Labrador keratopathy; lipid droplet degeneration.
*See* **pinguecula; pterygium.**

**keratopathy, band** A disorder characterized by the deposition of calcium salts in the anterior layers of the cornea. They appear as opacities forming a more or less horizontal band with clear holes within the band giving it a Swiss cheese appearance. It is typically associated with rheumatoid arthritis but also with chronic iridocyclitis, interstitial keratitis, glaucoma, vitamin D intoxication, old age, etc. Symptoms include irritation and blurring of vision. Treatment may be necessary for cosmetic or visual reasons. It consists of removal of the calcium salts by scraping the corneal epithelium followed by irrigation with EDTA, or laser keratectomy. *Syn.* band-shaped corneal dystrophy.
*See* **ethylenediamine tetraacetic acid (EDTA); rheumatoid arthritis.**

**keratopathy, bullous** Degenerative condition of the cornea characterized by the formation of epithelial blebs or bullae which burst after a few days. This condition may follow cataract surgery, corneal trauma, severe corneal oedema, glaucoma, iridocyclitis, etc. Soft contact lenses have often been found useful to relieve pain in this condition by protecting the denuded nerve endings.
*See* **cornea; cornea guttata; dystrophy, Fuchs' endothelial; lens, therapeutic soft contact; oedema.**

**keratopathy, climatic droplet; Labrador** *See* **keratopathy, actinic.**

**keratopathy, neurotrophic** Condition characterized by an anaesthesia of the cornea. It results in a breakdown of the corneal epithelial layer allowing trauma, desiccation and infection. It is believed to occur as a result of the loss of trophic influence of the nerve supply to the cornea and/or of reduced blinking and the loss of lacrimation. Causes include herpes virus, herpes zoster, lattice dystrophy, fifth nerve lesion and diabetes mellitus. Treatment mainly

consists of tear substitute and intermittent or constant lid taping, but anti-infective regimen, punctal occlusion, tarsorrhaphy or neurosurgical intervention may be necessary. *Syn.* neurotrophic keratitis (although this term is incorrect as inflammation is only a likely consequence of the disease).
*See* **keratomalacia; occlusion, punctal.**

**keratophakia** A surgical procedure on the cornea aimed at curing ametropia. A donor corneal disc (or lenticule) that was previously frozen and reshaped is inserted into the host cornea to modify the anterior corneal curvature. There are many complications and technical difficulties associated with this procedure. *Syn.* refractive keratoplasty and keratorefractive surgery (both terms also include epikeratoplasty, keratomileusis and radial keratotomy).
*See* **epikeratoplasty; Intacs; keratomileusis; keratotomy, radial; LASIK; lenticule.**

**keratoplasty** Excision of corneal tissue and its replacement by a cornea from a human donor. This can be done either over the entire cornea (**total keratoplasty**) or over a portion of it (**partial keratoplasty**). Two main techniques are used: (1) the **penetrating keratoplasty** in which the entire thickness of the cornea is removed and replaced by transparent corneal tissue; (2) the **lamellar keratoplasty** in which a superficial layer is removed and replaced by healthy tissue. Common indications to perform keratoplasty are therapeutic (e.g. keratoconus, corneal ulcer) or cosmetic (e.g. removing an unsightly opacity). *Syn.* corneal transplant.
*See* **dystrophy, granular; eye bank; graft, corneal.**

**keratoplasty, laser refractive; refractive** *See* **keratotomy, radial.**

**keratoreformation** The process of improving vision following radial keratotomy by correcting a residual ametropia and an irregular corneal topography. This is usually accomplished by contact lenses.
*See* **keratotomy, radial.**

**keratorefractive surgery** *See* **epikeratoplasty; Intacs; keratomileusis; keratophakia; keratotomy, radial; LASIK.**

**keratoscleritis** Inflammation of both the cornea and the sclera.

**keratoscope** Instrument for examining the front surface of the cornea. It consists of a pattern of alternately black and white concentric rings reflected by the cornea and seen through a convex lens mounted in an aperture at the centre of the pattern. Such an instrument gives a qualitative evaluation of large corneal astigmatism, and is useful in cases of irregular astigmatism as in keratoconus, for example (Fig. K3). *Syn.* Placido disc.
*See* **keratoconus; photokeratoscopy.**

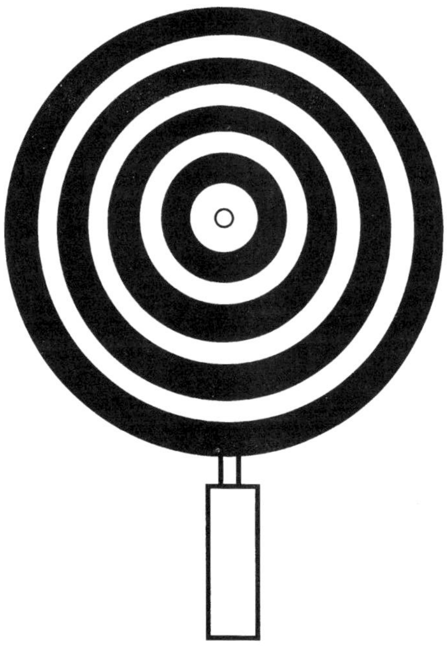

**Fig. K3** Keratoscope

**keratosis, seborrhoeic** Lesion of the skin appearing as brown or yellowish thickening of the skin of the face, eyelids and/or conjunctiva. It is common in the elderly and may be a precursor to squamous cell carcinoma. Management includes cryotherapy, local surgical excision or radiotherapy.
*See* **carcinoma; distichiasis.**

**keratotomy, radial (RK)** A surgical procedure on the cornea aimed at curing ametropia. It consists of making incisions in the anterior part of the cornea in order to flatten it and thereby produce a reduction of its power. The incisions are usually radial, extending from the limbus to about halfway towards the centre like the spokes of a wheel, but other patterns of incision are also used. In some cases, the procedure does not produce a perfect correction and vision is poor, especially in the dark. The use of the excimer laser provides greater accuracy and success. The technique is then called **laser refractive keratoplasty** (LRK) or **photorefractive keratectomy** (PRK). *Syn.* refractive keratoplasty and keratorefractive surgery (both terms also include epikeratoplasty, keratomileusis and keratophakia).
*See* **cornea; epikeratoplasty; keratomileusis; keratophakia; keratoreformation; laser, excimer; LASIK.**

**Kestenbaum's rule** *See* **rule, Kestenbaum's.**

**keyhole bridge; pupil; visual field** *See* under the nouns.

**kinescope** **1.** An instrument for determining the refraction of the eye by having the subject observe the apparent 'with' or 'against' movement of a test object through a stenopaeic slit moved across the front of the eye. **2.** An instrument for recording television programmes.
*See* **disc, stenopaeic.**

**kinetic depth effect** *See* **effect, kinetic depth.**

**kinetic perimetry** *See* **perimetry, kinetic.**

**Kirschmann's law** *See* **law, Kirschmann's.**

**Knapp's law** *See* **law, Knapp's.**

**Koeppe lens; nodules** *See* under the nouns.

**Kollner's rule** *See* **rule, Kollner's.**

**König bars** Target used to measure visual acuity consisting of two bars on a white background. The length of each bar is usually three times its width but the space between the bars is always equal to the width of one bar. The smallest pair of bars that can be perceived as separate gives a measure of the acuity.
*See* **acuity, visual; optotype.**

**Krause's end bulbs** Nerve endings enclosed by a capsule from 0.02 mm to 0.1 mm in length. They probably act as cold receptors. Their regular presence in the corneal limbus has been questioned.
*See* **conjunctiva; limbus, corneal.**

**Krause, glands of** *See* **glands of Krause.**

**Krebs cycle** *See* **cycle, Krebs.**

**Krimsky's method** *See* **method, Krimsky's.**

**Krukenberg spindle** A more or less vertical spindle-shaped deposition of brownish pigment on the corneal endothelium. It is often accompanied by pigment deposits on the lens, zonule, anterior surface of the iris and trabecular meshwork and may form part of the **pigment dispersion syndrome**. The pigment comes from the iris pigment epithelium but the cause of its shedding is not established and may be strenuous exercise, mechanical rubbing by the zonules due to posterior bowing of part of the iris or degenerated pigment. It occurs in young to middle-aged myopic individuals and sometimes following uveitis.
*See* **syndrome, pigment dispersion.**

**krypton laser** *See* **laser, krypton.**

# L

**Labrador keratopathy** *See* **keratopathy, actinic.**

**lacquer cracks** *See* **Fuchs' spot.**

**lacrimal** Relating to tears.

**lacrimal apparatus** The system involved in the production and conduction of tears. It consists of the **lacrimal gland** and accessory lacrimal glands (glands of Krause and Wolfring); the **eyelid margins**; and the two **puncta lacrimal**. Each punctum is a small round or oval aperture situated on a slight elevation at the inner end of the upper and lower lid margin (**lacrimal papilla**) and forms the entrance to the **canaliculi**. Each canaliculus consists of a vertical portion of about 2 mm long and then bends inward for some 8 mm, the upper one being slightly shorter. The canaliculi pierce the **lacrimal fascia** (i.e. the periorbita covering the **lacrimal sac** or **tear sac**) and unite (forming the **common canaliculus)** to enter a small diverticulum of the sac called the **sinus of Maier**. The **lacrimal sac** is closed above and open below where it is continuous with the **nasolacrimal duct** which extends over some 1.5 cm in length to **Hasner's valve** (or **Bianchi's valve** or **plica lacrimalis**) (folds of mucous membrane) at the inferior meatus of the nose. The inferior opening of the duct is called the **ostium lacrimale** (Fig. L1).
*See* **dacryocystitis; epiphora; fossa for the lacrimal gland; fossa for the lacrimal sac; glands of Krause; glands of Wolfring; orbit; syndrome, Sjögren's; tear duct; tears; test, dye dilution; test, Jones II; valve of Hasner; valve of Krause.**

**lacrimal artery** *See* **artery, lacrimal.**

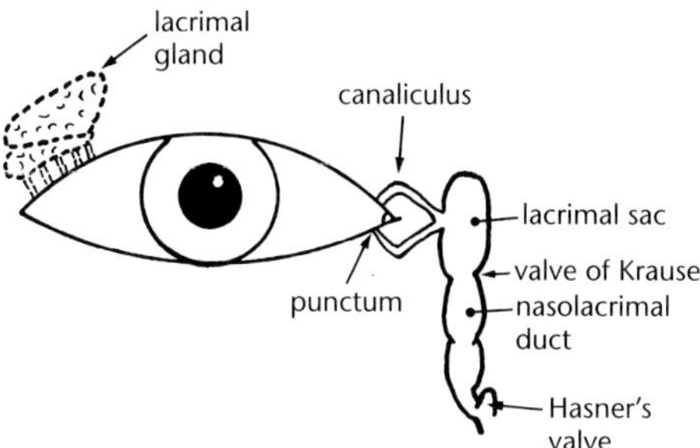


**Fig. L1** Lacrimal apparatus

**lacrimal bone** *See* **orbit.**

**lacrimal canaliculi** *See* **lacrimal apparatus.**

**lacrimal caruncle** *See* **caruncle, lacrimal.**

**lacrimal crest, anterior** The anterior margin of the fossa for the lacrimal sac located on the frontal process of the maxilla.
*See* **fossa for the lacrimal sac.**

**lacrimal crest, posterior** The posterior margin of the fossa for the lacrimal sac situated on the lacrimal bone.
*See* **fossa for the lacrimal sac.**

**lacrimal duct** *See* **tear duct.**

**lacrimal fascia** *See* **lacrimal apparatus.**

**lacrimal fluid** *See* **tears.**

**lacrimal gland** *See* **gland, lacrimal.**

**lacrimal lake** Accumulation of tears in the angle between the eyelids and the inner canthus prior to draining into the lacrimal puncta.
*See* **epiphora; tear meniscus.**

**lacrimal layer** *See* **film, precorneal.**

**lacrimal lens** *See* **lens, liquid.**

**lacrimal nerve** *See* **nerve, ophthalmic.**

**lacrimal papilla** *See* **lacrimal apparatus; papilla, lacrimal.**

**lacrimal prism** *See* **tear meniscus.**

**lacrimal punctum** *See* **lacrimal apparatus.**

**lacrimal reflex** *See* **reflex, lacrimal.**

**lacrimal sac** *See* **lacrimal apparatus.**

**lacrimal tubercle** *See* **tubercle, lacrimal.**

**lacrimation 1.** Secretion and flow of tears. **2.** Synonym for weeping.
*See* **epiphora; reflex, lacrimal; tears; weeping.**

**lacrimation, paradoxic** *See* **tears, crocodile.**

**laevoclination** Rotation of the upper pole of an eye towards the subject's left. *Syn.* laevocycloduction; laevotorsion.

**laevocycloduction** *See* **laevoclination.**

**laevocycloversion** Rotation of the upper poles of the vertical meridians of both eyes towards the subject's left.
*See* **dextrocycloversion.**

**laevodeorsumversion** Movement of the eyes down and to the left.

**laevoduction** Rotation of one eye to the left. *Note*: also spelt levoduction.
*See* **duction.**

**laevophoria** A tendency of the visual axes of both eyes to deviate to the left, in the absence of a stimulus to fusion.
*See* **dextrophoria; heterophoria.**

**laevosursumversion** Movement of the eyes up and to the left.

**laevotorsion** *See* **laevoclination; torsion.**

**laevoversion** Movement of both eyes to the left.
*See* **version.**

**lag of accommodation** *See* **accommodation, lag of.**

**lagophthalmos** Failure of the upper eyelid to close the eye completely. During sleep, about one-third of the population has a slight lagophthalmos.
*See* **ectropion; eyelids; keratitis, exposure.**

**Lagrange's law** *See* **law, Lagrange's.**

**lambert** Unit of luminance equal to 3183 candelas per m$^2$. *Symbol*: L.
*See* **luminance.**

**Lambert's cosine law** *See* **diffusion.**

**lamellar keratoplasty; cataract** *See* under the nouns.

**lamina cribrosa** *See* **cribriform plate.**

**lamina elastica** *See* **membrane, Bruch's.**

**lamina elastica anterior** *See* **membrane, Bowman's.**

**lamina elastica posterior** *See* **membrane, Descemet's.**

**lamina fusca** *See* **choroid.**

**lamina papyracea** Synonym for the orbital plate of the ethmoid bone which forms part of the medial wall of the orbit. It is thus named because it is as thin as paper and this may contribute to an infection of an ethmoidal sinus spreading into the orbit and resulting in orbital cellulitis.
*See* **cellulitis, orbital; orbit.**

**lamina vitrae** *See* **membrane, Bruch's.**

**laminated lens** *See* **lens, laminated.**

**lamp, Burton** Ultraviolet lamp, including some short wavelengths from the visible spectrum (e.g. Wood's light), mounted with a magnifying lens in a rectangular frame. It is used primarily in the evaluation of the fit of a hard contact lens, in conjunction with the instillation of fluorescein into the eye.
*See* **light, Wood's; staining; test, fluorescein.**

**lamp, filament** A lamp in which light is produced by electrically heating a filament, usually of tungsten. The filament is contained in a bulb in which there is either a vacuum or an inert gas. The emitted spectrum is continuous.
*See* **spectrum, continuous.**

**lamp, fluorescent** Discharge lamp in which most of the light is emitted by a layer of fluorescent material excited by the ultraviolet radiation from the discharge (CIE).
*See* **fluorescence.**

**lamp, halogen** A tungsten filament lamp in which the glass envelope is made of quartz and is filled with gaseous halogens. This permits a higher filament temperature and consequently provides a higher luminance and a higher colour temperature as well as a longer operating life than a conventional filament lamp of the same input power. Halogen lamps are used in some ophthalmoscopes and retinoscopes and as very bright sources for people with low vision. *Syn.* tungsten-halogen lamp.
*See* **colour temperature.**

**lamp, incandescent electric** Lamp in which light is produced by means of a body (filament of carbon or metal) heated to incandescence by the passage of an electric current (CIE).
*See* **illuminants, CIE standard; incandescence; luminescence.**

**lamp, Macbeth** A lamp used in testing colour vision. It contains a powerful tungsten filament bulb with a blue filter of specific absorption properties such that it produces a source of a colour temperature of about 6800 K, thus approximating the spectral characteristics of natural sunlight. The lamp is also fitted with a stand to hold the colour vision booklet (Fig. L2). *Syn.* Macbeth illuminant C.
*See* **illuminants, CIE standard; plates, pseudoisochromatic; test, Farnsworth.**

**lamp, slit-** *See* **slit-lamp.**

**lamp, tungsten-halogen** *See* **lamp, halogen.**

**Landolt ring** A test object used for measuring visual acuity consisting of an incomplete ring resembling the letter C. The width of the break and of the ring are each one-fifth of its overall diameter. The subject must indicate where the break is located, the break being positioned in any direction. The minimum angle of resolution corresponds to the angular subtense of the just noticeable break at the eye (Fig. L3). *Syn.* Landolt broken ring; Landolt C; Landolt test type.
*See* **acuity, visual; chart, Landolt broken ring.**

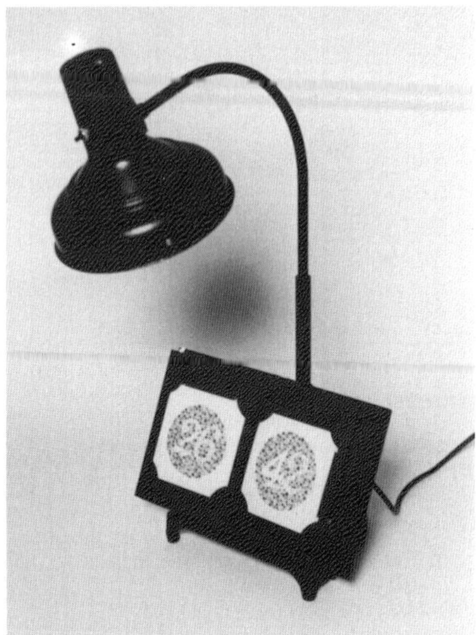

**Fig. L2** Macbeth lamp

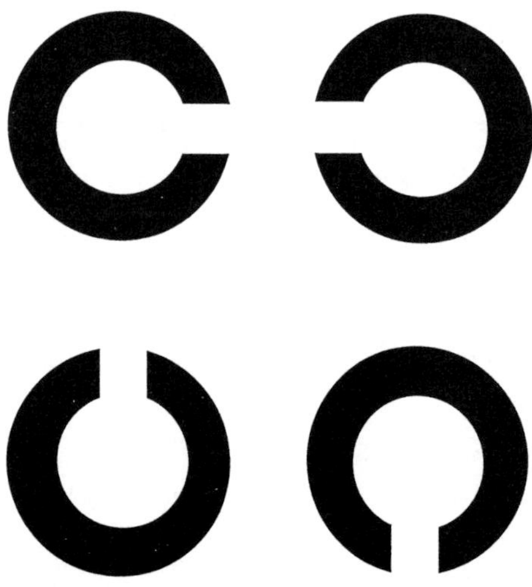

**Fig. L3** Landolt ring

**Lang stereotest** *See* **stereotest, Lang.**

**Langerhans' cells** *See* **cells, Langerhans'.**

**lantern test** *See* **Edridge–Green lantern; test, lantern.**

**L'Anthony desaturated D-15 test** *See* **test, Farnsworth.**

**laser** An intense luminous source of coherent and monochromatic light. The term is an acronym for Light Amplification by Stimulated Emission of Radiation. Lasers are used in the treatment of a variety of ocular conditions, especially of the cornea, the retina (e.g. detached retina, diabetic retinopathy) and glaucoma.
*See* **iridectomy; keratotomy, radial; ophthalmoscope, scanning laser; photocoagulation.**

**laser, argon** A laser with ionized argon gas as the active medium which emits a blue-green light beam with a wavelength of 514 nm. It may be used to perform iridectomy, iridoplasty, iridotomy, photocoagulation or trabeculoplasty.

**laser, excimer** A gas laser which emits pulses of light in the ultraviolet region (at 193 nm). All the energy is absorbed by the superficial layers (e.g. the corneal epithelium) which are then exploded away or ablated without any change to the underlying or adjacent tissue or material.
*See* **keratotomy, radial; LASIK.**

**laser interferometry** *See* **maxwellian view system, clinical.**

**laser iridotomy** *See* **iredectomy.**

**laser, krypton** A laser with krypton gas ionized by electric current as the active medium which emits a light beam in the yellow-red region of the visible spectrum (521 nm, 568 nm or 647 nm). It may be used to perform photocoagulation or trabeculoplasty.

**laser, neodymium-yag (Nd-Yag)** A solid-state laser whose active medium is a crystal of yttrium, aluminium and garnet doped with neodymium ions. It emits an infrared light beam with a wavelength of 1064 nm. It is typically used with a slit-lamp and in conjunction with a helium-neon laser which produces a red beam of light (633 nm) to allow focusing. It may be used to perform capsulotomy, iridotomy or trabecular surgery. Yag is an acronym for **y**ttrium-**a**luminium-**g**arnet.

**laser refraction** *See* **refraction, laser.**

**laser trabeculoplasty** *See* **trabeculoplasty, laser.**

**LASIK** A surgical procedure on the cornea aimed at correcting ametropia. A suction ring is applied to the globe and an increase in intraocular pressure to approximately 65 mmHg is induced for a maximum of 2 minutes. During that time an automated microkeratome advances across the cornea creating a corneal flap of about 8.5 mm in diameter. The vacuum is then switched off and the suction ring removed. The corneal flap which is hinged on one side of the cornea is turned round onto the conjunctiva and the exposed stroma is ablated with the excimer laser. On completion of the laser ablation, the corneal flap is repositioned and left to adhere without sutures. There are some complications associated with this procedure, but it gives rise to less post-operative pain and more rapid visual rehabilitation than other similar surgical procedures. LASIK is an acronym made from the following italic letters '*la*ser *i*n situ *k*eratomileusis' or '*la*ser *as*sisted *i*ntrastromal *k*eratoplasty'.
*See* **epikeratoplasty; Intacs; keratoconus, posterior; keratome; keratomileusis; keratophakia; keratotomy, radial; laser, excimer.**

**latanoprost** *See* **prostaglandin analogues.**

**latent hypermetropia** *See* **hypermetropia, latent.**

**lateral geniculate body** *See* **geniculate bodies, lateral.**

**lateral inhibition** *See* **inhibition, lateral.**

**lateral rectus muscle** *See* **muscle, lateral rectus; muscles, extraocular.**

**lateral rectus paralysis** *See* **paralysis of the sixth nerve.**

**lathe-cut contact lens** *See* **lens, lathe-cut contact.**

**lattice degeneration of the retina** *See* **retina, lattice degeneration of the.**

**lattice dystrophy** *See* **dystrophy, lattice.**

**lattice theory** *See* **theory, Maurice's.**

**Laurence–Moon–Bardet–Biedl syndrome** *See* **syndrome, Laurence–Moon–Bardet–Biedl.**

**law, Abney's** The total luminance of an area is equal to the sum of the luminances which compose it.

**law, all or none** The response in a nerve fibre to any stimulus strong enough to produce a response is always of the same amplitude. However, different nerve fibres have action potentials with different amplitudes. An increase in the intensity of the stimulus yields only an increase in the frequency of nerve impulses (or action potentials). *Syn.* all or nothing law.
*See* **potential, action.**

**law, Bloch's** The luminance *L* of a stimulus required to produce a threshold response is inversely proportional to the duration of exposure $t$ of the stimulus, i.e.

$$Lt = C$$

where C is a constant. This law is only valid for exposure $t$ below about 0.1 s.

**law, Bunsen–Roscoe** In photochemistry, the product of the intensity of the light stimulus and the duration of exposure is a constant. *Syn.* **law of reciprocity.**
*See* **law, Bloch's.**

**law, cosine** *See* **diffusion**

**law, Descartes'** *See* **law of refraction.**

**law, Donders'** For any determinate position of the line of fixation with respect to the head there corresponds a definite and invariable angle of torsion.
*See* **torsion.**

**law, Draper's** An effect is produced in a medium, only by that portion of the spectrum which is absorbed by the medium. The effect may be thermal, chemical or the production of fluorescence. *Syn.* Grotthus' law.

**law, Emmert's** The apparent size of a projected after-image varies in proportion to the distance of the surface on which it is projected. The law can be expressed by the following relationship $h/H = d/D$, where $h$ is the linear size of the object, $H$ the apparent size of the projected after-image, $d$ the object's distance from the observer and $D$ the distance between the observer and the surface on which the after-image is projected. It follows from the above expression that $H = hD/d$, i.e. the greater the distance of the projected image the larger its apparent size.

**law of equal innervation** *See* **law of equal innervation, Hering's.**

**law of equal innervation, Hering's** Innervation to the extraocular muscles is equal to both eyes. Thus, all movements of the two eyes are equal and symmetrical. *Syn.* Hering's law; law of equal innervation.
*See* **muscles, yoke.**

**law, Fechner's** The intensity of a sensation $S$ varies as the logarithm of the intensity $I$ of the stimulus, i.e.

$$S = \text{k} \log I$$

where k is a constant. However, in some conditions this law is not valid and Stevens' law (or power law) is more appropriate. This stipulates that the intensity of a sensation $S$ varies as the intensity of the stimulus $I$ to the power of $x$, i.e.

$$S = \text{k}I^x$$

where $x$ is a constant which depends on the stimulus.
*See* **magnitude estimation.**

**law, Fermat's** The path taken by a light ray in going from one point to another is that route which takes the least time. *Syn.* Fermat's principle.

**law, Ferry–Porter** The critical flicker frequency $F$ is directly proportional to the logarithm of the luminance $L$ of the stimulus, i.e.

$$F = \text{a} \log L + \text{b}$$

where a and b are constants.
*See* **frequency, critical fusion.**

**law, Granit–Harper** The critical fusion frequency increases with the logarithm of the retinal area stimulated.
*See* **frequency, critical fusion.**

**law, Grotthus'** *See* **law, Draper's.**

**law, Hering's** *See* **law of equal innervation, Hering's.**

**law of identical visual directions** An object stimulating corresponding retinal points is localized in the same apparent monocular direction in each eye. *Syn.* law of oculocentric visual direction.
*See* **line of direction; retinal corresponding points.**

**law of illumination, inverse square** The illuminance $E$ of a surface by a point source is directly proportional to the luminous intensity $I$ of a point source and to the cosine of the angle θ of incidence and inversely proportional to the square of the distance $d$ between the surface and the source, i.e.

$$E = \frac{I \cos(\theta)}{d^2}$$

*Syn.* law of illumination.
*See* **illuminance.**

**law, Imbert–Fick** Applied to applanation tonometry, this law states that the intraocular pressure $P$ (in mmHg) is equal to the tonometer weight $W$ (in g) divided by the applanated area $A$ (in $\text{mm}^2$), hence,

$$P = \frac{W}{A}$$

Strictly speaking, this law is correct only for infinitely thin, dry, elastic, spherical membranes.
*See* **pressure, intraocular; tonometer, applanation.**

**law, Kirschmann's** The greatest contrast in colour is seen when the luminosity difference is small.

**law, Knapp's** A correcting lens placed at the anterior focal plane of an axially ametropic eye forms an image equal in size to that formed in a standard

emmetropic eye. Knapp's law applies to the relative spectacle magnification but not to the spectacle magnification. *Syn.* Knapp's rule.
*See* **magnification, relative spectacle.**

**law, Kollner's** *See* **rule, Kollner's.**

**law, Lagrange's** In paraxial optics, the product of the index of refraction of image space $n'$, the image size $h'$ and the half-angle of the refracted cone in image space $u'$ is equal to the product of the index of refraction of object space $n$, the object size $h$ and the half-angle of the incident cone in object space $u$, i.e.

$$n'h'u' = nhu$$

*Syn.* Helmholtz's law of magnification; Lagrange's relation; Smith–Helmholtz law.
*See* **sign convention.**

**law, Lambert's** *See* **cosine diffusion.**

**law, Listing's** When an eye moves to any position from the primary position, it may be considered to have made a single rotation about an axis that is perpendicular to both the initial and final lines of fixation at their point of intersection.
*See* **position, primary.**

**law of magnification, Helmholtz's** *See* **law, Lagrange's.**

**law of oculocentric visual direction** *See* **law of identical visual directions.**

**law, Piéron's** *See* **law, Ricco's.**

**law, Piper's** *See* **law, Ricco's.**

**law, Planck's** Law giving the energy distribution of a black body as a function of wavelength, for a specified temperature.
*See* **body, black.**

**law, power** *See* **law, Fechner's.**

**law, Prentice's** The prismatic effect $P$ in prism dioptres at a point on a lens is equal to the product of the distance $c$ in centimetres of the point from the optical centre of the lens, and the dioptric power $F$ of the lens, i.e.

$$P = cF$$

*Syn.* Prentice's rule.
*See* **dioptre, prism; effect, differential prismatic; power, prism; prism, induced.**

**law of reciprocal innervation, Sherrington's** The contraction of a muscle is accompanied by simultaneous and proportional relaxation of its antagonist. For example, if the superior oblique muscle contracts, its antagonist, the inferior oblique muscle, relaxes. The validity of this law has been established by electromyography.
*See* **electromyogram; muscle, antagonistic.**

**Table L1** Approximate amount of spectacle lens decentration (in mm) of its optical centre away from the pupillary centre of the eye to produce 5 prismatic effects (in prism dioptres) for distance vision. The results ignore the effect of spherical aberration

| lens power + or − | prismatic effect required | | | | |
|---|---|---|---|---|---|
| | 1 Δ | 2 Δ | 3 Δ | 4 Δ | 5 Δ |
| 20 D | 0.5 | 1.0 | 1.5 | 2.0 | 2.5 |
| 16 D | 0.6 | 1.3 | 1.9 | 2.5 | 3.1 |
| 14 D | 0.7 | 1.4 | 2.1 | 2.9 | 3.6 |
| 12 D | 0.8 | 1.7 | 2.5 | 3.3 | 4.2 |
| 10 D | 1.0 | 2.0 | 3.0 | 4.0 | 5.0 |
| 9 D | 1.1 | 2.2 | 3.3 | 4.4 | 5.6 |
| 8 D | 1.3 | 2.5 | 3.8 | 5.0 | 6.3 |
| 7 D | 1.4 | 2.9 | 4.3 | 5.7 | 7.1 |
| 6 D | 1.7 | 3.3 | 5.0 | 6.7 | 8.3 |
| 5 D | 2.0 | 4.0 | 6.0 | 8.0 | 10.0 |
| 4 D | 2.5 | 5.0 | 7.5 | 10.0 | 12.5 |
| 3 D | 3.3 | 6.7 | 10.0 | 13.3 | 16.7 |
| 2 D | 5.0 | 10.0 | 15.0 | 20.0 | 25.0 |
| 1 D | 10.0 | 20.0 | 30.0 | 40.0 | 50.0 |

**law of reciprocity** *See* **law, Bunsen–Roscoe.**

**law of reflection** The incident and reflected rays and the normal to the surface at the point of incidence lie in the same plane and the angle of incidence is equal to the angle of reflection (Fig. L4).

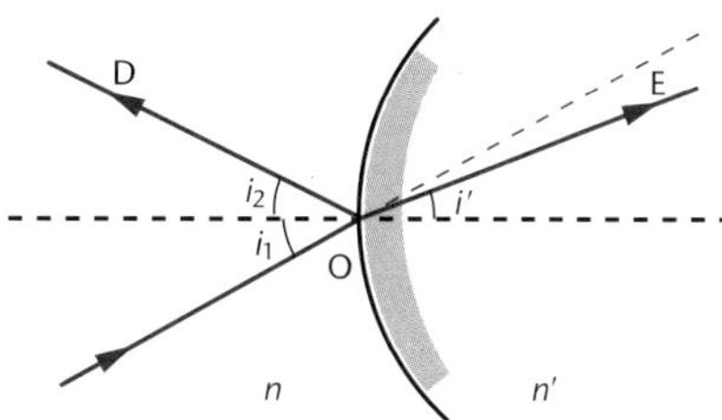


**Fig. L4** Light ray incident at O on a surface separating two media of different refractive indices, $n$ and $n'$. Some light is reflected along OD and most of the light is refracted along OE ($i_1$, angle of incidence = $i_2$, angle of reflection; $i'$, angle of refraction; $n' > n$)

**law of refraction** The incident and refracted rays and the normal to the surface at the point of incidence lie in the same plane and the ratio of the sine of the angle of incidence $i$ to the sine of the angle of refraction $i'$ is a constant for any two media, i.e.

$$\frac{\sin i}{\sin i'} = \frac{n'}{n} \text{ (or) } n \sin i = n' \sin i'$$

where $n$ and $n'$ are the refractive indices of the first and second medium, respectively. This constant ($n'/n$) is called the relative index of refraction for the two media. *Syn.* Descartes' law; Snell's law.
*See* **index of refraction; sign convention.**

**law, Ricco's** The product of the absolute threshold of luminance $L$ and the image area $A$ is a constant, i.e.

$LA = C$

This law is valid for small images subtending an angle of a few minutes of arc in the fovea and to one degree in the near macular region. For larger images in the macular area, **Piéron's law** applies; it states that the product of the luminance $L$ of the image at threshold and the cube root of the retinal area $A$ stimulated is a constant, i.e.

$L^3\sqrt{A} = C$

In the peripheral retina, **Piper's law** becomes valid. This law states that the product of the luminance of the stimulus $L$ and the square root of the area $A$ is a constant, i.e.

$L\sqrt{A} = C$

In the far periphery of the retina, $L$ tends to become independent of $A$.

**law, Smith–Helmholtz** *See* **law, Lagrange's.**

**law, Snell's** *See* **law of refraction.**

**law, Stevens'** *See* **law, Fechner's.**

**law, Talbot's** *See* **law, Talbot–Plateau.**

**law, Talbot–Plateau** The brightness of a light source presented at short intervals above the critical fusion frequency is equal to that which would be produced by a constant light source of an intensity equal to the mean value of the intermittent stimuli. *Syn.* Talbot's law.
*See* **frequency, critical fusion.**

**law, Weber's** The just noticeable difference (or difference threshold) in intensity of a stimulus $\Delta I$ varies as a constant ratio of the initial intensity of the stimulus $I$, i.e.

$\Delta I = kI$

where $k = \{\Delta I/I\}$ is a constant called **Weber's fraction** (or **Weber's constant**). *Example*: if the initial stimulus was a light source of 1000 cd/m$^2$ and k = 0.01 (or 1%), $\Delta I = 0.01 \times 1000 = 10$ cd/m$^2$. *Syn.* Weber–Fechner law.
*See* **threshold, differential.**

**law, Weber–Fechner** *See* **law, Weber's.**

**layer of Henle, fibre** Located in the macular region, it is formed by the cone and rod fibres which run parallel to the retinal surface within the outer molecular layer of the retina.
*See* **Haidinger's brushes; macular star; retina.**

**layers of the iris; of the retina** *See* under the nouns.

**lazy eye** *See* **eye, amblyopic.**

**leaf room** *See* **room, leaf.**

**Leber's congenital amaurosis** A hereditary, bilateral blindness present at birth or in early childhood. Initially, the ocular fundus appears normal although the ERG is markedly reduced. A salt and pepper fundus and optic atrophy appear later. The condition is often accompanied by nystagmus and photophobia.
*See* **fundus, salt and pepper.**

**Leber's disease** *See* **Leber's hereditary optic atrophy.**

**Leber's hereditary optic atrophy** A hereditary, bilateral condition which appears suddenly in healthy people, primarily males, of about the age of 20 and results in a marked loss of vision and ultimately optic atrophy. A very small percentage of people recover some visual acuity in one or both eyes after the disease has run its course. *Syn.* Leber's disease; Leber's hereditary optic neuropathy.
*See* **atrophy, optic; cataract, complicated.**

**Lees screen** *See* **screen, Lees.**

**legibility** Term referring to the difference in the ease of difficulty with which optotypes can be read. Some letters are easier to recognize (e.g. L, T, U, V, Z and C) than others (e.g. S, G, H, F, R and B). Test charts either mix these letters or use letters of similar difficulty; the latter facilitates standardization of charts.

**length, equivalent focal** In an optical system composed of more than one lens, it is the linear distance separating the principal focus from the corresponding principal point. It is usually the most important quantity in the specification of an optical system as in objectives, eyepieces, etc.
*See* **focus, principal; power, equivalent.**

**length of the eye, axial** The distance between the anterior and posterior poles of the eye. In vivo, it is typically measured by ultrasonography (although strictly speaking, that measurement represents the distance between the anterior pole and the anterior surface of the retina, in most eyes). The axial length of the eye at birth is approximately 17 mm and reaches approximately 24 mm in adulthood.
*See* **poles of the eyeball; ultrasonography.**

**length, focal** The linear distance separating the principal focal point (or focus) of an optical system from a point of reference (e.g. vertex, principal point, nodal point). The **first** (or **anterior**) **focal length** is the distance from the lens (or first principal point) to the first principal focus. The **second** (or **posterior**) **focal length** is the distance from the lens (or second principal point) to the second principal focus. *Symbol*: *f*. In a spherical mirror the focal length *f*, i.e. the distance between the focal point and the pole of the mirror, is equal to half its radius of curvature *r*,

$$f = \frac{r}{2}$$

*Syn.* focal distance.
*See* **focus, principal; mirror; points, cardinal; points, principal; power, equivalent; power, refractive; sign convention.**

**lens** A piece of transparent glass, crystal, plastic or similar substance (e.g. liquid) having two opposite regular surfaces which can be plane or curved and which alter the vergence of pencils of light transmitted through it. There are many types of lenses which are described below.
*See* **coquille; glass; moulding; surfacing.**

**lens, absorptive** A lens which absorbs a proportion of the incident radiation. Some lenses absorb mostly in the infrared region of the spectrum, others absorb mostly in the ultraviolet region and others absorb more or less equally throughout the visible spectrum.
*See* **CR-39; filter; infrared; lens, coated; light; pterygium; ultraviolet.**

**lens, achromatic** A compound lens designed to reduce or eliminate chromatic aberrations. The most common type is called a doublet. *Syn.* achromat.
*See* **doublet; lens, apochromatic; lens, hyperchromatic.**

**lens, achromatizing** Lens aimed at reducing or eliminating the chromatic aberration of the eye. It consists of either a doublet or a triplet which possesses longitudinal chromatic aberration opposite to that of the eye and thereby neutralizes it. Thus the lens system has negative power for short wavelengths and positive power for long wavelengths of an amount similar to that of the eye for those wavelengths.
*See* **aberration, longitudinal chromatic; doublet; triplet.**

**lens adherence 1.** Refers to a contact lens being firmly fixed to the cornea. **2.** Attachment of bacteria (e.g. pseudomonas, staphylococcus) to a contact lens, particularly soft lens materials (although the amount and strength vary with the material). *Syn.* lens binding.
*See* **keratitis; lens, silicone hydrogel; tear stasis.**

**lens, afocal** A lens of zero power (Fig. L5). *Syn.* plano lens.
*See* **afocal; lens, aniseikonic.**

**lens, Alvarez** A variable power lens composed of two elements that can be moved with respect to each other along two mutually perpendicular axes. When the two lenses are in exact register with each other the Alvarez lens provides zero power. Moving one of the elements either laterally or vertically in relation to the other provides increasing spherical or cylindrical power. Moving both elements produces a combined spherocylindrical power. Such a lens is used in the Humphrey Vision Analyser.
*See* **Analyser, Humphrey Vision.**

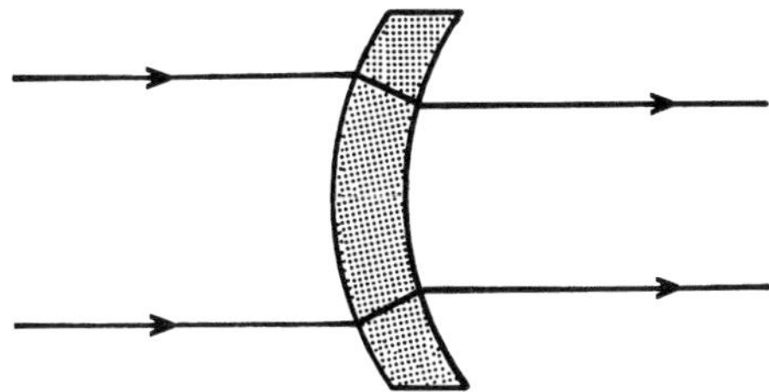

**Fig. L5** Afocal size lens

**lens, anastigmatic 1.** A lens which has a single focal point. **2.** A lens which is corrected for oblique astigmatism and minimum curvature of field. *Syn.* stigmatic lens.
*See* **lens, astigmatic; Petzval surface.**

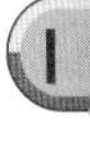

**lens, anti-actinic** A lens which absorbs ultraviolet radiations to a much greater extent than a white spectacle lens.
*See* **actinic; ultraviolet.**

**lens, aniseikonic** Lens designed to correct aniseikonia. It can have power like a regular ophthalmic lens but also produces a magnification of the image. A lens which only produces magnification but has zero power is called an **overall size lens** and if it magnifies in only one meridian it is called a **meridional size lens**. *Syn.* iseikonic lens; eikonic lens; size lens.
*See* **aniseikonia; lens, afocal; magnification, shape; room, leaf.**

**lens, anti-reflection coated** *See* **lens, coated.**

**lens, aphakic** A lens used for the correction of aphakia. It is of high dioptric power, usually above +10 D. Due to their thickness, these lenses are usually made of plastic to reduce weight and because of the aberrations, aspherical surfaces are used.
*See* **aphakia; lens, lenticular; phenomenon, jack-in-the-box.**

**lens, aplanatic** A lens designed to correct for spherical aberration and coma.

**lens, apochromatic** A compound lens designed to correct chromatic and spherical aberrations.

It uses three or more kinds of glass. This lens corrects chromatic aberration more thoroughly than an achromatic lens.
*See* **lens, achromatic.**

**lens, aspheric** A lens in which one or both surfaces are not spherical, so designed to minimize certain optical aberrations.

**lens, astigmatic** A toric or cylindrical lens which produces two separate focal lines at right angles, instead of a single focal point. Hence it has two principal powers. One of these powers may be zero (**cylindrical lens**).
*See* **axis, cylinder; lens, anastigmatic; lens, cylindrical; lens, spherocylindrical; lens, toric; protractor; Sturm, interval of; transposition.**

**lens, back toric contact** A contact lens used to correct corneal astigmatism in which the surface of the lens facing the cornea is not spherical but toroidal in order to obtain a good physical fit on the cornea. To create better stability of the lens on the eye it usually incorporates a prism ballast.
*See* **ballast.**

**lens, Bagolini's** *See* **glass, Bagolini's.**

**lens, balancing** A lens fitted to a spectacle frame or mount, to balance the weight of the other lens, its power being unspecified or unimportant.

**lens, bandage** *See* **lens, therapeutic soft contact.**

**lens, bent** *See* **lens, meniscus.**

**lens, best-form** A curved lens whose curvatures are calculated to eliminate or minimize aberrations when viewing through the peripheral portions of the lens. *Syn.* corrected lens; point-focal lens.
*See* **ellipse, Tscherning.**

**lens, biconcave** A lens which has two concave surfaces.

**lens, biconvex** A lens which has two convex surfaces.

**lens, bifocal** A lens having two portions of different focal power. Usually the upper portion is larger and is used for distance vision while the lower portion is smaller and used for near vision. There are, however, many types of bifocals: those in which the use of the two portions is the opposite of that described above, others in which the shape of the **near portion** (or **segment**) differs; in certain types the near segment is fused onto the surface of the glass (**fused bifocal**); in others the near portion is produced by grinding or moulding a different curvature on one surface (**solid bifocal** or **one-piece bifocal**). There is also a one-piece bifocal in which there is a gradual transitional zone between the two portions instead of a clear line of demarcation (**blended bifocal**). In addition, several other bifocals are known by their tradename (Fig. L6).
*See* **button; jump; lens, high index; lens, progressive; monocentric; segment height; segment of a bifocal lens; wafer.**

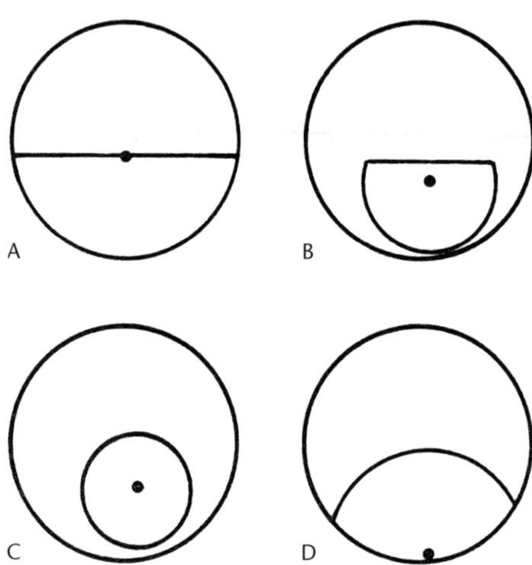


**Fig. L6** Examples of bifocal types. In each case the dot indicates the optical centre of the near portion (A, executive-type segment; B, flat-top segment; C, round segment; D, curved segment)

**lens binding** *See* **lens adherence.**

**lens blank** A moulded piece of ophthalmic glass before completion of the surfacing processes.
*See* **glass; lens, semi-finished; surfacing.**

**lens capsule** *See* **capsule; lens, crystalline.**

**lens carrier** *See* **lens, lenticular; telescope, bioptic.**

**lens, cast-moulding contact** A contact lens produced by pressing a concave female mould filled with liquid monomer against a male mould. The concave mould determines the front surface of the lens. The edge is formed when the two sides of the mould come together. The assembled moulds are irradiated with ultraviolet light to cause polymerization and a dry contact lens, which is then hydrated in saline water. Cast-moulding has been used to manufacture hard and soft lenses, especially mass production of the latter.
*See* **lens, lathe-cut contact; lens, spin-cast contact.**

**lens, Chavasse** A lens with an irregular surface used to depress the visual acuity while permitting the eye to be seen from the front (British Standard).

**lens, ChromGen** Tradename of a tinted, soft contact lens worn with the aim of enhancing colour perception in individuals with colour vision deficiencies, especially red-green defects. It is fitted on either one or both eyes. The lenses exist in a variety of tints and are chosen by the patient by trial and error. Some patients with dyslexia or migraine have also claimed to benefit from wearing these lenses.
*See* **lens, X-Chrom.**

**lens clock** *See* **lens measure.**

**lens, coated** A lens upon which is deposited an evaporated film consisting of a metallic salt such as magnesium fluoride, about one-quarter as thick as a wavelength of light. This film reduces, by interference, the amount of light reflected by the surfaces and to some extent the amount of stray light reflected inside the lens. With **multilayer coating** the lens can selectively reflect radiations and increase transmission. All coated lenses show some residual colour. *Syn.* anti-reflection (AR) coated lens; bloomed lens.
*See* **anti-reflection coating; coating; filter, bandpass; Fresnel's formula; image, ghost.**

**lens, cobalt** A lens which absorbs the central region of the visible spectrum and only transmits the red and blue ends of the spectrum. It is sometimes used in the testing of ametropia, since a light source located at 1.4 m from the eye will form, in an emmetropic eye viewing it through a cobalt lens, two equal circles superimposed on the retina and the subject will report seeing a purple circle. A hyperope will see a blue spot surrounded by a red annulus and a myope will see a red spot surrounded by a blue annulus. An appropriate spherical lens placed in front of the eye which changes the appearance to a purple circle represents the spherical refractive correction. *Syn.* cobalt-blue glass.
*See* **test, duochrome.**

**lens, collimating** *See* **collimator.**

**lens, combination** A lens made from two different materials; usually a rigid centre portion made from gas-permeable material surrounded by a soft peripheral flange of HEMA material. It is used in the management of keratoconus, irregular astigmatism, etc. Few such lenses exist at present.
*See* **lens, piggyback.**

**lens, composite** A contact lens composed of two or more different materials.

**lens, compound 1.** A lens which functions as a combination of a spherical lens and a cylindrical lens. *Example*: a spherocylindrical lens. **2.** A system composed of several refracting surfaces or lenses placed along the same axis. *Examples*: doublet; triplet.
*See* **doublet; lens, spherocylindrical; triplet.**

**lens, concave** *See* **lens, diverging.**

**lens, condensing** *See* **condenser.**

**lens, contact** A small lens usually made of a plastic material, worn in contact with the cornea or sclera and used to correct refractive errors of the eye. There are many types of contact lenses. Lenses that rest on the sclera are called **scleral** (or **haptic**) contact lenses whereas lenses that rest on the cornea are called **corneal** contact lenses, or, more commonly, contact lenses. Lenses that are made of a hard plastic material which is impermeable to oxygen, such as those made of polymethyl methacrylate (PMMA), are called **hard** or **rigid** contact lenses. Hard contact lenses which transmit oxygen are called **gas permeable** contact lenses (GP, GPL, GPCL, HGP or RGP). Other lenses made of a soft plastic material which transmit a certain amount of oxygen are called **soft** (or **hydrophilic** or **hydrogel** or **gel** or **flexible**) contact lenses (SCL) whose water content varies; the greater the water content the more oxygen is transmitted (for equal thickness). Very high water content lenses are used for **extended wear** (EW). There are also **bifocal contact lenses** consisting of two segments with different focal powers which provide either **simultaneous** vision (light from both the distance and near portions enters the eye at the same time) or **alternating** vision (the lens must be moved to see through either portion). Other bifocal contact lenses have a zone of variable power between the two portions and others are **diffractive** in which light from both distance and near objects can be focused on the retina (without moving the lens) owing to diffraction produced by a series of rings in the centre of the back surface of the lens (the higher the near addition the greater the number of rings). There are also **toric** contact lenses in which the back optic surface is toroidal; they are used to improve the physical fit. **Bitoric** contact lenses are lenses in which both surfaces are toroidal; they are used to improve the physical fit and correct the induced astigmatism. **Disposable** contact lenses are worn for about 1 week continuously (or 2 weeks on a daily basis) and then discarded.
*See* **lens adherence; lens, back toric contact; lens, cast-moulding; lens, ChromGen; lens, cosmetic contact; lens, extended wear; lens, fenestrated; lens, flare; lens, flat; lens, flexure; lens, lathe-cut contact; lens, liquid; lens, piggyback; lens, scleral contact; lens, sealed scleral contact; lens, silicone hydrogel; lens, spin-cast contact; lens, steep; lens, therapeutic soft contact; lens, X-Chrom; water content.**

**Table L2** Relationship between object and image formed in a converging and in a diverging lens. The object is moved from left to right. *F* and *F'* are the first and second focal points, respectively

| position of the object | type of object | type of image | position of the image |
|---|---|---|---|
| **converging lens** | | | |
| infinity | — | real (inverted) | *F'* |
| between infinity and *F* | real | real (inverted) | between *F'* and infinity |
| *F* | real | — | infinity |
| between *F* and lens | real | virtual (erect) | between infinity and lens |
| between lens and infinity | virtual | real (erect) | between lens and *F'* |
| **diverging lens** | | | |
| infinity | — | virtual (erect) | *F'* |
| between infinity and lens | real | virtual (erect) | between *F'* and lens |
| between lens and *F* | virtual | real (erect) | between lens and infinity |
| *F* | virtual | — | infinity |
| between *F* and infinity | virtual | virtual (inverted) | between infinity and *F'* |

**lens, converging** A lens which causes incident rays of light to converge. *Syn.* convex lens; plus lens; positive lens.

**lens, convex** *See* **lens, converging.**

**lens, corrected** *See* **lens, best-form.**

**lens cortex** *See* **lens, crystalline.**

**lens, cosmetic contact** A contact lens designed to improve the appearance of the eye, to conceal a disfigurement (e.g. a scar), or to change the colour of the eye. *Examples*: a tinted lens; an opaque lens with an artificial pupil and iris.
*See* **aniridia; lens, tinted.**

**lens, cross-cylinder** An astigmatic lens consisting of a minus cylinder ground on one side and a plus cylinder ground on the other side, the two axes being located 90° apart. The dioptric power in the principal meridians is equal. Usual cross-cylinder lenses are provided in three powers: ±0.25 D, ±0.37 D and ±0.50 D (higher values are also available for use with low vision patients). This lens is used in the subjective measurement of the power and axis of astigmatism, or to refine the cylindrical correction determined otherwise (Fig. L7). *Syn.* Jackson cross-cylinder lens.
*See* **astigmatism; test for astigmatism, cross-cylinder.**

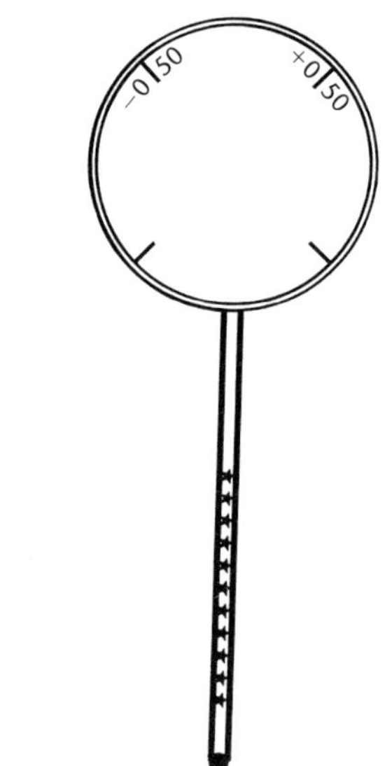


Fig. L7 Cross-cylinder lens

**lens, crystalline** The biconvex, usually transparent body, situated between the iris and the vitreous body of the eye and suspended from the ciliary body by the zonular fibres (**zonule of Zinn**) which are attached to the equator of the lens. The diameter of the lens is equal to 9–10 mm and its thickness 3.6 mm, being greater when the eye accommodates. The radii of curvature of the anterior and posterior surfaces are 10.6 mm and −6.2 mm, respectively in the unaccommodated eye, while maximum accommodation alters these values to about 6 mm and −5.3 mm, respectively. The crystalline lens displays a complex gradient of refractive index (averaging 1.42), and a power of 21 D. It consists of the **capsule** which envelops the lens, the anterior epithelium and the **cortex** which surrounds the **nucleus**, the latter two containing the lens fibres. With age, there is an increase in light scatter originating in the nucleus, as well as some light absorption and yellowing of the nucleus (Fig. L8). *Syn.* lens of the eye.
*See* **accommodation; capsule; capsulectomy; constants of the eye; disease, Wilson's; fissure,**

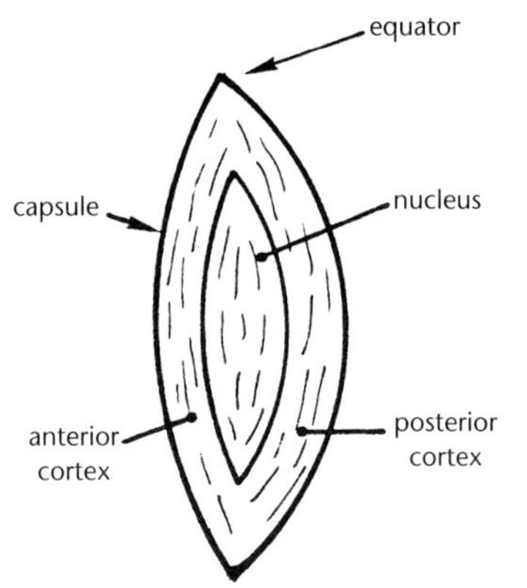


**Fig. L8** Cross-section of the crystalline lens

**optic; implant, intraocular lens; lens paradox; luxation; myopia, lenticular; phakic; shagreen; suture, lens; Zinn, zonule of.**

**lens, curved** *See* **lens, meniscus.**

**lens, cylindrical** A lens in which one of the principal meridians has zero refractive power. It usually consists of one plano surface and one cylindrical surface (Fig. L9).
*See* **lens, astigmatic.**

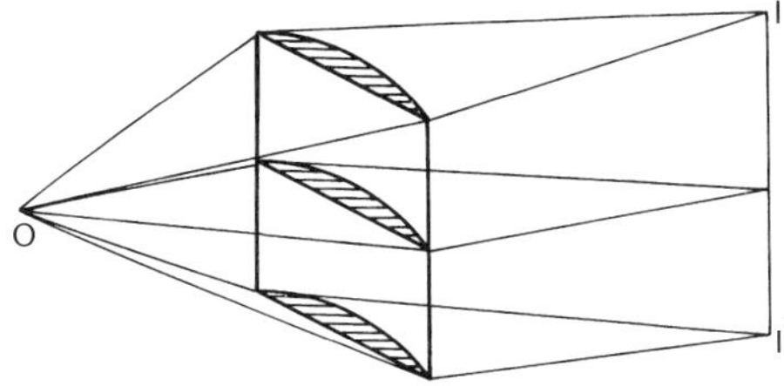


**Fig. L9** Cylindrical lens (O, object; II′, image)

**lens deposits, contact** *See* **deposits, contact lens.**

**lens dislocation** *See* **luxation of the lens.**

**lens, disposable** *See* **lens, contact.**

**lens, diverging** A lens which causes incident rays of light to diverge. *Syn.* concave lens; minus lens; negative lens.

**lens, eikonic** *See* **lens, aniseikonic.**

**lens, equi-concave** A lens having two concave surfaces of the same power.

**lens, equi-convex** A lens having two convex surfaces of the same power.

**lens, equivalent** *See* **equivalent, spherical.**

**lens exfoliation** *See* **exfoliation of the lens.**

**lens, extended wear** A contact lens designed to be worn continuously for more than one day and, usually, no more than seven days before cleaning and sterilization. It is, typically, a soft lens, with high oxygen transmissibility.
*See* **cornea guttata; corneal infiltrates; lens, silicone hydrogel; microcysts, epithelial; microscope, specular; oxygen transmissibility; pannus; ulcer, corneal.**

**lens extraction** *See* **cataract extraction.**

**lens, fenestrated** A hard contact lens having one or more small holes to aid tear exchange and corneal oxygenation. It was essential with PMMA scleral contact lenses, but with the advent of gas permeable materials, fenestration is rarely necessary. *Syn.* ventilated lens.
*See* **lens, scleral contact.**

**lens, finished** A spectacle lens that has been surfaced on both sides to the required power and thickness and is still in uncut form. *syn.* uncut lens.
*See* **lens, semi-finished; surfacing.**

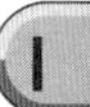

**lens, fisheye** A camera lens with a very wide angle of view. The angle can be as wide as 220°. To achieve this the lens has a large diameter that produces image distortion (especially barrel-shaped distortion); thus the image magnification varies across the picture causing some fishbowl effects.
*See* **distortion; lens, wide-angle.**

**lens flare** Type of blur characterized by the presence of a secondary or ghost image. Flare may be caused by a contact lens with an optic zone diameter that is smaller than the pupil diameter or when the lens decentres so that part of the edge of the optic zone is within the pupil area. Flare is usually more apparent under conditions of reduced illumination as the pupil is larger. Management consists in refitting the patient with a lens with a larger optic zone diameter or with better centration.
*See* **image, ghost; optic zone diameter.**

**lens, flat 1.** Any lens that is not of curved form. **2.** A contact lens in which the back optic zone radius is longer than the flattest meridian of the cornea. This definition may not be valid for a soft lens that may have a back optic zone radius longer than the flattest meridian of the cornea and yet not be flat fitting. *Syn.* loose lens (it is preferable to use this term for soft lenses).
*See* **fitted on K; lens, steep.**

**lens flexure** Characteristic of a spherical contact lens to adopt a toroidal curvature when placed on an astigmatic cornea. Flexure depends upon the material and its thickness, being more common with thin lenses. As it occurs during blinking, it sometimes results in fluctuating vision.

**lens flippers** Two pairs of lenses mounted on a central bar, one pair on each side. One pair can be held in front of the patient's eyes and then quickly changed for the other pair by twisting the bar extension handle. The lenses may be one pair of minus lenses of equal power and the other pair of plus lenses of equal power. The most common pairs are ±2.00 D, although ±1.00 D, ±1.50 D and ±2.50 D are also available. These are used in the testing and training of accommodative facility. **Prisms** may also be used, as for example base-in for one pair and base-out for the other. They are used in the testing and training of vergence facility (Fig. L10). *Syn.* flippers; flipper bar; flip lenses; flip prisms; prism flippers.
*See* **accommodative facility; vergence facility.**

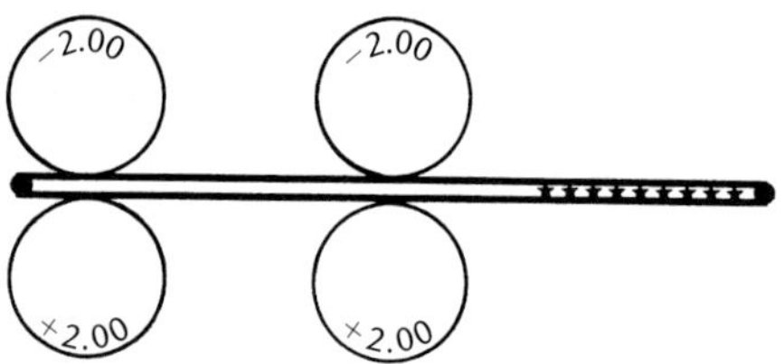


**Fig. L10** Lens flippers

**lens, Fresnel** A plastic lens consisting of one flat surface which can adhere to a clean lens surface and another surface on which there is a series of concentric prismatic rings or elements. The same focusing effect can be obtained in an optical element if the lens surface is divided into small elements and these elements are brought together in a common plane normal to the optical axis. The apical angles of these prismatic elements increase ring by ring towards the lens periphery. Thus, the Fresnel lens has the same power as a continuous spherical lens surface but without the thickness and the weight. However, owing to the imperfect surface of the lens a slight reduction in acuity is obtained. These lenses are primarily used for temporary correction in orthoptics therapy, or following eye surgery and as condensers in overhead projectors, headlights, etc. Fresnel lenses are also made in vinyl material called **Fresnel Press-On** lenses which can adhere to a standard lens surface. (Fig. L11)
*See* **prism, Fresnel Press-On.**

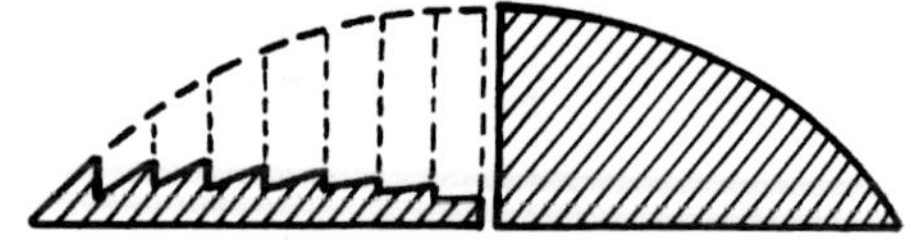

**Fig. L11** Cross-section of a Fresnel lens of approximately the same refractive power as the planoconvex lens next to it

**lens, frosted** A lens made translucent by having one or both surfaces smoothed but not polished.
*See* **glass, ground; surfacing; translucent.**

**lens, Goldmann three mirror** *See* **gonioscope; slit-lamp.**

**lens, gonioscopic** A lens placed in contact with the cornea for the purpose of viewing the angle of the anterior chamber. It may be a prismatic lens or a lens with mirrors, or merely a thick convex contact lens. Some, like the Goldmann three-mirror goniolens, enables visualization with a slit-lamp of the ciliary body and peripheral retina, as well as the angle of the anterior chamber. Other goniolenses (e.g. Zeiss) have four mirrors. *Syn.* goniolens.
*See* **gonioscope; lens, Koeppe; lens, Zeiss.**

**lens, gradient-index** A lens with an index of refraction that changes continuously through the whole material, or part of, thus providing an area of progressive power. However, there are still problems in manufacturing these lenses reliably and without unwanted astigmatism.
*See* **lens, progressive.**

**lens groove** An indentation on the edge of a lens designed to accommodate a cord (usually a nylon thread) which retains the lens in a rimless mounting.
*See* **rimless fitting; spectacles, rimless; spectacles, supra.**

**lens, high index** A specialized lens made with higher refractive material than crown glass. Included in these are flint and titanium glasses in which the refractive index can be as high as 1.8. However, as the index increases there is usually a decrease in the constringence. For example, Zenlite (a tradename) has a refractive index of 1.805 and a constringence of 25.4. Recently, technical advances have made it possible to manufacture high index progressive lenses. High index lenses are used for high prescriptions as they can be made much thinner than crown glass lenses of equivalent power. As high index lenses have very reflective surfaces it is valuable to have them coated.
*See* **constringence; glass, flint.**

**lens, high water content** A contact lens whose water content is greater than 50%.
*See* **water content.**

**lens, honey bee** A compound magnifying lens consisting of three to six small telescopes mounted in the upper portion of a spectacle lens. The telescopes are so arranged as to resemble the multifaceted eye of the honey bee. They have their axes converging on the eye as well as prismatic objectives to provide an approximately continuous field of view.

**lens, Hruby** A spherical diverging lens of −55 D mounted on a slit-lamp and biomicroscope in such a way that it can be placed very close to the patient's cornea. It is used, coupled with the microscope, to examine internal ocular structures including the retina.
*See* **biomicroscope; slit-lamp.**

**lens, hydrogel** *See* **lens, contact.**

**lens, hyperchromatic** A compound lens designed to have a large amount of chromatic aberration. It may be of use in the correction of presbyopia by extending the depth of focus of the eye; the eye receives a clear red image of distant objects and a clear blue image of near objects without having to change its focus. However, because of the reduced information in the retinal image, such a lens would be more beneficial with high contrast objects.
*See* **depth of focus; lens, achromatic.**

**lens, immersion** Objective of a high power microscope in which the space between its front lens and the cover plate of the microscope slide is filled with an immersion liquid, e.g. water, cedar wood oil, etc.
*See* **microscope; objective.**

**lens implant, intraocular** *See* **implant, intraocular lens.**

**lens, Irlen** *See* **syndrome, Meares–Irlen.**

**lens, iseikonic** *See* **lens, aniseikonic.**

**lens, isochromatic** A tinted lens which absorbs all radiations equally.

**lens, Koeppe** A diagnostic goniolens designed to be placed on the anaesthetized cornea for a direct view (without a mirror) of the angle of the anterior chamber. It consists of a high-plus (50 D) lens with a back concave surface and a flange that retains the lens in place. Like all goniolenses its overall power more or less neutralizes the refractive power of the cornea. Its image magnification is about half that of goniolenses with mirrors but its field of view is wider. The lens is typically used with a hand-held biomicroscope, in surgery and with children in whom it can be used to examine the fundus as well. *Syn.* Koeppe contact lens; Koeppe gonioscopic lens.
*See* **lens, gonioscopic; gonioscope.**

**lens, lacrimal** *See* **lens, liquid.**

**lens, laminated** A lens consisting of a thin layer of plastic (e.g. cellulose acetate) cemented between two layers of glass. Such a lens protects the eye because in case of breakage the glass pieces remain attached to the plastic layer.
*See* **glass, safety; lens, safety.**

**lens, lathe-cut contact** A contact lens in which the optic radii of the surfaces are cut into a block of plastic mounted in a lathe and then polished. Hydrophilic polymers are cut in a solid state with shorter radii and thinner centre thickness than is desired in the hydrated state, and they are polished with an oil-based compound as water cannot be used.
*See* **lens, cast-moulding contact; lens, spin-cast contact.**

**lens, lenticular** An ophthalmic lens with a central zone finished to prescription surrounded by a supporting margin (or **carrier**), generally made in order to reduce the weight of lenses of high power. They can be made either as one solid piece or the power element may be cemented on a plano carrier.
*See* **aperture of a lenticular lens; lens, aphakic.**

**lens, liquid** The lens formed by the tear layer lying between the back surface of a contact lens and the cornea. It must be taken into account when fitting contact lenses. If the back surface of the lens is steeper than the cornea, the liquid lens is positive and the eye is made more myopic. If the back surface of the lens is flatter than the cornea, the liquid lens is negative and the eye is made more hyperopic. (Fig. L12) *Syn.* fluid lens; lacrimal lens; tear lens.
*See* **keratometer; lens, contact.**

**lens, loose** *See* **lens, flat.**

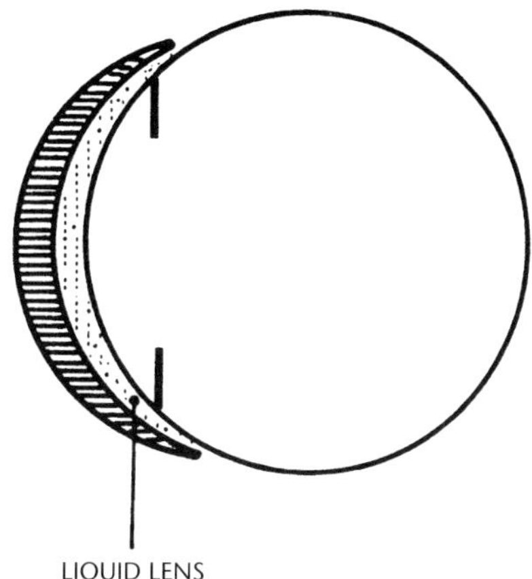


**Fig. L12** Liquid lens between a contact lens and the cornea (it is positive in this diagram)

**lens, low water content** A contact lens whose water content is less than 50%.
*See* **water content.**

**lens, luxation of the** *See* **luxation.**

**lens, magnifying** A converging lens used to magnify an object without image inversion. *Syn.* magnifying glass.
*See* **magnifier.**

**lens measure** Instrument for determining the radius of curvature of a spherical or cylindrical surface, based on measuring the sag of the curve. The instrument shaped like a pocket watch consists of two fixed, pointed prongs attached to the edge and a movable one located halfway between the two. The sag of the surface in the meridian containing all three prongs is measured by the linear displacement of the central one. The instrument is calibrated to give a reading in dioptres of the surface power for that meridian which has been calculated usually using the refractive index of crown glass ($n = 1.523$). If the material has a different refractive index, the true surface power, $F_T$, in dioptres, is given by the following formula,

$$F_T = \frac{n-1}{0.523} \times F_{LM}$$

where $n$ is the refractive index and $F_{LM}$ is the reading, in dioptres, shown on the lens measure (Fig. L13). *Syn.* lens clock; spherometer (the old models had three outer fixed prongs instead of two).
*See* **focimeter; neutralization; sag; vertex depth.**

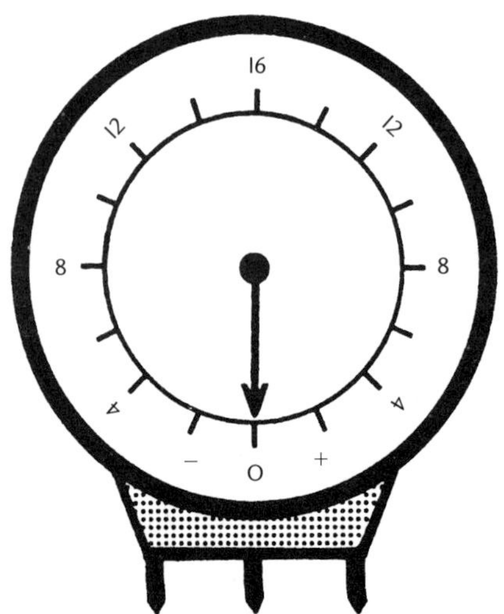


**Fig. L13** Lens measure

**lens, meniscus** Lens having a spherical convex surface and a spherical concave surface. Meniscus lenses often have a base of 6 D for the surface of lesser curvature. *Syn.* curved lens; bent lens.
*See* **curve, base; lens, periscopic; lens, toric.**

**lens, meridional size** *See* **lens, aniseikonic.**

**lens, microscopic** *See* **lens, telescopic.**

**lens, mid-water content** A contact lens whose water content is between 50% and 65%.
*See* **water content.**

**lens, minus** *See* **lens, diverging.**

**lens, monocentric** *See* **monocentric.**

**lens, multifocal** A lens with various dioptric powers such as a bifocal, a trifocal, or a progressive lens.

**lens, negative** *See* **lens, diverging.**

**lens nucleus** *See* **lens, crystalline.**

**lens, objective** *See* **objective.**

**lens, ophthalmic** Any lens used to correct refractive errors of the eye. Sometimes it also includes lenses used to measure the refractive error.
*See* **focimeter; lens, spectacle; refractive error.**

**lens, orthoscopic** A lens corrected for peripheral aberrations.
*See* **ellipse, Tscherning.**

**lens paradox** A change of the ametropia of the eye towards hypermetropia (or less myopia) in old eyes, although the crystalline lens increases in size and the anterior and posterior surfaces become more curved. This is paradoxical since this should lead to an increase in lens power and a change towards myopia. This paradox is attributed to a reduction in the index of refraction occurring within the various layers of the lens, as well as to an increase in the refractive index of the vitreous humour which would result in a reduction of the total lens power.
*See* **index of refraction; lens, crystalline.**

**lens pattern** *See* **former.**

**lens, periscopic** A spherical lens in which the minus lenses have base curves of +1.25 D and the plus lenses have base curves of −1.25 D. Meniscus lenses are more curved.
*See* **curve, base; lens, meniscus.**

**lens, photochromatic** *See* **lens, photochromic.**

**lens, photochromic** A lens used either in sunglasses or as an ophthalmic lens. It is made up of a glass material which changes in colour and/or in light transmission as a result of changes in incident light intensity or heat. The changes are reversible and relatively rapid. There exist several types which are known by their

tradename (e.g. Photogray Extra, Reactolite Rapide). *Syn.* photochromatic lens.
*See* **vignetting.**

**lens, piggyback** A combination of two contact lenses; usually a rigid contact lens (preferably gas-permeable) over a hydrogel lens. The soft lens is used for comfort and the rigid lens for best visual results. Piggyback lenses can be used after corneal surgery, corneal scarring and in the management of severe keratoconus or irregular astigmatism. *Syn.* combination system.
*See* **lens, combination; lens, therapeutic soft contact.**

**lens, plano** *See* **lens, afocal.**

**lens, planoconcave** A lens with one plane and one concave surface.

**lens, planoconvex** A lens with one plane and one convex surface.
*See* **vertex depth.**

**lens, plastic** Lens made of transparent plastic. It is approximately 50% lighter than a glass lens of equal power but more liable to scratching. Plastic lenses do not shatter like glass lenses and therefore give better protection.
*See* **CR-39; glass, safety; lens, safety; plastic.**

**lens, plus** *See* **lens, converging.**

**lens, point-focal** *See* **lens, best-form.**

**lens, polarizing** A lens which transmits light waves vibrating in one direction only. In the other direction perpendicular to it, the light waves are absorbed. In this way reflected glare is reduced. Common polarizing materials include herapathite crystal, calcite crystal or a stretched sheet of polyvinyl alcohol containing iodine.
*See* **glare; light, polarized.**

**lens, positive** *See* **lens, converging.**

**lens, prismatic** A lens with prism power.

**lens, prism ballast** *See* **ballast.**

**lens, prismatic effect of a** *See* **convergence, correction induced; prism, induced.**

**lens, progressive addition (PAL)** A spectacle lens having a gradual and progressive change in power either over the whole lens or over a region intermediate between areas of uniform power. The **progression** is produced by a complex aspheric shape of one of the surfaces. This lens is used to correct presbyopia. (Fig. L14) *Syn.* varifocal lens.
*See* **distance, interpupillary; lens, bifocal; lens, gradient-index; lens, multifocal.**

**lens, reading** A lens prescribed for near vision (or a magnifying glass).

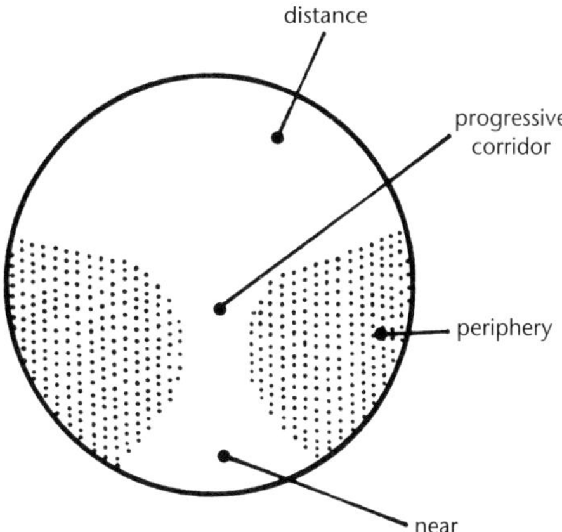


**Fig. L14** Typical positions of the various portions of a progressive addition lens (PAL). The periphery has unwanted astigmatism and distortion

**lens, rigid** *See* **lens, contact.**

**lens rim artifact** An apparent reduction in the extent of the visual field when perimetry is carried out with the patient's correction. The greatest reduction is usually found with the standard trial case lens. It is even more noticeable in the elderly, possibly because many of them have deep-set eyes that increases the distance from the lens to the eye. With the patient's own spectacles the artifact is less extensive. It is usually non-existent when wearing contact lenses.

**lens, safety 1.** A lens made of safety glass. **2.** A general term referring to any lens that protects the eyes against injury due to impact and which is more resistant to fracture and less likely to splinter than an ordinary glass lens. *Examples*: plastic lenses (especially polycarbonate); toughened lenses; laminated lenses. Plastic lenses have the greatest impact resistance of all these lenses.
*See* **glass, safety; lens, laminated; lens, plastic; lens, toughened.**

**lens, scleral contact** A contact lens which fits over both the cornea and the surrounding sclera. It is divided into an optical zone and a scleral (or haptic) zone. When made of PMMA material it includes small holes (called fenestrations) to aid tear exchange and corneal oxygenation. Modern scleral contact lenses are made of gas-permeable material and do not require fenestration. Scleral contact lenses are used mainly therapeutically for corneal protection, tear retention and pain relief in ocular surface disorders, vision improvement as in keratoconus and after penetrating keratoplasty or occasionally for theatrical and sports purposes.

**lens, sealed scleral contact** A scleral contact lens made up of gas permeable material. The optic portion of the lens has a curvature such that there is no contact between the lens and the cornea and that space (called corneal clearance) is filled with saline water forming a fluid pre-corneal reservoir. There is no tear exchange and corneal oxygenation is essentially provided through the lens matrix, as there is no fenestration. This lens is used in patients with corneal ectasia, such as keratoconus, keratoglobus and pellucid marginal degeneration, dry eyes of various aetiologies, etc.

**lens, semi-finished** An ophthalmic lens of which only one surface is completely polished. The other side can be surfaced to any required curvature. If it is a bifocal lens, the side with the segment is usually the one which is completely surfaced. *Syn.* semi-finished lens blank.
*See* **lens, blank; lens, finished.**

**lens, silicone hydrogel** A contact lens made of a combination of silicone rubber and hydrogel polymer to form a co-polymer that has the properties of both. Such a lens has a high oxygen permeability, adequate wettability, good optical properties and acceptable lens movement on the eye (unlike basic silicone rubber material, which tends to adhere to the cornea). This type of lens can be used for extended wear as contact lens-induced oedema is virtually eliminated. Transmissibility ($Dk/t$) of such lenses exceeds 100.

**lens, single-vision (SV)** An ophthalmic lens having only one power.

**lens, size** *See* **lens, aniseikonic.**

**lens, slab-off** A lens in which a portion of one surface has been ground with the same radius of curvature as the rest of the surface, but with separated centres of curvature. That portion of the lens produces a prismatic effect. Slab-off lenses are used most commonly to correct an induced vertical imbalance as, for example, in a patient with anisometropia looking through the lower part of the spectacle lenses when reading.

**lens, spectacle** Any lens used as a correction or protection and mounted a short distance from the eye, usually in a frame but also as a lorgnette, pince-nez, monocle, etc.
*See* **lens, ophthalmic; lorgnette; monocle; pince-nez.**

**lens speed** *See* **f number.**

**lens, spherical** A lens in which the two surfaces are spherical.

**lens, spherocylindrical** A lens with one surface spherical and the other cylindrical. It has two different refractive powers in its two principal meridians.
*See* **lens, astigmatic; lens, cylindrical; lens, toric.**

**lens, spin-cast contact** A contact lens produced by placing a quantity of liquid mixture into a concave spinning mould with polymerization taking place during rotation. The curvature of the mould determines the front optic zone radius, whereas the speed of rotation and other factors determine the curvature of the back optic zone.
*See* **lens, cast-moulding contact; lens, lathe-cut contact; moulding.**

**lens stalk** *See* **cup, optic.**

**lens, steep** A contact lens in which the back optic zone radius is shorter than the flattest meridian of the cornea. This definition may not be valid for a soft lens which may fit steeply even when its back optic zone radius is not shorter than the flattest meridian of the cornea. *Syn.* tight lens (it is preferable to use this term for soft lenses).
*See* **blanching, limbal; contact lens acute red eye; fitted on K; lens, flat.**

**lens, stigmatic** *See* **lens, anastigmatic.**

**lens, Stokes** A lens consisting of two planocylinders of equal and opposite power mounted with their flat surfaces almost in contact with each other in a cell, and geared to rotate equally in opposite directions from a zero setting. At that setting, the two cylinder axes coincide and produce the minimum astigmatic value. When the lenses are rotated so that the two cylinder axes are at right angles to each other the lens produces the maximum astigmatic value. Intermediate settings of the two cylinder axes result in intermediate astigmatic values. This lens is used in some ophthalmic instruments.

**lens suture** *See* **suture, lens.**

**lens, tear** *See* **lens, liquid.**

**lens, telescopic** A thick lens system forming a galilean telescope used to magnify the image. It is mounted in some form of frame and is lighter than an actual telescope. It is used to help low vision patients for either distance or near vision, although for the latter the lens system (or sometimes a single lens) is often referred to as a **microscopic lens**.
*See* **telescope, galilean; vision, low.**

**lens, therapeutic soft contact** A hydrophilic contact lens used as a protective device for the cornea, as in entropion, trichiasis, or damage by application of a tonometer; as a pressure bandage to relieve pain, as in bullous keratopathy; to facilitate corneal healing, as in corneal erosion due to trauma; to improve vision during the healing process; and as a delivery mechanism for drugs, since soft contact lenses placed on the eye can slowly release a drug which was previously absorbed. Because of the risks associated with this type of lens, it is important to follow the patient very assiduously. *Syn.* bandage lens. *See* **dystrophy, Cogan's microcystic epithelial; entropion; keratitis, Thygeson's superficial punctate; keratopathy, bullous; lens, combination; lens, piggyback; trichiasis.**

**lens, thick** *See* **lens, thin.**

**lens thickness caliper** *See* **caliper.**

**lens, thin** A lens or combination of lenses in which the refracting surfaces are regarded as coincident, that is in which the separation between surfaces does not appreciably alter the total power of the system. Most ophthalmic lenses are thin lenses, but the crystalline lens of the eye is considered to be a **thick lens**. For optical purposes contact lenses are also regarded as thick lenses.
*See* **plane, principal.**

**lens, Thorpe four mirror fundus** *See* **slit-lamp.**

**lens, tight** *See* **lens, steep.**

**lens, tinted** An absorptive lens having a noticeable colour and absorbing certain radiations more than others.
*See* **bleaching; glass; lens, absorptive; lens, cosmetic contact; photophobia; sunglasses; transmission curve.**

**lens, toric** This is usually a meniscus-type lens with a toroidal convex or concave surface. A toroidal surface is a surface with meridians of least and greatest curvature located at right angles to each other.
*See* **lens, astigmatic; lens, meniscus; lens, spherocylindrical.**

**lens, toughened** A lens made of glass which has been either thermally or chemically strengthened.
*See* **glass, safety; lens, safety.**

**lens, trial** **1.** A lens used in a trial case. **2.** A trial contact lens.
*See* **trial case.**

**lens, trifocal** A multifocal lens consisting of three portions of different focal power usually for distance, intermediate and near vision (Fig. L15).
*See* **lens, multifocal; portion, intermediate.**

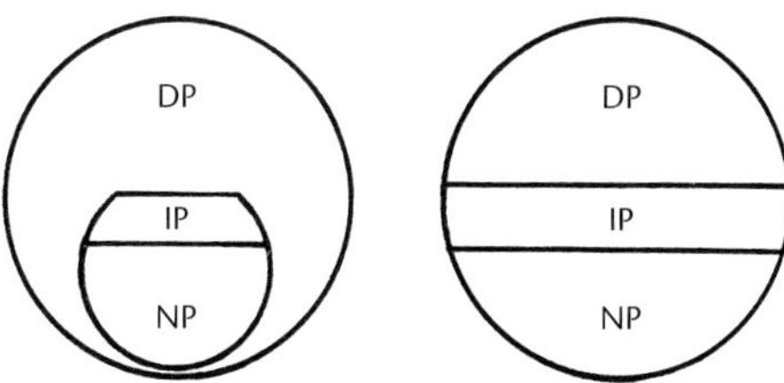


**Fig. L15** Examples of trifocal types (DP, distance portion; IP, intermediate portion; NP, near portion)

**lens, uncut** *See* **lens, finished.**

**lens, varifocal** *See* **lens, progressive.**

**lens, ventilated** *See* **lens, fenestrated.**

**lens, Volk** *See* **slit-lamp.**

**lens, wide-angle** A lens giving good resolution over a wide field of view, usually used in better quality cameras.
*See* **lens, fisheye.**

**lens, Wilson three mirror fundus** *See* **slit-lamp.**

**lens, Wollaston** Lens based on the values provided by Wollaston of the Tscherning ellipse.
*See* **ellipse, Tscherning.**

**lens, X-Chrom** Tradename for a dyed hard corneal contact lens aimed at enhancing colour perception in red-green deficient people. It is usually fitted on the non-dominant eye. The lens has maximum transmission above 575 nm with some additional transmission below 480 nm. Wearing this lens shifts the original absorption spectrum of the eye with the contact lens towards longer wavelengths. Objects may thus appear slightly different than with the other eye. This difference between the two eyes may, in certain conditions, improve colour discrimination.
*See* **colour vision, defective; lens, ChromGen.**

**lens, Zeiss** A type of goniolens, which when placed over the eye allows viewing of the anterior chamber angle. The Zeiss lens differs from other goniolenses in so much that it contains four mirrors, allowing visualization of the entire anterior chamber angle without the need to rotate the lens.
*See* **gonioscopy, indentation; lens, gonioscopic.**

**lens, zoom** A lens in which the components can be adjusted to provide continuously variable magnification while the image remains constantly in focus.

**Lenscorometer** *See* **distometer.**

**Lensometer** *See* **focimeter.**

**lenticele** *See* **phacocele.**

**lenticonus** A conical projection of either the anterior or posterior surface of the crystalline lens of the eye, occurring as a rare congenital anomaly. The anterior lenticonus is the most common and most often associated with Alport's syndrome. If the bulging is spherical, instead of conical, the condition is referred to as **lentiglobus**. It produces a decrease in visual acuity and irregular refraction which cannot be corrected by either spectacle or contact lenses.
*See* **keratoconus; syndrome, Alport's.**

**lenticular astigmatism** *See* **astigmatism, lenticular.**

**lenticular fossa** *See* **fossa, hyaloid.**

**lenticular lens** *See* **lens, lenticular.**

**lenticular progressive degeneration** *See* **disease, Wilson's.**

**lenticular stereoscope** *See* **stereoscope, Brewster's.**

**lenticule** A disc-shaped piece of corneal tissue or a piece of synthetic material manufactured to produce a given curvature and thickness. It is implanted into or on top of the cornea to change its anterior curvature.
*See* **epikeratoplasty; keratophakia.**

**lentiglobus** *See* **lenticonus.**

**letter acuity** *See* **acuity, visual.**

**leucocorea** *See* **leukocoria.**

**leucokeratosis** *See* **dyskeratosis.**

**leucoma** *See* **leukoma.**

**leucoplakia** *See* **dyskeratosis.**

**leukocoria** A condition characterized by a whitish reflex within the pupil. It is secondary to cataract, Coats' disease, retinoblastoma, retrolental fibroplasia, persistent hyperplastic primary vitreous, etc. *Syn.* white pupil; white pupillary reflex. *Note*: also spelt leucocorea, leukocorea or leukokoria.

**leukoma** Dense, white, corneal opacity caused by scar tissue. A localized leukoma appears as a whitish scar surrounded by normal cornea. A generalized leukoma involves the entire cornea which appears white, often with blood vessels coursing over its surface. Visual impairment depends on the location and extent of the leukoma. If the opacity is faint, it is called a **nebula.** *Note*: also spelt leucoma.
*See* **cornea; hyperacuity; ulcer, corneal.**

**levator aponeurosis; palpebrae superioris** *See* **muscle, levator palpebrae superioris.**

**levo** Terms with this prefix can be found at laevo-.

**levobunolol hydrochloride** *See* **beta-blocker.**

**levocabastine** *See* **antihistamine.**

**library spectacles** *See* **spectacles, library.**

**lid** *See* **eyelids.**

**lid eversion** *See* **eversion, lid.**

**lid lag** *See* **disease, Graves'.**

**lid retractors** Term used to refer to the muscles that open the eyelids. In the upper eyelid it is the levator palpebrae muscle and its two divisions; the striated levator aponeurosis and the smooth Müller's muscle (or superior tarsal muscle). In the lower eyelid it is the smooth fibre bundle derived from the inferior rectus muscle which forms the inferior tarsal muscle.
*See* **muscle, levator palpebrae superioris; muscles, Müller's palpebral.**

**lidocaine hydrochloride (lignocaine hydrochloride)** A local anaesthetic of the amide type used in eye surgery. It is used in 1–4% solution. Its action starts in less than 1 minute and lasts about 1 hour.
*See* **anaesthetics; bupivacaine; procaine.**

**ligament, check** A strong band of connective tissue which leaves the surface of the sheath of the extraocular muscles and attaches to the surrounding tissues, so as to limit the action of the muscle. The medial rectus is attached to the lacrimal bone (**medial check ligament**) and the lateral rectus to the zygomatic bone (**lateral check ligament**). There are also check ligaments restricting the vertical movements but the expansions of these muscles are thinner and less distinct than those of the horizontal recti muscles.
*See* **muscle, lateral rectus; muscle, medial rectus.**

**ligament, hyaloideocapsular** *See* **ligament of Wieger.**

**ligament of Lockwood** The lower part of the capsule of Tenon and parts of the tendons of the inferior rectus and oblique muscles which are thickened to form a hammock-like structure on which the eyeball rests.
*See* **muscles, extraocular; Tenon's capsule.**

**ligament, palpebral** Strong connective tissue attaching the extremities of the tarsal plates of the upper and lower eyelids to the orbital margin. There are two sets: (1) the **lateral palpebral ligament** (or **lateral canthal tendon**) about 7 mm long and 2.5 mm wide which constitutes the deeper portion of the lateral palpebral raphe of the orbicularis muscle and attaches the tarsal plates to the lateral orbital tubercle (or **Whitnall's** tubercle) on the zygomatic bone and (2) the **medial palpebral ligament** (or **medial canthal tendon**) which attaches the medial ends of the tarsal plates to the frontal process of the maxilla and another insertion into the posterior lacrimal crest. It lies anterior to the canaliculi and the lacrimal sac.
*See* **eyelids; tarsus.**

**ligament, suspensory** A ligament whose principal function is to support another structure, e.g. ligament of Lockwood, the zonule of Zinn.
*See* **Zinn, zonule of.**

**ligament of Wieger** An attachment of the anterior surface of the vitreous humour to the posterior lens capsule in the shape of a ring about 8–9 mm in diameter. It forms a line called

**Egger's line**. This adherence is strong in youth but weakens with age enabling intracapsular cataract extraction without pulling the vitreous. *Syn.* hyaloideocapsular ligament.
*See* **cataract extraction, intracapsular.**

**light** Electromagnetic vibration capable of stimulating the receptors of the retina and of producing a visual sensation. The radiations that give rise to the sensation of vision are comprised within the wavelength band 380–780 nm. This band is called the **visible spectrum** or **visible light**. The borders of this band are not precise but beyond these radiations the visual efficacy of any wavelength becomes very low indeed (less than $10^{-5}$). For an older subject, the lower boundary of the visible spectrum is closer to 420 nm than 380 nm.
*See* **blue; green; infrared; lens, absorptive; orange; red; spectroscope; spectrum, electromagnetic; theory, quantum; theory, wave; ultraviolet; violet; wavelength; yellow.**

**light, achromatic** *See* **achromatic light stimulus.**

**light adaptation** *See* **adaptation, light.**

**light, artificial** Any light other than natural light.

**light, beam of** A collection of pencils arising from an extended source or object. *Syn.* bundle of light.
*See* **light, pencil of; object, extended; source, extended.**

**light, bundle of** *See* **light, beam of.**

**light chaos** *See* **light, idioretinal.**

**light, compound** Light composed of more than one wavelength.

**light, diffuse** Light coming from an extended source and having no predominant directional component. Illumination is thus relatively uniform with a minimum of shadows.
*See* **diffusion; source, extended.**

**light, fluorescent** Light emitted by fluorescence as in a fluorescent lamp.
*See* **lamp, fluorescent.**

**light, frequency of** *See* **hertz; spectrum, electromagnetic; wavelength.**

**light, idioretinal** A visual sensation occurring in total darkness which is attributed to spontaneous nervous impulses in the neurons of the visual pathway. *Syn.* intrinsic light; light chaos.

**light, incandescent** Light emitted by incandescence as in an incandescent lamp.
*See* **lamp, incandescent electric.**

**light, infrared** *See* **infrared.**

**light, intrinsic** *See* **light, idioretinal.**

**light, monochromatic** Light consisting of a single wavelength or, more usually, of a narrow band of wavelengths (a few nanometres).
*See* **wavelength.**

**light, natural** Light received from the sun and the sky.

**light, pencil of** A narrow cone of light rays coming from a point source or from any one point on a broad source after passing through a limiting aperture. A pencil of light may be either convergent, divergent or parallel. The ray passing through the centre of the aperture is the chief ray. *Syn.* homocentric bundle of rays; homocentric pencil of rays.
*See* **light, beam of; ray, chief; object, point; source, point.**

**light, polarized** Ordinary light is composed of transverse wave motions uniform in all directions in a plane perpendicular to its direction of propagation. Polarized light is composed of transverse wave motions in only one direction, called the **plane of vibration**. Polarized light can be obtained by using a polarizer (e.g. tourmaline crystals, polarizing material such as Polaroid, Nicol prism, etc.).
*See* **analyser; angle of polarization; crystal, dichroic; lens, polarizing; polarizer; prism, Nicol; prism, Wollaston; vectogram.**

**light, quantity of** Product of luminous flux and its duration. *Unit*: lumen-second.
*See* **lumen.**

**light reflex** *See* **reflex, corneal; reflex, pupil light.**

**light, solar** Light from the sun or having identical properties as the sun.
*See* **blindness, eclipse; light, white.**

**light source** Any source of visible radiant energy such as a candle flame, a lamp, the sky or the sun.
*See* **coherent sources; illuminants, CIE standard; lamp, fluorescent; lamp, incandescent electric; light, natural; light, solar; source, extended.**

**light, speed of** The currently accepted figure is 299 792.5 km/s (in a vacuum). This velocity decreases, differentially with wavelength, when the radiation enters a medium.
*See* **index of refraction; spectrum, electromagnetic; wavelength.**

**light stop** *See* **diaphragm.**

**light, stray** Light reflected or passing through an optical system but not involved in the formation of the image such as that reflected by the surfaces of a correcting lens. *Syn.* parasitic light.
*See* **image, ghost.**

**light-stress test** *See* **test, photostress.**

**light threshold** *See* **threshold, light absolute.**

**light, ultraviolet** *See* **ultraviolet; light, Wood's.**

**light, visible** *See* **light.**

**light, white** Light perceived without any attribute of hue. Any light produced by a source having an equal energy spectrum will appear white after the eye is adapted. Some of the CIE illuminants are often used as a source of white light, e.g. B, C and D. Sunlight is a source of white light. *See* **chromaticity diagram; illuminants, CIE standard; spectrum, equal energy.**

**light, Wood's** Ultraviolet light near the visible spectrum which, when used with certain dyes such as fluorescein, causes fluorescence. It is produced by a special type of glass (called **Wood's glass** or **Wood's filter**) which contains nickel oxide and transmits ultraviolet radiations near the visible spectrum. It is used to detect corneal abrasions and to evaluate the fit of hard contact lenses. It is available in a slit-lamp or in a Burton lamp.
*See* **fluorescein; fluorescence; lamp, Burton.**

**lightness** Attribute of visual sensation in accordance with which a body seems to transmit or reflect diffusely a greater or smaller fraction of the incident light. This attribute is the psychosensorial correlate, or nearly so, of the photometric quantity luminance factor (CIE).
*See* **luminance.**

**lignocaine hydrochloride** *See* **lidocaine.**

**limbus, corneal** The transition zone, about 1.5 mm wide, between the conjunctiva and sclera on the one hand, and the cornea on the other. *Syn.* corneoscleral junction.
*See* **blanching, limbal; cornea.**

**limen** *See* **threshold.**

**liminal** Pertaining to a threshold.

**limit of resolution** *See* **resolution, limit of.**

**line, base** The line joining the centres of rotation of the two eyes. It is approximately equal to the interpupillary distance (Fig. L16).
*See* **distance, interocular; distance, interpupillary.**

**line, demand** The line in Donders' diagram which represents the perfect amount of convergence required for each level of accommodation, for single binocular vision. *Syn.* orthophoria line; Donders' line.
*See* **Donders' diagram.**

**line of direction** Line joining an object in space with its image on the retina (allowing for the optical properties of the eye). The line joining the fixation point to the fovea is called the **principal line of direction**. However, the object appears to lie along a **visual direction** and that direction in visual space associated with the fovea is called the **principal visual direction**. All other visual directions associated with other retinal points are called **secondary visual directions**. The principal line of direction and the principal visual direction coincide, but the former indicates the direction towards the eye, while the latter indicates the direction away from the eye.
*See* **law of identical visual directions.**

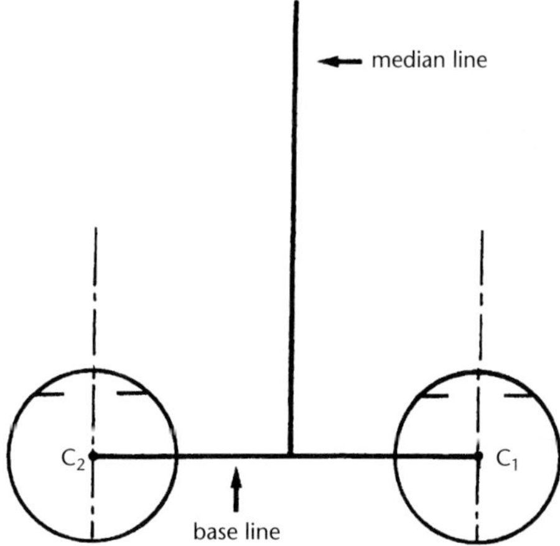


**Fig. L16** Base line $C_1$ $C_2$ and median line. The base line is situated about 13.5 mm behind the vertex of the cornea in the straight ahead position

**line, Donders'** *See* **line, demand.**

**line, Egger's** *See* **ligament of Wieger.**

**line of fixation** *See* **axis, fixation.**

**line, focal** Any astigmatic optical system produces two mutually, usually perpendicular, focal lines of a point object. The focal lines are situated at different image distances. Each focal line lies parallel to its associated cylinder axis. *Syn.* image line; line focus; Sturm's line.
*See* **astigmatism; circle of least confusion; distance, image; focus; Sturm, conoid of; Sturm, interval of.**

**line focus** *See* **line, focal.**

**line of Gennari** *See* **area, visual.**

**line, Hudson–Stähli** A yellowish-brown, more or less horizontal line containing iron which runs across the cornea below the centre. It occurs in normal corneas, more frequently in the elderly, or in association with corneal opacities.

**line, iron** Deposits of iron within the corneal epithelium appearing as a brown rust line. They often subside with time leaving a nebulous scar. Several eponymous types have been described depending on the cause and location.
*See* **line, Hudson–Stähli; line, Stocker's; ring, Coat's white; ring, Fleischer's; siderosis bulbi.**

**line, median** Line formed by the intersection of the median plane and the plane of regard (Fig. L16). *Syn.* midline.
*See* **plane, median; plane of regard.**

**line, orthophoria** *See* **line, demand.**

**line, phoria** On Donders' diagram, it is the line joining all the points representing the passive position of the eyes corresponding to various levels of accommodation.
*See* **Donders' diagram; position, passive.**

**line, retinal** Operationally, the collection of retinal elements that are activated in response to a line stimulus.

**line, Sampaolesi's** A pigmented, wavy line anterior to Schwalbe's ring and found mainly in the periphery of the inferior cornea. It may be noted in pigmentary dispersion syndrome.
*See* **ring of Schwalbe, anterior limiting; syndrome, pigmentary dispersion.**

**line of Schwalbe** *See* **ring of Schwalbe, anterior limiting.**

**line of sight** Line joining the point of fixation to the centre of the entrance pupil. This line is more practical than the visual axis. *Syn.* principal line of vision.
*See* **axis, visual.**

**line spectrum** *See* **spectrum, line.**

**line-spread function** *See* **function, line-spread.**

**line, Stocker's** An abnormal line containing iron located in the corneal epithelium which may appear in front of the advancing edge of a pterygium.
*See* **line, iron; pterygium.**

**line, Sturm's** *See* **line, focal.**

**line of vision, principal** *See* **line of sight.**

**linear magnification** *See* **magnification, lateral.**

**linear perspective** *See* **perspective, linear.**

**lines, Fraunhofer's** Fine dark lines distributed throughout the length of the solar spectrum due to the absorption of specific wavelengths by elements in the atmosphere of the sun and the earth. Fraunhofer observed about 600 of these lines and denoted the most prominent ones by letters from A in the extreme red to K in the violet. *Examples*: A corresponds to 759.4 nm, C to 656.3 nm, D to 589.3 nm, F to 486.1 nm, etc.
*See* **constringence; index of refraction; spectrum, solar.**

**Table L3** Common spectral lines of the visible spectrum

| designation | origin | wavelength (nm) |
|---|---|---|
| A | oxygen | 759.4 |
| C | hydrogen | 656.3 |
| C′ | cadmium | 643.8 |
| D | sodium | 589.3 |
| d | helium | 587.6 |
| e | mercury | 546.1 |
| F | hydrogen | 486.1 |
| F′ | cadmium | 480.0 |
| G | calcium | 430.8 |
| h | hydrogen | 410.2 |

**lipid droplet degeneration** *See* **keratopathy, actinic.**

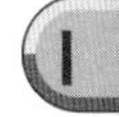

**liquid lens** *See* **lens, liquid.**

**Lisch nodule** A small, abnormal, lightly pigmented swelling which develops on the surface of the iris in almost all patients with neurofibromatosis type 1 during the second or third decades of life.
*See* **disease, von Recklinghausen's.**

**lissamine green** A vital stain with dyeing quality similar to that of rose bengal, but which causes less discomfort. It stains dead or degenerated epithelial cells green and is used to facilitate the diagnosis of keratitis sicca, xerophthalmia, etc. It has a molecular weight of 577.
*See* **keratitis sicca; rose bengal; xerophthalmia.**

**Listing's law; plane** *See* under the nouns.

**Listing's reduced eye** *See* **eye, reduced.**

**lithiasis, conjunctival** *See* **concretions, conjunctival.**

**lobe, occipital** Portion of each cerebral hemisphere posterior to the parietal lobe where visual information is received and processing begins.
*See* **area, visual.**

**local sign** *See* **direction, oculocentric.**

**localization** Perception of the location of an object in space with respect to either the eye (**oculocentric localization**) or the self (**egocentric localization**).
*See* **egocentre; oculocentre; pointing, past-.**

**lock, binocular; fusion** *See* **heterophoria, associated.**

**Lockwood's ligament** *See* **ligament of Lockwood.**

**lodoxamide tromethamine** *See* **mast cell stabilizers.**

**log MAR chart** *See* **chart, log MAR.**

**lomefloxacin** *See* **antibiotic.**

**long ciliary nerve** *See* **nerve, long ciliary.**

**long sight** *See* **hypermetropia.**

**loop, Archambault's** *See* **loop, Meyer's.**

**loop, Axenfeld's intrascleral nerve** An anomalous loop of the long ciliary nerve, often accompanied by the anterior ciliary artery, which has pierced the sclera a few millimetres behind the limbus and then re-enters the sclera and supplies the ciliary body. It is usually pigmented giving rise to a 1–2 mm black dot on the sclera. It appears only in a small percentage of individuals (10–15%). Treatment is not necessary. *Syn.* Axenfeld's pigmented nerve loop.

**loop, Meyer's** A bundle of inferior nerve fibres that originate from the lateral portion of the lateral geniculate body, extend forward around the anterior tip of the temporal horn of the lateral ventricle and then swing backward toward the occipital lobe. A lesion in this loop may cause a superior homonymous quadrantanopsia. *Syn.* Archambault's loop.
*See* **radiations, optic.**

**loratidine** *See* **antihistamine.**

**lorgnette** Eyeglasses for occasional use, held before the eyes by a handle, into which the lenses may fold when not in use (British Standard).
*See* **lens, spectacle; spectacles.**

**lorgnon** A spectacle lens for occasional use, mounted on a handle (British Standard).

**loteprednol etabonate** *See* **antiinflammatory drug.**

**Lotmar Visometer** *See* **maxwellian view system, clinical.**

**Lotze's local sign** *See* **direction, oculocentric.**

**loupe** *See* **magnifier.**

**loupe magnification** *See* **magnification, apparent.**

**loupe, Berger's** A binocular loupe fitted with a headband.

**low tension glaucoma** *See* **glaucoma, low tension.**

**low vision** *See* **vision, low.**

**lumen** SI unit of luminous flux. It is equal to the flux emitted within a unit solid angle of one steradian by a point source with a luminous intensity of one candela. *Symbol*: lm.
*See* **flux, luminous; light, quantity of; lux; SI unit.**

**luminance** Photometric term characterizing the way in which a surface emits or reflects light in a given direction. It is equal to the luminous intensity measured in a given direction divided by the area of this surface projected on a perpendicular to the direction considered. *Symbol*: L. *Units*: candela per square metre (SI unit); footlambert; lambert, etc.
*See* **brightness; candela per square metre; footlambert; lambert; lightness; millilambert; nit; photometry; SI unit.**

**Table L4** Approximate luminance (in cd/m$^2$) of some objects

| | |
|---|---|
| sun | $10^9$ |
| car headlight | $10^7$ |
| incandescent lamp (tungsten) | $10^6$–$10^7$ |
| fluorescent lamp | $10^4$–$10^5$ |
| clear sky at noon | $10^4$ |
| cloudy sky at noon | $10^3$ |
| shady street by day | $10^3$–$10^4$ |
| full moon | $10^3$ |
| book print under artificial light | $>10^2$ |
| photopic vision | $>10$ |
| street illumination | $1$–$10^{-1}$ |
| mesopic vision | $10$–$10^{-3}$ |
| cloudless night sky with full moon | $10^{-2}$ |
| scotopic vision | $<10^{-3}$ |
| moonless and cloudless night sky | $10^{-3}$–$10^{-6}$ |

**luminescence** Emission of light by certain substances resulting from the absorption of energy (e.g. from electrical fields, chemical reaction, or other light) which is not due to a rise in temperature (unlike incandescence). The emitted radiation is characteristic of the particular substance. When the light emitted is due to exposure to a source of light the process is usually called **photoluminescence**. When the light emitted is due to either a high-frequency discharge through a gas, or to an electric field through certain solids such as **phosphor** which is used in fluorescent lamps, television picture tubes, etc., it is called **electroluminescence.**
*See* **bioluminescence; fluorescence; incandescence; lamp, fluorescent; phosphorescence.**

**luminosity** *See* **brightness.**

**luminous efficiency, spectral** *See* **efficiency.**

**luminous flux** *See* **flux, luminous.**

**luminous intensity** *See* **intensity, luminous.**

**lumirhodopsin** *See* **rhodopsin.**

**Luneburg's theory** *See* **theory, Luneburg's.**

**lustre 1.** The effect of one colour appearing to be situated behind and through another. This can occur when looking in a haploscope when it is called **binocular lustre**. **2.** Appearance of glossiness on a metallic surface.

**lux** SI unit of illuminance. It is the illuminance produced by a luminous flux of one lumen uniformly distributed over a surface area of one square metre. *Symbol*: lx.
*See* **footcandle; illuminance; lumen; SI unit.**

**luxation of the lens** Pathological and complete dislocation of the lens relative to the pupil. If the luxation is incomplete it is called **subluxation** of the lens (or **dislocation** or **ectopia lentis**). Subluxation is one of the causes of monocular diplopia. If the luxation is complete the eye becomes markedly hyperopic and is unable to accommodate. Luxation occurs in contusion of the globe, in many ocular (e.g. buphthalmos) and other diseases (e.g. syphilis) or it can be inherited (e.g. the bilateral, symmetrical, superior subluxation commonly found in Marfan's syndrome). It is sometimes associated with ectopic pupils and keratoconus. Unless there are complications (e.g. secondary glaucoma) or monocular diplopia the lens is left in place and management is optical. (Fig. L17)
*See* **astigmatism; corectopia; diplopia, monocular; glaucoma, congenital; iridodonesis; pupillary block; syndrome, Ehlers–Danlos; syndrome, Marfan's.**

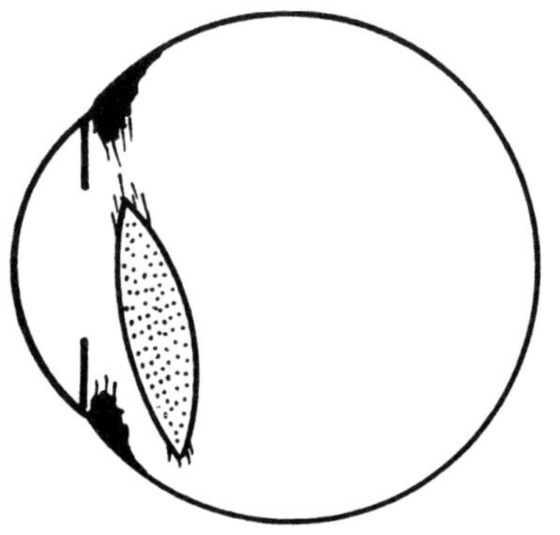

Fig. L17 Dislocation of the lens (usually in the vitreous humour)

**luxometer** *See* **photometer.**

**lymphadenopathy** An enlargement of a lymph gland. The preauricular lymph node located 1 cm in front of the external ear drains the orbital region and is sometimes involved with eyelid and conjunctival infection (e.g. adult inclusion conjunctivitis, follicular conjunctivitis). *Syn.* adenopathy (although strictly speaking this term refers to the enlargement of any gland).
*See* **conjunctivitis, adult inclusion; conjunctivitis, follicular.**

**lymphoma, B cell** A malignant tumour found predominantly within the orbit and conjunctiva. Orbital lymphomas are the most common form of ocular lymphomas and cause proptosis and diplopia. They affect mainly adults and are primarily of the B cell/non-Hodgkins type. Conjunctival lymphomas, also mainly of the B cell/non-Hodgkins type, are seen in approximately 10% of systemic lymphoma patients. Clinically, conjunctival lymphomas appear salmon-pink in colour and have flat and smooth surfaces. There are several types of B cell lymphoma, one of them being **Burkitt's lymphoma**. Treatment is by radiotherapy.

**lysozyme** An antibacterial enzyme present in the tears (as well as other tissues). In human tears, lysozyme makes up 21–25% of the total protein.
*See* **film, precorneal; gland, lacrimal; tears.**

# M

**M cell** *See* **cell, ganglion.**

**M Units** *See* **acuity, near visual.**

**Mach bands** When a light area is separated from a dark area by a transition zone in which the brightness increases or decreases regularly and rapidly, two bands are seen: one light band next to the dark area and another dark band next to the light area. The appearance of these two bands, known as Mach bands, is attributed to lateral inhibition processes occurring in the retina. The phenomenon is usually demonstrated with a rotating disc with black and white areas separated by a zone of brightness gradient. *Syn.* Mach rings.
*See* **inhibition, lateral.**

**Mackay–Marg tonometer** *See* **tonometer, Mackay–Marg.**

**macrocornea** *See* **keratoglobus.**

m

**macropsia** Anomaly of visual perception in which objects appear larger than they actually are. It may occur as a result of abnormal accommodation (less than required for the fixation distance) or because of various retinal anomalies in which the visual receptors are crowded together, or because of the recent wear of either base-in prisms or a presbyopic correction, etc. *Syn.* megalopsia.
*See* **dysmegalopsia; micropsia; metamorphopsia.**

**macula** *See* **fovea centralis; macula lutea**.

**macula, ectopia of the** Anomaly characterized by displacement of the macula, which can be either of acquired or congenital origin. It may follow some forms of retinal scarring, retinal detachment surgery, previous inflammation, etc. It may result in reduced acuity, metamorphopsia or strabismus. *Syn.* dystopia of the macula; heterotopia macula.

**macula, false** The retinal area of the deviating eye of a strabismic subject which corresponds to the fovea of the fixating eye.
*See* **retinal correspondence, abnormal.**

**macula lutea** An oval area of the retina 3–5 mm in diameter, with the foveal depression at its centre, slightly below the level of the optic disc and temporal to it (its centre lies 3.5 mm from the edge of the disc). The side wall of the depression slopes gradually towards the centre where the fovea centralis is located and where the best photopic visual acuity is obtained. Around the fovea, the ganglion cells are much more numerous than elsewhere, being arranged in five to seven layers. The outer molecular layer is also thicker than elsewhere and forms the outer fibre layer of Henle and there is a progressive disappearance of rods so that at the foveola only cones are found. The area of the macula lutea is impregnated by a yellow pigment (macular pigment) in the inner layers and for that reason is often called the **yellow spot**. *Syn.* area centralis (although that area is considered to be slightly larger, about 5.5 mm in diameter); punctum luteum.
*See* **acuity, central visual; entoptoscope, blue field; fovea centralis; layer of Henle, fibre; maculopathy, age-related; pigment, macular.**

**macula, sparing of the** Retention of macular function in spite of losses in the adjacent visual field as, for example, in homonymous hemianopsia due to a cortical lesion. This is due to the wide distribution of macular fibres.
*See* **hemianopsia, homonymous.**

**macular cyst** A swelling in the macular area in which oedema fluid has accumulated. It may eventually burst into the vitreous producing a macular hole. It usually results from an injury to the eye.
*See* **macular hole.**

**macular degeneration, senile** *See* **maculopathy, age-related.**

**macular dystrophy** *See* **dystrophy, macular.**

**macular epiretinal membrane** *See* **fibrosis, preretinal macular.**

**macular hole** A condition in which there is a partial or full thickness absence of the retina in the macular area. It may occur as a result of trauma, degeneration, old age, preretinal macular fibrosis or pathological myopia. It appears ophthalmoscopically as a round or oval, well defined, reddish spot at the macula. There is metamorphopsia, loss of visual acuity and a central scotoma. An operculum of retinal tissue may overlie the hole. The vitreous in front of the hole eventually condenses and separates from the retina. In partial macular hole a layer of photoreceptors may still be attached to the retinal pigment epithelium (**lamellar hole**), as in cystoid macular oedema. Treatment usually consists

of reattaching the retina, if detached, and possibly vitrectomy.
*See* **fibrosis, pretinal macular; metamorphopsia; oedema, cystoid macular; retinal tear; retinopathy, solar.**

**macular oedema** *See* **oedema, cystoid macular.**

**macular pigment** *See* **pigment, macular.**

**macular pucker** *See* **fibrosis, preretinal macular.**

**macular star** Deposits of lipid material in Henle's fibre layer radiating out in a star-like pattern. It may follow retinal oedema (e.g. in the late stage of hypertensive retinopathy).
*See* **layer of Henle, fibre.**

**maculopathy, age-related (ARM)** Condition found in a large percentage of elderly patients (and sometimes middle-aged ones), in which there is a degeneration of the photoreceptors of the macular area of the retina. This degeneration is characterized by the presence of fine pigment stippling with the later appearance of gross pigment clumps and white-yellowish spots (drusen) in the macular region while the surrounding retinal area remains usually relatively healthy. This condition is due to either an atrophy of the retinal pigment epithelium (RPE) and photoreceptors or a collapse of the RPE. Visual acuity becomes markedly reduced and the condition usually becomes bilateral developing over several years. Management of this condition is essentially by the use of low vision aids. *Syn.* non-neovascular or non-exudative 'dry' age-related maculopathy. There exists another less common form which is known as **disciform or neovascular** or **exudative 'wet' age-related maculopathy** in which the clinical picture is the same initially but is followed by the formation of new blood vessels (**choroidal neovascularization** (CNV)) and fibrous tissue in the macular region resulting in total loss of central vision. If detected early (usually with an Amsler chart), treatment with laser photocoagulation will reduce the risk of further visual loss. **Photodynamic therapy** (PDT) is another method of reducing the risk of visual loss. It allows selective destruction of the choroidal neovascularization with minimal damage to the overlying retinal tissue. It consists of injecting a photosensitizing agent (e.g. verteprofin) that is taken up by the abnormal vessels and when activated by a laser light of a given wavelength (e.g. 689 nm) it damages and shrivels up the vessels. *Syn.* senile macular degeneration (SMD); age-related macular degeneration (ARMD or AMD).
*See* **angiography, fluorescein; chart, Amsler; drusen; macula lutea; photocoagulation; rule, Kollner's; test, photostress; retinal pigment epithelium; vision, low.**

**maculopathy, bull's eye** An ocular condition in which degeneration of the retinal pigment epithelium in the macular area causes alternating ring-like light and dark zones of pigmentation, as in a target. It may result from drug toxicity or hereditary conditions (e.g. cone dystrophy, Laurence–Moon–Bardet–Biedl syndrome). The main symptoms are a loss of visual acuity, reduced colour vision and aversion to bright sunlight.

**madarosis** Loss of, either or both, the eyebrows and the eyelashes.

**Maddox cross** A scale for measuring the angle of heterophoria and heterotropia consisting of one horizontal and one vertical line in the form of a cross with a light source placed at the centre of intersection. The lines are graduated in prism dioptres or degrees and calibrated for use at a given distance (usually 6 metres). *Syn.* Maddox tangent scale.
*See* **dioptre, prism; Maddox rod.**

**Maddox double prism** *See* **test, double prism.**

**Maddox rod** This is not a rod but a series of cylindrical grooves ground usually into a coloured piece of glass and mounted in a rim. (Originally it consisted of a single cylindrical rod.) It is used to measure heterophoria by placing it in front of one eye of a subject viewing a spot of light binocularly. The Maddox rod and eye together form a long streak of light perpendicular to the axis of the grooves and this retinal image is so unlike the image formed in the other eye that the fusion reflex is not stimulated. The eyes will then stay in the passive position. If there is a phoria the streak of light will not intersect the spot of light. For horizontal phorias the rod axis is placed horizontally and for vertical phorias, vertically. The amount and type of the phoria can be quantified by placing a prism of appropriate power and direction in front of either eye such that the streak appears superimposed on the spot of light. Alternatively, the angle of the phoria could be determined using a Maddox cross and placing a rod in front of one eye; the phoria can be read directly by the patient who indicates where the streak of light appears to cross the scale. The Maddox rod is also used to detect or measure cyclophoria. (Fig. M1)
*See* **cyclophoria; heterophoria; Maddox cross; position, passive; test, Maddox rod; test, Thorington.**

**Maddox rod test** *See* **test, Maddox rod.**

**Maddox wing** Hand-held device used to measure heterophoria at near. It consists of a septum and two slit apertures, one for each eye. One eye sees a double tangent scale (vertical and horizontal) calibrated to read in prism dioptres, while the other eye sees a white arrow pointing

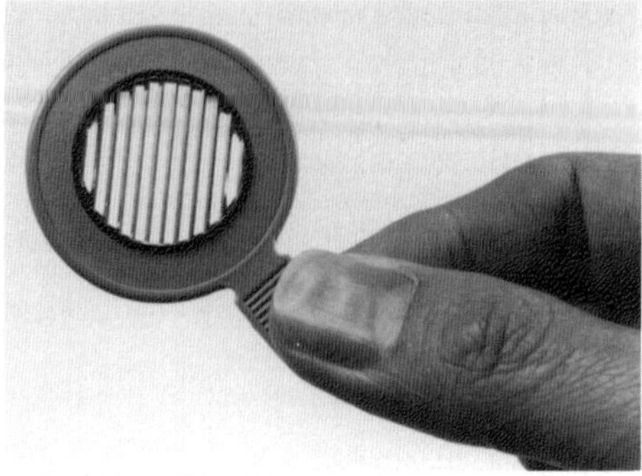

**Fig. M1** Maddox rod

upward and a red arrow pointing horizontally to the left. As the two retinal images are quite different there is no attempt at fusion and the eyes stay in the passive position. The arrows seen by the left eye point to the numbers seen by the right eye. The numbers represent the vertical and horizontal components of the phoria, which can be read directly by the observer. (Fig. M2)
*See* **heterophoria; position, passive.**

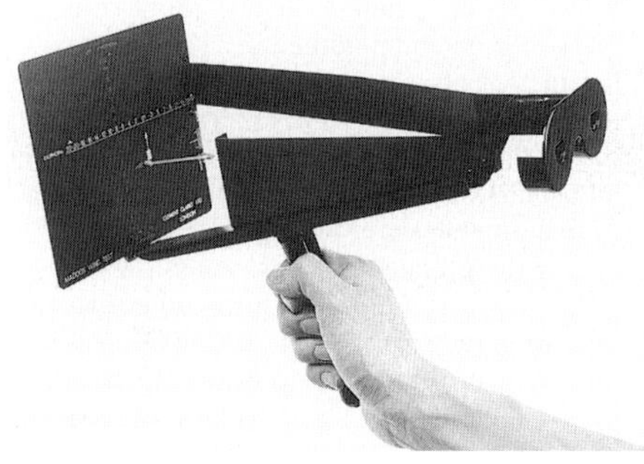

**Fig. M2** Maddox wing

**magenta 1.** Hue produced by the additive mixture of red and blue. **2.** Hue evoked by any combination of wavelengths which act as the complement of a wavelength of 515 nm.
*See* **colour, complementary.**

**magnetic resonance imaging (MRI)** Method of imaging part of the body to facilitate diagnosis and therapy. Unlike other radiological methods, this technique does not expose the patient to ionizing radiations. It depends instead on atoms within the body (e.g. hydrogen atoms) which when exposed to a strong magnetic field produce energy which is detected and analysed to determine the characteristics of that structure. This technique provides better image contrast than computerized tomography in many instances (e.g. the patches of demyelination in the grey matter of patients with multiple sclerosis), while the reverse is true in other instances (e.g. a meningioma in the posterior visual pathway). This procedure takes longer than computerized tomography. **Functional MRI** can map and measure behaviour by detecting and analysing oxygen atoms in the brain, since oxygen consumption varies with behaviour (e.g. colour perception). *Syn.* nuclear magnetic resonance (NMR).
*See* **radiology; tomography, computerized.**

**magnification** An increase in the apparent size of an object.

**magnification, angular** Magnification expressed as the ratio of the angle $\alpha'$ subtended at the eye by the image to the angle $\alpha$ subtended at the eye by the object.

$$M = \frac{\tan\alpha'}{\tan\alpha}$$

**magnification, apparent** Magnification produced by a viewing instrument or lens expressed as the ratio of the angle $w'$ subtended at the nodal point of the eye by the image, to the angle $w$ subtended at the nodal point by the object, when at the least distance of distinct vision from the unaided eye. It is conventional to take this distance as 250 mm and to place the object in the anterior focal plane of the magnifying device. The magnification $M$ is, then, equal to

$$M = \frac{\tan w'}{\tan w} = \frac{250}{f'} = \frac{F}{4}$$

where $f'$ and $F$ are the second focal length (in mm) and power (in dioptres) of the magnifying device, respectively (Fig. M3). In this object location the magnification (and therefore the retinal image size) is constant and independent of the distance between the magnifier and the eye, but the field of view decreases as the distance between the eye and the magnifier increases. *Syn.* conventional magnification; effective magnification; loupe magnification; nominal magnification; standard magnification.
If the object is closer to the magnifying device than its anterior focal plane so that its image is formed at the least distance of distinct vision, and assuming that the eye is so close to the magnifier as to ignore the distance separating them, the magnification $M$ is, then, equal to

$$M = 1 + \frac{F}{4}$$

*Example:* a lens of + 16.00 D provides, in these conditions, a magnification of 5×. *Syn.* magnifying power; trade magnification.

**magnification, axial** The ratio of the distance along the optical axis between two points in image space $l'$ to the distance along the optical axis between the corresponding two points in object space $l$, i.e. $l'/l$. The axial magnification is approximately equal to the square of the lateral

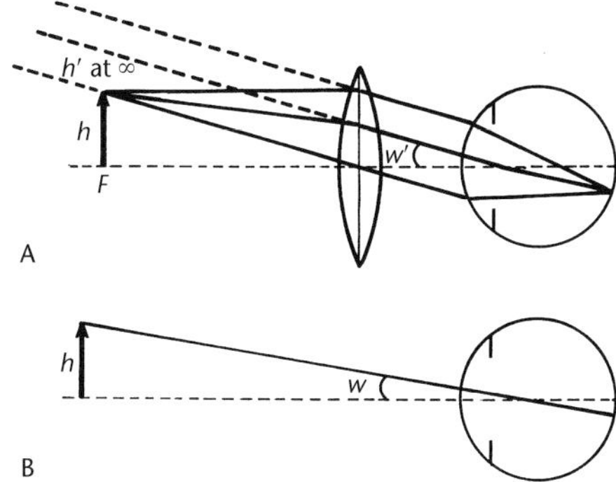


**Fig. M3** Object h viewed, A with a loupe and placed at its anterior principal focus F, and B without

**Table M1** Apparent magnification (or conventional magnification) of microscopic lenses of various powers used in the correction of low vision and their corresponding reading distance (assuming emmetropia or correction for distance and that no accommodation is exerted)

| magnification | lens power (D) | reading distance (cm) |
|---|---|---|
| 1× | +4.00 | 25 |
| 1.5× | +6.00 | 16.7 |
| 2× | +8.00 | 12.5 |
| 2.5× | +10.00 | 10 |
| 3× | +12.00 | 8.3 |
| 4× | +16.00 | 6.25 |
| 5× | +20.00 | 5 |
| 6× | +24.00 | 4.2 |
| 8× | +32.00 | 3.12 |
| 10× | +40.00 | 2.5 |

magnification when the object is far away from the optical system. This magnification is useful when considering an image in its three dimensions. Clinically, it is important when assessing the thickness of a retinal lesion in indirect ophthalmoscopy. *Syn.* longitudinal magnification. *See* **magnification, lateral.**

**magnification, conventional** *See* **magnification, apparent.**

**magnification, cortical** Term referring to the fact that the amount of cortical area devoted to processing visual information from the central area of the retina far exceeds the amount devoted to the peripheral retina. It is estimated that about 25% of the cells in the visual cortex are devoted to processing the central 2.5° of the visual field. *Syn.* magnification factor.
*See* **area, visual; pathway, visual.**

**magnification, distance** *See* **magnification, relative distance.**

**magnification, effective** *See* **magnification, apparent.**

**magnification factor** *See* **magnification, cortical.**

**magnification, lateral** Magnification of a lens or of an optical system, expressed as the ratio of the length of the image $h'$ to the length of the object $h$. It is usually denoted by

$$M = \frac{h'}{h}$$

*Syn.* linear magnification; transverse magnification.
*See* **plane, principal; sine condition.**

**Table M2** Approximate lateral magnification (in %) corresponding to various changes in spectacle lens distance and for various lens powers

| distance change | lens power (D) 1 | 2 | 4 | 6 | 8 | 10 |
|---|---|---|---|---|---|---|
| 1 mm | 0.1 | 0.2 | 0.4 | 0.6 | 0.8 | 1.0 |
| 2 mm | 0.2 | 0.4 | 0.8 | 1.2 | 1.6 | 2.0 |
| 3 mm | 0.3 | 0.6 | 1.2 | 1.8 | 2.4 | 3.0 |
| 4 mm | 0.4 | 0.8 | 1.6 | 2.4 | 3.2 | 4.0 |
| 5 mm | 0.5 | 1.0 | 2.0 | 3.0 | 4.0 | 5.0 |
| 10 mm | 1.0 | 2.0 | 4.0 | 6.0 | 8.0 | 10.0 |

minus lens: if moved closer to the eye magnification increases; if moved further from the eye magnification decreases
plus lens: if moved closer to the eye magnification decreases; if moved further from the eye magnification increases

**magnification, linear** *See* **magnification, lateral.**

**magnification, longitudinal** *See* **magnification, axial.**

**magnification, loupe** *See* **magnification, apparent.**

**magnification, negative** *See* **minification.**

**magnification, nominal** *See* **magnification, apparent.**

**magnification power** *See* **magnification, spectacle.**

**magnification, relative distance** The magnification which results from decreasing the distance between an object and the eye. It is expressed as

$$M_d = \frac{x}{x'}$$

where $x$ and $x'$ are the initial distance and the new distance, respectively. *Example*: if the viewing distance is decreased from 60 cm to 20 cm, $M_d = 60/20 = 3X$. *Syn.* distance magnification.

**magnification, relative size** The magnification which results from increasing the actual size of an object viewed. *Examples*: a larger TV screen; a larger print book than one used previously. It is expressed as

$$M_s = \frac{\tan\alpha_1}{\tan\alpha_2}$$

where $\alpha_1$ and $\alpha_2$ are the angles subtended at the eye by the enlarged object and the initial object, respectively. *Syn.* size magnification.

**magnification, relative spectacle (RSM)** The ratio of the retinal image size in the corrected ametropic eye to that in a standard emmetropic eye. *See* **law, Knapp's.**

**magnification, shape** Magnification resulting from a variation in the curvature of the front surface and thickness of an ophthalmic lens. In the treatment of aniseikonia it may be necessary to alter the magnification of a lens while leaving its dioptric power unchanged. *Syn.* shape factor. *See* **aniseikonia; lens, aniseikonic; magnification, spectacle.**

**magnification, size** *See* **magnification, relative size.**

**magnification, spectacle** The ratio of the retinal image of a distant object in the corrected ametropic eye to the blurred or sharp image formed in the same eye when uncorrected. It is greater than unity in the hyperopic eye, and less than unity in myopia. With a contact lens, though, this magnification is nearly equal to unity whatever the refractive error. Spectacle magnification *SM* depends both on the shape of the spectacle lens (i.e. the power of its front surface and its thickness) and on the power of the lens. Thus

$$SM = \left(\frac{1}{1-(t/n)F_1}\right)\left(\frac{1}{1-dF'_v}\right)$$

where $F_1$ is the power of the front surface, $F'_v$ the back vertex power of the lens, $t$ its thickness, $n$ the index of refraction and $d$ the distance from the back surface of the lens to the entrance pupil of the eye. The first term in the formula represents the **shape factor** (or **shape magnification**) and the second term the **power factor** (or **power magnification**). However, since the shape factor is very small for most common ophthalmic lenses (except for high plus lenses), it is often ignored in the above formula.

**magnification, trade** *See* **magnification, apparent.**

**magnification, transverse** *See* **magnification, lateral.**

**magnifier** An optical device, commonly used for close viewing, which produces an apparent magnification. It can be monocular or binocular, held in the hand (**hand magnifier**) or mounted in front of the eye (**stand magnifier**). It rarely exceeds a magnification of ×10 and does not produce an inversion of the image (Fig. M4). *Syn.* loupe. *See* **distance of distinct vision; lens, magnifying; magnification, apparent; vision, low.**

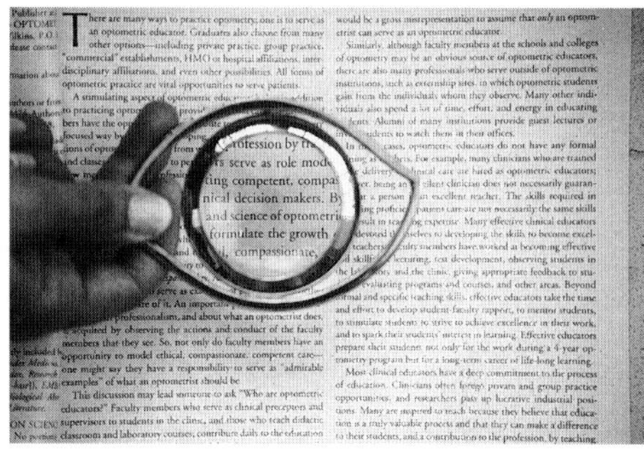


**Fig. M4** A hand magnifier

**Table M3** Approximate spectacle magnification of lenses of various back vertex powers ($F'_v$ in D) assuming d = 15 mm and the parameters of a typical spectacle lens of that power

| $F'_v$ | shape factor (S) | power factor (P) | spectacle magnification (SM) | percentage magnification |
|---|---|---|---|---|
| +12 | 1.08 | 1.22 | 1.32 | 32% increase |
| +10 | 1.06 | 1.18 | 1.25 | 25% " |
| +8 | 1.04 | 1.14 | 1.18 | 18% " |
| +6 | 1.03 | 1.10 | 1.13 | 13% " |
| +4 | 1.02 | 1.06 | 1.09 | 9% " |
| +2 | 1.01 | 1.03 | 1.04 | 4% " |
| 0 | 1.01 | 1.00 | 1.01 | 1% " |
| −2 | 1.00 | 0.97 | 0.97 | 3% decrease |
| −4 | 1.00 | 0.94 | 0.94 | 6% " |
| −6 | 1.00 | 0.92 | 0.92 | 8% " |
| −8 | 1.00 | 0.89 | 0.89 | 11% " |
| −10 | 1.00 | 0.87 | 0.87 | 13% " |
| −12 | 1.00 | 0.85 | 0.85 | 15% " |
| −14 | 1.00 | 0.83 | 0.83 | 17% " |
| −16 | 1.00 | 0.81 | 0.81 | 19% " |

**magnifying glass; lens** *See* **lens, magnifying.**

**magnifying power** *See* **magnification, apparent.**

**magnifying spectacles** *See* **spectacles, magnifying.**

**magnitude estimation** A psychophysical method of evaluating stimuli above threshold. The subject assigns numbers according to the apparent magnitudes of the stimuli. The results relating the magnitude of sensation $S$ and the stimulus intensity $I$ usually follow a **power law** (or **Stevens' power law**), that is $S = kI^n$ where k is a constant and $n$ the exponent which depends on the sensory modality. *Example*: the magnitude perceived brightness of a 5 degrees target viewed by a dark adapted subject follows the relation $S = kI^{0.33}$, that is the intensity of the light target needs to be increased some ten-fold to see it twice as bright. *Syn.* direct scaling.

**magno cells** *See* **geniculate bodies, lateral.**

**magnocellular layer** *See* **geniculate bodies, lateral.**

**magnocellular visual system** That part of the visual pathway from the photoreceptors in the retina to layer 4Cα (and to a lesser extent in layer 6) of the visual cortex, which is mainly responsible for transmitting information about movement, depth perception and high contrast targets. Action potentials are transmitted faster in this pathway because of the large diameter axons of these neurons than in the parvocellular pathway. *Syn.* dorsal pathway; parietal pathway; transient visual system; 'where' system.
*See* **cell, ganglion; cell, Y; dyslexia; geniculate bodies, lateral; parvocellular visual system; theory, two visual systems.**

**Maier, sinus of** *See* **lacrimal apparatus.**

**major amblyoscope** *See* **amblyoscope, Worth.**

**major arterial circle of the iris** *See* **arterial circle of the iris, major.**

**malar bone** *See* **orbit.**

**malingering** Feigning illness or disability (often for the purpose of gaining compensation or avoiding duty).
*See* **test, optokinetic nystagmus; vision, tunnel.**

**Mallett fixation disparity unit** Instrument used to measure the associated phoria (or compensating prism). It consists of a small central fixation letter X surrounded by two letters O, one on each side of X, the three letters being seen binocularly, and two coloured polarized vertical bars in line with the centre of the X which are seen by each eye separately. The instrument can be swung through 90° to measure any vertical fixation disparity. The associated phoria is indicated by the misalignment of the two polarized bars when the subject fixates the X through cross-polarized filters in front of the eyes. The amount of associated phoria is given by the value of the base-in or base-out prism power necessary to produce alignment. The unit can also be used to detect suppression.
*See* **disparity, retinal; Disparometer; heterophoria, associated; heterophoria, compensated; heterophoria, uncompensated.**

m

**Table M4** Approximate spectacle and contact lens magnification assuming d = 15 mm (vertex distance 12 mm plus 3 mm between cornea and entrance pupil) and negligible lens thickness. The percentage change in magnification going from spectacles to contact lenses was calculated using $(F_s/F_c - 1) \times 100$

| spectacle refraction ($F_s$) | equivalent power of contact lens ($F_c$) | percentage increased magnification spectacles | percentage increased magnification contact lens | % change in magnification from specs. to contact lens |
|---|---|---|---|---|
| +12 | +14.02 | 21.9 | 4.4 | −14.4 |
| +10 | +11.36 | 17.6 | 3.5 | −12 |
| +8 | +8.85 | 13.6 | 2.7 | −9.6 |
| +6 | +6.47 | 9.9 | 2.0 | −7.3 |
| +4 | +4.2 | 6.4 | 1.3 | −4.8 |
| +2 | +2.05 | 3.1 | 0.6 | −2.4 |
| −2 | −1.95 | −2.9 | −0.6 | 2.6 |
| −4 | −3.82 | −5.7 | −1.1 | 4.7 |
| −6 | −5.6 | −8.3 | −1.7 | 7.1 |
| −8 | −7.3 | −10.7 | −2.1 | 9.6 |
| −10 | −8.93 | −13 | −2.6 | 12 |
| −12 | −10.49 | −15.3 | −3 | 14.4 |
| −14 | −11.99 | −17.3 | −3.5 | 16.8 |
| −16 | −13.42 | −19.3 | −3.9 | 19.2 |

**malprojection** *See* **projection, false.**

**Mandelbaum effect** *See* **effect, Mandelbaum.**

**manifest hypermetropia; refraction** *See* under the nouns.

**mannitol** *See* **hyperosmotic agent.**

**manometer** An instrument for measuring the pressure of gases, vapour, blood or the intraocular pressure directly.
*See* **pressure, intraocular; tonometer.**

**manoptoscope** Apparatus for determining the dominant eye. It consists of a hollow truncated cone that subjects hold with the base against their face and over both eyes. Subjects will view a distant object through the hole at the end of the cone, using their dominant eye.
*See* **dominance, ocular.**

**Marcus Gunn phenomenon** *See* **phenomenon, jaw-winking.**

**Marcus Gunn pupil** *See* **pupil, Marcus Gunn.**

**Marfan's syndrome** *See* **syndrome, Marfan's.**

**marginal blepharitis; ray** *See* under the nouns.

**Mariotte's blind spot** *See* **blind spot.**

m

**mask** *See* **masking.**

**masking** A term describing any process whereby a detectable stimulus is made difficult or impossible to detect by the presentation of a second stimulus (called the **mask**). The main stimulus (typically called the **target**) may appear at the same time as the mask (**simultaneous masking**); or it may precede the mask (**backward masking**; *example*: metacontrast); or it may follow the mask (**forward masking**; *example*: paracontrast).
*See* **metacontrast.**

**masking, dichoptic** The masking of the visual function of one eye by the view presented to the other, as for example in a haploscope.
*See* **dichoptic; haploscope.**

**mast cell stabilizers** Prophylactic drugs used to treat allergic conjunctivitis, vernal conjunctivitis, giant papillary conjunctivitis, superior limbic keratoconjunctivitis. They act by stabilizing the membranes of mast cells thus preventing the release of histamine. Common agents are sodium cromoglycate (or cromolyn sodium), lodoxamide tromethamine, nedocromil sodium, olopatadine hydrochloride and pemirolast potassium.
*See* **allergic reactions; antihistamine.**

**matt surface** Surface which reflects light diffusely. *Example*: a magnesium oxide surface. *Syn.* diffusing surface.
*See* **diffusion; gloss; reflection, diffuse.**

**mature cataract** *See* **cataract, mature.**

**Maurice's theory** *See* **theory, Maurice's.**

**Maxwell, disc** *See* **disc, Maxwell.**

**maxwellian view** Method of observation in which a converging lens forms an image in the plane of the entrance pupil of the observer. If the observer's eye is focused on the lens it will appear as a disc filled with light of uniform intensity. This optical arrangement makes it possible to choose the point of incidence within the pupil, to minimize the effect of the optical aberrations of the eye and to avoid the effect of pupil size on the amount of light entering the eye (Fig. M5).
*See* **distances, conjugate; maxwellian view system, clinical.**

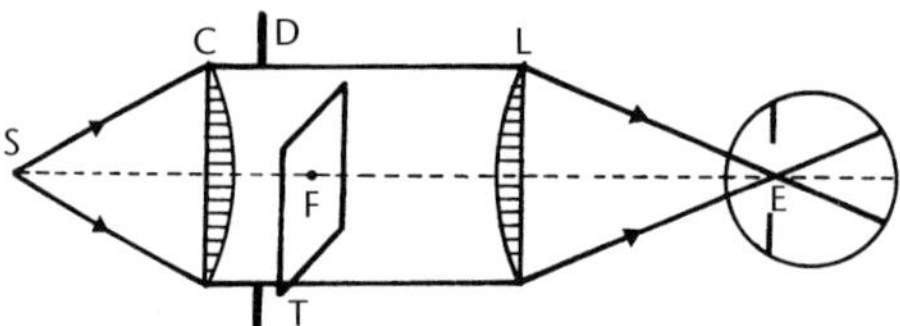


**Fig. M5** Maxwellian view system (S, source of light; C, collimator; D, diaphragm; T, target situated in the focal plane of lens L; F, first focal point of lens L and conjugate of the retina of an unaccommodated emmetropic eye; E, centre of the entrance pupil of the eye and conjugate of S

**maxwellian view system, clinical** Instrument designed to measure visual acuity by using a narrow beam or beams of light focused within the entrance pupil of the eye. The location of the beam or beams within the pupil can be controlled by the clinician. Such an instrument is valuable to assess acuity when part of the pupil is obstructed by a cataract or other opacity as the beam or beams of light can be directed to enter the eye through an area of the pupil where there is no opacity, thus providing an estimate of the visual acuity unaffected by optical image degradation. The results can contribute to the decision as to whether removal of a cataract will be beneficial. There are several types of these instruments: the **Potential Acuity Meter** (PAM) which focuses a single beam of light in the pupil and a letter chart onto the retina. Others focus two beams of light in the pupil and a grating which can be produced on the retina by interference (if the two sources are coherent). This method is called **laser interferometry**. Examples of these are the **Lotmar Visometer** and the **IRAS Randwal Interferometer** which are referred to as **clinical interferometers**. They tend to penetrate dense cataracts better than the PAM.
*See* **cataract; coherent sources; entoptoscope, blue field; hyperacuity; interferometer.**

**Maxwell's spot** Entopic phenomenon in which the subject can observe a dark or greyish spot in the visual field corresponding to his fovea. This is accomplished by viewing a diffusely illuminated field through a purple-blue or dark blue filter. (These are the best colours for this observation.) This phenomenon is used clinically to detect eccentric fixation by placing a fixation point in the diffusely illuminated field. The degree of eccentric fixation can thus be estimated by asking the subject to describe the position of the grey spot with respect to the fixation point. *See* **fixation, eccentric; image, entoptic.**

**McCollough effect** *See* **effect, McCollough.**

**Meares–Irlen syndrome** *See* **syndrome, Meares–Irlen.**

**mechanical optics** *See* **optics, mechanical.**

**media, ocular** The transparent substances of the eye, i.e. the cornea, the aqueous humour, the crystalline lens and the vitreous humour.

**medial rectus muscle** *See* **muscle, medial rectus.**

**median line; plane** *See* under the nouns.

**medium, optical** Any material, substance or space through which light can be transmitted.

**medullated nerve fibres** *See* **fibres, myelinated nerve.**

**Meesmann's dystrophy** *See* **dystrophy, Meesmann's.**

**megalocornea** A non-progressive enlargement of the cornea (more than 13 mm in diameter) without significant change in corneal thickness and normal clarity and function. Intraocular pressure is normal and high myopia and astigmatism often occur. It is usually transmitted as an X-linked recessive trait. Some systemic associations include Marfan's syndrome, Apert's syndrome, Down's syndrome, Weil–Marchesani syndrome and osteogenesis imperfecta. *See* **keratoglobus.**

**megalophthalmos** A condition in which the eye is abnormally large. It is an inherited condition and occurs mainly in males. *See* **keratoglobus.**

**megalopsia** *See* **macropsia.**

**meibometry** A method for quantifying the amount of lipids present in the tears. It may be used to facilitate the diagnosis of meibomian gland dysfunction. *See* **glands, meibomian.**

**meibomian cyst** *See* **chalazion.**

**meibomian gland dysfunction; glands** *See* **glands, meibomian.**

**meibomianitis** Inflammation of the meibomian glands. It is believed not to be a primary bacterial disease. It is characterized by the presence of a white, frothy secretion or 'foam' on the eyelid margin. Meibomianitis is often associated with blepharitis and conjunctivitis. Symptoms include mild itching of the lids and occasionally blurred vision due to the oily secretion spreading over the cornea. This condition may also result from hard contact lens wear. Management of this disease consists of tarsal massage and removal of the secretion with a moist cotton-tipped applicator. *Syn.* meibomitis.
*See* **blepharitis, marginal; glands, meibomian; hordeolum, internal.**

**meibomitis** *See* **meibomianitis.**

**melanin** Dark brown to black pigment normally present in the skin, the hair, the choroid, the iris, the retina, the ciliary body, the cardiac tissue, the pia mater and the substantia nigra of the brain. It is absent in albinos.
*See* **albinism; fuscin; melanocyte; melanosis; naevus, choroidal; retinal pigment epithelium.**

**melanocyte** A pigment-bearing cell. It is found in the iris, the choroid, the retina, the sclera, the skin, etc.
*See* **melanin; naevus, choroidal; naevus, iris.**

**melanocytosis** A unilateral lesion characterized by slate grey areas of increased pigmentation. The pigment is curiously not found in the conjunctival epithelium, but is located in the uvea and episcleral tissues. It may predispose the individual to uveal melanoma. *Syn.* congenital melanosis oculi.
*See* **naevus of Ota.**

**melanoma** Tumour derived from cells that are capable of forming melanin.

**melanoma, choroidal** The most common primary malignant tumour in the eye in adults. It appears under ophthalmoscopic examination as a pigmented, elevated mass, usually brown in colour and sometimes with orange pigment. The tumour may cause a decrease in vision or a defect in the visual field, or be asymptomatic, depending on its size or location. The condition is typically unilateral. Differential diagnosis with retinal detachment or choroidal naevus is essential. Treatment may include radiotherapy or photocoagulation, or enucleation if the melanoma is large and vision irreversibly lost. *Syn.* malignant melanoma of the choroid.
*See* **naevus, choroidal; retinal detachment.**

**melanosis** An abnormal accumulation of melanin pigment in the skin or other tissues. If there is a larger quantity than normal of pigment in the tissues of the eye, the condition is referred to as **melanosis bulbi** (or **melanosis oculi**) or **primary**

**acquired melanosis** when on the conjunctival epithelium. It may be benign or become malignant, in which case nodules appear and excision or cryotherapy is required.
*See* **naevus of Ota.**

**melanosis bulbi; oculi** *See* **melanosis.**

**membrane, Bowman's** Thin layer of the cornea (about 12 μm) located between the anterior stratified epithelium and the stroma. This membrane is acellular; it is a modified superficial stromal layer found only in primates. It is composed of a randomly orientated array of fine collagen fibrils, primarily of collagen types I, III and V. *Syn.* anterior limiting layer; Bowman's layer; lamina elastic anterior.

**membrane, Bruch's** Thin (about 1.5 μm), shiny, non-vascular layer of the choroid located on the inner side next to the pigment epithelium of the retina. It consists of two contiguous layers; the inner one called the **lamina vitrea** (or basement membrane of the pigment epithelium) and the outer one called the **lamina elastica.**
*See* **angioid streaks; choroid; retinal pigment epithelium.**

**membrane, Descemet's** Strong, resistant, thin (about 8 μm) layer of the cornea located between the endothelium (from which it is secreted) and the stroma. It is practically the last corneal structure to succumb to disease processes and it can regenerate after injury. *Syn.* lamina elastica posterior; posterior limiting layer.
*See* **descemetocele; ring, Kayser–Fleischer.**

**membrane, hyaloid** This is not really a membrane, but a concentration of cells and fibres at the front surface of the vitreous body.
*See* **humour, vitreous.**

**membrane, intermuscular** A thin, elastic membrane originating from the muscle sheath of each rectus muscle and connecting it to the neighbouring rectus muscle. The membrane fuses with the capsule of each muscle, as well as with Tenon's capsule.

**membrane, nictitating** A fold of the conjunctival mucous membrane that can be drawn over part or all of the cornea in a winking-like action to clean and lubricate the cornea. It is present in many birds, reptiles, fishes and some mammals and is normally hidden in the inner canthus. *Syn.* third eyelid.
*See* **plica semilunaris.**

**membrane of the retina, external limiting** This layer has the form of a wire netting through which pass the processes of the rods and cones of the retina. It is located between the latter and the outer nuclear layer. It is believed to be formed by the fibres of Mueller.
*See* **cell, Mueller's; retina.**

**membrane of the retina, internal limiting** Glass-like membrane lying between the retina and the vitreous body and forming a boundary for both. For that reason it has sometimes also been considered to be the hyaloid membrane of the vitreous. The feet of the fibres of Mueller are attached to this membrane but do not form it. *Syn.* internal limiting layer of the retina.
*See* **cell, Mueller's; retina.**

**membrane, preretinal** *See* **fibrosis, preretinal macular.**

**membrane, pupillary** Embryonic mesodermal tissue which is present in the centre of the iris and normally disappears by the eighth fetal month to form the pupil. Some strands of the membrane may remain in adults; this is referred to as a **persistent pupillary membrane.**

**meniscus lens** *See* **lens, meniscus.**

**meridional accommodation** *See* **accommodation, astigmatic.**

**meridional amblyopia** *See* **amblyopia, meridional.**

**meridional size lens** *See* **lens, aniseikonic.**

**meshwork, trabecular** Meshwork of connective tissue located at the angle of the anterior chamber of the eye and containing endothelium-lined spaces (the **intertrabecular spaces**) through which passes the aqueous humour to Schlemm's canal. It is usually divided into two parts: the **corneoscleral meshwork** which is in contact with the cornea and the sclera and opens into Schlemm's canal and the **uveal meshwork** which faces the anterior chamber.
*See* **angle of the anterior chamber; canal, Schlemm's; glaucoma, phacolytic; humour, aqueous; iris, plateau; ring of Schwalbe, anterior limiting; syndrome, pigment dispersion.**

**mesopic vision** *See* **vision, mesopic.**

**metacontrast** This is an apparently paradoxical phenomenon because it consists of a reduction in subjective brightness of a flash of light which is caused by a second flash following shortly afterward in an adjacent region of the visual field. The effect depends upon the duration, intensity, surface areas of the two flashes, the retinal area stimulated, and particularly the interval of time between the two flashes. The phenomenon appears most clearly with an interval of about 0.1 s and disappears when that interval reaches 0.3–0.4 s. *Syn.* backward masking (this term is used to indicate when the test stimulus and the masking stimulus overlap spatially). A flash of light can also be made to appear slightly less bright when it is preceded by another flash in an adjacent region of the visual field and the interval of time is of the

order of 0.05 s. This second phenomenon is called **paracontrast**. *Syn.* forward masking (this term is used when the test stimulus and the masking stimulus overlap spatially).
*See* **masking.**

**metal spectacle frame** *See* **spectacle frame, metal.**

**metameric colour** *See* **colour, metameric.**

**metamers** *See* **colour, metameric.**

**metamorphopsia** An anomaly of visual perception in which objects appear distorted in shape or of different size or in a different location than the actual object. It may be due to a displacement of the visual receptors as a result of inflammation, tumour or retinal detachment, or it can be of central origin (e.g. migraine, drug intoxication, neurosis), or it can be induced by recently prescribed myopic correction (e.g. micropsia) or presbyopic correction (e.g. macropsia) etc. Metamorphopsia can be detected with an Amsler chart.
*See* **accommodation, spasm of; chart, Amsler; dysmegalopsia; macropsia; macular hole; micropsia; pelopsia; teleopsia.**

**metarhodopsin** *See* **rhodopsin.**

**method, Bruckner's** An objective method of detecting the presence of strabismus. The examiner illuminates both eyes of the patient simultaneously with an ophthalmoscope from a distance of about 1 metre. Looking through the ophthalmoscope the examiner focuses on the fundus reflexes seen in the two pupils. If one pupil appears brighter it is considered that this eye may be strabismic and perhaps amblyopic. The reason may be due to the fact that this eye will be deviated and optical aberrations will make the pupil area appear brighter and whiter. The examiner may also note the position of the corneal reflexes when carrying out this test. This test is more reliable when patients are wearing their correction. *Syn.* Bruckner's test.
*See* **method, Hirschberg's.**

**method, cross-cylinder** *See* **test for astigmatism, cross-cylinder.**

**method, Donders'** *See* **method, push-up.**

**method, Drysdale's** A method which has been applied for the determination of the radius of curvature of hard contact lenses. The principle consists of placing a light source in a modified microscope in focus at the surface of the lens and at the centre of curvature of the surface, the distance between the two being recorded on a dial as the radius of curvature.
*See* **optic zone radius, back; Radiuscope.**

**method, duochrome** *See* **test, duochrome.**

**method, fogging** Method of relaxing accommodation during the subjective measurement of (astigmatic) ametropia. This is achieved by placing enough plus lens power (or less minus lens power) in front of an eye so as to form an image in front of the retina. In this condition, any effort to accommodate will produce a poorer image and relaxation of accommodation is thus achieved (Fig. M6). Then, plus lens power is decreased (or minus lens power increased) until the patient reports no further improvement in visual acuity. This point represents the maximum positive lens power (or minimum negative lens power) and it is called the **best vision sphere** (BVS).
*See* **refraction; refractive error; test, fan and block; test, plus 1.00 D blur.**

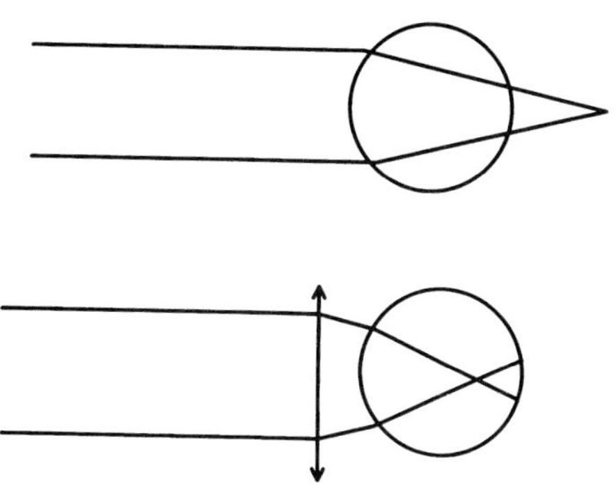

**Fig. M6** Principle of the fogging method: the eye is rendered artificially myopic

**method, von Graefe's** *See* **test, diplopia.**

**method, van Herick, Shaffer and Schwartz** A technique for estimating the angle of the anterior chamber. It is based on the fact that the width of the angle of the anterior chamber is correlated to the distance between the posterior corneal surface and the anterior iris as viewed near the corneal limbus. This is done using a slit-lamp with a narrow slit beam perpendicular to the temporal or nasal corneal surface, viewing from the straight-ahead position and comparing the depth of the anterior chamber to the thickness of the cornea. If the AC depth is equal to or greater than the corneal thickness, the angle is considered to be **grade 4** (corresponding to a wide open angle). If the AC depth is equal to one-half the corneal thickness, the angle is considered to be **grade 3** (this is the most common angle width). If the AC depth is equal to one-fourth the corneal thickness, it is considered to be **grade 2**, and if the AC depth is less than one-fourth the corneal thickness, it is considered to be **grade 1** (corresponding to a very narrow angle). **Grade 0** is considered to be a closed angle. The method is most useful for predicting the possibility of angle-closure glaucoma.

*See* **angle of the anterior chamber; glaucoma, angle-closure; gonioscope; test, shadow.**

**method, Hirschberg's** Method for estimating the objective angle of strabismus. The examiner's eye is placed directly above a small penlight source fixated by the subject and observes the position of the corneal reflex of the deviating eye. The angle of strabismus can be estimated on the basis that each mm of displacement, relative to the corneal reflex in the fixating eye, represents approximately 22 Δ of strabismus. *Syn.* Hirschberg's test.
*See* **method, Bruckner's; method, Krimsky's.**

**method, Humphriss** Method of binocular subjective refraction in which the eye not being refracted is blurred by means of a +0.75 D (or +1.0 D) spherical lens above the correcting lens. This lens produces a suppression of foveal vision while allowing peripheral fusion to maintain binocular alignment of the two eyes during refinement of the correction to the other eye. *Syn.* Humphriss immediate contrast test (HIC). However, HIC differs somewhat from the above method because it relates only to one specific procedure: a +0.25 D sphere is followed by a −0.25 D sphere in front of the unfogged eye and the patient has to indicate which is the clearest. The above method can be used for many types of refractive procedures.
*See* **refraction; refractive error; test, balancing.**

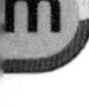

**method, Javal's** Method for determining the objective angle of strabismus using a perimeter. The patient is seated before a perimeter arc with the deviating eye at the centre of the arc while the other eye fixates a distant point straight ahead. The examiner moves both a light source and his eye directly above it, until the corneal reflex appears centred in the entrance pupil of the deviating eye. The position of the source on the arc can be read to give the objective angle of strabismus. Angle lambda must be added in convergent and subtracted in divergent strabismus as the criterion used was the pupillary axis which makes an angle with the line of sight. Strictly speaking, angle kappa, rather than lambda, should be taken into account.
*See* **angle of deviation; strabismus.**

**method, Krimsky's** Method used to determine the objective angle of strabismus. The examiner's own eye is placed directly above a small penlight source fixated by the subject and observes the position of the corneal reflexes. Prisms are placed in front of the deviating eye until the examiner finds the prism power that makes the corneal reflex appear to occupy the same relative position as that in the fixating eye. *Syn.* prism reflex test.
*See* **method, Hirschberg's; strabismus.**

**method, minus lens** Method of measuring the monocular amplitude of accommodation which consists in placing minus lenses in front of one eye while the subject fixates the smallest optotypes (usually subtending about one minute of arc, that is the 6/6 or 20/20 line). Progressively stronger lenses are used until the patient reports that the test appears blurred. The determination of the amplitude must take into account the vergence at the eye of the fixation point and the test must be carried out with the patient's distance correction. If the minus lens to blur is − 4 D and the fixation distance 40 cm, the amplitude will be equal to 6.5 D.
*See* **accommodation, amplitude of; accommodation, subjective.**

**method, preferential looking (PL)** A method of assessing visual acuity in infants. It consists of presenting two stimuli on a uniform background, one of which contains a pattern (e.g. a checkerboard or a grating) and the other a plain field of equal shape, size and luminance, and observing the infant's eyes. If the infant can resolve the pattern he or she tends to fixate that stimulus for a larger percentage of time. By reducing the size of the detail in the pattern, a threshold can be obtained when the infant fixates at either stimulus for the same length of time.
*See* **acuity, objective visual; acuity cards, Teller; test, Cardiff acuity.**

**method, push-out** *See* **method, push-up.**

**method, push-up** Method of determining the near point of accommodation by moving a test object (made up of small optotypes subtending one minute of arc (that is the 6/6 or 20/20 line) at the eye and uniformly illuminated) closer to the patient's eye. It is usually done monocularly and then binocularly. The near point is achieved when the small test object yields a sustained blur and not just begins to blur. Alternatively, the card is moved back after appearing blurred until the small test object just appears to clear again. This is often called the **push-out method**. In older patients, plus lenses may be needed to carry out the test and the power of the lens is subtracted from the reading. The amplitude of accommodation is deduced by taking into account the vergence at the eye of the far point (it is at infinity in emmetropes and corrected ametropes). *Syn.* Donders' method.
*See* **accommodation, amplitude of; accommodation, near point of; accommodation, subjective; rule, near point.**

**method of stabilizing the retinal image** *See* **stabilized retinal image.**

**methylcellulose** A highly viscous, water-soluble, non-irritating compound used as a thickening, lubricating and clinging agent in drugs such as artificial tears, wetting and contact lens solutions. *See* **alacrima; keratitis sicca; tears, artificial; wetting solution.**

**methyl methacrylate** *See* **polymethyl methacrylate.**

**metipranolol hydrochloride** *See* **beta-blocker.**

**metre angle** *See* **angle, metre.**

**miconazole** *See* **antifungal agent.**

**microaneurysm** Tiny swelling in the wall of a blood vessel. It appears in the retinal capillaries as a small, round, red spot. It is commonly found in diabetic retinopathy, retinal vein occlusion or absolute glaucoma.
*See* **retinopathy, diabetic.**

**microcoria** Abnormally small pupils, usually congenital and due to an absence of the dilator pupillae muscle.

**microcornea** An abnormally small cornea. It may be accompanied by hypermetropia.
*See* **keratoglobus.**

**microcysts, epithelial** Very small, round vesicles containing fluid and cellular debris observed on the surface of the cornea under slit-lamp examination in some types of corneal dystrophy and in wearers of extended wear contact lenses, due to chronic hypoxia. They appear to originate in the basal layer of the corneal epithelium as a result of cellular necrosis. They can be seen by slit-lamp examination using a magnification of at least ×20. If caused by extended wear contact lenses, the patient should be advised to change to daily wear contact lenses of high oxygen transmissibility. *Syn.* microepithelial cysts.
*See* **lens, extended wear; slit-lamp.**

**microfluctuations of accommodation** *See* **accommodation, microfluctuations of.**

**micrometre** An SI unit of length equal to one millionth of a metre ($10^{-6}$ m). *Symbol*: μm. *Syn.* micron (obsolete term).
*See* **nanometre.**

**micron** *See* **micrometre.**

**micronystagmus** *See* **movements, fixation.**

**micropachometer** *See* **pachometer.**

**microphthalmia** Congenital anomaly in which the eyeball is abnormally small and often deeply set in a small orbit. *Syn.* microphthalmus. When there is no other abnormality, the condition is called **nanophthalmos.**
*See* **anophthalmia; monophthalmia; pseudoptosis.**

**micropsia** Anomaly of visual perception in which objects appear smaller than they actually are. It may be due to a retinal disease in which the visual cells are spread apart, or to paresis of accommodation or to uncorrected presbyopia, or to the recent wear of either base-out prisms or a correction for myopia, etc.
*See* **dysmegalopsia; macropsia; metamorphopsia.**

**microsaccades** *See* **movements, fixation.**

**microscope** An optical instrument for magnifying small near objects. It can consist of a single converging lens such as a loupe (**simple microscope**) or of two or more lenses or lens systems (**compound microscope**) (Fig. M7). In this latter case, one lens or lens system serves as an objective to form real and magnified images of the object while the other lens or lens system serves as an eyepiece to examine the aerial image formed by the objective. The final image is inverted with respect to the object. It can use light or a beam of electrons (**electron microscope**) which produces magnification some 50 to 100 times greater than with light. The magnification, $M$, of a light microscope, adjusted for a final image at infinity, is equal to

$$M = M_o \times M_e$$

where $M_o$ is the lateral magnification of the objective, and $M_e$ the angular magnification of the eyepiece.
*See* **eyepiece; lens, immersion; magnification; magnifier; objective; slit-lamp; stage.**

**microscope, confocal** A microscope which allows viewing of cells, organisms (such as bacteria or fungi) and other structures within various tissues, in living patients. The instrument has been used to investigate and diagnose corneal disease processes, including dystrophies and infectious keratitis, or to follow corneal healing after laser or traditional surgery. It is based on focusing on a single illuminated corneal plane while the out-of-focus light above and below the plane of focus is greatly reduced. In addition, the instrument scans the object of interest by varying the plane of focus to form an image in three dimensions, of higher contrast and resolution than provided by a specular microscope.
*See* **microscope, specular.**

**microscope, slit-lamp** Compound microscope used in conjunction with a slit-lamp. It is designed to have a working distance of about 90–125 mm to allow room for the clinician or for placing certain accessories such as a tonometer or pachometer. Slit-lamp microscopes have a magnification which varies usually within the range of ×6 to ×40.
*See* **distance, working; slit-lamp.**

m

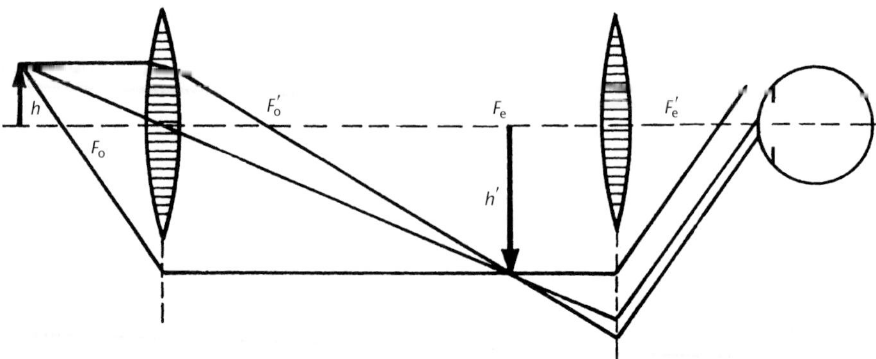


**Fig. M7** Optical principle of a compound microscope ($F_o$, $F'_o$, first and second principal focus of the objective; $F_e$, $F'_e$, first and second principal focus of the eyepiece; $h$, $h'$, object and image formed by the objective)

**microscope, specular** A light microscope utilizing specular reflection to view the component layers of the cornea and particularly to observe and photograph the endothelium. It consists of an objective which is divided longitudinally. Light in the form of a slit beam is directed down one half and is reflected from the cornea–aqueous interface to the other half of the objective to form a visible and photographic image of the endothelium. The microscope is usually fitted with a ×40 water immersion objective which has a **working distance** of 1.6 mm. The cornea is covered with silicone fluid into which the objective tip is immersed. Good resolution is achieved provided that the width of the slit beam is kept small, to reduce the light scatter from the overlying corneal layers. This microscope allows examination of the corneal endothelium in vitro. For clinical measurements, the specular microscope is mounted horizontally using an objective with less magnification (usually ×20). The tip of the microscope has a glass-windowed, fluid-filled, screw-on cap, which applanates the cornea over a very small area. The field of view is usually increased by the insertion of a +10 D into the incident light path before the objective. Photomicrography is accomplished with a flash unit, as otherwise eye movements make photography with long exposure impossible. However, corneal anaesthesia is necessary and clear images of the endothelium are not possible if the cornea is oedematous. For these reasons new systems have been developed which fit on a slit-lamp and facilitate photography. Their magnification is greater than other slit-lamps, being ×40 to ×70, and they do not require contact with the cornea as they have long working distances. Specular microscopy is used to monitor changes in corneal endothelium in contact lens wearers, especially those wearing extended wear lenses.
*See* **corneal endothelium; distance, working; lens, extended wear; microscope, confocal; polymegethism, endothelial; reflection, regular.**

**microspherophakia** A congenital, usually bilateral condition in which the crystalline lens is smaller than normal and spherical in shape. It may give rise to lenticular myopia, subluxation or glaucoma. It may occur independently or it may be associated with the Weill–Marchesani syndrome or more rarely with Marfan's syndrome, Peter's anomaly or congenital rubella.

**microsquint** *See* **microtropia.**

**microstrabismus** *See* **microtropia.**

**microtropia** A small-angled (usually less than 6–8 Δ in angle) inconspicuous strabismus which is not usually detected by cover test, either because the deviation is too small or because the angles of abnormal retinal correspondence and eccentric fixation coincide with the angle of deviation. There is usually amblyopia in the deviated eye and there may also be anisometropia. The patient with this condition displays nearly normal binocular vision without symptoms. Management usually consists of correcting the refractive error. *Syn.* microsquint; microstrabismus; small angle strabismus.
*See* **strabismus; test, four prism dioptre base out.**

**middle third technique** *See* **criterion, Percival.**

**midline** *See* **line, median.**

**migraine** An intense and recurring pain usually confined to one side of the head and often accompanied by vertigo, nausea and vomiting, photophobia and scintillating appearances of light and even hemianopsia.
*See* **aura, visual; metamorphopsia; scotoma, scintillating.**

**Mikulicz's syndrome** *See* **syndrome, Mikulicz's.**

**millilambert** Non-metric unit of luminance. It is equal to 3.183 cd/$m^2$.

**millimicron** *See* **nanometer.**

**miner's nystagmus** *See* **nystagmus.**

**minification** A reduction in the apparent size of an object. *Example*: viewing a distant object through the objective of a galilean telescope. *Syn.* negative magnification.
*See* **telescope, galilean.**

**minimum cognoscible** The threshold of recognition of shapes or contours.

**minimum legible** The threshold for the recognition of letters or numbers.

**minimum separable** Perception of the least distance separating two objects, yet being still distinguished as two.
*See* **resolution, limit of.**

**minimum visible** Perception of the smallest area of light.

**minus lens** *See* **lens, diverging.**

**minus lens method** *See* **method, minus lens.**

**miosis** Contraction of the pupil or condition in which the pupil is very small (2 mm or less in diameter). It can be brought about by a spasm of the sphincter muscle or by the effect of a miotic drug (e.g. eserine, neostigmine, pilocarpine), or in certain spinal diseases or any stimulation of the parasympathetic supply to the eye. Miosis occurs naturally when doing close work or when stimulated by light. *Note*: also spelt myosis.
*See* **blind spot, baring of the; glaucoma, open-angle; mydriasis; reflex, pupil light; syndrome, Horner's.**

**miotics** Drugs which constrict the pupil. They may be used in the treatment of glaucoma and accommodative esotropia and, sometimes, after a mydriatic examination. Miotics are either **parasympathomimetic** (or **cholinergic-stimulating**) drugs which have a direct muscarinic action, such as pilocarpine and carbachol, or **anticholinesterase** drugs which block the effect of acetylcholinesterase thus letting acetylcholine produce its effect, such as physostigmine, neostigmine, echothiophate and demecarium. There are also some miotics which act by blocking α- or β-adrenergic receptors. For example, dapiprazole and thymoxamine block the α-adrenergic receptors and propranolol blocks the β-adrenergic receptors.
*See* **adrenergic receptors; glaucoma, open-angle; muscle, sphincter pupillae; mydriatic.**

**mire** A pattern used in an optical instrument to guide the observer. *Examples*: the luminous pattern seen in a keratometer; the two half-circles seen in an applanation tonometer.
*See* **keratometer.**

**mirror** A surface capable of reflecting light rays and forming optical images. Such surfaces are smooth or polished, made of highly polished metal, or a thin film of metal (e.g. aluminium) on glass, quartz or plastic. Object distance $l$ and image distance $l'$ relate to the focal distance $f$ or the radius of curvature $r$ of the mirror, as follows

$$\frac{2}{r} = \frac{1}{f} = \frac{1}{l'} + \frac{1}{l}$$

$2/r$ represents the refractive power of the mirror, in air. If the medium which contains the incident and reflected rays is $n$, the power becomes $F = 2n/r$ and the focal length, $f = r/2n$. (Fig. M8)
*See* **catadioptric system; distance, image; distance, object; length, focal; paraxial equation, fundamental.**

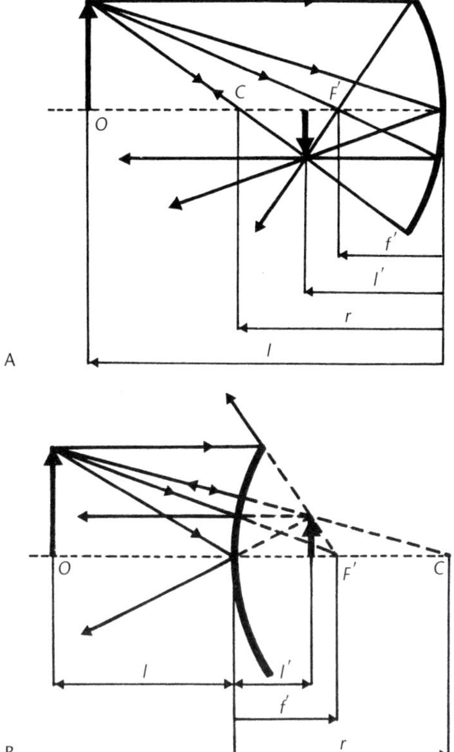


Fig. M8 Image of an object O formed in A, a concave mirror and B, a convex mirror. Four rays are drawn in each case for completeness, but two would suffice (C, centre of curvature; F', focal point; f', focal length; l and l', object and image length; r, radius of curvature). Aberrations are ignored in this diagram

**mirror, back surface** A mirror which reflects from the back surface of a refracting layer, usually glass. *See* **mirror, front surface.**

**mirror, concave** A mirror with a spherical concave surface forming an erect, magnified, virtual image when the distance from the mirror is less than the focal distance and an inverted real image when the object distance is greater than the focal distance (Fig. M8).

**mirror, convex** A mirror with a spherical convex surface forming a virtual, erect and diminished image (Fig. M8).

**mirror, front surface** A mirror which reflects directly from its front surface. The advantages of this type are that, unlike back surface mirrors, there is no chromatic effect as the glass is not used optically, therefore ultraviolet rays can be used which would otherwise be absorbed in the glass and there is no ghost reflection from the front surface. However, these mirrors can be easily scratched and the coating may tarnish. Often a coating of silicon monoxide is evaporated on top of the surface, but this causes a loss of reflectivity.
*See* **image, ghost; mirror, back surface.**

**mirror, plane** A mirror whose surface is plane and forms a virtual image of the same size as the object. Object and image distances are equal.
*See* **distance, image; distance, object.**

**mirror, semi-silvered** *See* **beam-splitter.**

**mirror writing** Writing backward, Latin letters being written from right to left and the details of the letters reversed. The writing thus appears normal when viewed in a mirror. *Syn.* retrography.

**mitosis** Process by which a cell nucleus divides into two nuclei with chromosome numbers and genetic make-up identical to that of the parent cell. Mitosis is inhibited by anaesthetics and thus tissue repair is delayed. It is also slowed by hypoxia. *Example*: the mitosis of the basal cells of the corneal epithelium.
*See* **corneal abrasion; corneal epithelium; cycle, Krebs.**

**Mittendorf's dot** *See* **hyaloid remnant.**

**mixed astigmatism** *See* **astigmatism, mixed.**

**mixture, colour** *See* **colour mixture.**

**Mizuo's phenomenon** *See* **phenomenon, Mizuo's.**

**Mobius syndrome** *See* **syndrome, Mobius.**

**modality** One of the types of sensation (e.g. vision). The term is usually used to specify the sense (e.g. the visual modality, the touch modality).

**modulation transfer function** *See* **function, modulation transfer.**

**modulus of elasticity** The ratio of a force applied to a material to the increment of change (e.g. increase in length; angular deformation) in that material. Materials with low modulus of elasticity are less resistant to stress, while materials with high modulus of elasticity resist stress and hold their shape better. *Examples*: the modulus of elasticity of the crystalline lens capsule decreases progressively with age, being about $6 \times 10^7$ dyne/cm$^2$ in childhood to $1.5 \times 10^7$ dyne/cm$^2$ in very old age; the modulus of elasticity of a contact lens is about $2000 \times 10^5$ dyne/cm$^2$ in PMMA lenses, $500–1500 \times 10^5$ dyne/cm$^2$ in siloxane acrylate gas-permeable lenses and $65–75 \times 10^5$ dyne/cm$^2$ in high water hydrogel lenses. *Syn.* coefficient of elasticity; Young's modulus of elasticity.

**moiré effect** An illusory shimmering movement produced by moving one pattern superimposed on another pattern very similar to it. The phenomenon occurs because parts of the periodic patterns are in phase in some locations, and out of phase in other locations. *Examples*: passing by a set of railings; if a transilluminated square wave grating is superimposed on an identical grating but cross each other at an angle of less than 45°, moiré fringes will appear at the intersections. *Syn.* moiré pattern.
*See* **Toposcope.**

**Moll's glands** *See* **glands of Moll.**

**mondrian** A complex visual display used in studies of colour perception. It consists of rectangles of various dimensions with all sides parallel or perpendicular to each other, and each rectangle of a colour or brightness different from the adjacent rectangles.

**monoblepsia** Condition in which monocular vision is more distinct than binocular vision.

**monocentric** Pertaining to a lens with only one optical centre. A **monocentric bifocal lens** is one in which the optical centres of the distance and near portions coincide and jump is eliminated.
*See* **jump; lens, bifocal.**

**monochromasia** *See* **achromatopsia.**

**monochromasy** *See* **achromatopsia.**

**monochromat** Person who has a condition of monochromatism (total colour blindness). There are two types of monochromats: the **cone monochromat** whose photopic luminosity curve resembles the normal and who has normal visual acuity and dark adaptation; and the **rod monochromat** whose retina does not contain functional cones and, therefore, has poor vision, photophobia and sometimes associated nystagmus and myopia. Monochromats are very rare: estimated at about three persons in 100 000. *See* **achromatopsia; colour vision, defective; dystrophy, cone; nystagmus.**

**monochromatic light** *See* **light, monochromatic.**

**monochromatism** *See* **achromatism; achromatopsia; colour vision, defective; monochromat.**

**monochromator** A modified spectroscope for producing nearly monochromatic light. *See* **spectroscope.**

**monocle** A single ophthalmic lens, with or without a frame, which is worn by holding it between the brow and the cheek.

**monocular** Pertaining to one eye. *Syn.* uniocular.

**monocular cues; depth perception** *See* **perception, depth.**

**monocular diplopia; vision** *See* under the nouns.

**monofixation** **1.** Monocular fixation. **2.** *See* **syndrome, monofixation.**

**monophthalmia** A rare, abnormal development in which one eye is absent. The remaining eye is often microphthalmic. *Syn.* unilateral anophthalmia. *See* **anophthalmia; microphthalmia.**

**monoptic** Relating to the presentation of different stimuli to one eye. *See* **dichoptic.**

**monovision** Term referring to a method of correcting presbyopia by using a contact lens corrected for distance in one eye (usually the dominant one) and a contact lens corrected for near in the other eye. Binocular vision is impaired with this method; however, it has been found to be relatively successful in many cases.

**moon illusion** *See* **illusion, moon.**

**Mooren's ulcer** *See* **ulcer, Mooren's.**

**Morax–Axenfeld, diplobacillus of** *See* **conjunctivitis.**

**morgagnian cataract** *See* **cataract, morgagnian.**

**morning glory disc** *See* **disc, morning glory.**

**mosaic, retinal** The pattern formed by the distribution of the retinal visual cells and their interspaces.

**motility test** *See* **test, motility.**

**motion after-effect** *See* **after-effect, waterfall.**

**motion parallax** *See* **parallax, motion.**

**motor cortex** *See* **cortex, motor.**

**motor end-plate** *See* **muscles, extraocular.**

**motor field** *See* **field of fixation.**

**motor fusion** *See* **fusion, motor.**

**motor neuron** *See* **neuron.**

**motor pathway** Pathway from the cortex to the muscles that control the movements of the eyes enabling them to act as a unit.

**motor unit** A group of muscle fibres which respond to a stimulus from a single motor neuron. In the extraocular muscles a motor unit consists of less than a dozen small fibres, that is considered to be a small unit. It produces a finer degree of neural control over contraction than a larger unit, which produces more powerful gross movements when activated. *See* **neuron.**

**mouches volantes** *See* **image, entoptic; muscae volitantes.**

**mould** *See* **impression, eye.**

**moulding** A process for making a lens in which a hot piece of glass (called a **parison** or **gob**) or liquid polymer (for contact lenses) is pressed to a predetermined shape. Frames can also be manufactured by pouring a soft material (plastic or molten metal) into a mould which takes on the desired shape after cooling (or drying). The technique is useful for large volume production. *Note*: also spelt molding. *See* **lens, spin-cast contact; surfacing.**

**movement, after-effect** *See* **after-effect, waterfall.**

**movement, against** **1.** Apparent movement of an object seen through a lens in a direction opposite to that in which the lens is moved. This occurs when looking through a plus lens. **2.** *See* **retinoscope.** *See* **movement, with.**

**movement, apparent** The perception of movement induced by stationary objects, under certain circumstances. *Example*: phi movement. *See* **movement, phi.**

**movement, autokinetic** *See* **illusion, autokinetic visual.**

**movement, following** *See* **movement, pursuit.**

**movement, fusional** *See* **fusional movements.**

**movement, optokinetic** *See* **nystagmus.**

**movement, phi** Illusion of movement created when one object disappears and an identical object appears in a neighbouring region of the

same plane. If the time interval between the two sources is between 0.06 s and 0.2 s, the observer will see an apparent movement of the object from the first to the second position. The illusion of movement obtained in the cinema is based on this phenomenon. The phi phenomenon has been applied to test patients with convergent and divergent strabismus. This is the **phi phenomenon test of Verhoeff:** two light sources, separated by the angle of strabismus, are placed in front of the patient, as in a major amblyoscope. The two foveas are stimulated with a short time interval between stimulations and patients with normal retinal correspondence do not see a movement whereas those with abnormal retinal correspondence do. *Syn.* phi phenomenon.
*See* **retinal correspondence, abnormal; strabismus; test, cover; threshold, movement.**

**movement, pursuit** Movement of an eye fixating a moving object. The fixation can remain locked on the target as long as the movement is smooth and the velocity below about 40°/s. *Syn.* following movement.
*See* **test, motility.**

**movement, saccadic eye** A short rapid and abrupt movement of the eye as occurring in reading a line of printed words or in fixating from one point to another. The peak velocity of a saccade of 10° amplitude can exceed 400°/s and be completed in 40 ms.
*See* **movements, fixation; reading.**

**movement, scissors 1.** Apparent change in the angle between two lines seen through a rotating astigmatic lens. **2.** *See* **retinoscope.**

**movement threshold** *See* **threshold, movement.**

**movement, torsional** *See* **torsion.**

**movement, with 1.** Apparent movement of an object seen through a lens in the same direction as that in which the lens is moved. This occurs when looking through a minus lens. **2.** *See* **retinoscope.**
*See* **movement, against.**

**movements, compensatory eye** *See* **reflex, static eye.**

**movements, conjugate eye** *See* **version.**

**movements, cyclofusional eye** *See* **cyclofusion.**

**movements, disjugate eye** *See* **movements, disjunctive eye.**

**movements, disjunctive eye** Movements of the two eyes in which the eyes move in opposite directions, as in convergence or divergence. They are known as vergence movements. *Syn.* disconjugate movements; disjugate eye movements.
*See* **vergence.**

**movements, eye** *See* **electro-oculogram; fusion, motor; movement, pursuit; movement, saccadic eye; movements, disjunctive eye; movements, fixation; movements, rapid eye; reflex, vestibulo-ocular; vergence; version.**

**movements, fixation** Involuntary movements of the eye occurring when actually fixating an object. Three types of movements have been observed: the **drifts**, the **micronystagmus** (or **tremors** or **microsaccades**) and the **saccades.** These movements are too subtle to be seen by direct observation. The drifts are characterized by a small amplitude (1–7 minutes of arc) and a low frequency (2–5 Hz). The micronystagmus movements are characterized by a very small amplitude (10–20 seconds of arc) and a higher frequency (30–100 Hz) and the saccadic movements by a small amplitude (1–25 minutes of arc) and low frequency (0.1–1 Hz). *Syn.* involuntary eye movements; physiological nystagmus.
*See* **hypermetria; movement, saccadic eye; muscles, extraocular; stabilized retinal image.**

**movements, rapid eye (REM)** Fast eye movements that occur periodically during sleep and are associated with dreaming.

**moxisylyte (thymoxamine)** *See* **alpha-adrenergic antagonist.**

**mucin** Glycoprotein produced by the goblet cells and the subsurface vesicles of the conjunctiva which forms the basis of the mucous layer of the precorneal film. Mucin (or more likely **glycocalyx** which is another type of glycoprotein) is adsorbed by the epithelium of the cornea to convert it from a hydrophobic into a wettable hydrophilic surface. A deficiency in the production of mucin leads to an abnormally short precorneal film break-up time and to desiccation of the ocular surface. In addition, the mucous layer prevents microbial invasion of the cornea. In some contact lens wearers (especially of silicone hydrogel lenses) collapsed mucin, as well as lipids and tear proteins, accumulate behind the lens and form small, discrete spheres (called **mucin balls** or **mucin plugs**). These mucin balls cause neither discomfort nor loss of vision.
*See* **cell, goblet; conjunctiva; eye, dry; film, precorneal; gland, lacrimal; keratitis sicca; lens, silicone hydrogel; test, break-up time; xerophthalmia.**

**mucocele** An abnormal enlargement of a cavity, such as the lacrimal sac when the nasolacrimal sac is blocked (or obstructed). The obstruction may occur as a result of infection, allergy, trauma or tumour, or it may cause the infection as is often the case with dacryocystitis. The patient may present with epiphora, eyelid or periorbital swelling, proptosis but rarely pain unless there is an infection. Treatment involves removal of the mucocele and perhaps construction of a new drainage channel.

**Mueller's cells** *See* **cell, Mueller's.**

**Müller–Lyer illusion** *See* **illusion, Müller–Lyer.**

**Müller's muscle** *See* **muscle, ciliary.**

**Müller's palpebral muscles** *See* **muscles, Müller's palpebral.**

**multifocal lens** *See* **lens, multifocal.**

**multiple sclerosis** *See* **sclerosis, multiple.**

**multiple vision** *See* **polyopia.**

**Munsell colour system** A system of classification of colours composed of about 1000 colour samples, each designated by a letter and number system. The letter and number of each sample indicate its hue, saturation (called **chroma** in this system) and brightness (called **value**). They are represented by a three-dimensional polar coordinate system in which the hue is represented along the circumference, the value along the vertical axis and the chroma along a radius (Fig. M9). *See* **colorimetry; test, Farnsworth.**

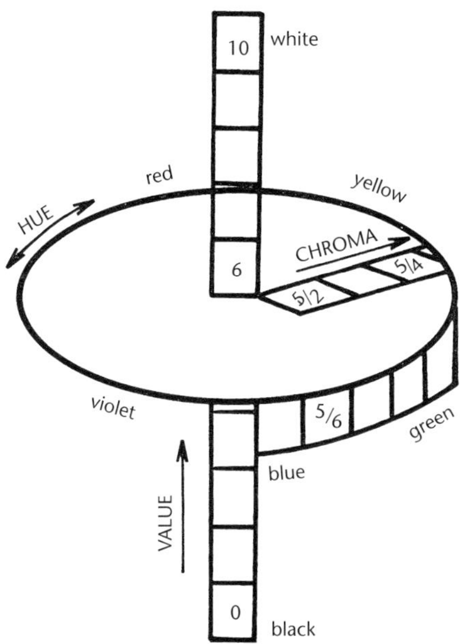


**Fig. M9** Schematic representation of the three coordinates of the Munsell colour system

**Munson's sign** *See* **sign, Munson's.**

**muscae volitantes** An entoptic phenomenon produced by the presence of remnants of embryonic structures floating within the vitreous humour. They appear like floating spots on a bright uniform background. As they are lighter than the vitreous body they tend to float upward but appear to the patient to move downward because of the reversal of the retinal image. *Syn.* mouches volantes.
*See* **floaters; image, entoptic; opacity.**

**muscarine** *See* **acetylcholine.**

**muscle** A contractile organ of the body which produces movements of the various parts or organs. Typically it is a mass of fleshy tissue, attached at each extremity by means of a tendon to a bone or other structure. Muscles are classified according to structure as non-striated (or unstriated or unstriped or smooth) or striated (or striped), by control as voluntary or involuntary, or by location as cardiac, skeletal or visceral.

**muscle, abducens** *See* **muscle, lateral rectus.**

**muscle, adducens** *See* **muscle, medial rectus.**

**muscle, agonistic** A muscle which performs the desired movement, or does the opposite to an antagonistic muscle. *Example*: the left lateral rectus is the agonistic muscle when the left eye turns to the left.
*See* **muscle, antagonistic.**

**muscle, antagonistic** A muscle which opposes the action of another. *Example*: the right superior rectus muscle is the contralateral antagonist of the left superior oblique.
*See* **muscle, agonistic; muscles, synergistic.**

**muscle, Brücke's** *See* **muscle, ciliary.**

**muscle, ciliary** The smooth (or unstriated and involuntary) muscle of the ciliary body. In a meridional section of the eye it has the form of a right-angled triangle, the right angle being internal and facing the ciliary processes. The posterior angle is acute and points to the choroid, the hypotenuse runs parallel with the sclera. Some of its fibres have their origin in the scleral spur at the angle of the anterior chamber, while other fibres take origin in the trabecular meshwork. The fibres radiate backward in three directions: (1) Fibres coursing **meridionally** or **longitudinally** more or less parallel to the sclera and can be traced posteriorly into the suprachoroid to the equator or even beyond. They end usually in branched stellate figures known as muscle stars with three or more rays to each. These fibres represent **Brücke's muscle**. (2) Other fibres course **radially**. These fibres lie deep in the longitudinal fibres from which they are distinguished by the reticular character of their stroma but are often very difficult to separate from the circular fibres. (3) The **circular** fibres (or **Müller's muscle**)

**Table M5** Agonistic, antagonistic and synergistic extraocular muscles

| agonist | ipsilateral antagonist | ipsilateral synergist(s) | contralateral synergist |
|---|---|---|---|
| lateral rectus | medial rectus | superior oblique<br>inferior oblique | medial rectus |
| medial rectus | lateral rectus | superior rectus<br>inferior rectus | lateral rectus |
| superior rectus | inferior rectus | inferior oblique | inferior oblique |
| inferior rectus | superior rectus | superior oblique | superior oblique |
| superior oblique | inferior oblique | superior rectus | inferior rectus |
| inferior oblique | superior oblique | inferior rectus | superior rectus |

occupy the anterior and inner portion of the ciliary body and run parallel to the limbus. As a whole, these fibres form a ring.

Innervation to the ciliary muscle (mainly parasympathetic fibres derived from the oculomotor nerve) is provided through the short ciliary nerves and stimulation causes a contraction of the muscle. However, a small amount of sympathetic supply is also believed to act and relax the muscle. Blood supply to the ciliary muscle is provided by the anterior and long posterior ciliary arteries. Contraction of the ciliary muscle causes a reduction in its length thus causing the whole muscle to move forward and inward. Consequently the zonule of Zinn, which suspends the lens, relaxes. This leads to a decrease in the tension in the capsule of the lens allowing it to become more convex and thereby providing accommodation. *Syn.* Bowman's muscle.

*See* **accommodation, mechanism of; accommodation, resting point of; adrenergic receptors; ciliary body; limbus; scleral spur; theory, Helmholtz's of accommodation; Zinn, zonule of.**

**muscle cone** A structure formed by the sheath of the four recti muscles as they pass forward from their common origin at the apex of the orbit in the fibrous ring called the annulus of Zinn (and around the optic nerve) to be inserted into the sclera around the eyeball. Some authors consider the muscle cone to include the superior oblique muscle.

*See* **annulus of Zinn.**

**muscle, dilator pupillae** Smooth (or unstriated and involuntary) muscle whose fibres constitute the posterior membrane of the iris. This muscle extends from the ciliary body close to the margin of the iris where it fuses with the sphincter pupillae muscle. Contraction of the dilator pupillae muscle draws the pupillary margin towards the ciliary body and therefore dilates the pupil. This muscle is supplied by the sympathetic fibres in the long ciliary nerves and by a few parasympathetic fibres.

*See* **adrenergic receptors; iris; muscle, sphincter pupillae; mydriatic.**

**muscle, external rectus** *See* **muscle, lateral rectus.**

**muscle, Horner's** A thin layer of fibres which originates behind the lacrimal sac from the upper part of the **posterior lacrimal crest** (a ridge on the lacrimal bone which borders the fossa for the lacrimal sac). The muscle passes outward and forward and divides into two slips surrounding the canaliculi. It then becomes continuous with the pretarsal portions of the orbicularis muscle of the upper and lower lids and with the muscle of Riolan. Horner's muscle may be involved in tear drainage through action on the lacrimal sac. *Syn.* pars lacrimalis muscle; tensor tarsi muscle.

*See* **muscle of Riolan; tears.**

**muscle, inferior oblique (IO)** One of the extraocular muscles, it takes its origin at the anteromedial corner of the floor of the orbit. It passes underneath the inferior rectus in a backward direction (making an angle of about 50° with the sagittal plane of the eye), then under the lateral rectus to be inserted by the shortest tendon of all extraocular muscles on the posterior, temporal portion of the eyeball, for the most part below the horizontal meridian, some 5 mm away from the optic nerve. It is innervated by the oculomotor nerve and it extorts (main action), elevates and abducts the eyeball when the eye is in the primary position. Combined with the action of the superior rectus muscle, it directs the eye upward.

*See* **muscles, extraocular; position, primary; test, Bielschowsky's head tilt; test, three-step.**

**muscle, inferior rectus (IR)** This is the shortest of the four recti muscles. It arises from the lower part of the annulus of Zinn, runs forward, downward and outward (making an angle of about 23° with the sagittal plane) and inserts into the inferior portion of the sclera about 6.5 mm from the corneal limbus. It is innervated by the inferior division of the oculomotor nerve and it depresses (main action), adducts and extorts the eyeball when the eye is in the primary position.

*See* **annulus of Zinn; muscles, extraocular; muscles, Müller's palpebral; position, primary; test, Bielschowsky's head tilt.**

**muscle, inferior tarsal** *See* **muscles, Müller's palpebral.**

**muscle, internal rectus** *See* **muscle, medial rectus.**

**muscle, lateral rectus (LR)** One of the extraocular muscles, it arises from both the lower and upper parts of the annulus of Zinn which bridge the superior orbital fissure. The muscle passes forward along the lateral wall of the orbit, crosses the tendon of the inferior oblique muscle and inserts into the sclera about 6.9 mm from the corneal limbus. It is innervated by the abducens nerve and it abducts the eyeball when the eye is in the primary position (Fig. M10). *Syn.* external rectus muscle; abducens muscle.
*See* **annulus of Zinn; ligament, check; muscles, extraocular; position, primary.**

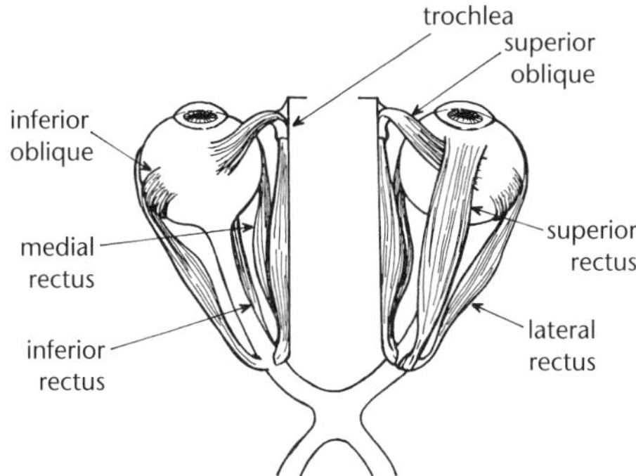


**Fig. M10** Extraocular muscles of the eye (the left superior rectus muscle is not shown to allow a clearer view of the muscles underneath)

**muscle, levator palpebrae superioris** Striated muscle that arises from the under surface of the lesser wing of the sphenoid bone above and in front of the optic canal. It passes forward below the roof of the orbit and above the superior rectus muscle and terminates in a tendinous expansion or **aponeurosis** (also called **levator aponeurosis**) that spreads out in a fan-shaped manner so as to occupy the whole breadth of the orbit and thus gives the whole muscle the form of an isosceles triangle. From the inferior surface of the aponeurosis arises a thin sheet of smooth muscle fibres called **Müller's palpebral muscle** (or **superior tarsal muscle**) which inserts into the posterior margin of the superior tarsal plate and into the superior fornix of the conjunctiva. These smooth muscle fibres are innervated by sympathetic nerves from the superior cervical sympathetic ganglion and assist in elevating the upper eyelid. The fibres of the aponeurosis are attached to the anterior margin of the superior tarsal plate while some fuse with bundles of the orbicularis oculi muscle to attach to the skin. These latter sets of fibres produce the horizontal skin crease of the upper eyelid. The striated levator aponeurosis is innervated by the superior division of the oculomotor nerve and elevates the upper eyelid. Its antagonist is the orbicularis muscle.
*See* **muscle, orbicularis; muscles, Müller's palpebral.**

**muscle, medial rectus (MR)** The largest of the extraocular muscles, it arises from the medial part of the annulus of Zinn. It passes forward along the medial wall of the orbit and is inserted into the sclera about 5.5 mm from the corneal limbus. It is innervated by the inferior division of the oculomotor nerve and it adducts the eyeball when the eye is in the primary position (Fig. M10). *Syn.* internal rectus muscle; adducens muscle.
*See* **annulus of Zinn; ligament, check; muscles, extraocular; position, primary.**

**muscle, Müller's** *See* **muscle, ciliary.**

**muscle, Müller's palpebral** *See* **muscles, Müller's palpebral.**

**muscle, oculorotary** *See* **muscles, extraocular.**

**muscle, orbicularis** A thin oval sheet of striated muscle which surrounds the palpebral fissure, covers the eyelids and spreads out for some distance onto the temple, forehead and cheek. It consists of two portions: (1) The palpebral portion which is the essential part of the muscle and is confined to the lids and may itself be divided into pretarsal and ciliary (muscle of Riolan) portions. The palpebral portion (also called the **pars palpebralis muscle**) is used in closing the eye without effort or in reflex blinking. (2) The orbital portion (also called the **pars orbitalis muscle**) which is found in the eyebrow, the temple, the forehead and the cheek. This portion of the muscle is used to close the eye tightly and the skin of the forehead, temple and cheek is drawn towards the inner side of the orbit. The orbicularis muscle is innervated by the facial nerve. *Syn.* sphincter oculi muscle.
*See* **ectropion; myokymia.**

**muscle, pars ciliaris** *See* **muscle of Riolan.**

**muscle, pars lacrimalis** *See* **muscle, Horner's.**

**muscle, pars orbitalis** *See* **muscle, orbicularis.**

**muscle, pars palpebralis** *See* **muscle, orbicularis.**

**muscle of Riolan** The ciliary portion of the orbicularis muscle, it consists of very fine striated muscle fibres which lie in the dense tissue of the

eyelids near their margin. It is continuous with Horner's muscle and encircles the eyelid margins mainly between the tarsal glands and the eyelash follicles. Its action is to bring the eyelid margins together when the eyes are closed. *Syn.* pars ciliaris muscle.
*See* **muscle, Horner's; muscle, orbicularis.**

**muscle, sphincter oculi** *See* **muscle, orbicularis.**

**muscle, sphincter pupillae** Smooth, circular muscle about 1 mm broad, forming a ring all round the pupillary margin near the posterior surface of the iris. It is innervated by parasympathetic fibres of the oculomotor nerve that synapse in the ciliary ganglion and by a few sympathetic fibres. Its contraction produces a reduction in the diameter of the pupil.
*See* **miotics; muscle, dilator pupillae; reflex, pupil light.**

**muscle spindle** *See* **muscles, extraocular.**

**muscle, superior oblique (SO)** This is the longest and thinnest of the extraocular muscles. It arises above and medial to the optic foramen on the small wing of the sphenoid bone. It passes forward between the roof and medial wall of the orbit to the **trochlea** (which is in the form of a pulley made of fibrocartilage) located at the front of the orbit where it loops over and turns sharply backward, downward and outward (making an angle of about 55° with the sagittal plane), passes under the superior rectus and inserts into the sclera just behind the equator on the superior temporal portion of the eyeball. It is innervated by the trochlear nerve and it intorts (main action), depresses, and also abducts the eyeball when the eye is in the primary position (Fig. M10).
*See* **fossa, trochlear; muscles, extraocular; position, primary; test, Bielschowsky's head tilt; test, three-step.**

**muscle, superior rectus (SR)** The longest rectus muscle, it arises from the upper part of the annulus of Zinn. It passes forward and outward (making an angle of about 23° with the sagittal plane) and inserts into the sclera about 7.7 mm from the corneal limbus. It is innervated by the superior division of the oculomotor nerve and elevates (main action), adducts, and also intorts the eyeball when the eye is in the primary position (Fig. M10).
*See* **annulus of Zinn; muscles, extraocular; position, primary; test, Bielschowsky's head tilt.**

**muscle, superior tarsal** *See* **muscles, Müller's palpebral.**

**muscle, tensor tarsi** *See* **muscle, Horner's.**

**muscles, extraocular** The striated (or voluntary) muscles that control the movements of the eyes. There are six such muscles: four recti muscles (lateral rectus, medial rectus, superior rectus and inferior rectus) which move the eye more or less around the transverse and vertical axes, and two oblique muscles (inferior oblique and superior oblique) which move the eyes obliquely. The muscles are composed of striated fibres of varying length, mostly running parallel to the direction of the muscle and united by fibrous connective tissue. They have a greater ratio of nerve fibres to muscle fibres than other striated muscles of the body. The fibre thickness varies from 3 to 50 μm, although functionally there seem to be two main types of fibres, the fast and the slow fibres. The former are the thickest and probably responsible for the fast movements of the eyes (saccades) and the latter consist of thin fibres. The **tendons** (bands of connective tissue) at one end of each extraocular muscle are attached to bones. This is the origin of the muscle. At the other end of the muscle the tendon is attached to the eye and this area is called the **insertion**. The substance proper of the muscle is called the **belly**. Contraction of a muscle occurs in the direction of its constituent fibres and causes a shortening of the muscle. Consequently the eye turns in a given direction depending upon which extraocular muscle is contracting. Contraction results from nervous impulses arriving at the **motor end-plate** (the junction between an axon and a striated muscle fibre) of the muscle through one of the ocular motor nerves. This causes a transmitter substance to be discharged in the microscopic gap between the end-plate and a muscle fibre. These muscles also possess specialized receptors called **muscle spindles** which are small groups of muscle fibres that are provided with both a sensory and a motor nerve supply. There are between 12 and 50 in each muscle. The muscle spindles provide a constant and continuous monitoring of the degree of tension of the muscle itself (Fig. M10). *Syn.* extrinsic muscles; oculorotary muscles.
*See* **cholinergic; fibres, felderstruktur; motor unit; movements, fixation; orbit; recession; resection; test, motility; test, three-step.**

**muscles, extrinsic** *See* **muscles, extraocular.**

**muscles, intraocular** The smooth (or unstriated and involuntary) muscles found within the eye. They are the ciliary, the dilator pupillae and the sphincter pupillae muscles. *Syn.* intrinsic muscles.
*See* **cholinergic.**

**muscles, Müller's palpebral** Smooth muscles of the eyelids. The superior one (also called **superior tarsal muscle**) originates from the under surface of the levator palpebrae superioris muscle and passes below to insert into the upper margin of the tarsal plate of the upper eyelid. The inferior one (also called **inferior tarsal muscle**)

| Table M6 Innervation and action of the 6 extraocular muscles | | |
|---|---|---|
| **muscle** | **innervation** | **action in the primary position** |
| medial rectus | oculomotor (III) | adduction |
| lateral rectus | abducens (VI) | abduction |
| inferior rectus | oculomotor (III) | **depression*** adduction extorsion |
| superior rectus | oculomotor (III) | **elevation** adduction intorsion |
| inferior oblique | oculomotor (III) | **extorsion** elevation abduction |
| superior oblique | trochlear (IV) | **intorsion** depression abduction |

*Bold characters indicate main action.

| Table M7 Intraocular muscles of the eyeball (unstriated muscles) | | |
|---|---|---|
| **name of muscle** | **nerve supply** | **action** |
| sphincter pupillae | parasympathetic via oculomotor nerve | constricts pupil |
| dilator pupillae | sympathetic via trigeminal nerve | dilates pupil |
| ciliary | parasympathetic via oculomotor nerve | controls shape of lens in accommodation |

originates from the muscular fascia covering the inferior rectus muscle. It extends upward and inserts into the bulbar conjunctiva and the lower margin of the tarsal plate of the lower eyelid. Müller's palpebral muscles are innervated by sympathetic fibres and help in lifting the upper eyelid and depressing the lower eyelid.
*See* **muscle, inferior rectus; muscle, levator palpebrae superioris.**

**muscles, pupillary** The dilator pupillae and the sphincter pupillae muscles.

**muscles, synergistic** Muscles having a similar and mutually helpful action as, for example, the inferior rectus and superior oblique muscles in depressing the eyeball.
*See* **Table M5.**

**muscles, tarsal** *See* **muscles, Müller's palpebral.**

**muscles, yoke** Muscles of the two eyes which simultaneously contract to turn the eyes in a given direction. *Example*: the medial rectus of the right eye and the lateral rectus of the left eye when turning the eyes to the left.
*See* **law of equal innervation, Hering's; test, motility; version.**

**muscular imbalance** *See* **imbalance, muscular.**

**myasthenia gravis** A disorder of neuromuscular transmission marked by severe, fluctuating muscle weakness. It is due to a reduction of acetylcholine receptors in the postsynaptic membrane of the neuromuscular junction. In the eye it may result in ptosis, diplopia, keratitis sicca due to improper blinking and consequent dryness of the cornea and eyelid twitch due to a paresis of the extraocular muscles.
*See* **diplopia; keratitis sicca; ptosis; sign, Cogan's lid twitch.**

**mydriasis 1.** Dilatation of the pupil. **2.** The condition of an eye having an abnormally large pupil diameter (5 mm in daylight). The condition may be due to a paralysis of the sphincter pupillae muscle, to an irritation of the sympathetic pathway, to a drug (e.g. atropine, homatropine), or to adaptation to darkness.
*See* **miosis; muscle, dilator pupillae; mydriatic; pupil.**

**mydriatic 1.** Causing mydriasis of the pupil. **2.** A drug which produces mydriasis. Mydriatics are used to carry out a thorough inspection of the fundus and lens, especially in elderly patients in whom the pupils are usually smaller. However, in older people it must be ascertained that the patient does not have glaucoma. There are two classes of mydriatics: (1) **antimuscarinic**

| Table M8 Yoke muscles | | |
|---|---|---|
| **right eye** | **left eye** | **version*** |
| lateral rectus | medial rectus | to the right |
| medial rectus | lateral rectus | to the left |
| superior rectus | inferior oblique | up and to the right |
| inferior rectus | superior oblique | down and to the right |
| superior oblique | inferior rectus | down and to the left |
| inferior oblique | superior rectus | up and to the left |

*The directions refer to those of the patient.

(or **parasympatholytic** or **anticholinergic** or **atropine-like**) **drugs** which antagonize the muscarinic action of acetylcholine, such as cyclopentolate, homatropine, hyoscine (or scopolamine) and tropicamide. Antimuscarinic drugs produce cycloplegia as well; (2) **sympathomimetic drugs** which directly or indirectly stimulate the dilator pupillae muscle which is innervated by the sympathetic division of the autonomic nervous system. These include cocaine, ephedrine hydrochloride, adrenaline (epinephrine), naphazoline and phenylephrine hydrochloride.
*See* **acetylcholine; adrenaline (epinephrine); adrenergic receptors; cholinergic; cocaine; cycloplegia; homatropine; miotics; muscle, dilator pupillae; mydriasis; reflex, pupil light; thymoxamine.**

**myectomy** The excision of a portion of a muscle. It is done to decrease the effective action of an extraocular muscle in the correction of strabismus.
*See* **myotomy.**

**myelinated nerve fibres** *See* **fibres, myelinated nerve.**

**myiasis** An infection or infestation of tissues or cavities by larvae of flies. In the eye (called **ophthalmomyiasis** or **ocular myiasis**) the larvae may affect the ocular surface, the conjunctival sac, the intraocular tissues or occasionally the deeper orbital tissues. Treatment consists of the mechanical removal of the larvae following topical anaesthesia.

**myoclonus, ocular** Bursts of pendular eye movements normally associated with lesions in the midbrain.
*See* **flutter, ocular; opsoclonus.**

**myodioptre** The contractile power of the ciliary muscle such that it induces an increase in the accommodation of the eye of 1 D.
*See* **dioptre.**

**myoid** *See* **ellipsoid.**

**myokymia** Twitching of a few bundles of fibres of the eyelid muscle. It occurs most commonly when fatigued, sometimes on exposure to cold, and in some pathological cases (e.g. multiple sclerosis) in which case the entire muscle is involved. **Superior oblique myokymia** can often be diagnosed by noting fine torsional nystagmus of the affected eye on slit-lamp examination. In cases where no nystagmus is noted, a patient's history of monocular episodic oscillopsia, associated with vertical diplopia may be sufficient to make a diagnosis. The use of carbamazepine or propranolol has been suggested as possible treatments in stopping the myokymia.
*See* **eyelids; muscle, orbicularis; sclerosis, multiple.**

**myopathy, ocular** *See* **ophthalmoplegia.**

**myopathy, restrictive** *See* **disease, Graves'.**

**myope** A person who has myopia.

**myopia (M)** Refractive condition of the eye in which the images of distant objects are focused in front of the retina when the accommodation is relaxed. Thus distance vision is blurred. In myopia the point conjugate with the retina, that is the far point of the eye, is located at some finite point in front of the eye (Fig. M11). *Syn.* nearsight; short sight.
*See* **epikeratoplasty; keratotomy, radial; orthokeratology; retina, lattice degeneration of the; syndrome, Marfan's; theory, use-abuse.**

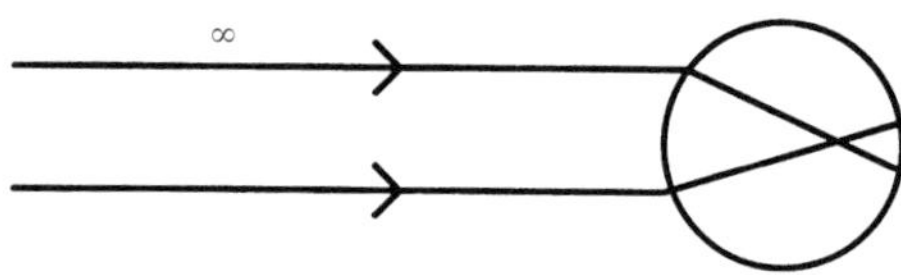


**Fig. M11** A myopic eye looking at a distant axial point

**myopia, acquired** Myopia appearing after infancy, or in adulthood. Almost all myopias are acquired. Those myopias developing in the late teens and adulthood are usually referred to as **late-onset myopia** (or **adult-onset myopia**), whereas those occurring earlier are often referred to as **early-onset myopia** (or **juvenile-onset myopia**).

**Table M9** Approximate relationship between uncorrected myopia and visual acuity

| | Snellen visual acuity | |
|---|---|---|
| **myopia** | **(m)** | **(ft)** |
| −10.0 D | 6/600 | 20/2000 |
| −6.00 D | 6/232 | 20/775 |
| −5.00 D | 6/170 | 50/565 |
| −4.00 D | 6/126 | 20/420 |
| −3.00 D | 6/85 | 20/285 |
| −2.50 D | 6/68 | 20/225 |
| −2.00 D | 6/50 | 20/165 |
| −1.50 D | 6/33 | 20/110 |
| −1.00 D | 6/20 | 20/65 |
| −0.50 D | 6/9 | 20/30 |

**myopia, degenerative** *See* **myopia, pathological.**

**myopia, early-onset** *See* **myopia, acquired.**

**myopia, empty-field** *See* **myopia, space.**

**Table M10** Common ocular and systemic diseases with myopia as an associated sign

| | |
|---|---|
| Marfan's syndrome | retinopathy of prematurity |
| Ehlers–Danlos syndrome | Stargardt's disease |
| Down's syndrome | homocystinuria |
| Cornelia de Lange syndrome | choroideraemia |
| Weil–Marchesani syndrome | gyrate atrophy |
| Laurence–Moon–Bardet–Biedl syndrome | rod monochromat |
| Riley–Day syndrome | ectopia lentis |
| Turner's syndrome | Fabry's disease |
| Wagner's disease | |

**myopia, false** *See* **accommodation, spasm of.**

**myopia, high** Myopias above 6.0 D or more are usually considered as high myopias.
*See* **glaucoma, open-angle; lens, high index; myopia, pathological.**

**myopia, hypertonic** *See* **accommodation, spasm of.**

**myopia, index** *See* **myopia, lenticular.**

**myopia, instrument** A temporary increase in accommodation induced by looking through an optical instrument.
*See* **accommodation, resting state of.**

**myopia, juvenile-onset; late-onset** *See* **myopia, acquired.**

**myopia, lenticular** Myopia attributed to an increase in the index of refraction of the lens. As a result there is an increase in refractive power. Such a change usually accompanies the development of some cataracts. This type of myopia may also accompany or follow an increase in blood sugar level, in which case it is usually of a transient nature, i.e. the power of the crystalline lens diminishes after the blood sugar level returns to normal. *Syn.* index myopia.
*See* **cataract, nuclear; diabetes; microspherophakia.**

**myopia, low** Myopias of 3.0 D or less are usually considered as low myopias.

**myopia, malignant** *See* **myopia, pathological.**

**myopia, medium** Myopias between 3.0 and 6.0 D are usually considered as medium myopias.

**myopia, night** An increase in ocular refraction (essentially accommodation) occurring at low levels of illumination.
*See* **accommodation, resting state of.**

**myopia, pathological** Myopia attributed to any degenerative changes in the choroid or retina. The myopia usually exceeds 8–10 D, tends to increase rapidly during adolescence and continues to increase during adulthood. Visual acuity is usually subnormal after correction. *Syn.* degenerative myopia; malignant myopia; progressive myopia.
*See* **crescent, myopic; Fuchs' spot; retinal detachment; staphyloma; vitreous detachment.**

**myopia, physiological** This is the most common type of myopia. It occurs because of a failure in correlation of the refractive power of lens and cornea, and the length of the eye. Thus, the power of the eye is too great for its length. Unlike pathological myopia, this myopia usually stabilizes when the growth process has been completed. It is associated with normal visual acuity after correction. *Syn.* simple myopia; typical myopia.
*See* **theory, biological–statistical.**

**myopia, progressive** *See* **myopia, pathological.**

**myopia, pseudo** *See* **accommodation, spasm of.**

**myopia, senile lenticular** *See* **sight, second.**

**myopia, simple** *See* **myopia, physiological.**

**myopia, space** An increase in accommodation occurring when viewing a field without any stimuli to accommodation as, for example, a clear sky. *Syn.* empty-field myopia.
*See* **accommodation, resting state of.**

**myopia, spurious** *See* **accommodation, spasm of.**

**myopia, typical** *See* **myopia, physiological.**

**myopic conus; crescent** *See* **crescent, myopic.**

**myopigenic** Pertains to factors causing myopia. They are: genetic predisposition which includes ethnicity and a family history of high myopia; visual experiences, such as prolonged reading and extensive near work; and diseases such as congenital cataract, congenital ptosis and haemangiomas of the eyelids and orbit.

**myosis** *See* **miosis.**

**myotomy** The surgical division or dissection of a muscle. It is done to reduce the pull of an extraocular muscle in the correction of strabismus.
*See* **myectomy.**

**myotonic pupil** *See* **pupil, Adie's.**

# N

**naevus** Any localized area of pigmentation or vascularization of the skin or eye tissues, usually benign and congenital. *Note*: also spelt nevus. *Plural*: naevi.

**naevus, choroidal** A benign accumulation of melanocytes in the choroid. It affects some 10% of the population. Ophthalmoscopically it appears as a slate-grey lesion, flat or minimally elevated, oval or circular. With time drusen may also appear.
*See* **choroid; drusen; melanocyte; melanoma, choroidal.**

**naevus, conjunctival** A naevus located on the conjunctiva, most often near the limbus. It appears as a yellowish-red area or deeply pigmented mass usually before the age of 20. A pigmented conjunctival naevus must be distinguished from an acquired melanoma of the conjunctiva which occurs later in life (after the third decade, is typically unilateral and may become malignant). A conjunctival naevus rarely becomes malignant. It can be excised if cosmetically undesirable or has enlarged to such a degree as to irritate the eye.

**naevus, flammeus** *See* **syndrome, Sturge–Weber.**

**naevus, iris** Benign accumulation of melanocytes in the iris.
*See* **melanocyte; syndrome, ICE.**

**naevus of Ota** A benign, usually congenital, accumulation of melanocytes on the cheek, eyelids, forehead, nose or sclera. Some naevi may become malignant melanoma. *Syn.* oculocutaneous melanosis; oculodermal melanocytosis.
*See* **melanocyte; melanosis.**

**Nagel anomaloscope** *See* **anomaloscope.**

**nanometre (nm)** SI unit of length equal to one-millionth of a millimetre (or 10 ångströms or $10^{-9}$m). *Syn.* millimicron (obsolete).
*See* **ångström; micrometre.**

**nanophthalmos** *See* **microphthalmia.**

**naphazoline hydrochloride** A sympathomimetic vasoconstrictor which may be used as a topical decongestant in 0.1% eyedrops. It causes slight mydriasis. It also comes as naphazoline nitrate.
*See* **adrenaline (epinephrine); decongestant, ocular.**

**narrow-angle glaucoma** *See* **glaucoma, angle-closure.**

**nasal step** *See* **Roenne nasal step.**

**nasolacrimal duct** *See* **lacrimal apparatus.**

**natamycin** *See* **antifungal agent.**

**nativism** The belief that knowledge or behaviour is inborn.
*See* **empiricism; theory, nativist.**

**nativist theory** *See* **theory, nativist.**

**Nd-Yag laser** *See* **laser, neodymium-yag.**

**near addition** *See* **addition, near.**

**near point of accommodation** *See* **accommodation, near point of.**

**near point of convergence** *See* **convergence, near point of.**

**near point retinoscopy** *See* **retinoscopy, dynamic.**

**near point rule; point sphere** *See* under the nouns.

**near point stress** *See* **asthenopia.**

**near reflex** *See* **reflex, accommodative.**

**near sight** *See* **myopia.**

**near triad** *See* **reflex, accommodative.**

**near vision** *See* **vision, near.**

**near visual acuity** *See* **acuity, near visual.**

**nearsightedness** *See* **myopia.**

**nebula** *See* **leukoma.**

**Necker cube** Perspective drawing of the outline of a cube which can induce two perceptions, either a three-dimensional cube orientated upward or a three-dimensional cube orientated downward (Fig. N1).
*See* **figure, Blivet; Schroeder's staircase; vase, Rubin's.**

**necrosis** Death of some or all of the cells in an organ or tissue. It is caused by disease, trauma or interference with blood supply.

**necrotizing scleritis** *See* **scleritis, necrotizing.**

**nedocromil sodium** *See* **mast cell stabilizers.**

**negative after-image** *See* **after-image, negative.**

**negative convergence** *See* **divergence.**

**negative eyepiece** *See* **eyepiece, negative.**

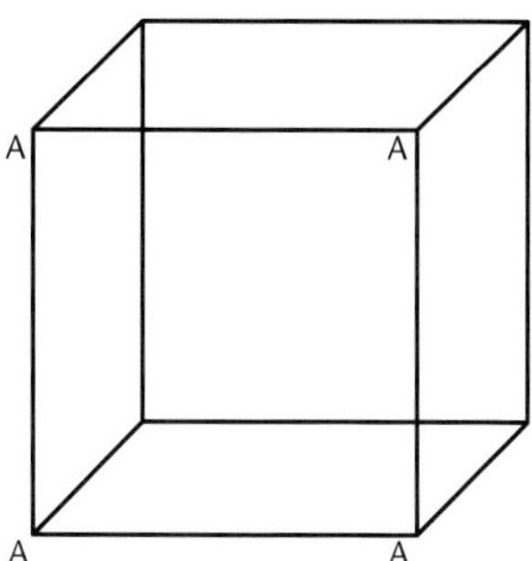


**Fig. N1** Necker cube. This ambiguous figure can appear with the plane AAAA, either in front or at the back

**negative lens** *See* **lens, diverging.**

**negative relative accommodation** *See* **accommodation, relative amplitude of.**

**negative relative convergence** *See* **convergence, relative.**

**negative scotoma** *See* **scotoma, negative.**

**negative spherical aberration** *See* **aberration, spherical.**

**neodymium-yag laser** *See* **laser neodymium-yag.**

**neomycin** A broad-spectrum antibiotic agent effective against gram-negative and gram-positive organisms, although it is not effective against *Pseudomonas aeruginosa*. It may be applied topically as eyedrops or eye ointment, but it is most commonly combined with bacitracin and polymyxin B. *Syn.* framycetin (a mixture of neomycin A, neomycin B and neomycin C).
*See* **antibiotic; sulfacetamide sodium.**

**neonatal conjunctivitis** *See* **ophthalmia neonatorum.**

**neostigmine** A reversible anticholinesterase drug which neutralizes the effect of acetylcholinesterase and thereby allows the prolonged action of acetylcholine on the iris and ciliary muscle. Its action is similar to physostigmine but it is not so irritating a miotic. Both are occasionally used in the treatment of glaucoma.
*See* **acetylcholine; parasympathomimetic; physostigmine; miosis; miotics.**

**neovascular glaucoma** *See* **glaucoma, neovascular.**

**neovascularization, choroidal** *See* **maculopathy, age-related.**

**neovascularization, corneal** *See* **pannus.**

**neovascularization, iris** Abnormal formation of new blood vessels on the anterior surface of the iris. It is commonly associated with many conditions that have led to retinal ischaemia, such as diabetic retinopathy, occlusion of the central retinal vein, carotid arterial disease, retinal and choroidal tumours, long-standing retinal detachment, etc. The neovascularization begins at the pupil margin and often at the same time in the angle of the anterior chamber and spreads over the whole surface. New vessels are associated with fibrous tissue membranes which may block the passage of aqueous humour through the trabecular meshwork (neovascular glaucoma) and ectropion uveae near the pupillary margin. Treatment typically includes photocoagulation to prevent the formation of new blood vessels.
*See* **ectropion uveae; glaucoma, neovascular; retinal vein occlusion; retinopathy, diabetic.**

**nerve** A whitish cord made up of myelinated or unmyelinated nerve fibres held together by connective tissue sheath in bundles and through which stimuli are transmitted from the central nervous system to the periphery or vice versa.

**nerve, abducens** Sixth cranial nerve. It has its origin from the abducens nucleus at the lower border of the pons and at the lateral part of the pyramid of the medulla and enters the orbit through the superior orbital fissure. It supplies motor innervation to the ipsilateral lateral rectus muscle. Additionally, interneurons leave the abducens nucleus and project to the contralateral medial rectus sub nucleus to allow conjugate gaze. A lesion in the nuclear region will cause gaze palsy, whereas an abducens nerve lesion will produce only an abduction deficit.
*See* **muscle, lateral rectus; paralysis of the sixth nerve.**

**nerve fibre layer** *See* **retina.**

**nerve, fifth cranial** *See* **nerve, trigeminal.**

**nerve, fourth cranial** *See* **nerve, trochlear.**

**nerve, frontal** *See* **nerve, ophthalmic.**

**nerve impulse** *See* **potential, action.**

**nerve, infratrochlear** *See* **nerve, ophthalmic.**

**nerve, lacrimal** *See* **nerve, ophthalmic.**

**nerve, long ciliary** One of a pair of nerves that comes off the nasociliary nerve and runs with the short ciliaries, pierces the sclera and, passing between this and the choroid, supplies sensory fibres to the iris, cornea, and ciliary muscle and sympathetic motor fibres to the dilator pupillae muscle (Fig. N2).
*See* **muscle, dilator pupillae; nerve, ophthalmic.**

**nerve, nasociliary** *See* **nerve, ophthalmic.**

**nerve, oculomotor** Third cranial nerve. It is classified as a motor nerve. Its origin lies in the

**Table N1** Cranial nerves

| nerve | type | function (sensory is in italic, the rest is motor) |
|---|---|---|
| olfactory (I) | sensory | *smell* |
| optic (II) | sensory | *vision* |
| oculomotor (III) | mixed, primarily motor | movement of eye and eyelids, regulation of pupil size, accommodation, *proprioception* |
| trochlear (IV) | mixed, primarily motor | eye movements, *proprioception* |
| trigeminal (V) | mixed | chewing movements, *sensations from head and face, proprioception* |
| abducens (VI) | mixed, primarily motor | abduction, *proprioception* |
| facial (VII) | mixed | facial expression, secretion of saliva and tears, taste, *proprioception* |
| vestibulo-cochlear (VIII) | sensory | |
| 1. auditory (or cochlear) branch | | *hearing* |
| 2. vestibular branch | | *sense of balance* |
| glossopharyngeal (IX) | mixed | secretion of saliva, *taste, control of blood pressure and respiration, proprioception* |
| vagus (X) | mixed | smooth muscle contraction and relaxation (e.g. heart) *sensations* from *organs supplied, proprioception* |
| accessory (XI) | mixed, primarily motor | movements of head, swallowing movements and voice production, *proprioception* |
| hypoglossal (XII) | mixed, primarily motor | tongue movements, *proprioception* |

tegmentum of the midbrain. Just before it enters the orbit it divides into a small superior and a larger inferior division. Both divisions penetrate into the orbit through the superior orbital fissure. In the orbit the superior division passes inward above the optic nerve to supply the superior rectus and the levator palpebrae superioris muscles. The inferior division sends branches to the medial rectus, the inferior rectus and inferior oblique muscles, as well as providing parasympathetic fibres to the sphincter pupillae and ciliary muscles via a branch to the ciliary ganglion. *See* **ganglion, ciliary; paralysis of the third nerve.**

**nerve, ophthalmic** This is the smallest of the three divisions of the trigeminal nerve, the other two being the maxillary and mandibular branches. It comes off the medial and upper part of the convex anterior border of the gasserian ganglion and just behind the superior orbital fissure it divides into three branches, the **lacrimal**, **frontal** and **nasociliary**, which pass through the fissure to enter the orbit. (1) The smallest of the three, the **lacrimal** nerve, supplies sensory fibres to the lacrimal gland, the skin of the upper eyelid and the conjunctiva. Just before reaching the gland the nerve communicates with the zygomaticotemporal nerve (itself a branch of the zygomatic nerve). This branch contains parasympathetic fibres from the facial nerve that pass to the lacrimal gland. (2) The **frontal nerve**, which is the largest of the three divisions, divides into the **supratrochlear** and **supraorbital** nerves. The supratrochlear further anastomoses with the **infratrochlear** nerve and supplies the lower part of the forehead, the upper eyelid and the conjunctiva. The infratrochlear supplies sensory fibres to the skin and conjunctiva round the inner angle of the eye, the root of the nose, the lacrimal sac and canaliculi and caruncle. The supraorbital nerve sends sensory fibres to the forehead, the upper eyelid and conjunctiva. (3) The **nasociliary** nerve gives origin to several nerves: the long ciliary nerves, the long or sensory root (ramus communicans) to the ciliary ganglion, the posterior ethmoidal nerve and the infratrochlear nerve. (Fig. N2)
*See* **ganglion, gasserian; nerve, trigeminal.**

**nerve, optic** Second cranial nerve. It forms a link in the visual pathway. It takes its origin at the retina and is made up of nearly 1.2 million fibres from the ganglion cells and some efferent fibres that end in the retina. The nerve runs backward from the eyeball and emerges from the orbit through the optic foramen, and then forms the optic chiasma. The total length of the optic nerve is 5 cm; the portion before the chiasma called intracranial being about 1 cm, the intracanalicular 6 mm, the intraorbital 3 cm and the intraocular

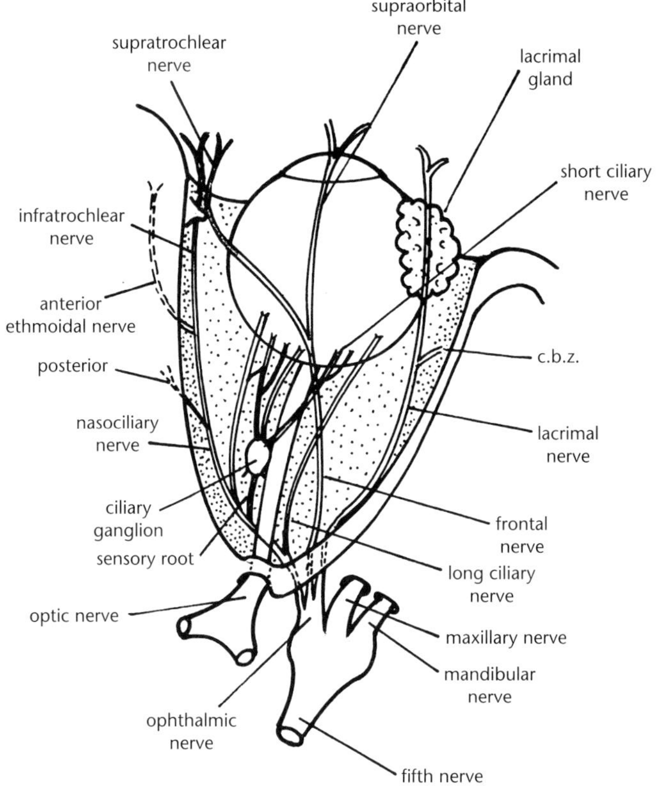


**Fig. N2** Diagram of the ophthalmic division of the trigeminal nerve (fifth). This is a view of the right eye from above (c.b.z, communicating branch to the zygomatic nerve). *Note*: the ciliary ganglion is usually situated lateral to the optic nerve

0.7 mm. The optic nerve is more often divided into only two portions: the **intraocular** (or **bulbar**) portion and the **orbital** (or **retrobulbar**) portion. (Fig. N2)
*See* **atrophy, optic; canal, optic; chiasma, optic; fibres, pupillary; neuritis, optic; neuropathy, anterior ischaemic optic; papilloedema.**

**nerve, sixth cranial** *See* **nerve, abducens.**

**nerve, supraorbital; supratrochlear** *See* **nerve, ophthalmic.**

**nerve, third cranial** *See* **nerve, oculomotor.**

**nerve, trigeminal** Fifth cranial nerve. It is the largest of the cranial nerves. It originates above the middle of the lateral surface of the pons as two divisions, a larger sensory root and a motor root. The sensory root passes to the gasserian ganglion and from that ganglion the three divisions of the fifth nerve are given off: the **ophthalmic**, **maxillary** and **mandibular** nerves. The fifth nerve is sensory to the face, the eyeball, the conjunctiva, the eyebrow, the teeth, the mucous membranes in the mouth and nose. The motor root of the nerve has no connection with the ganglion. It joins the mandibular nerve and is motor to the muscles of mastication.
*See* **ganglion, gasserian.**

**nerve, trochlear** Fourth cranial nerve. It is the most slender of the cranial nerves but with the longest intracranial course (75 mm). It is the only motor nerve which originates from the dorsal surface of the brain between the midbrain and the cerebellum. It enters the orbit through the superior orbital fissure and supplies motor fibres to the superior oblique muscle.
*See* **paralysis of the fourth nerve.**

**nerve, zygomatic** A branch of the maxillary division of the trigeminal nerve, it enters the orbit by the inferior orbital fissure and soon divides into the **zygomaticotemporal** and **zygomaticofacial** branches. The former gives a twig to the lacrimal nerve and is thought to conduct autonomic fibres to the lacrimal gland and the latter supplies the skin over the zygomatic bone.
*See* **gland, lacrimal; nerve, trigeminal.**

**nerves, short ciliary** Six to ten nerves which arise from the ciliary ganglion and are derived from the oculomotor nerve. They run a course with the short ciliary arteries, above and below the optic nerve, anastomose with each other and with the long ciliary nerves and pierce the sclera around the optic nerve. They run anteriorly between the choroid and sclera and innervate the ciliary muscle, the cornea, the iris and the sphincter pupillae muscle.
*See* **ganglion, ciliary; reflex, pupil light.**

**neural rim** A term used in describing the area of the optic disc which contains the neural elements and is located between the edge of the disc and the physiological cup. When describing the neural rim, as is often done in cases of glaucoma, one must include its colour, size, slope and uniformity.
*See* **cup, physiological; disc, optic.**

**neuritis, optic** Inflammation of the optic nerve which can occur anywhere along its course from the ganglion cells in the retina to the synapse of these cell fibres in the lateral geniculate body. If the inflammation is restricted to the optic nerve head the condition is called **papillitis** (or **intraocular optic neuritis**) and if it is located in the orbital portion of the nerve it is called **retrobulbar optic neuritis** (or **orbital optic neuritis**).
In **papillitis** the optic nerve head is hyperaemic with blurred margins and slightly oedematous. Haemorrhages and exudates may also appear. In retrobulbar optic neuritis, there are usually no visible signs in the fundus of the eye until the disease has advanced and optic atrophy may appear. However, both types are accompanied by a loss of visual acuity along with a central scotoma and impairment of colour vision. The loss of vision may occur abruptly over a few hours and recovery may be equally rapid but in other patients the loss may be slow. In **retrobulbar optic neuritis**, there is also pain on movement of the eyes and sometimes tenderness on palpation. The disease is usually unilateral although the second eye may become involved later. The disease is usually transient and full or partial recovery takes place within weeks. The primary cause of optic neuritis is multiple sclerosis but it may also be associated with severe inflammation of the retina or choroid, vitamin B deficiency, diabetes mellitus, thyroid disease, lactation, infectious diseases and toxicity.
*See* **disease, Devic's; nerve, optic; papilloedema; pupil, Marcus Gunn; rule, Kollner's; sclerosis, multiple; test, photostress.**

**neurofibromatosis type I** *See* **disease, von Recklinghausen's.**

**neuromyelitis optica** *See* **disease, Devic's.**

**neuron** Structural unit of the nervous system consisting of the nerve cell body and its various processes, the dendrites, the axon and the ending. There are many types of neurons within the nervous system; some transmit sensory **afferent** nerve impulses (e.g. those forming the visual pathway), others transmit **efferent** motor nerve impulses to a muscle (**motor neuron**). Other neurons carry nerve impulses from one neuron to another (**internuncial neurons**). *Note*: also spelt neurone.
*See* **potential, action; synapse.**

**neuroparalytic keratitis** *See* **keratitis, neuroparalytic.**

**neuropathy, ischaemic optic** An obstruction of the blood supply to the optic nerve, usually to its anterior part. It causes a sudden loss of vision. It may be due to arteriosclerosis, temporal arteritis or emboli of the ciliary circulation. Treatment depends on the cause.
*See* **arteries, ciliary; arteriosclerosis; arteritis, temporal.**

**neuropathy, Leber's optic** *See* **Leber's hereditary optic atrophy.**

**neuropathy, optic** A non-inflammatory or degenerative disease of the optic nerve.
*See* **neuritis, optic; ophthalmopathy.**

**neuroprotection** A therapeutic strategy aimed at preventing the ultimate result of a neurodegenerative disease process. *Example*: in current glaucoma therapy, the principal objective is to lower the intraocular pressure, but that appears to be only one of the risk factors that lead ultimately to death of retinal ganglion cells and visual field loss. Neuroprotection is aimed at preventing that secondary ganglion cell degeneration in glaucomatous eyes, which may have been caused as a result of inflammatory or toxic mediators released by the primary degenerative event. Neuroprotective strategies presently being evaluated include glutamate antagonists, calcium channel blockers, nitric oxide synthase inhibitors and neurotrophins.

**neurosensory retina** *See* **retina, neurosensory.**

**neurotransmitter** A substance stored in the synaptic vesicles that is released when the axon terminal is excited by a nervous impulse. The substance then travels across the synaptic cleft to either excite or inhibit another neuron. This is accomplished by either decreasing the negativity of postsynaptic potentials (excitation), or increasing the negativity of postsynaptic potentials (inhibition). Common neurotransmitters include acetylcholine, dopamine, endorphins, adrenaline (epinephrine), gamma-aminobutyric acid

(GABA), glutamic acid, noradrenaline (norepinephrine), serotonin and substance P.

**neurotrophic keratitis; keratopathy** *See* **keratopathy, neurotrophic.**

**neutral density filter** *See* **filter.**

**neutral point** *See* **point, neutral.**

**neutralization** **1.** A technique for determining the power of an ophthalmic lens. It is accomplished by placing lenses of known power and opposite sign in contact with it until the observation of movements (against or with) of the distant image seen through the lenses, which are moved back and forth in a plane perpendicular to the line of sight, disappear. The unknown lens will have the opposite power to that which neutralizes this apparent movement. **2.** A method of breaking down hydrogen peroxide from a contact lens (mostly soft) following contact lens disinfection to avoid possible irritation to ocular tissues. This can be accomplished either by rinsing and dilution or by using a platinum catalyst or with agents such as sodium pyruvate or sodium sulphite or sodium thiosulphate.
*See* **antiseptic; focimeter; lens measure.**

**nevus** *See* **naevus.**

**New Aniseikonia Test** *See* **test, New Aniseikonia.**

**Newton's formula** An expression relating the focal lengths of an optical system ($f$ and $f'$) and the object $x$ and image $x'$ distances measured from the respective focal points. Thus,

$$ff' = xx'$$

If the optical system is a lens in air $-f = f'$ and the formula becomes

$$-f^2 = xx'$$

*Syn.* Newton's equation; Newton's relation.
*See* **paraxial equation, fundamental; sign convention; theory, gaussian.**

**Newton's rings** Circular, concentric interference fringes surrounding a point of contact when two glass surfaces are pressed together. The thicker the air film separating the two surfaces the greater the number of concentric rings.

**Newton's theory** *See* **theory, Newton's.**

**newtonian telescope** *See* **telescope.**

**Nicol prism** *See* **prism, Nicol.**

**nicotine** An alkaloid which has pharmacological actions similar to those of acetylcholine at autonomic ganglia and skeletal neuromuscular junctions.
*See* **acetylcholine; cholinergic.**

**nictitating membrane** *See* **membrane, nictitating.**

**Niemann–Pick disease** *See* **disease, Niemann–Pick.**

**night blindness** *See* **hemeralopia.**

**night vision** *See* **vision, scotopic.**

**nit** *See* **candela per square metre.**

**nocturnal vision** *See* **vision, scotopic.**

**nodal plane; points** *See* under the nouns.

**nodules, Busacca's** Nodules often found in the iris stroma of an eye affected by granulomatous uveitis (up to about 30% of cases). *Syn.* floccules of Busacca.
*See* **nodules, iris; nodules, Koeppe's.**

**nodules, Dalen–Fuchs** Multiple, small yellow-white mounds consisting mainly of epithelial cells protruding through the retinal pigment epithelium. They are seen in the fundus of an eye with sympathetic ophthalmia, Vogt–Koyanagi–Harada syndrome or some other granulomatous inflammations.
*See* **ophthalmia, sympathetic; syndrome, Vogt–Koyanagi–Harada.**

**nodules, iris** Small, solid elevations found on the iris and epithelial cells and lymphocytes. They are usually whitish or grey, depending on their location.
*See* **nodules, Busacca's; nodules, Koeppe's.**

**nodules, Koeppe's** Small nodules frequently found on the iris around the pupillary margin of an eye affected by granulomatous uveitis.
*See* **nodules, iris; nodules, Busacca's; uveitis.**

**nomogram** *See* **tonography.**

**non-concomitance** *See* **incomitance.**

**non-contact tonometer** *See* **tonometer, non-contact.**

**non-invasive break-up time test** *See* **test, non-invasive break-up time.**

**non-steroidal antiinflammatory drug** *See* **anti-inflammatory drug.**

**nonius horopter** *See* **horopter, nonius.**

**noradrenaline (norepinephrine)** A neurohumoral transmitter for most postganglionic sympathetic fibres. It is produced with adrenaline (epinephrine) in the adrenal medulla. It is a powerful excitator of α-adrenergic receptors.
*See* **adrenaline (epinephrine); adrenergic receptors; miotics; mydriatic; neurotransmitter.**

**norepinephrine** *See* **noradrenaline.**

**norfloxacin** *See* **antibiotic.**

**normal retinal correspondence** *See* **retinal corresponding points.**

**normal saline** *See* **saline, physiological.**

**Norn's test** *See* **test, Norn's.**

**nose pad** *See* **pad.**

**nuclear cataract** *See* **cataract, nuclear.**

**nuclear layer, inner retinal** *See* **retina.**

**nucleus 1.** A mass of grey matter composed of nerve cell bodies in any part of the brain or spinal cord and dealing with a common function. **2.** Core or central portion of the cell body of a neuron, containing cellular DNA in particular. *See* **geniculate bodies, lateral.**

**nucleus, abducens** Nucleus of the abducens nerve (sixth cranial nerve) located in the lower part of the pons and whose axons supply the lateral rectus muscle.
*See* **nerve, abducens.**

**nucleus, accessory oculomotor** *See* **nucleus, Edinger–Westphal.**

**nucleus of the crystalline lens** *See* **lens, crystalline.**

**nucleus, Edinger–Westphal** Part of the oculomotor nucleus, it is situated posterior to the main nucleus and contains the parasympathetic component of the complex. Axons from the Edinger–Westphal pass out along the third (or oculomotor) nerve to synapse in the ciliary ganglion. Postganglionic fibres pass through the short ciliary nerves to the sphincter pupillae and ciliary muscles. The nucleus also receives fibres concerned with accommodation and fibres from the pretectal nucleus dealing with pupil light reflexes. *Syn.* accessory oculomotor nucleus; accessory parasympathetic nucleus.
*See* **ganglion, ciliary; muscle, ciliary; muscle, sphincter pupillae; nerve, oculomotor; nucleus, oculomotor; nucleus, pretectal; reflex, pupil light.**

**nucleus, lateral** Part of the oculomotor nucleus which supplies, via the oculomotor nerve, all the extraocular muscles except the superior oblique and the lateral rectus muscles.
*See* **nerve, oculomotor.**

**nucleus, oculomotor** This is the nucleus of the oculomotor nerve (third cranial nerve). It is a complex mass of cells located in the midbrain, beneath the cerebral aqueduct (of Sylvius) which connects the third and fourth ventricles. It is divided into several subnuclei.
*See* **nerve, oculomotor; nucleus, Edinger–Westphal; nucleus, Perlia's; nucleus, trochlear.**

**nucleus, Perlia's** Midline part of the oculomotor nucleus. It is rudimentary in man and primates and may provide part of the innervation of the superior rectus muscle.
*See* **nucleus, oculomotor.**

**nucleus, pretectal** A complex group of nerve cells in the midbrain anterior to the superior colliculi. One of these, the pretectal olivary nucleus, receives retinal inputs via the optic tract and superior brachium and sends axons to both Edinger–Westphal nuclei. It constitutes a centre of the pupil light reflex. Another, the nucleus of the optic tract, may be involved in the control of reflex eye movements. Other fibres from the pretectal nucleus innervate the cornea, the iris, the ciliary muscle and the extraocular mucles (except the lateral rectus and superior oblique muscles), as well as the levator palpebrae muscle. *See* **nucleus, Edinger–Westphal; reflex, pupil light.**

**nucleus, trochlear** A nucleus of the trochlear nerve (fourth cranial nerve) located at the posterior end of the oculomotor nerve nucleus, it sends fibres to the contralateral superior oblique muscle.
*See* **muscle, superior oblique; nerve, trochlear.**

**nyctalopia** *See* **hemeralopia.**

**nystagmograph** Instrument for recording the movements of the eyes in nystagmus.

**nystagmoid** Resembling nystagmus.

**nystagmus** A regular, repetitive, involuntary movement of the eye whose direction, amplitude and frequency are variable. Nystagmus can be induced, acquired or congenital. (In a very small percentage of people it can even be induced voluntarily.) These eye movements characteristically appear as one of two types: one in which there is a slow and fast phase and the nystagmus is conventionally defined by the direction of the fast phase. Such nystagmus is called a **jerk nystagmus**. A feature of jerk nystagmus is the **null zone** (or **null point**) which represents the direction of gaze at which the nystagmus has the smallest amplitude. A jerk nystagmus is usually due to a motor defect that may be induced by brainstem or cerebellar lesions, drug intoxication (**upbeat nystagmus** in which the fast phase is in the upward direction or **downbeat nystagmus** in which the fast phase is downward); associated with a lesion of the central nervous system or the vestibular nerve or nuclei (**central nystagmus** and **vestibular nystagmus**); or to disease or injury to the labyrinth (**labyrinth nystagmus**); or to multiple sclerosis. Jerk nystagmus can also be induced physiologically, as for example **optokinetic nystagmus** (OKN) or **train nystagmus** which occurs when watching objects which traverse the visual field

rapidly, or as a result of thermal stimulation of the labyrinth of the inner ear by cold or hot water (**caloric nystagmus** or **Barany's nystagmus**), or when the eyes of a fatigued person are turned into an extreme position of gaze (**end-point nystagmus**), or when a person who had been spinning round is stopped (**vestibular nystagmus**).
The other type is a nystagmus which is characterized by movements of equal velocity in each direction and this is called a **pendular nystagmus**. A pendular nystagmus usually occurs as a result of poor central vision (**sensory deprivation nystagmus**) as in bilateral chorioretinitis, total colour blindness, albinism, congenital cataract, corneal scarring, amblyopia (**amblyopic nystagmus**) or in coal miners after many years of working in the dark (**miner's nystagmus**). In some cases one eye rotates upward and intorts while the other rotates downward, and extorts (**see-saw nystagmus** as a result of brainstem stroke, chiasmal lesion or multiple sclerosis). In some cases there is a mixture of the two main types; pendular in the primary position and jerk on lateral gaze (**mixed nystagmus**). The movements of the eyes are usually the same in both eyes (**conjugate nystagmus**) but in other cases they may be unrelated as a result of internuclear ophthalmoplegia (**dissociated nystagmus**). Examples of the latter are **end-gaze nystagmus, convergence-retraction nystagmus** and **see-saw nystagmus**. Or the eye movements are of equal amplitude and type but in opposite or different directions (**disjunctive nystagmus**), also commonly associated with internuclear ophthalmoplegia. There are also cases of unknown origin (**idiopathic nystagmus**).
*See* **ataxia, hereditary spinal; disease, Wernicke's; monochromat; optokinetic; oscillopia; prisms, yoke; reflex, vestibulo-ocular; syndrome, Down's; test, optokinetic nystagmus.**

**nystagmus blockage syndrome** *See* **syndrome, nystagmus blockage.**

**nystagmus, caloric** *See* **caloric testing.**

**nystagmus, congenital** A motor nystagmus which is present at birth or soon after. It may be inherited as X-linked recessive or autosomal dominant, or induced in the uterus, and results from decreased vision due to corneal opacity, cataract, albinism, aniridia, macular disease or optic atrophy. It is typically a horizontal jerk nystagmus and it may be associated with abnormal head movement and decreases in intensity with convergence. The visual prognosis is reasonably good, but if the head turn is excessive, extraocular muscle surgery may be needed.

**nystagmus, convergence-retraction** A jerk nystagmus which appears on attempted upward gaze and in which the fast phase brings the two eyes towards each other in a convergent movement with retraction of the globes into the orbit. It may result from a lesion affecting the tectum or dorsal midbrain or a pineal tumour, or form part of Parinaud's syndrome.
*See* **pinealoma; syndrome, Parinaud's; tectum of the mesencephalon.**

**nystagmus, occlusion** A form of nystagmus occurring when one eye is covered, or which increases in intensity when one eye is covered. The nystagmus is typically of the horizontal, jerk variety, with the fast phase occurring in the direction of the occluded eye.

**nystagmus, physiological** *See* **movements, fixation.**

**nystagmus, rotary** A very rare form of nystagmus in which the eyeball makes a movement about the visual axis. It may result from a lesion to the vestibular nerve.
*See* **nystagmus, vestibular.**

**nystagmus, sensory** A form of nystagmus thought to be due to an abnormality in the afferent mechanism. It is most often due to inadequate image stimulation of the macula, leading to abnormal development of the ocular fixation reflex. Causes include congenital cataracts, optic nerve hypoplasia, aniridia, albinism, achromatopsia, as well as Leber's congenital amaurosis.

**nystagmus, vestibular** There are two main types of vestibular nystagmus: **Peripheral vestibular nystagmus** results from stimulation, injury or disease (e.g. Menière's disease) of the labyrinth or of the vestibulo-cochlear nerve (VIII). It presents as a jerk, mainly horizontal, nystagmus with a torsional component. It may be accompanied by vertigo, tinnitus and hearing loss. Fixation inhibits the nystagmus. **Central vestibular nystagmus** results from stimulation, injury, disease of the central vestibular pathways of the brainstem or the cerebellum, or lesion of the vestibular nuclei. It is typically a jerk nystagmus, which can be purely horizontal, vertical or torsional. It is not inhibited by fixation.

**nystatin** *See* **antifungal agent.**

# O

**object** **1.** Something that has a fixed shape or form that you can touch or see. **2.** Anything from which an image is formed by an optical system. *See* **image; object, extended.**

**object, extended** An object consisting of many point objects separated laterally to form a certain shape (e.g. trees, people).
*See* **light, beam of; light, pencil of; object, point; size, angular; source, extended.**

**object plane** *See* **plane, object.**

**object, point** A small component of an extended object, in relation to an optical system. If the point object is situated on the axis of an optical system it gives rise to the axial ray and it is referred to as the **axial point object.**
*See* **light, pencil of; object, extended; ray, axial.**

**object, real** An object from which emergent rays diverge.
*See* **image, real.**

**object of regard** *See* **fixation, point of.**

**object space** Region on one side of an optical system or a lens in which the object is situated.
*See* **image space.**

**object, virtual** One towards which incident rays are converging after refraction or reflection. *Example*: a positive lens forms an image of an object placed beyond its anterior focal point. Introducing a mirror between the lens and the image makes that image become a virtual object.
*See* **image, virtual.**

**objective** An optical system or a lens used to provide a real image of an object. In cameras this image is situated on the film but in viewing instruments (telescopes, microscopes, etc.) this image is seen through an eyepiece. *Syn.* objective lens.
*See* **aperture, numerical; eyepiece; microscope; telescope.**

**objective refraction** *See* **refraction, objective.**

**oblique astigmatism; effect** *See* under the nouns.

**oblique illumination shadow test** *See* **test, shadow.**

**oblique muscles** *See* **muscle, superior oblique; muscle, inferior oblique.**

**occipital cortex; lobe** *See* under the nouns.

**occluder** A device placed before an eye to block vision or to partially obscure vision. *Syn.* eye shield.

**occlusion** The act of blocking vision with an occluder.

**occlusion amblyopia** *See* **amblyopia; occlusion treatment.**

**occlusion nystagmus** *See* **nystagmus, occlusion.**

**occlusion, punctal** Sealing of the lacrimal punctum, temporarily (e.g. with a plastic plug) or permanently (e.g. by heat cauterization), to preserve the natural tears or prolong the effect of artificial tears. This method is commonly used in the management of keratoconjunctivitis sicca.
*See* **keratitis sicca; keratopathy, neurotrophic.**

**occlusion, retinal arterial** *See* **retinal arterial occlusion.**

**occlusion, retinal vein** *See* **retinal vein occlusion.**

**occlusion test** *See* **test, cover.**

**occlusion treatment** A method of treating amblyopia or strabismus by covering the good eye or preferred eye. Such a method is most effective below the age of 4 years and with little effect after the age of 9 years. However, this technique must be used with caution as prolonged occlusion in very young children can lead to a reversal of eye dominance in which the previously good eye becomes amblyopic (called **occlusion amblyopia**). Alternate occlusion is preferred as both eyes are thus stimulated.
*See* **amblyopia; dominance, ocular; penalization; pleoptics; strabismus.**

**octave** The interval between two frequencies having a ratio of two to one. *Example*: from 4 to 8 c/deg. Two octaves is a quadrupling of frequencies, and so on. Octaves are commonly used in specifying the bandwidth of the frequencies (e.g. spatial frequencies) to which cells in the visual pathway respond.
*See* **cycle per degree.**

**ocular** **1.** *See* **eyepiece. 2.** Appertains to eye.

**ocular adnexa** *See* **appendages of the eye.**

**ocular albinism; appendages; apraxia; bobbing; column; cup; decongestant; dominance; dysmetria; flutter; fundus; headache; hypertension; hypotonia; impression; media;**

**myoclonus; pathology; pemphigoid; prosthesis** *See* under the nouns.

**ocular myopathy** *See* **ophthalmoplegia.**

**ocular refraction** *See* **refractive error.**

**ocular tension** *See* **pressure, intraocular.**

**ocular tremors of fixation** *See* **movements, fixation.**

**ocularist** One who designs and fits artificial eyes. *See* **eye, artificial; prosthesis, ocular.**

**oculist** *See* **ophthalmologist.**

**oculocardiac reflex** *See* **reflex, oculocardiac.**

**oculocentre** Pertaining to the eye as a centre of reference.
*See* **direction, oculocentric; egocentre; localization.**

**oculocentric direction; localization** *See* under the nouns.

**oculocutaneous albinism** *See* **albinism.**

**oculocutaneous melanosis; melanocytosis** *See* **naevus of Ota.**

**oculogyric** Pertaining to movement of the eye about the anteroposterior axis.

**oculogyric crisis (OCG)** Sudden involuntary contractions of some eye muscles resulting in repetitive, conjugate ocular deviations, usually, though not always, in an upward direction. The attack or crisis may last from seconds to minutes. It occurs most frequently after the use of neuroleptic medication, but it may be precipitated or accompany, emotional stress, alcohol or general fatigue.

**oculomotor** Pertaining to movement of the eyes, or to the oculomotor nerve.

**oculomotor nerve** *See* **nerve, oculomotor.**

**oculomotor paralysis** *See* **paralysis of the third nerve.**

**oculomycosis** Any disease of the eye caused by a fungus.
*See* **antifungal agent; keratitis; keratomycosis.**

**oculorotary muscles** *See* **muscles, extraocular.**

**oculus** Latin for eye. *Plural*: oculi.

**oculus dexter (OD)** Latin for right eye.

**oculus sinister (OS)** Latin for left eye.

**oculus uterque (OU)** Latin for both eyes.

**oedema** The presence of an excessive amount of fluid in or around cells, tissues or serous cavities of the body. In the eye oedema can occur in the cornea, the conjunctiva, the uvea, the retina, the choroid, and the ciliary body. Corneal oedema usually accompanies eye diseases, or contact lens wear with low oxygen transmissibility. Corneal oedema is easily seen with a slit-lamp using retroillumination or sclerotic scatter illumination. Quantitatively, it can be assessed with the addition of a pachometer that measures corneal swelling. Beyond about 4% swelling, there appear **striae** (wispy greyish-white lines usually vertical) in the stroma. Beyond about 8% swelling, there appear **folds** (dark lines) believed to represent physical buckling of the posterior corneal layers. Corneal swelling of 15% or greater, which indicates a gross separation of the collagen fibres of the stroma, results in a hazy or cloudy appearance of the cornea. There is a physiological oedema occurring during sleep in every human cornea amounting to an increase in thickness of about 4%. Corneal oedema gives rise to the appearance of haloes around lights, photophobia, spectacle blur, losses in corneal transparency and sometimes stinging. Management depends on the cause and tissue involved. If due to contact lenses, refitting with daily wear lenses of higher oxygen transmissibility and reducing wearing time usually solves the problem. *Note*: also spelt edema.
*See* **blebs, endothelial; clouding, central corneal; hypoxia; lens, silicone hydrogel; oxygen permeability; oxygen requirement, critical; pachometer; stria; syndrome, overwear.**

**oedema, cystoid macular (CMO)** Oedema and cyst formation of the macular area of the retina. It may occur as a result of, or be associated with, systemic vascular disease, retinal vein occlusion, diabetic retinopathy, uveitis, retinitis pigmentosa and following some ocular surgery such as vitreoretinal, photocoagulation, glaucoma procedures and especially cataract surgery. When cystoid macular oedema follows cataract surgery it is called the **Irvine–Gass syndrome** and it is sometimes accompanied by intraoperative vitreous loss or vitreous adhesion to the iris or to the corneoscleral wound. Visual acuity is affected initially but recovers in the majority of cases. In some cases antiinflammatory therapy may help in restoring visual acuity and in other cases the vitreous adhesion may be disrupted with a Nd-Yag laser.

**ofloxacin** *See* **antibiotic.**

**Oguchi's disease** *See* **disease, Oguchi's.**

**olopatadine hydrochloride** *See* **mast cell stabilizers.**

**ommatidium** One of the visual elements of the compound eye of arthropods.
*See* **eye, compound.**

**onchocerciasis** A disease caused by infestation with the filarial worm (*Onchocerca volvulus*) spread by blackflies. It is common in tropical Africa and Central America, especially in areas near rivers. Large numbers of microfilariae are present on the skin and often enter the eye. The patient initially complains of itching, but blindness occurs as a result of chorioretinitis and optic neuritis. The disease is treated successfully with ivermectin. *Syn.* onchocercosis; river blindness.

**'one and one half' syndrome** *See* **syndrome, 'one and one half'.**

**opacity** The condition of a tissue or structure which is not transparent, or being opaque. The location of an opacity within the eye can be determined with a slit-lamp. It can also be determined using an ophthalmoscope and asking the patient to look up or down. If the opacity moves very little, or not at all, it is situated in the lens. If the opacity moves in the same direction as the eye it is situated in front of the lens and if it moves in the opposite direction it is situated in the vitreous humour.
*See* **cataract; density, optical; muscae volitantes; transparent; ulcer, corneal.**

**opaque** Impervious to the passage of light.
*See* **transparent.**

**open-angle glaucoma** *See* **glaucoma, open-angle.**

**operculum** A flap of detached retina which projects forward, or is totally free in the vitreous.

**ophryosis** Spasmodic twitching in the region of the eyebrow.
*See* **eyebrow.**

**ophthalmagra** A sudden pain in the eye.

**ophthalmia** Inflammation of the eye, particularly of the conjunctiva.
*See* **conjunctivitis.**

**ophthalmia neonatorum** An acute conjunctivitis that occurs in the first month of life as a result of infection acquired in the birth canal. The most common causes are *Chlamydia trachomatis, Streptococcus pneumoniae, Neisseria gonorrhoeae, Staphylococcus aureus* and herpes simplex virus. The eyelids are swollen and stuck together by purulent discharge. If the cause is gonococcal, loss of the eye is a real and immediate threat. A gonococcal infection develops within 2–4 days after birth, whereas a chlamydial infection normally appears 5–14 days after birth. Differential diagnosis is facilitated by laboratory tests (e.g. Gram staining of conjunctival scrapings). Management depends on the cause: systemic erythromycin and topical tetracycline for chlamydial infection, ceftriaxone or cefotaxime for gonococcal infection, and eye irrigation with saline solution. *Syn.* blennorrhoea neonatorum; gonococcal ophthalmia; neonatal conjunctivitis.
*See* **conjunctivitis, acute; conjunctivitis, adult inclusion.**

**ophthalmia, sympathetic** A rare, bilateral inflammation of the uveal tract that usually follows perforation of one eye. The inflammation occurs first in the injured eye (called the **exciting eye**) and soon follows in the other eye (called the **sympathetic eye**). *Syn.* sympathetic ophthalmitis.
*See* **enucleation; eye, sympathetic.**

**ophthalmic** Pertaining to the visual apparatus and its function.

**ophthalmic artery** *See* **artery, ophthalmic.**

**ophthalmic crown** *See* **glass, crown.**

**ophthalmic cup** *See* **cup, optic.**

**ophthalmic Graves' disease** *See* **disease, Graves'.**

**ophthalmic lens; nerve** *See* under the nouns.

**ophthalmic optician** *See* **optician; optometrist.**

**ophthalmic optics** *See* **optics, ophthalmic.**

**ophthalmic zoster** *See* **herpes zoster ophthalmicus.**

**ophthalmitis, sympathetic** *See* **ophthalmia, sympathetic.**

**ophthalmodynamometer (ODM)** **1.** Instrument for measuring the near point of convergence of the eyes. **2.** Instrument for measuring the blood pressure of the central retinal artery. There are two types: the compression type (e.g. Bailliart's ophthalmodynamometer) in which the pressure is raised by pressing on the eye, the force being produced by a spring-loaded plunger resting on the temporal bulbar conjunctiva of the anaesthetized eye, while the examiner observes the optic nerve through an ophthalmoscope. The other type is by suction in which negative pressure is applied to the eye using a scleral vacuum cup near the limbus (e.g. Doppler's ophthalmodynamometer). The diastolic pressure is read from the gauge provided with the instrument when the central retinal artery is seen to pulsate on the optic disc and the systolic pressure is read when all arterial pulsations just cease (the instrument should be removed immediately afterwards). A low systolic pressure is indicative of an occlusive disease of the carotid artery (a comparison between the two eyes is also very informative) as such disorders are responsible for a significant percentage of ocular symptoms and strokes.
*See* **amaurosis fugax; plaques, Hollenhorst's.**

**ophthalmologist** A medical specialist who practises ophthalmology. *Syn.* oculist (this term is rarely used nowadays); ophthalmic surgeon.

**ophthalmology** Part of medical science concerned with the medical and surgical care of the eye and its appendages.

**ophthalmometer** *See* **keratometer.**

**ophthalmopathy** Any eye disease. **External ophthalmopathy** refers to any disease of the conjunctiva, cornea, eyelids or the appendages of the eye. **Internal ophthalmopathy** refers to any disease of the lens, retina or other internal structures of the eye.

**ophthalmopathy, thyroid** Disease of the thyroid gland which leads to ocular manifestations. There are two main types: mild and severe. The mild type occurs in Graves' disease in which most or some of the typical signs may be present and to a different extent. The severe type is much less common and affects the sexes equally in middle age. All the signs of Graves' disease are present but are more pronounced with the addition of oedema of the eyelids and of the conjunctiva, conjunctival injection, enlargement of the extraocular muscles and in a few cases there is also optic neuropathy due to compression of the optic nerve or its blood supply with consequent visual loss, colour vision impairment and often diplopia. *Syn.* dysthyroid eye disease; thyroid eye disease.
*See* **accommodative insufficiency; disease, Graves'; keratoconjunctivitis, superior limbic; neuropathy, optic.**

**ophthalmophakometer** Optical instrument modified from the keratometer using the principle of Purkinje images and designed to measure the radii of curvature and positions of the surfaces of the crystalline lens and the cornea.
*See* **images, Purkinje–Sanson; keratometer; phacoscope.**

**ophthalmoplegia** Paralysis of the ocular muscles. **External ophthalmoplegia** refers to paralysis of one or more extraocular muscles. If the levator palpebrae muscle is also involved, the condition is usually referred to as **ocular myopathy**. **Internal ophthalmoplegia** refers to a paralysis of the muscles of the iris and the ciliary muscle. **Total ophthalmoplegia** refers to a paralysis of all the muscles in the eye which results in ptosis, immobility of the eye and pupil, and loss of accommodation.
*See* **disease, Graves'; muscles, extraocular; paralysis of the third nerve.**

**ophthalmoplegia, internuclear (INO)** An eye movement disorder resulting from a lesion in the medial longitudinal fasciculus which disrupts the coordination between the oculomotor nucleus and the abducens nucleus. It is characterized by a limited adduction by the eye on the same side of the body as the lesion, and a jerky, horizontal nystagmus by the other eye on abduction, when moving the eyes towards the side of the body opposite to that of the lesion. Convergence is usually intact, unless the lesion is widespread. Vertical gaze gives rise to nystagmus and oscillopia. The condition is associated with multiple sclerosis, vascular disease, tumour of the brainstem or encephalitis.
*See* **palsy, supranuclear gaze; syndrome, 'one and one half '.**

**ophthalmorrhagia** Ocular haemorrhage.

**ophthalmorrhoea** A discharge of mucus, pus or blood from the eye. *Note*: also spelt ophthalmorrhea.

**ophthalmoscope** An instrument for viewing the media and fundus of the eye. It consists essentially of: (1) a light source (a halogen or tungsten bulb), a condenser system, a lens and a reflector (a prism, mirror, or metallic plate) to illuminate the interior of the eye, and (2) a viewing system comprising a sight hole and focusing system (usually a rack of lenses of different powers) to compensate for the combined errors of refraction of the patient and the practitioner.
*See* **ophthalmoscope, direct; ophthalmoscope, indirect; transillumination; Visuscope.**

**ophthalmoscope, binocular indirect (BIO)** An indirect ophthalmoscope with a binocular viewing system for obtaining a magnified, inverted, stereoscopic image of the fundus. It consists of a light source mounted above and between the examiner's eyes on a headset. This illuminates a hand-held condensing lens of high positive power close to the patient's eyes which forms an image of the patient's pupil in both of the examiner's pupils. An aerial image of the patient's fundus is formed between the condensing lens and the examiner (if the patient is emmetropic the image will be formed in the focal plane of the condensing lens). It appears inverted and stereoscopically through the oculars attached to the headset. Stereopsis is obtained by reducing the interpupillary distance by means of mirrors or prisms within the headset of the instrument. This ophthalmoscope allows examination of a wide area of fundus and perception of depressed and raised areas.

**ophthalmoscope, direct** An ophthalmoscope that provides a virtual, erect image with a magnification of about ×15 of the fundus, formed by the patient's eye in combination with whatever focusing lenses are needed to correct for the refractive errors of the observer and patient. The instrument is held at close range to the patient's eye and the field of view is small (less

**Table O1** Comparison between direct and indirect ophthalmoscopes

| ophthalmoscope | form | image | field of view (in degrees) | magnification |
|---|---|---|---|---|
| direct | monocular | erect | 8 | ×15 |
| indirect | monocular | inverted | 20 | ×5 to × 7 |
| indirect | binocular | inverted | 40–75 | ×1.5 to × 4.5* |

*Varies according to the power of the condensing lens.

than 10°) (Fig. O1). The magnification $M$ of a direct ophthalmoscope is equal to

$$M = \frac{F_e}{4}$$

where $F_e$ is the power of the eye. *Example*: the magnification of the fundus of an aphakic eye of +40.00 D is equal to 40/4 = 10X.

**ophthalmoscope, indirect** An ophthalmoscope that provides an aerial image of the fundus (and not the fundus itself as with a direct ophthalmoscope) which is real, inverted, with a magnification of ×5 to ×7 and formed at approximately arm's length from the practitioner. This aerial image is usually produced by a strong positive lens ranging in power from + 13 D to + 30 D that is held in front of the patient's eye. The practitioner views this aerial image through a sight hole with a focusing lens to compensate for ametropia and accommodation. This instrument provides a large field of view (25–40°) and allows easier examination of the periphery of the retina. This instrument has been supplanted by the binocular indirect ophthalmoscope. The magnification of an indirect ophthalmoscope $M$ is equal to

$$M = \frac{F_e}{F_c}$$

where $F_e$ and $F_c$ are the powers of the eye and of the condensing lens, respectively. *Example*: using a condensing lens of +15.00 D to view the fundus of an emmetropic eye yields a magnification of 60/15 = 4X.
*See* **camera, fundus; image, aerial; image, inverted; ophthalmoscope, binocular indirect.**

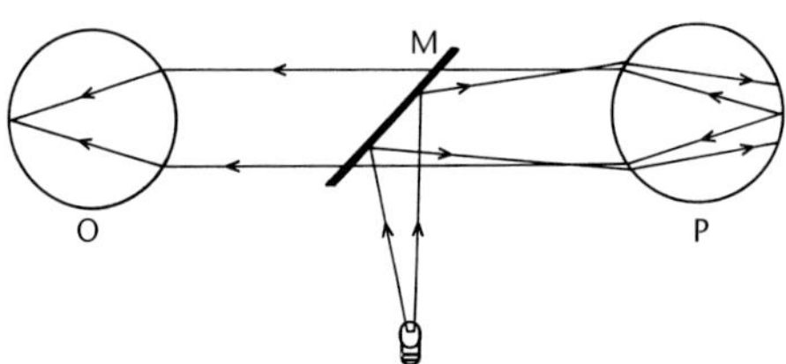


**Fig. O1** Optical principle of the simplest form of direct ophthalmoscope (O, observer's eye; P, patient's eye; M, semi-silvered mirror)

**ophthalmoscope, scanning laser (SLO)** An ophthalmoscope which provides a continuous image of the ocular fundus on a TV monitor. It consists of a narrow laser beam which is scanned horizontally and vertically to produce a rectangular area (called a raster) on the retina. A small beam of light is reflected back out of the eye to a light detector which monitors the brightness of each point on the raster and relays the information to the corresponding element on a TV monitor where the image can be viewed and/or stored. Low illumination is used to make this procedure more comfortable than conventional photography and mydriatics are usually unnecessary. The field of view extends up to 40 degrees. The instrument has been especially valuable in diagnosing glaucoma and research.

**ophthalmoscopy** Method of examination of the interior of the eye with an ophthalmoscope.

**ophthalmoscopy, red-free** Method of ophthalmoscopy using a blue-green filter in the illumination system. This gives a better contrast between the retinal vessels and the background and helps to differentiate more easily between retinal and choroidal lesions: retinal lesions appear black while choroidal ones appear grey. However, in most ophthalmoscopes which use tungsten filament bulbs, the amount of light of short wavelength is so small that the observation is difficult and a filter which lets more long wavelengths pass is used, such as a yellow-green one. As a result of this compromise there is only a slight increase in contrast between the retinal vessels and the background.

**Oppel–Kundt visual illusion** *See* **illusion, Oppel–Kundt visual.**

**opponent-colour cells** *See* **cells, colour-opponent.**

**opponent-colour theory** *See* **theory, Hering's of colour vision.**

**opsin** *See* **rhodopsin.**

**opsoclonus** Involuntary, chaotic movements of both eyes in horizontal and vertical directions. It may be a sign of cerebellar disease.
*See* **flutter, ocular; myoclonus, ocular.**

**optic** Pertaining to light or to vision.

**optic atrophy; canal; chiasma; cup; disc; disc coloboma** *See* under the nouns.

**optic fibre** *See* **optics, fibre.**

**optic foramen** *See* **canal, optic.**

**optic nerve** *See* **nerve, optic.**

**optic nerve head** *See* **disc, optic.**

**optic neuritis; neuropathy; neuropathy, ischaemic; pit** *See* under the nouns.

**optic portion of a scleral lens** *See* **transition.**

**optic radiations** *See* **radiations, optic.**

**optic stalk** *See* **cup, optic.**

**optic sulcus** *See* **pit, optic.**

**optic tracts; vesicle** *See* under the nouns.

**optic tectum** *See* **tectum of the mesencephalon.**

**optic zone, central** Central region of a contact lens that has a prescribed optical effect where there is a peripheral optic zone or zones (British Standard).
*See* **diameter, total; lens, contact; optic zone diameter.**

**optic zone diameter** Diameter of the optic zone (front or back) of a contact lens measured to the surrounding junction. It is commonly specified in millimetres. Specifically, there are the **back optic zone diameter** (BOZD), formerly called back central optic diameter (BCOD), and the front optic zone diameter (FOZD). It is often difficult to measure these dimensions due to the blending of the line separating the zones, especially for the back optic zone diameter. The region surrounding the central optic zone is the **peripheral zone**. If there is more than one, the zones will be numbered first, second, etc., beginning with the zone immediately surrounding the central optic zone. The diameter of each peripheral zone is referred to as the **back** (or front) **peripheral zone diameter** (BPZD).
*See* **blending; diameter, total; edge lift; optic zone, central; optic zone radius, back.**

**optic zone radius, back (BOZR)** Radius of curvature of the back optic zone of a contact lens. (It was formerly called the back central optic radius (BCOR or BC) or posterior central curve radius (PCCR).) If the optic zone is surrounded by a peripheral zone there will be a radius of curvature of a back peripheral zone (BPR). If there are several zones there will be $BPR_1$, $BPR_2$, etc., beginning with the zone immediately surrounding the central optic zone.
*See* **method, Drysdale's; optic zone, central; optic zone diameter; radiuscope; Toposcope.**

**optical aid** *See* **appliance, optical.**

**optical anisotropy; axis; centre** *See* under the nouns.

**optical centre position, standard** *See* **centre, standard optical position.**

**optical density; dispensing; illusion** *See* under the nouns.

**optical interface** A plane or surface forming a common boundary between two optical media.

**optical medium** *See* **medium, optical.**

**optical microspherometer** *See* **radiuscope.**

**optical surface** Surface at which light is either refracted or reflected, or both simultaneously.

**optical system** *See* **system, optical.**

**optical system, compound** *See* **system, compound optical.**

**optical wedge** *See* **wedge, optical.**

**optical zone of cornea** A theoretical zone of about 4 mm in diameter in the centre of the cornea. It is assumed to be spherical for clinical purposes.
*Syn.* corneal cap.
*See* **apex, corneal.**

**optician 1.** One who designs and makes optical instruments or lenses. **2.** Dispensing optician. **3.** Ophthalmic optician.

**optician, dispensing** One who fits and adapts spectacles and contact lenses on the basis of a prescription by an ophthalmologist or optometrist (or ophthalmic optician). In many countries dispensing opticians cut and edge lenses and fit them into a frame.
*See* **dispensing, optical; glazing.**

**optician, manufacturing** One who makes optical or ophthalmic instruments, lenses, prisms or spectacles.

**optician, ophthalmic** *See* **optometrist.**

**optician–optometrist** *See* **optometrist.**

**optics** Branch of physics which deals with the phenomena of light and/or the elements of an optical system. It also includes, sometimes, the phenomenon of vision.
*See* **theory, gaussian; theory, Newton's; theory, quantum; theory, wave.**

**optics, dispensing** *See* **optics, ophthalmic.**

**optics, fibre** A fine flexible glass or plastic rod which transmits light longitudinally by repeated total internal reflection. By using a bundle of such fibres in a fixed array, a complete image

can be transmitted. As total internal reflection can occur even if the fibres are curved, the system is of great value for viewing or photographing inaccessible objects, such as internal organs of the body. *Syn.* fibre optic (although strictly this term is an adjective, e.g. a fibre optic cable, whereas the term fibre optics is a noun).
*See* **angle, critical; endoscope.**

**optics, first-order** *See* **optics, paraxial.**

**optics, gaussian** *See* **optics, paraxial.**

**Table O2** Common optical symbols

| Symbol | Meaning |
|---|---|
| *f, f'* | primary and secondary focal lengths |
| *h, h'* | object and image sizes |
| *i, i'* | angles of incidence or reflection and refraction |
| *k, k'* | distances from the corneal pole to the far point and to the retina, respectively |
| *l, l'* | distances of object and image from the optical system |
| *n, n'* | refractive indices of object and image space |
| *u, u'* or *w, w'* or *α, α'* | angular size of object and image |
| *x, x'* | distances between object and first focal point, and image and second focal point, respectively |
| *r* | radius of curvature |
| *C* | centre of curvature |
| *A* | ocular accommodation |
| $A_s$ | spectacle accommodation |
| *Amp* | amplitude of accommodation |
| Add | addition for near vision |
| B | dioptric distance to near point of accommodation, measured from the eye |
| D | dioptre |
| *d* | vertex distance |
| *d* or *dec* | decentration |
| *F* | power |
| $F_c$ | power of a contact lens correction |
| $F_e$ | equivalent power; power of the eye |
| $F_{sp}$ | power of a spectacle lens correction |
| $F_v$, $F'_v$ | front and back vertex power |
| *K* | ocular correction |
| *K'* | vergence of the retina or dioptric length of the eye |
| *E, E'* | centres of entrance and exit pupils |
| *L, L'* | object and image vergences |
| *M* or *m* | magnification |
| *F, F'* | first and second focal points |
| *N, N'* | first and second nodal points |
| *P, P'* | first and second principal points |
| *RSM* | relative spectacle magnification |
| *SM* | spectacle magnification |
| *ε* or *P* | refractive power of a prism |
| Δ | prism dioptre |

**optics, geometrical** The branch of optics which deals with the tracing of light rays through optical systems.
*See* **sign convention; theory, gaussian.**

**optics, mechanical** *See* **optics, ophthalmic.**

**optics, ophthalmic 1.** The branch of optics which deals with the design, measurement, assembly and fitting of lenses, spectacles, contact lenses, as well as optical aids for low vision patients. *Syn.* dispensing optics; mechanical optics. **2.** In the UK and the Republic of Ireland it is used as a synonym for optometry.
*See* **dispensing, optical; optometry.**

**optics, paraxial** A simplified representation of geometrical optics which deals only with paraxial rays and in which the law of refraction and the fundamental paraxial equation are applicable. *Syn.* first-order optics; gaussian optics.
*See* **law, Lagrange's; law of refraction; paraxial equation, fundamental; ray, paraxial.**

**optics, physical** The branch of optics which deals with the nature of light and with the phenomena of diffraction, interference, polarization and velocity of light.
*See* **theory, quantum; theory, wave.**

**optics, physiological** The branch of optics concerned with physiological, psychological and optical aspects of visual perception.

**optics, visual** Branch of optics and optometry which deals with the dioptric system of the eye and its correction.

**optogram** Trace left on the retina by a retinal image due to the bleaching of rhodopsin.

**optokinetic** Term referring to movements of the eyes in response to the movement of objects across the visual field. *Example*: optokinetic nystagmus.
*See* **nystagmus; reflex, vestibulo-ocular.**

**optokinetic drum** *See* **test, optokinetic nystagmus.**

**optokinetic nystagmus** *See* **nystagmus.**

**optokinetic nystagmus test** *See* **test, optokinetic nystagmus.**

**optokinetic reflex** *See* **reflex, vestibulo-ocular.**

**optokinetoscope** *See* **test, optokinetic nystagmus.**

**optometer** Instrument for measuring the refractive state of the eye. There are two main types of optometers: subjective and objective. **Subjective** optometers rely upon the subject's judgement of sharpness or blurredness of a test object while **objective** ones contain an optical system which determines the vergence of light reflected from

the subject's retina. Electronic optometers in which all data appear digitally within a brief period of time after the operator has activated a signal can be of either type. Objective types (also called **autorefractors** or **autorefractometers**) have become very popular and many of these autorefractors are now providing both objective and subjective systems within the same instrument. *Syn.* refractometer.
*See* **accommodation, objective; Analyser, Humphrey Vision; autorefraction; optometer, infrared; photorefraction; refractive error.**

**optometer, Badal's** A simple, subjective optometer consisting of a single positive lens and a movable target. The vergence of light from the target, after refraction through the lens, depends upon the position of the target. The patient is instructed to move the target towards the lens from a position where it appears blurred until it becomes clear. That point (converted in dioptric value) represents the refraction of the patient's eye. This is a crude and inaccurate instrument, in which the measurement is marred by accommodation, variation in retinal image size with target distance, large depth of focus, non-linearity of the scale, etc. Badal's improvement was to place the lens so that its focal point coincides with either the nodal point of the eye or the anterior focal point of the eye or the entrance pupil of the eye, thus overcoming the problems of the non-linear scale and the changing retinal image size (Fig. O2).
*See* **refractive error.**

**optometer of Fincham, coincidence** An objective optometer which forms the image of an illuminated fine line target on the retina by passing through a small, peripheral portion of the pupil. The examiner views through a telescope with an optical doubling system which splits the visual field into two. If the incident beam of light is not in focus on the retina the reflected beam will not be along the optical axis and the two half-lines will be seen out of alignment. Adjusting the dioptric value of the target in order to obtain alignment gives a measure of the ametropia.

**optometer, infrared** An optometer which uses infrared light rather than visible light. This is done so that the target used in the optometer is invisible to the patient. Otherwise when it is altered it tends to become a stimulus to accommodation. However, the instrument must be corrected for the chromatic aberration of the eye. Most modern optometers use infrared light. They are based on one of three principles: (1) retinoscopy, (2) Scheiner's experiment, (3) ophthalmoscopy (indirect).
*See* **experiment, Scheiner's; optometer; ophthalmoscopy; retinoscope.**

**optometer, objective; subjective** *See* **optometer.**

**optometer, Young's** A simple optometer consisting of a single positive lens and using the Scheiner's disc principle. The target is either a single point of light or a thread which is moved back and forth until it is seen singly by the observer. When the target is out of focus, it is seen double and slightly blurred.
*See* **experiment, Scheiner's.**

**optometric physician** *See* **optometrist**.

**optometrist** A person trained in the practice of optometry. The **World Council of Optometry** defines optometrists as 'the primary healthcare practitioners of the eye and visual system who provide comprehensive eye and vision care, which includes refraction and dispensing, the detection/diagnosis and management of diseases in the eye, and the rehabilitation of conditions of the visual system'. *Syn.* ophthalmic optician (term used principally in the UK and the Republic of Ireland); optician–optometrist (term used in some European countries); optometric physician (term used in some US states, especially where therapeutic drugs are used).

**optometry** An autonomous, healthcare profession involved in the services and care of the eye and visual system, and the enhancement of visual performance. *Syn.* ophthalmic optics (term used principally in the UK and the Republic of Ireland).
*See* **optometry, primary care.**

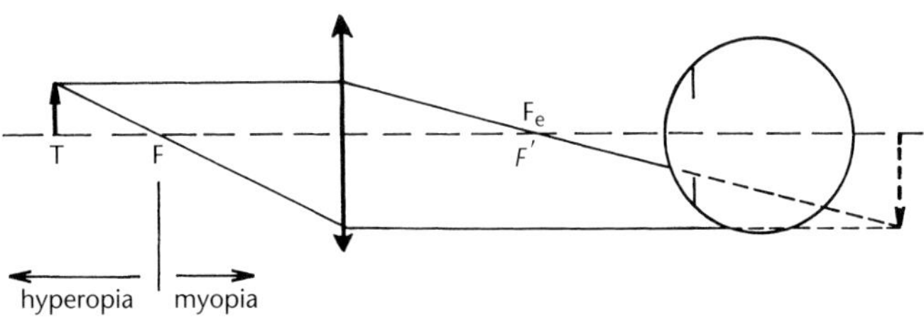


**Fig. O2** Optical principle of the Badal optometer ($F$, $F'$, first and second principal focus of the lens; $F_e$, anterior focal point of the eye; T, target)

**optometry, behavioural** A branch of optometry concerned with the diagnosis and treatment of visual problems taking into account not only the ocular history, signs and symptoms but the whole person and his or her environment.

**optometry, experimental** The branch of optometry concerned with the scientific investigation of optometric problems by experimentation upon humans or animals, or by clinical research.
*See* **psychophysics.**

**optometry, geriatric** A branch of optometry concerned with the prevention, diagnosis and treatment of visual problems in old age.

**optometry, paediatric** A branch of optometry concerned with the prevention, development, diagnosis and treatment of visual problems in children.

**optometry, primary care** Term referring to the basic field of optometry to which patients usually come directly and are not usually referred by other professionals. Primary care optometric practitioners may refer some of their patients to other practitioners such as ophthalmologists, neurologists or to other optometric specialists for specialized services such as paediatric optometry, low vision aids or highly specialized aspects of contact lens fitting.

**optotype** Test type used for measuring visual acuity.
*See* **acuity, monotype visual; chart, Snellen; Jaeger test types; König bars; Landolt ring.**

**ora serrata** The serrated anterior boundary of the retina located some 8 mm from the limbus. At the ora serrata, the retina is firmly adherent to the choroid which is the reason why a retinal detachment ends here.
*See* **ciliary body; retina; retinal dialysis; stria.**

**orange** Hue corresponding to wavelengths between 590 and 630 nm.
*See* **colour; light.**

**orbicularis muscle** *See* **muscle, orbicularis.**

**orbicularis ciliaris** *See* **ciliary body.**

**orbit** A rigid bony cavity in the skull which contains an eyeball, orbital fat, the extraocular muscles, the optic nerve, nerves and blood vessels and fibrous tissue of various kinds. This packing serves to keep the eyeball reasonably well fixed in place as it rotates. The walls of the orbital cavity are formed by seven bones. The *medial* wall of the orbit consists of: (1) the frontal process of the **maxilla** (or **maxillary**); (2) the **lacrimal bone**; (3) the lamina papyracea of the **ethmoid**; and (4) a small part of the body of the **sphenoid**. The *floor* of the orbit consists of: (1) the orbital plate of the maxilla; (2) the orbital surface of the **zygomatic** (or **malar**) bone and (3) the orbital process of the **palatine** bone. The *lateral* wall of the orbit consists of (1) the orbital surface of the great wing of the **sphenoid**, and (2) the orbital surface of the **zygomatic**. The *roof* of the orbit is made up mainly by the **frontal** bone and behind this by the lesser wing of the **sphenoid**. The orbit is lined with a membrane of tissue called the **periorbita** (or **orbital periosteum**) which extends to the **orbital margin** (anterior rim of the orbit) where it becomes continuous with the periosteum covering the facial bones. The periorbita is loosely attached to the bones except at sutures, foramina and the orbital margin where it is firmly attached.
*See* **axis, orbital; canal, optic; fat, orbital; fissure, inferior orbital; fissure, superior orbital; lamina papyracea.**

**Table O3** Bones forming the walls of the orbit

| roof | medial wall |
|---|---|
| 1. frontal | 1. maxilla |
| 2. lesser wing of sphenoid | 2. lacrimal |
| | 3. ethmoid |
| | 4. sphenoid |
| **floor** | **lateral wall** |
| 1. maxilla | 1. great wing of sphenoid |
| 2. zygomatic | 2. zygomatic |
| 3. palatine | |

**orbital cellulitis** *See* **cellulitis, orbital.**

**orbital fat** *See* **fat, orbital.**

**orbital fissure** *See* **fissure, inferior orbital**; **fissure, superior orbital.**

**orbital inflammatory syndrome** *See* **syndrome, orbital inflammatory.**

**orbital margin** *See* **orbit.**

**orbital optic neuritis** *See* **neuritis, optic.**

**orbital septum** A thin membrane containing collagenous and elastic fibres which is attached to the orbital margin at a thickening called the **arcus marginale**. It is continuous with the tarsal plates of the upper and lower eyelids except where it is pierced by the fibres of the levator palpebrae superioris muscle in the upper lid and the expansion from the inferior rectus in the lower lid. *Syn.* palpebral fascia; septum orbitale.
*See* **dermatochalasis; eyelids; tarsus.**

**orbital tubercle** A small elevation on the orbital surface of the zygomatic bone which serves as a point of attachment to the cheek ligament of the lateral rectus muscle, the ligament of Lockwood, the lateral palpebral ligament and aponeurosis of the levator palpebrae muscle.

**orbitotomy** A surgical incision made into the orbit to allow the removal of a tumour or foreign body, to treat a lesion, or to drain an abscess.

**ordinary ray** *See* **birefringence.**

**organ of sight; organ, visual** *See* **eye.**

**organic amblyopia** *See* **amblyopia.**

**orientation column** *See* **column, cortical.**

**orthokeratology** Method of fitting contact lenses for the purpose of altering the curvature of the cornea, especially to reduce the eye's refractive power in myopia.

**orthophoria** The case when the two visual axes are directed towards the point of binocular fixation, in the absence of an adequate stimulus to fusion. It represents a perfect balance of the oculomotor system; and the active and passive positions coincide, unlike in heterophoria. *Syn.* phoria.
*See* **heterophoria; orthophorization; position, active; position, passive.**

**orthophorization** A process that is presumed to operate to produce a greater frequency of nearly orthophoric conditions (in distance vision) than would otherwise occur on the basis of chance. This process may also operate after prolonged occlusion of one eye or after the introduction of prisms in front of one eye or both eyes.
*See* **adaptation, vergence; emmetropization; orthophoria.**

**orthopic fusion** *See* **fusion, orthopic.**

**orthoptics** The study, diagnosis and nonoperative treatment of anomalies of binocular vision, strabismus and monocular functional amblyopia.
*See* **training, visual.**

**orthoptist** A person who practises orthoptics.

**orthoscope** A device by which water is held in contact with the cornea and thereby neutralizes the refractive power of the front surface of the cornea.

**orthoscopic eyepiece** *See* **eyepiece, orthoscopic.**

**orthoscopic lens** *See* **lens, orthoscopic.**

**orthotropia** **1.** Absence of strabismus. **2.** The term is sometimes used following successful surgery or prism compensation of a strabismus, or when there is a vertical deviation with no deviation in the horizontal plane.

**oscillopsia** Vision in which objects appear to oscillate. It may be due to acquired nystagmus, neurosis, multiple sclerosis, in superior oblique myokymia, etc.
*See* **myokymia; nystagmus.**

**osmotic pressure** *See* **pressure, osmotic.**

**osteogenesis imperfecta** *See* **sclera, blue.**

**ostium lacrimale** *See* **lacrimal apparatus.**

**Ostwalt curve** *See* **ellipse, Tscherning.**

**Ota's naevus** *See* **naevus of Ota.**

**otitis media** *See* **syndrome, Gradenigo's.**

**outer segment** *See* **cell, cone; cell, rod.**

**overaction** Term referring to the excessive action of an extraocular muscle as a consequence of palsy or limitation to the ipsilateral antagonist or the contralateral synergist.
*See* Table M5.

**over-refraction** Determination of a residual error of refraction of the eye while the patient is wearing spectacles or contact lenses.

**overall size lens** *See* **lens, aniseikonic.**

**overcorrected spherical aberration** *See* **aberration, spherical.**

**overcorrection, post-operative** *See* **strabismus, consecutive.**

**overwear syndrome** *See* **syndrome, overwear.**

**oxyblepsia** *See* **oxyopia.**

**oxybuprocaine hydrochloride** *See* **benoxinate hydrochloride.**

**oxygen permeability** The degree to which a polymer allows the passage of a gas or fluid. *Symbol*: *Dk*. Oxygen permeability (*Dk*) of a material is a function of the **diffusivity** (*D*) (that is the speed at which oxygen molecules traverse the material) and the **solubility** (*k*) (or the amount of oxygen molecules absorbed, per volume, in the material). Values of oxygen permeability (*Dk*) typically fall within the range $10–100 \times 10^{-11}$ (cm$^2$ ml $O_2$)/(s ml mmHg). A semi-logarithmic relationship has been demonstrated between hydrogel water content and oxygen permeability. *Unit*: Barrer.
*See* **Barrer; CAB; oedema; oxygen pressure, equivalent; oxygen requirement, critical; refractometer; siloxane.**

**oxygen pressure, equivalent (EOP)** A percentage value of the assumed oxygen pressure existing behind a contact lens. The oxygen pressure in the air corresponds to about 20.9% (or about 159 mmHg; that value is actually close to 155 mmHg because of the presence of water vapour) and each percentage point is equal to a pressure of about 7.4 mmHg.

**oxygen requirement, critical (COR)** The minimum oxygen pressure at the epithelial surface required to prevent corneal swelling during the

O

day. This value was initially assumed to be between 11 and 19 mmHg but it is nowadays considered to be at least 74 mmHg near the centre of the cornea (or 10% EOP or a *Dk/L* of about $25 \times 10^{-9}$ (cm$^2$ ml $O_2$)/(s ml mmHg) at 25°C) for daily wear. This figure increases to at least $90 \times 10^{-9}$ for overnight wear. *Syn.* critical oxygen tension.
*See* **hypoxia; oxygen pressure, equivalent.**

**oxygen tension, critical** *See* **oxygen requirement, critical.**

**oxygen toxicity** *See* **retinopathy of prematurity.**

**oxygen transmissibility** The degree to which oxygen may pass through a particular material of a given thickness. It is equal to the oxygen permeability divided by the thickness of the measured sample under specific conditions. *Symbol*: *Dk/t*; *Dk/L*. *Unit*: Barrer/cm.
*See* **hypercapnia; oedema; oxygen permeability; syndrome, corneal exhaustion.**

**oxyopia** Extreme acuteness of vision. *Syn.* oxyblepsia.

**oxyphenbutazone eye ointment** A non-steroidal antiinflammatory agent usually used in 10% concentration for non-purulent inflammatory anterior eye conditions. It does not have the side-effects of topical steroid therapy.
*See* **antiinflammatory drugs.**

# P

**P cell** *See* **cell, ganglion.**

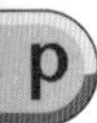

**pachometer** A device that, mounted on a slit-lamp, is used for measuring corneal thickness (or the depth of the anterior chamber). It consists of an optical system which provides two half-fields by means of two glass plates with parallel sides placed in front of one objective of the microscope, the other being occluded. These plates rest one on top of the other with the junction between them situated so as to horizontally bisect the objective. The top plate can be rotated while the bottom one is fixed. The observer viewing through the microscope sees two corneal optical sections and adjusts the top plate until the outer surface of the epithelium appears aligned with the inner surface of the endothelium. The corneal thickness is then read directly from a scale attached to the pachometer and calibrated in millimetres. To increase the accuracy of the measurement a special eyepiece is used with the microscope. It has a magnification of ×10 and has two additional components: a horizontal slit and a biprism. The role of the eyepiece is to remove from the field of view half of the two optical sections. The measurement of the depth of the anterior chamber is made with a similar device but with a different scale. *Note*: also spelt pachymeter.
An instrument with greater magnification (called a **micropachometer**) has been devised, principally for research purposes, using a projection system which incorporates variable doubling plates and forms two slit images on the cornea in conjunction with the viewing system of a slit-lamp and a magnification of up to ×100, mounted on another arm. This instrument allows the measurement of the thickness of the corneal epithelium alone with a precision which can reach ±1 μm. The above pachometers are referred to as **optical pachometers** to differentiate them from **ultrasonic pachometers** which use high-frequency ultrasound waves which are reflected from the anterior and posterior corneal surfaces.
*See* **corneal epithelium; ultrasonography.**

**pad** One of a pair of protuberances attached to the bridge of a spectacle frame or mounting which rests against the side of the nose. *Syn.* nose pad.
*See* **bridge, pad; pince-nez; spectacle frame, metal.**

**Paget's disease** *See* **disease, Paget's.**

**palinopsia** Visual persistence of the image of an object in the absence of its original stimulus. There is usually a latent period which may amount to several minutes between the visual stimulation and the corresponding mental image. The latter typically disappears within seconds, although it may persist in some cases for several minutes. The subsequent mental image is quite faithful to the original stimulus. It is usually associated with a lesion in the parieto-occipital or temporal-occipital areas as a result of a cerebral infarction, epilepsy, tumour, or brain injury. *Syn.* visual perseveration.

**palisades of Vogt** The crests of epithelium folds that run radially towards the cornea, at the limbus, from the bulbar conjunctiva. They are often seen in slit-lamp examination, especially in pigmented individuals and clearly in fluorescein angiography. They may contain stem cells that play a role in the regeneration of corneal epithelium cells.
*See* **corneal epithelium.**

**palpebrae** *See* **eyelids.**

**palpebrae muscle, levator** *See* **muscle, levator palpebrae.**

**palpebral aperture; conjunctiva** *See* under the nouns.

**palpebral, elephantiasis** *See* **elephantiasis oculi.**

**palpebral fissure** *See* **aperture, palpebral.**

**palpebral ligament** *See* **ligament, palpebral.**

**palsy** Synonym for paralysis, although it often implies partial paralysis.
*See* **paralysis; paresis.**

**palsy, abducens nerve** *See* **paralysis of the sixth nerve.**

**palsy, Bell's** A paralysis of the upper and lower muscles of the face on one side, due to an inflammation of the facial nerve. It results in a wider palpebral aperture and inability to close the eye on the affected size and drying of the cornea.
*See* **sign, Bell's; tears, artificial; tears, crocodile.**

**palsy, double elevator** A condition characterized by limited or complete inhibition of the upward rotation of an eye, due to, either paresis of its superior rectus and inferior oblique muscles, or entrapment of the inferior orbital tissues. It may be congenital or acquired (e.g. a lesion in the pretectum). Treatment is principally surgical.

**palsy, gaze** Inability of the eyes to make conjugate movements due to a lesion in the cortical or subcortical oculomotor centres.
*See* **paralysis of the fourth nerve; paralysis of the sixth nerve; paralysis of the third nerve.**

**palsy, supranuclear gaze** A disturbance of the conjugate movements of the eye. If the lesion is in the frontal lobe the patient is unable to direct the eyes to the contralateral side of the lesion (**frontal gaze palsy**). In bilateral lesion the patient is unable to voluntarily turn the eyes in any direction but is able to maintain fixation and perform pursuit movements. If the lesion is in the midbrain it produces Parinaud's syndrome in which there is an inability to elevate (and sometimes depress) the eyes on command and the pupils are large and may not react to light. If the lesion is in the paramedian pontine reticular formation there is an ipsilateral horizontal gaze palsy while lesions in the medial longitudinal fasciculus produce internuclear ophthalmoplegia.
*See* **ophthalmoplegia, internuclear; syndrome, Parinaud's.**

**pannus** Abnormal superficial vascularization of the cornea covering the upper half, or sometimes the entire cornea. It is characterized by a thick plexus of vessels. It is found in some cases of contact lens wear, mainly soft lenses. Pannus following contact lens wear is referred to as **corneal vascularization**. If induced by soft lenses, it can be reduced by changing to lenses of high oxygen transmissibility or ceasing contact lens wear. Deep corneal vascularization involving the stroma is usually the result of a disease process (e.g. interstitial keratitis, phlyctenular keratitis, severe long-standing trichiasis, trachoma).

**panophthalmitis** Acute inflammation of the eyeball involving all its structures and extending into the orbit. The disease develops very rapidly. The eyelids are red and swollen and there is severe chemosis of the conjunctiva. The cornea is often a whitish mass of necrotic tissue and there may be severe ocular pain.
*See* **endophthalmitis.**

**panoramic vision** *See* **vision, panoramic.**

**pantoscopic angle** *See* **angle, pantoscopic.**

**Panum's area** *See* **area, Panum's.**

**Panum's fusional space** An area in space corresponding to Panum's area within which there is fusion and stereopsis of a non-fixated target.
*See* **area, Panum's; horopter.**

**papilla** Any small elevation shaped like a nipple.
*Plural*: papillae.
*See* **follicle, conjunctival.**

**papilla, Bergmeister's** *See* **glial veil.**

**papilla, lacrimal** A small elevation at the inner canthus of each eyelid containing a punctum lacrimale.
*See* **lacrimal apparatus.**

**papilla lacrimalis** *See* **tubercle, lacrimal.**

**papilla, optic** *See* **disc, optic.**

**papillary conjunctivitis, giant** *See* **conjunctivitis, giant papillary.**

**papillitis** *See* **neuritis, optic.**

**papilloedema** A non-inflammatory oedema of the optic nerve head produced by raised intracranial

Table P1 Differential diagnosis between papilloedema and papillitis

| | papilloedema | papillitis |
|---|---|---|
| **Signs** | | |
| disc elevation | raised | slightly raised |
| disc hyperaemia | present | present |
| disc margins | blurred | blurred |
| retinal veins | congested | congested |
| haemorrhages | near disc | some in late stage |
| pupil light reflex | normal | impaired |
| venous pulsation | absent | present |
| secondary optic atrophy | present in late stage | may appear in late stage |
| **Symptoms** | | |
| visual acuity | normal, except in late stage | reduced |
| visual field | enlarged blind spot | central scotoma |
| diplopia | present | absent |
| colour vision | normal | impaired |
| pain | absent | present on moving the eyes |
| headache | present | absent |

pressure, and due most commonly to a cerebral tumour. It can also result from cerebral abscesses, meningitis, encephalitis, subarachnoid haemorrhages, head injury, hydrocephalus, etc. The optic disc appears raised above the level of the retina and its margins are blurred, the central vessels on the surface of the disc are displaced forward, the retinal veins are dilated and there is nearly always a loss of induced venous pulsation. The swollen disc displaces the retina and this causes an enlargement of the blind spot on visual field measurement. In the early stages visual acuity is not affected (unlike in papillitis), although if the condition persists there will be some loss. In advanced stages, there may be haemorrhages around the disc, secondary optic atrophy, exudates, as well as headaches and vomiting. The condition is usually bilateral. *Note*: also spelt papilledema. *Syn.* choked disc.
*See* **atrophy, optic; neuritis, optic; syndrome, Foster Kennedy.**

**papilloma** A tumour most commonly found on the conjunctiva, the limbus or the lid margins. It is usually benign. It should be excised but it is likely to recur.

**papillomacular bundle; fibres** *See* **fibres, papillomacular.**

**paracontrast** *See* **metacontrast.**

**paradoxical ARC** *See* **retinal correspondence, abnormal.**

**paradoxical diplopia** *See* **diplopia, incongruous.**

**parallax, binocular** The difference in angle subtended at each eye by an object which is viewed first with one eye and then with the other.

**parallax, chromatic** Apparent lateral displacement of two monochromatic sources (e.g. a blue object and a red object) when observed through a disc with a pinhole placed near the edge of the pupil. When the pupil is centred on the achromatic axis (in some people the pinhole may have to be placed away from the centre of the pupil), the two images appear superimposed. The relative displacement of the two images becomes reversed when the pinhole is on the other side of that axis. This phenomenon is attributed to the chromatic aberration of the eye.
*See* **axis, achromatic; chromostereopsis; aberration, longitudinal chromatic.**

**parallax, monocular** The apparent change in the relative position of an object when the eye is moved from one position to another.

**parallax, motion** Apparent difference in the direction of movement or speed produced when the subject moves relative to his environment (Fig. P1). *Example*: when viewing the landscape through the window of a moving train near objects appear to move much more quickly than distant objects.
*See* **perception, depth; stereopsis.**

**parallax, relative binocular** *See* **acuity, stereoscopic visual.**

**paralysis** Loss of action of a muscle due to injury or disease of that muscle or its nerve supply.
*See* **palsy.**

**paralysis, abducens** *See* **paralysis of the sixth nerve.**

**paralysis of accommodation** *See* **accommodation, paralysis of.**

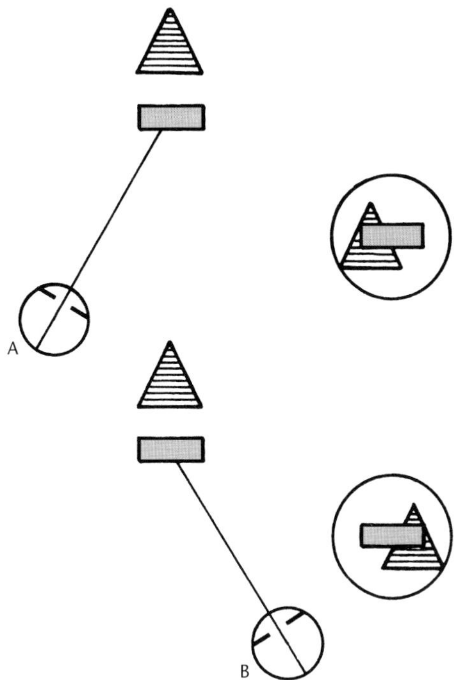


**Fig. P1** An example of motion parallax. As the eye moves from A to B, the more distant object (triangle) appears to move in the same direction while the near object (rectangle) appears to move in the opposite direction, as shown in the circles on the right

**paralysis of convergence** A condition characterized by an inability of the eyes to converge while all other monocular eye movements are unaffected. The patient notices diplopia in near vision, which usually occurs suddenly. It is presumably due to some lesion in the nuclei responsible for convergence as may happen in tabes dorsalis or Parkinson's disease.

**paralysis, divergence** A condition characterized by an inability of the eyes to diverge while all other monocular eye movements are unaffected. It is characterized by a sudden development of diplopia with marked esotropia at distance and sometimes headaches. The key difference with divergence insufficiency is the sudden onset of symptoms. Its association includes encephalitis, multiple sclerosis, head trauma, cerebral haemorrhage, brain tumour and vascular lesions of the brainstem.

**paralysis of the fourth nerve** A condition characterized by a hypertropia of the eye with the affected superior oblique muscle. It may be due to a lesion of the fourth cranial nerve or its nucleus as a result of injury (the most common cause), disease (e.g. diabetes, hypertension), aneurysm (especially of the internal carotid artery), or tumour. The patient usually presents with an abnormal head posture to avoid diplopia. If the condition does not recover by itself following therapy of the underlying cause, surgery is usually the only alternative treatment. *Syn.* trochlear paralysis.
*See* **head posture, abnormal; nerve, trochlear; strabismus, paralytic.**

**paralysis, oculomotor** *See* **paralysis of the third nerve.**

**paralysis of the sixth nerve** A condition characterized by an esotropia of the eye with the affected lateral rectus muscle. It may be due to a lesion of the sixth cranial nerve or its nucleus as a result of a vascular disease (e.g. diabetes, hypertension), injury, aneurysm (especially of the internal carotid artery), or tumour. The patient presents with an abnormal head turn to avoid diplopia. If the condition does not recover by itself following therapy of the underlying cause, surgery is usually the only alternative treatment. *Syn.* abducens paralysis; lateral rectus palsy.
*See* **head posture, abnormal; nerve, abducens; strabismus, paralytic; syndrome, Gradenigo's.**

**paralysis of the third nerve** A condition which leads to a wide impairment of motor function, as this nerve innervates most of the muscles of the eye. It may be due to a vascular disease (e.g. diabetes, hypertension), aneurysm (especially of the internal carotid artery), injury or tumour. In total paralysis only the lateral rectus and the superior oblique muscles will be spared and the eye will be in a position of abduction, slight depression and intorsion. Ptosis will also be present and the pupil will be dilated and non-reactive, and there will also be paralysis of accommodation. If the condition does not recover by itself following therapy of the underlying cause, surgery is usually the only alternative. *Syn.* oculomotor paralysis.
*See* **circle of Willis; muscles, extraocular; nerve, oculomotor; ophthalmoplegia; pupil; strabismus, paralytic; syndrome, Benedikt's; syndrome, Weber's; test, forced duction.**

**paralysis, trochlear** *See* **paralysis of the fourth nerve.**

**parastriate area** *See* **areas, visual association.**

**parasympatholytic** *See* **acetylcholine; mydriatic.**

**parasympathomimetic drug** A drug that has an action resembling that caused by stimulation of the parasympathetic nervous system. *Example*: a miotic of which there are two types: a direct-acting cholinergic, such as pilocarpine or carbachol; and the other, indirect-acting anticholinesterase, such as physostigmine, neostigmine, echothiophate iodide, demecarium bromide. *Syn.* cholinergic drug.
*See* **miotics; pilocarpine.**

**paraxial** Pertains to light rays situated near enough to the axis of an optical system for the gaussian theory to apply.
*See* **theory, gaussian.**

**paraxial approximation** *See* **ray, paraxial.**

**paraxial equation, fundamental** Equation based on gaussian theory and dealing with refraction at a spherical surface:

$$\frac{n'}{l'} - \frac{n}{l} = \frac{n' - n}{r} \quad \text{(or)} \quad L' - L = \frac{n' - n}{r}$$

where $n$ and $n'$ are the refractive indices of the media on each side of the spherical surface, $r$ is the radius of curvature of the surface and $l$ and $l'$ the distances of the object and the image from the surface, respectively. $n/l$ and $n'/l'$ are the **vergences** (or **reduced vergences**) of the incident and refracted light rays respectively. $L' - L$ corresponds to the change produced by the surface in the vergence of the light and is called the **focal power** (or **vergence power**, or **refractive power**) $F$ of the surface. Thus

$$L' - L = F$$

Focal power is usually expressed in dioptres and can be either positive or negative.
At a **reflecting** surface or a **mirror** the equation becomes

$$L' - L = \frac{2}{r}$$

where $r$ is the radius of curvature of the surface or mirror. *Syn.* general refraction formula.
*See* **dioptre; distance, image; distance, object; mirror; power, refractive; sign convention; theory, gaussian; vergence.**

**paraxial optics** *See* **optics, paraxial.**

**paraxial ray** *See* **ray, paraxial.**

**paraxial region** The hypothetical cylindrical narrow space surrounding the optical axis within

**Table P2** Clinical manifestations of lesions in the visual pathway

| site of lesion | clinical manifestations |
|---|---|
| macula | central scotoma |
| papillomacular bundle | central or centrocaecal scotoma |
| other part of the retina | scotoma on the opposite side of the central fixation point |
| complete section of one optic nerve | total blindness of that eye<br>absence of direct light reflex<br>presence of consensual light reflex<br>other eye: normal pupil reaction, direct but not consensual |
| pituitary enlargement pressing on inferior part of chiasma | bitemporal hemianopsia or bitemporal superior quadrantanopsia |
| aneurysm pressing on lateral part of the chiasma | binasal hemianopsia |
| sagittal section in the middle of the chiasma | bitemporal hemianopsia<br>normal pupil reflexes if light falls on temporal retina |
| optic tract | contralateral incongruous homonymous hemianopsia<br>Wernicke's pupillary reflex |
| lateral geniculate body | contralateral incongruous homonymous hemianopsia<br>normal pupil reflexes |
| anterior optic radiations on one side | contralateral incongruous homonymous hemianopsia<br>often sparing of the macula<br>normal pupil reflexes |
| visual cortex on one side | contralateral congruous homonymous hemianopsia<br>often sparing of the macula<br>normal pupil reflexes |

which rays of light are still considered paraxial. *Syn.* gaussian space.
*See* **ray, paraxial; theory, gaussian.**

**paraxial theory** *See* **theory, gaussian.**

**paresis** Slight or partial paralysis.
*See* **palsy; paralysis.**

**Parinaud's syndrome** *See* **syndrome, Parinaud's.**

**pars ciliaris muscle** *See* **muscle of Riolan.**

**pars plana; plicata** *See* **ciliary body.**

**partial sight** *See* **vision, low.**

**parvo cells** *See* **geniculate bodies, lateral.**

**parvocellular layer** *See* **geniculate bodies, lateral.**

**parvocellular visual system** That part of the visual pathway from the photoreceptors in the retina to layer 4Cβ, (and to a lesser extent in layers 4A and 6) of the visual cortex, which is mainly responsible for transmitting information about visual acuity, form vision, colour vision and low contrast targets. *Syn.* sustained visual system; 'what' system.
*See* **cell, ganglion; cell, X; geniculate bodies, lateral; magnocellular visual system; theory, two visual systems.**

**passive position** *See* **position, passive.**

**past-pointing** *See* **pointing, past-.**

**pathological myopia** *See* **myopia, pathological.**

**pathology, ocular** The discipline which deals with the nature of diseases of the eye and its surrounding structures, their effect on the ocular tissues and on ocular functions, as well as the causes and management.

**pathway, magnocellular** *See* **magnocellular visual system.**

**pathway, motor** Pathway from the cortex to the muscles that control the movements of the eyes enabling them to act as a unit.

**pathway, parvocellular** *See* **parvocellular visual system.**

**pathway, retinotectal** **1.** The nervous pathway connecting the retina to the pretectal region (anterior to the superior colliculi) and from there to the Edinger–Westphal nucleus. It is involved in the pupillary light reflexes. **2.** The nervous pathway between the retina and the superior colliculus. It is involved in the involuntary blink reflex to a dazzling light and in the eye movements occurring in response to the sudden appearance of a novel or a threatening stimulus.
*See* **blind sight; fibres, pupillary; reflex, pupil light; tectum of the mesencephalon.**

**pathway, visual** Neural path starting in the receptors of the retina and travelling through the following structures: the optic nerve, the optic chiasma, the optic tract, the lateral geniculate bodies, the optic radiations and the visual cortex where the pathway ends. The fibres of the optic nerve of one eye meet with the fibres from the other eye at the optic chiasma, where approximately half of them (the nasal half of the retina) cross over to the other side. Thus, there is semi-decussation in the visual pathway (Fig. P2).
*See* **area, visual; chiasma, optic; decussation; geniculate bodies, lateral; magnification, cortical; radiations, optic; retinotopic map; tracts, optic.**

**patient** Term originating from the Latin *patior* meaning to suffer; one who suffers or is ill and requires treatment.

**pattern, A** A neuromuscular anomaly of the eyes characterized by an increase in exotropia when the eyes fixate downward, or increase in esotropia when the eyes fixate upward. Upgaze and downgaze are usually measured at 25 degrees from the horizontal. *Syn.* A syndrome.
*See* **strabismus, convergent; strabismus, divergent.**

**pattern, checkerboard** A square set of equal size black and white squares placed adjacent to one another. It is used to test visual acuity. The common way of using this pattern is to present it in

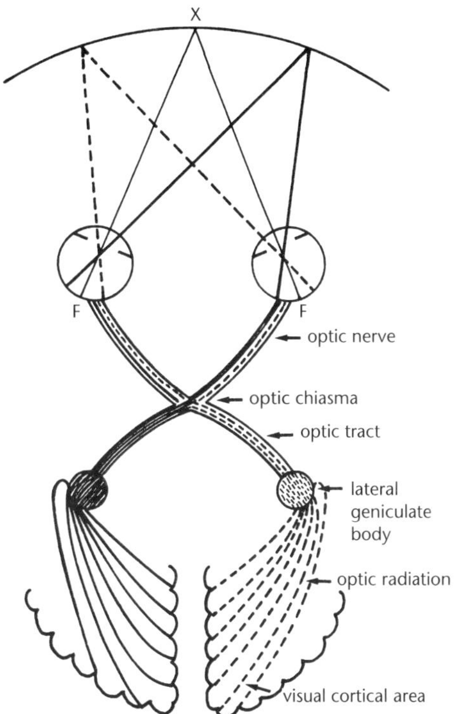


**Fig. P2** Visual pathway and nerve fibres distribution (X, fixation point; F, fovea)

the form of a square diamond made up of four smaller diamonds. Three of these are composed of a pattern of much smaller squares than the fourth. Resolution of the pattern with larger squares consists in indicating where it is located (top, bottom, right or left) while the other three squares appear as a uniform grey. This acuity test is less dependent on cognitive factors than letters. (Fig. P3).
*See* **acuity, visual; test type.**

**pattern, V** A neuromuscular anomaly of the eyes characterized by an increase in exotropia when the eyes rotate upward, or increase in esotropia when the eyes rotate downward. *Syn.* V syndrome.
*See* **strabismus, convergent; strabismus, divergent.**

**pattern, X** A neuromuscular anomaly in which the visual axes are more divergent when the eyes fixate upward and downward, as compared to the primary position of gaze.

**paving-stone degeneration** *See* **degeneration, paving-stone.**

**PD** Abbreviation for interpupillary distance and also, but more rarely, for prism dioptre.
*See* **dioptre, prism; distance, interpupillary; rule, PD.**

**PD gauge; meter** *See* **pupillometer.**

**PD rule** *See* **rule, PD.**

**pedicle, cone** The foot of a cone located in the outer molecular (or plexiform) layer of the retina.
*See* **cell, cone; retina.**

**Pelli–Robson chart** *See* **chart, Pelli–Robson.**

**pellucid** Allowing maximum passage of light.

**pellucid marginal corneal degeneration** *See* **degeneration, pellucid marginal corneal.**

**pelopsia** Anomaly of visual perception in which objects appear to be much nearer than they actually are. It may be due to vision in a very clear atmosphere, recent wear of an optical correction, neurosis, etc.
*See* **metamorphopsia.**

**pemirolast potassium** *See* **mast cell stabilizers.**

**pemphigoid, cicatricial** A rare, idiopathic, chronic systemic disease, most commonly of the elderly and characterized by recurrent blisters and bullae of the skin and mucous membranes, with subsequent scarring and shrinkage. The disease may affect only the conjunctiva (**ocular pemphigoid**). In this case, the clinical picture is a conjunctivitis with hyperaemia, mucous discharge and small vesicles which on bursting result in ulceration, pseudomembranes,

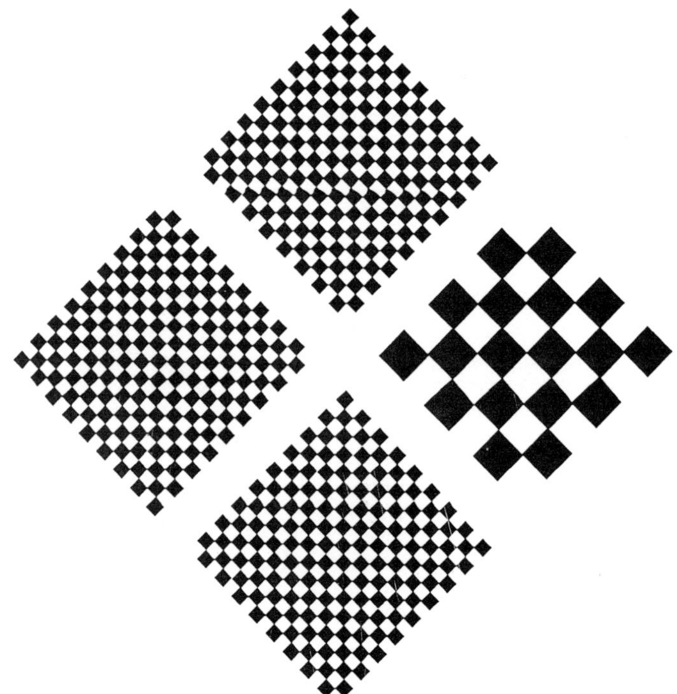

Fig. P3 Checkerboard pattern

conjunctival subepithelial fibrosis and conjunctival shrinkage. The disease may give rise to the following complications: adhesion between the palpebral and bulbar conjunctiva (symblepharon), ankyloblepharon, xerophthalmia, keratoconjunctivitis sicca, entropion, trichiasis and dry eye with corneal ulcer. There is pain or irritation and blurred vision. Treatment includes corticosteroids, surgery for entropion and trichiasis, and keratoprosthesis if vision is affected. *Syn.* benign mucous pemphigoid.
*See* **conjunctivitis, pseudomembranous; syndrome, Stevens–Johnson.**

**pemphigoid, ocular** *See* **pemphigoid, cicatricial.**

**penalization** A clinical method of treating amblyopia and eccentric fixation in which vision by the fixating eye is decreased by various means (optical overcorrection, atropinization for near vision especially, and neutral density filters) in order to compel the amblyopic eye to fixate. Sometimes the treatment consists of using the amblyopic eye for near vision and the fixating eye for distance vision.
*See* **amblyopia; attenuation; fixation, eccentric; occlusion treatment; pleoptics.**

**pencil of light** *See* **light, pencil of.**

**pencil push-up** *See* **convergence insufficiency.**

**pencil-to-nose exercise** *See* **convergence insufficiency.**

**penetrating keratoplasty** *See* **keratoplasty.**

**pendular nystagmus** *See* **nystagmus.**

**penumbra** **1.** Region of very low illumination on a dark background. **2.** Zone in which the brightness varies from some illumination to zero (**umbra**) in the shadow cast by an opaque object intercepting light from an extensive light source.
*See* **shadow.**

**Pepper test** *See* **test, Pepper.**

**percept** The complete mental image of an object obtained in response to sensory stimuli.

**perception** The mental process of recognizing and interpreting an object through one or more of the senses stimulated by a physical object. Thus one recognizes the shape, colour, location and differentiation of an object from its background.
*See* **sensation.**

**perception, anorthoscopic** *See* **anorthoscope.**

**perception, binocular** Perception obtained through simultaneous use of both eyes.

**perception, depth** Perception of the distance of an object from the observer (**absolute distance**) or of the distance between two objects (**relative distance**). Our ability to judge the latter is much more precise than the former. There are many factors which contribute to depth perception. Most importantly is the existence on the two retinae of different images of the same object (called **binocular disparity** or **retinal disparity**). There are also many other contributing factors, such as the characteristics of the stimulus (called **cues**), binocular parallax and, to a smaller extent, the muscular proprioceptive information due to the efforts of accommodation and convergence. Depth perception is more precise in binocular vision but is possible in monocular vision using the following **cues**: interposition, relative position, relative size, linear perspective, textural gradient, aerial perspective, light and shade, shadow and motion parallax (Fig. P4). *Syn.* spatial vision.
*See* **acuity, stereoscopic visual; cliff, visual; illusion, moon; parallax, motion; perspective; perspective, aerial; perspective, linear; relief; room, Ames; room, leaf; shadow; stereopsis.**

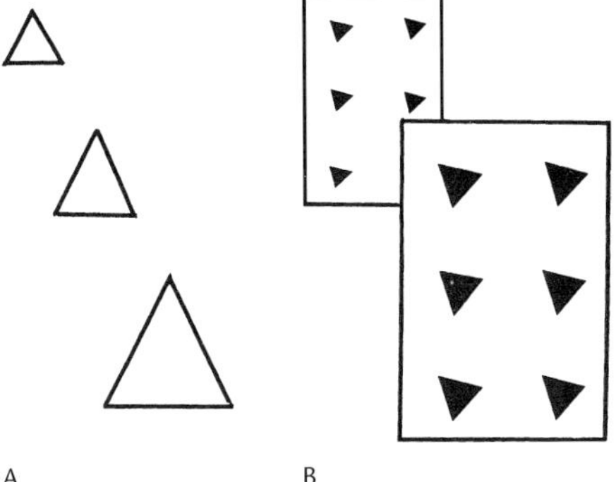


**Fig. P4** Examples of monocular cues to depth perception; A, relative size; B, interposition and relative size

**perception, dermo-optical** *See* **perception, extrasensory.**

**perception, extrasensory** Perception obtained by means other than through the ordinary senses as, for example, telepathy (mind reading) or reading by moving a finger over a printed text (**dermo-optical perception**).

**perception, light (LP)** Term used to indicate a barely seeing eye which can just see light but not the form of objects. Loss of light perception represents blindness.

**perception, subliminal** Stimuli below the threshold of sensation (i.e. subliminal) may, in rare circumstances (e.g. exposure of 40 ms duration masked by another stimulus), unconsciously arouse perception. The effect is then of extremely short duration (less than 200 ms).

**perception, visual** Perception obtained through the sense of vision.

**perceptual span** *See* **reading.**

**Percival criterion** *See* **criterion, Percival.**

**pericorneal plexus** *See* **plexus, pericorneal.**

**perimeter** An instrument for measuring the angular extent and the characteristics (e.g. presence of scotoma) of the visual field.
*See* **campimeter; field, visual; isopter; screen, tangent.**

**perimeter, arc** Perimeter consisting of a semicircular arc, the inside surface of which is painted matt black or grey. The patient's head is placed such that the eye under investigation is located at the centre of curvature of the arc. The visual field is determined by moving a target along the black surface of the perimeter until the patient either just sees it or just no longer sees it. The targets are small discs of varying colour and size attached to the end of black wands or may be projected on the arc which can be rotated around the fixation point located at its centre. Thus the visual field can be tested along any meridian.
*See* **field, visual.**

**perimeter, automated** An instrument to test the visual field in which the presentation of the stimuli and the recording are carried out electronically and under the control of a built-in computer. There exist many types (e.g. Henson CFA, Humphrey Field Analyzer, Octopus, Dicon). Computerized perimeters have the following advantages: the examination strategy is reproducible; they can be operated by non-specialists; the testing routine (e.g. number of stimuli or their location) can be altered by modifying the program; each instrument can contain several examination routines aimed at testing various pathologies (e.g. one for glaucoma and another for hemianopic defects); the computer capacity can be used for quantifying the results as, for example, in the Henson CFA where the visual fields can be classified as normal, suspect or defective on the basis of a system included in the instrument (Fig. P5). *Syn.* computerized perimetry.
*See* **analyser, Friedmann visual field; field, visual; perimetry, frequency doubling; perimetry, short wavelength automated.**

**perimeter, bowl** *See* **perimeter, Goldmann.**

**perimeter, Goldmann** Perimeter consisting of a hemispherical bowl, the inside radius of which is 30 cm. Targets of varying intensity and size are projected onto the inside white surface. The background luminance of the bowl is also controlled. In addition there is a telescope attached to the back of the bowl through which the practitioner can verify that the patient maintains fixation. Goldmann perimeter can be used either for kinetic or static perimetry, although it is more appropriately designed for the former. *Syn.* bowl perimeter.
*See* **perimetry, kinetic; perimetry, static.**

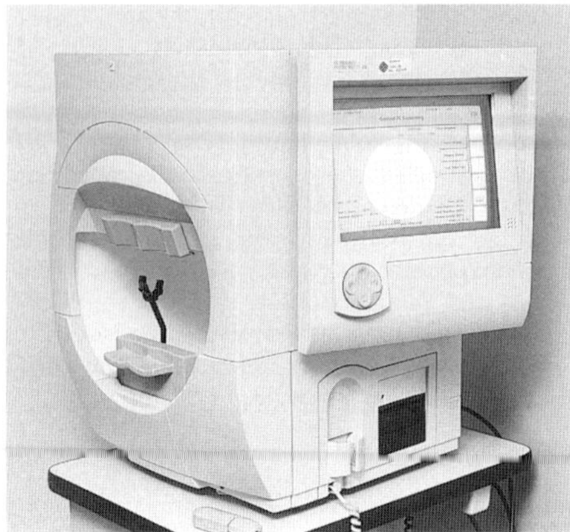

**Fig. P5** Computerized perimeter (Humphrey Field Analyzer, Humphrey Instruments, Inc.)

**perimeter, projection** A perimeter in which the target is projected either onto an arc or a bowl such as the Goldmann perimeter.
*See* **perimeter, Goldmann.**

**perimetry** The determination of the extent of the visual field, usually for the purpose of detecting anomalies in the visual pathway.
*See* **field, visual; glaucoma; lens rim artifact; perimeter; pathway, visual.**

**perimetry, frequency doubling (FDP)** A method of testing the visual field based on the frequency doubling illusion and thus assessing the functional integrity of the large-diameter retinal ganglion M cells which are very susceptible to early glaucomatous damage. A commercial version of this method which provides rapid and efficient visual field testing is available (Humphrey Instruments/Welch Allyn). It is a computerized perimeter in which the stimulus display consists of a low spatial frequency (0.25 c/deg) sinusoidal grating which flickers in a counterphase fashion (i.e. light bars become dark and vice versa) at a rate of 25 Hz. The grating is presented in many locations throughout the visual field and the patient's task is to detect it.
*See* **cell, ganglion; glaucoma, open-angle; illusion, frequency doubling.**

**perimetry, kinetic** Measurement of the visual field with a moving target of fixed luminance.

**perimetry, short wavelength automated (SWAP)** A valuable procedure for detecting and monitoring visual defects in patients with ocular

hypertension and patients with early glaucomatous visual field losses. It uses a blue stimulus on a yellow background, as may be arranged in an automated perimeter. It is a more sensitive and efficient method of detecting and monitoring early visual field losses than standard white-on-white automated perimetry (white stimulus on a white background).
*See* **glaucoma, open-angle.**

**perimetry, static** Measurement of the visual field with a target that can be varied in dimension and luminance. The target can be presented in any part of the visual field.

**period, critical** A time after birth during which neural connections can still be modified by interference with normal visual experience or lesion of the visual pathway. If a person has an anomaly (e.g. amblyopia), the treatment is most likely to be effective during the earliest part of the critical period. In man it lasts up to about 8–10 years of age. *Syn.* plastic period (However, this term relates more specifically to the time course during which the visual system is still responsive to treatment. This may differ from the critical period of development); sensitive period.

**periocular** Situated around the eye.

**periorbita** *See* **orbit.**

**peripapillary** Situated around the optic disc.

**peripheral clearance** *See* **edge lift.**

**peripheral vision; visual acuity** *See* under the nouns.

**peripheral zone** *See* **optic zone diameter.**

**periphoria** *See* **cyclophoria.**

**periscope** An optical instrument using two right angle reflectors in order to allow observation of an object from behind a shield or around an obstruction where direct vision is impossible. It has many applications, especially in the military forces (e.g. in tanks, submarines).

**periscopic lens** *See* **lens, periscopic.**

**peristriate area** *See* **areas, visual association.**

**Perkins tonometer** *See* **tonometer, applanation.**

**Perlia's nucleus** *See* **nucleus, Perlia's.**

**persistent hyaloid artery** *See* **hyaloid remnant.**

**persistent hyperplastic primary vitreous** *See* **vitreous, persistent hyperplastic primary.**

**persistent pupillary membrane** *See* **membrane, pupillary.**

**perspective** Perceptual attribute of the third dimension in space or in graphic representation on a plane, as in a drawing (Fig. P6).

**perspective, aerial** Perspective influenced by the state of clarity of the atmosphere. Far away objects appear less distinct and desaturated in colour due to the diffusion of light by the air in between the object and the eye. However, a very pure atmosphere may lead to underestimation of the distance of objects as they retain their distinctness and colour in this case. Aerial perspective is used by artists who soften and blur the colour and outlines of objects which they wish to appear as far away.
*See* **perception, depth; shadow.**

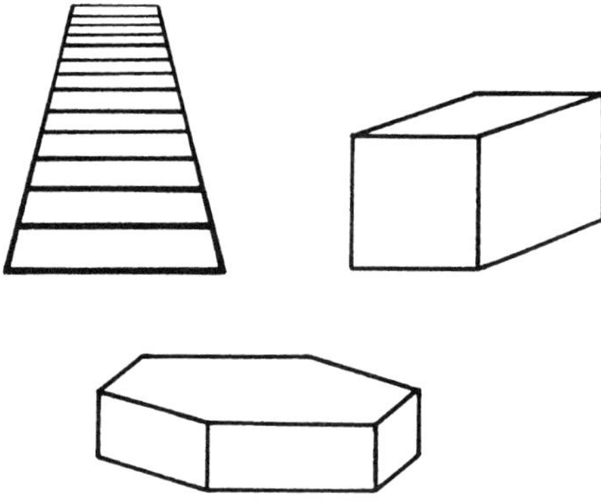

**Fig. P6** Examples of perspective drawings

**perspective, geometrical** *See* **perspective, linear.**

**perspective, linear** Perspective conveyed by drawing images in different sizes. For example, parallel lines receding into the distance are made to converge. (Fig. P6) *Syn.* geometrical perspective.
*See* **perception, depth.**

**Peter's anomaly** A rare, congenital anomaly of the anterior segment of the eye. It is characterized by a central corneal opacity, usually accompanied by the adhesion of strands of iris tissue to the margins of the corneal opacity. It is frequently associated with glaucoma. *Syn.* anterior chamber cleavage syndrome.
*See* **syndrome, Axenfeld's; syndrome, Rieger's.**

**Petit, canal of** *See* **canal of Petit.**

**Petzval surface** The imaginary curved surface upon which images would be formed if curvature of field were the only aberration present. It is the curved surface in which the tangential and sagittal image shells of a point-focal lens coincide.
*See* **astigmatism, oblique; curvature of field; lens, anastigmatic.**

**pH** Symbol for the logarithm to base 10 of the reciprocal of the hydrogen (H) ion concentration measured in gram molecular weight in an aqueous solution. A solution with a pH 7.0 is neutral, one with a pH of more than 7.0 is alkaline, one with a pH lower than 7.0 is acid. It is a convenient way of expressing the acidity or alkalinity of solutions, particularly of contact lens buffer solutions. Alkaline ophthalmic solutions generally cause less discomfort than acidic ones. *Note*: pH stands for *p*ower (or *p*otency) of *H*.

**phacocele** Hernia of the crystalline lens through a rupture of the sclera near the limbus. It lodges underneath the conjunctiva. *Syn.* lenticele.

**phacodonesis** A tremulous condition of the crystalline lens.
*See* **iridodonesis.**

**phacoemulsification** Procedure for removal of the crystalline lens in cataract surgery which consists of emulsifying and aspirating the contents of the lens with the use of a low frequency ultrasonic needle inserted into the eye near the limbus. This technique usually produces more rapid wound healing and early stabilization of refractive error with less astigmatism, due to the small incision. However, this technique may damage the corneal endothelium if excessive ultrasound is used. Following removal of the lens cortex and nucleus, an intraocular lens may be implanted within the remaining lens capsule. The lens is folded and inserted through a small incision (e.g. 3.2 mm) using a special injector. This procedure is preferred over other cataract extraction techniques due to both the rapid wound healing and the lower incidence of potentially vision threatening side effects (e.g. retinal detachment).
*See* **after-cataract; cataract extraction; implant, intraocular lens; iridectomy.**

**phacolytic glaucoma** *See* **glaucoma, phacolytic.**

**phacoscope** Instrument for observing the crystalline lens and measuring accommodative changes using the Purkinje–Sanson images, as in the ophthalmophakometer.
*See* **images, Purkinje–Sanson; ophthalmophakometer.**

**phakic** Refers to an eye possessing its crystalline lens or an intraocular lens implant.
*See* **aphakia; eye, pseudophakic; lens, crystalline; implant, intraocular lens.**

**phase** The state of vibration of a light wave at a particular time. Light waves vibrating with the same frequency are said to be **in phase** if their peaks and troughs occur at the same time; otherwise they are said to be **out of phase** and one wave lags or precedes another by a **phase difference** (e.g. a fraction of a wavelength, or one wavelength, or a number of wavelengths). For waves exactly out of phase the phase difference is half a wavelength and for waves exactly in phase it is 0.
*See* **wavelength.**

**phenomenon, Abney's** A slight change in hue resulting from a change in saturation. This is especially noticeable when white light is added to a monochromatic blue or green light.

**phenomenon, Aubert's** If, in the dark the head is tilted slowly to one side while looking at a bright vertical line, this line will appear to tilt in the opposite direction. This phenomenon is due to the absence of compensatory postural changes. *Syn.* Aubert's effect.

**phenomenon, Bell's** An outward and upward rolling of the eyes when closing, or attempting to close the eyelids.
*See* **sign, Bell's.**

**phenomenon, Bezold–Brücke** A change in perceived hue of some spectral colours with a change in intensity. However, some wavelengths, such as 478, 503 and 578 nm, remain a constant hue with varying intensity. These are called **invariant wavelengths** or **unique hues**. *Syn.* Bezold–Brücke effect.

**phenomenon, Bielschowsky's** In alternating hypertropia, occluding one eye leads to its rotation upward, and then placing a neutral density filter in front of the other eye gives rise to a downward movement of the occluded eye. Using a wedge rather than a filter, and thus gradually increasing the light absorption, the eye behind the cover performs a gradual downward movement and a gradual upward movement if the wedge is moved in the other direction.
*See* **hypertropia, alternating; wedge, optical.**

**phenomenon, Broca–Sulzer** *See* **effect, Broca–Sulzer.**

**phenomenon, Brücke–Bartley** *See* **effect, Brücke–Bartley.**

**phenomenon, crowding** A difficulty or inability to discriminate small visual acuity tests when they are presented next to each other in a row, whereas the same sized acuity symbols presented singly against a uniform background are resolved. Although this phenomenon may be experienced by normal patients, it is most often characteristic of amblyopic eyes and of people with reading difficulties. *Syn.* crowding effect.
*See* **acuity, morphoscopic visual; amblyopia.**

**phenomenon, doll's head** Reflex movement of the eyes in a direction opposite to that in which the head is suddenly moved, followed by a return towards the original position. If the eye movements do not accord with the above, it may indicate a brainstem defect. *Syn.* doll's eye sign.

**phenomenon, entoptic** *See* **image, entoptic.**

**phenomenon, extinction** A condition in which individual stimuli placed in the visual field are seen, but when the nasal field of one eye and the temporal field of the other eye are stimulated simultaneously the subject fails to see one of the stimuli. This condition is common following a stroke. *Syn.* pseudo-hemianopia.

**phenomenon, jack-in-the-box** When wearing very high positive lenses (e.g. in aphakia) there exists an area in the periphery situated between the outer extent of the field seen through the lens and the field beyond the edge of the lens which is not seen (**ring scotoma**). This phenomenon refers to the disappearance and sudden reappearance of an object when the eye moves from the periphery to the centre passing over the ring scotoma. This phenomenon can be avoided by turning the head rather than the eye for peripheral viewing or by correcting with contact lenses. Modern aspheric lenses minimize this phenomenon as they have reduced peripheral power.
*See* **field of view, real; scotoma, ring.**

**phenomenon, jaw-winking** An abnormal condition associated with congenital ptosis which is characterized by the elevation of the ptotic eyelid when the mouth is opened or the jaw is moved laterally to the side opposite to the ptosis. The eyelid droops again if the jaw maintains its new position or is closed. The condition often diminishes with time, otherwise surgery is the main treatment. *Syn.* Marcus Gunn phenomenon; Marcus Gunn jaw-winking syndrome.
*See* **ptosis.**

**phenomenon, Marcus Gunn** *See* **phenomenon, jaw-winking.**

**phenomenon, Mizuo's** The appearance of a golden brown colour of the retina as it adapts to light, in Oguchi's disease. When adapted to darkness the fundus has the normal red appearance. *Syn.* Mizuo's sign.
*See* **disease, Oguchi's.**

**phenomenon, phi** *See* **movement, phi.**

**phenomenon, Pulfrich** *See* **stereophenomenon, Pulfrich.**

**phenomenon, Purkinje's** *See* **Purkinje shift.**

**phenomenon, Riddoch** Ability to perceive the motion of an object while being unable to detect any other features of that object, such as its colour or its form. This may occur in a scotomatous area of the visual field caused by a lesion somewhere in the visual pathway from the lateral geniculate body to the occipital cortex.

**phenomenon, Troxler's** An image in the periphery of the retina tends to fade or disappear during steady fixation of another object. This phenomenon is rarely noticed due to the involuntary eye movements. When these are neutralized optically, as in stabilized retinal imagery, the phenomenon occurs readily even in central vision. *See* **movements, fixation; stabilized retinal image.**

**phenomenon, Uhthoff's** *See* **Uhthoff's symptom.**

**phenylephrine hydrochloride** *See* **alpha-adrenergic antagonist; mydriatic.**

**phi movement** *See* **movement, phi.**

**phlyctenular keratitis** *See* **keratitis, phlyctenular.**

**phoria** Synonym for heterophoria as well as orthophoria.
*See* **heterophoria; orthophoria.**

**phoria line** *See* **line, phoria.**

**phorometer** An instrument for measuring heterophoria consisting usually of Maddox rods and rotary prisms mounted on a phoropter or trial frame.
*See* **heterophoria.**

**phoropter** An instrument for measuring the ametropias, phorias and the amplitude of accommodation of the eyes. It consists of a large unit placed in front of the patient's head in which there are three rotating discs containing convex and concave spherical and cylindrical lenses, as well as occluders, Maddox rods, pinholes, Polaroids, prisms and coloured filters. An attachment on the instrument allows sets of rotary prisms and cross-cylinders to be swung in front of each sight hole (Fig. P7). *Syn.* refracting unit; refractor; refractor head.
*See* **Simultantest; trial case.**

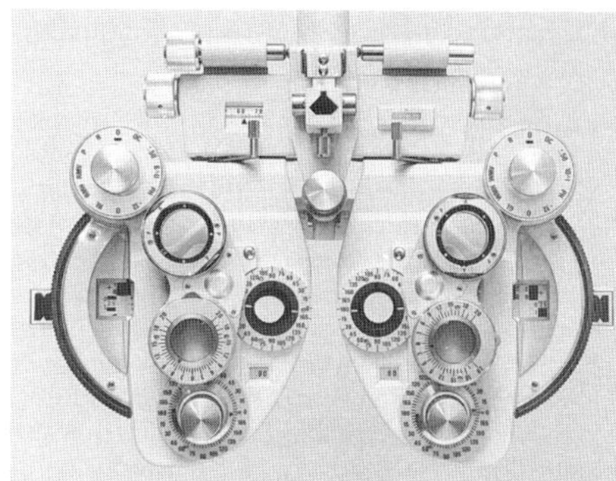

**Fig. P7** Phoropter (Topcon)

**phosphene** A visual sensation arising from stimulation of the retina by something other than light. The stimulation can be either electrical, mechanical (e.g. a blow to the head or pressure on the eyeball), or some electromagnetic waves such as X-rays.
*See* **image, entoptic; photopsia; stimulus, adequate.**

**phosphorescence** Luminescence which persists for some time after the exciting stimulus has ceased.
*See* **luminescence.**

**photic** Pertaining to light or the production of light.

**photocell** Physical receptor which produces electric current when light is incident upon it. *Syn.* photoelectric cell.

**photochemical** Relating to a chemical change as a result of the absorption of light. *Example*: The action of light on rhodopsin in the photoreceptors of the retina.
*See* **rhodopsin.**

**photochromatic interval** *See* **interval, photochromatic.**

**photochromatic lens** *See* **lens, photochromatic.**

**photocoagulation** Process of changing blood and tissue from a fluid to a clotted state produced by the heat of an intense beam of light (e.g. laser), as used in the treatment of retinal diseases (e.g. diabetic retinopathy, retinal detachments, haemorrhages).
*See* **laser; maculopathy, age-related; retinal detachment; retinopathy, diabetic.**

**photodynamic therapy** *See* **maculopathy, age-related.**

**photoelectric** Pertaining to the interaction between radiation and matter resulting in the absorption of photons and the consequent emission of electrons.

**photokeratitis** *See* **keratoconjunctivitis, actinic.**

**photokeratoconjunctivitis** *See* **keratoconjunctivitis, actinic.**

**photokeratoscopy** Determination of corneal curvatures and topography by photographing the corneal image of a target (usually black and white concentric rings) provided with the instrument. Measuring the size of the image and knowing the size of the object, it is possible to calculate the topography of the cornea. The theory is the same as that of the keratometer. A permanent photographic record is given with this method. The area of the cornea which is evaluated is much larger than with a keratometer.
*See* **keratometer; keratoscope; stereophotography; videokeratoscope.**

**photoluminescence** *See* **luminescence.**

**photometer** An instrument for measuring the luminous intensity of a light source or a surface, by comparing it with a standard source. The comparison can be done either with the human eye (as in the Lummer–Brodhun or SEI exposure photometers) or with a photoelectric cell (as in the Pritchard photometer). *Syn.* illuminometer; luxometer.
*See* **illuminance; luminance.**

**photometer, flicker** Visual photometer in which the observer sees a field illuminated alternately by two sources to be compared. When the sensation of flicker disappears, the intensity of the test source can be deduced by reading that of the reference standard source to which it is compared. For luminance difference, the frequency of alternation is chosen to be below the critical fusion frequency but for colour difference it is chosen above it.
*See* **frequency, critical fusion.**

**photometer, Lummer–Brodhun** A cube in which two adjacent or concentric portions of a comparison viewing screen are separately illuminated by the test source and a standard source. The instrument gives quite accurate readings when the two sources are of identical colour.

**photometer, Macbeth** Photometer using the Lummer–Brodhun cube, an eyepiece and a movable standard source illuminating a diffusing surface seen as an annulus by reflection within the cube. The portion of the source to be measured is seen through the cube as a spot within the annulus. The brightness of the annulus is adjusted until it matches that of the spot.

**photometer, objective** *See* **photometer, physical.**

**photometer, physical** A photometer employing a radiant energy sensitive element (e.g. a photoelectric cell, a thermopile) and an intensity indicator. *Example*: Pritchard photometer. *Syn.* objective photometer.

**photometer, Pritchard** *See* **photometer, physical.**

**photometer, SEI exposure; subjective** *See* **photometer, visual.**

**photometer, visual** A photometer in which the equality of brightness of a light source or a surface with a comparison standard source is made by visual observation. *Examples*: flicker photometer; Lummer–Brodhun photometer; Macbeth photometer; SEI photometer. *Syn.* subjective photometer.

**photometry** The measurement of light with a photometer.
*See* **candela per square metre; flux, luminous; footcandle; footlambert; illuminance; intensity, luminous; lambert; luminance; millilambert; photometer.**

**Table P3** Common photometric units

| |
|---|
| *luminous flux* |
| lumens |
| *luminous intensity (I)* |
| candela = lumens/steradian |
| *illuminance (E)* |
| lux = lumens/m$^2$ |
| footcandle = lumens/ft$^2$ |
| *luminance (L)* |
| candela/m$^2$ |
| candela/ft$^2$ |
| footlambert |
| lambert |
| millilambert |
| 1 footlambert (fL) = 3.426 cd/m$^2$ |
| 1 lambert = 3183 cd/m$^2$ |
| 1 millilambert = 3.183 cd/m$^2$ |
| 1 candela/m$^2$ = 0.2919 fL |
| 1 candela/ft$^2$ = 3.142 fL |

**photon** The basic unit of radiant energy defined by the equation

$$E = h\nu$$

where h is **Planck's constant** ($6.62 \times 10^{-34}$ joule × second), $\nu$ the frequency of the light and $E$ the energy difference carried away by the emission of a single photon of light. The term photon usually refers to visible light whereas the term **quantum** refers to other electromagnetic radiations.
*See* **theory, quantum; theory, wave; troland.**

**photonics** Term referring to all the methods, procedures and systems used to measure, transmit or utilize light.

**photophobia** Abnormal fear or intolerance of light. It can be physiological although it often accompanies inflammations of the anterior segment of the eye, especially anterior uveitis. It is also noted in patients with cone degeneration. Management is usually aimed at treating the primary cause (e.g. keratitis, uveitis), but in other cases (e.g. albinism, drug-induced mydriasis, recent aphakes, fear of light) tinted lenses will give relief.
*See* **albinism; iritis; keratitis; lens, tinted; monochromat; sunglasses; uveitis.**

**photophthalmia** *See* **keratoconjunctivitis, actinic.**

**photopic eye** *See* **eye, light-adapted.**

**photopic vision** *See* **vision, photopic.**

**photopigment** A pigment altered by the absorption of light energy.
*See* **pigment, visual; rhodopsin.**

**photopsia** Hallucinatory perceptions such as sparks, lights or colours arising in the absence of light stimuli and observed when the eyes are closed. They occur often as a result of diseases of the optic nerve, retina (e.g. retinal and vitreous detachment) or the brain, migraine, or they can also occur with pressure upon the closed eye.
*See* **floaters; Fuchs' spot; humour, vitreous; retinal detachment; retinitis, cytomegalovirus; vitreous detachment.**

**photoreceptor** A receptor capable of reacting when stimulated by light, such as the rods and cones of the retina.
*See* **cell, cone; cell, rod.**

**photorefraction** A family of photographic techniques which provide a rapid, objective method of measuring the refractive error and accommodative response of the eye. Light emitted from a small flash source placed close to the camera lens is reflected from the eye and returned to the camera. Three methods have been developed: **orthogonal**, **isotropic** and **eccentric** (also called **photoretinoscopy**). The optical design of each method results in a specific photographic pattern which varies with the degree to which the eye is defocused with respect to the plane of the camera. Photorefractive methods are not as accurate as retinoscopy but as they are entirely objective, much quicker and do not require prolonged fixation on the part of the patient, they are highly suited for testing infants and young children.
*See* **optometer; refractive error; retinoscope.**

**photorefractive keratectomy** *See* **keratotomy, radial.**

**photoretinoscopy** *See* **photorefraction.**

**photostress test** *See* **test, photostress.**

**phototransduction** *See* **transduction.**

**phototropism** Reaction of certain plants and animals to move towards (positive phototropism) or away from (negative phototropism) a source of light.

**phthiriasis** Infestation of the eyelid margin by lice. It causes itching along the eyelid margin. Removal of the parasites is relatively easy either with forceps or by **cryotherapy** (removal under cold or freezing conditions).
*See* **eyelids.**

**phthisis bulbi** Shrinkage and atrophy of the eyeball following a severe inflammation (e.g. uveitis), absolute glaucoma or trauma.

**phthisis corneae** Shrinkage and atrophy of the cornea following a severe inflammation of the cornea or trauma. It is associated with shrinkage of the globe.

**phycomycosis** A fungal infection caused by various microorganisms. These fungi may spread from the sinuses or the nasal tissue into the orbit, particularly in patients with diabetes, renal failure, malignant tumour or on steroid therapy. Therapy is aimed at the underlying disease, often accompanied by antifungal agents. *Syn.* zygomycosis.

**physical optics** *See* **optics, physical.**

**physiological astigmatism; blind spot; cup; diplopia; optics; position of rest; saline** *See* under the nouns.

**physostigmine** A reversible anticholinesterase drug used as a parasympathomimetic which, when used in the eye constricts the pupil. It may be used in solution of 0.25–1% or ointment 0.25–0.50% in the treatment of glaucoma, but because of its side-effects its usage is rare nowadays. It is sometimes combined with pilocarpine. *Syn.* eserine.
*See* **miotics; neostigmine; parasympathomimetic drug; pilocarpine.**

**pia mater** A delicate fibrous membrane closely enveloping the brain, spinal cord and the optic nerve. It terminates at the eye.

**Pickford–Nicholson anomaloscope** *See* **anomaloscope.**

**Piéron's law** *See* **law, Ricco's.**

**Pigeon–Cantonnet stereoscope** *See* **stereoscope, Pigeon–Cantonnet.**

**piggyback lens** *See* **lens, piggyback.**

**pigment dispersion syndrome** *See* **syndrome, pigment dispersion.**

**pigment epithelium** *See* **retinal pigment epithelium.**

**pigment in the macula, yellow** *See* **macula lutea.**

**pigment, macular** A yellow pigment, insensitive to light and located in the inner layers of the macular area of the retina. It extends over an area of about 12° in diameter. Its density declines markedly with eccentricity. The major components of this pigment are carotene-like pigments: lutein and zeaxanthin. These yellow pigments absorb blue light maximally. The macular pigment has been thought to mitigate the effect of chromatic aberration and to protect the retina against short wavelength radiations.
*See* **filter, red; image, retinal; macula lutea.**

**pigment, visual** Photosensitive pigment contained in the outer segments of both rods and cones. The pigment in the rods is called rhodopsin. The cones contain three other types of pigments (one in each cone) which have spectral absorption curves with a maximum around 420, 530 and 560 nm. These three pigments form the basis of normal trichromatic colour vision. *Syn.* for cone visual pigments: **cyanolabe**, **chlorolabe** and **erythrolabe**, names sometimes used for the short-wave, middle-wave and long-wave sensitive cone pigments, respectively. *Note*: erythrolabe, meaning red pigment, has, in fact, its maximum spectral absorption around 560 nm which is in the green-yellow portion of the visible spectrum.
*See* **bleaching; cell, cone; cell, rod; colour vision, defective; densitometry, retinal; iodopsin; porphyropsin; rhodopsin; test, photostress; trichromatism; theory, Young–Helmholtz.**

**pigmentary glaucoma** *See* **syndrome, pigment dispersion.**

**pigmentary reaction of the retina** *See* **disease, Batten–Mayou; fundus albipunctatus; fundus flavimaculatus; Leber's congenital amaurosis; retinitis pigmentosa; syndrome, Laurence–Moon–Bardet–Biedl; syndrome, Usher's.**

**pilocarpine** An alkaloid obtained from the leaves of *Pilocarpus microphyllus* and other species of *Pilocarpus*. It is a **parasympathomimetic** (or **direct-acting cholinergic) drug** which mimics the effect of acetylcholine causing miosis and accommodation. It counteracts sympathomimetic mydriatics. It is used in the treatment of glaucoma. Pilocarpine hydrochloride is most commonly applied to the eye as a 1% solution. Carbachol and bethanechol chloride are other parasympathomimetic drugs with similar effects to pilocarpine.
*See* **acetylcholine; glaucoma, angle-closure; glaucoma, open-angle; miotics; parasympathomimetic drug; physostigmine.**

**Table P4** Cone pigments in normal and congenital dichromatic colour vision defects (excluding cases due to anomalies of the central visual pathway)

| colour vision | long-wave sensitive (around 560 nm) | middle-wave sensitive (around 530 nm) | short-wave sensitive (around 420 nm) |
|---|---|---|---|
| normal | present | present | present |
| protanope | absent or abnormal | present | present |
| deuteranope | present | absent or abnormal | present |
| tritanope | present | present | absent or abnormal |

**pince-nez** Eyeglasses without sides, held on the nose by tension from springs attached to the nose pads.
*See* **lens, spectacle; pad.**

**pincushion distortion** *See* **distortion.**

**pinealoma** A tumour of the pineal body, a small glandular structure that lies between the two superior colliculi in a depression below the splenium of the corpus callosum. It may result in a loss of the pupil light reflex, vertical gaze palsy (especially in children), hydrocephalus, as well as a disturbance of the secretion of melatonin, which is related to the diurnal dark-light cycles. *Syn.* pineoblastoma.
*See* **nystagmus, convergence-retraction.**

**pinguecula** A benign degenerative tumour of the bulbar conjunctiva that appears as a slightly raised, yellowish-white, oval shaped thickening on either side of the cornea, but usually the nasal side. Histologically, it consists of a deposition of hyaline substance. It becomes more common in elderly people, especially those exposed to high levels of ultraviolet radiation, wind and dust. Although benign, surgical excision may be requested for cosmetic reasons.
*See* **pterygium.**

**pinhole disc; spectacles** *See* under the nouns.

**pinhole test** *See* **disc, pinhole.**

**pink eye** *See* **conjunctivitis, contagious.**

**Piper's law** *See* **law, Ricco's.**

**pit, optic** A depression on each side of the end of the neural ectoderm (or neural tube) of the embryo. The pit deepens to form the optic vesicle. *Syn.* optic sulcus.
*See* **vesicle, optic.**

**placebo** A substance or a prescription (e.g. plano lenses) devoid of any physiological effect which is given merely to satisfy a patient. It is also used in research as a control against which the real effect of another product (similar in appearance) can be established.
*See* **test, blind.**

**Placido disc** *See* **keratoscope.**

**Planck's constant** *See* **photon.**

**Planck's law** *See* **law, Planck's.**

**plane** A flat surface.

**plane, aperture** A plane which passes through the aperture of an optical system.

**plane, apparent frontoparallel (AFPP)** Plane passing through the fixation point and containing all other points judged to appear in the same frontal plane. At about 1 metre from the eye it more or less coincides with a frontal plane; this is the **abathic distance**. Closer to 1 metre it is often a concave surface with its concavity turned towards the observer and beyond 1 metre it is a convex surface with its convexity turned towards the observer.
*See* **deviation, Hering–Hillebrand; horopter.**

**plane, equatorial** Vertical plane passing through the centre of curvature of the large circle of the eyeball, perpendicular to the optical axis and which divides the eyeball into anterior and posterior halves.
*See* **anterior segment of the eye.**

**plane of the eye, horizontal** Plane, such as the *xy* plane, passing through the centre of rotation of the eye and dividing it into superior and inferior halves. When the eye is looking straight ahead this plane is horizontal.
*See* **plane, subjective horizontal; plane, *xy*.**

**plane of fixation** *See* **plane of regard.**

**plane, focal** A plane, perpendicular to the optical axis, which passes through one of the focal points of an optical system.
*See* **focus, principal.**

**plane, frontal** A vertical plane perpendicular to the median plane.

**plane, frontoparallel** The frontal plane passing through the fixation point.

**plane, image** A plane, perpendicular to the optical axis at any axial image point of an optical system.

**plane of incidence** The plane containing the incident and reflected rays, and the normal to the surface at the point of incidence.

**plane, Listing's** A frontal plane passing through the centre of rotation which corresponds to the equatorial plane of the eye when it is looking in the straight ahead position.

**plane, median** The vertical plane that divides the head into right and left halves.

**plane mirror** *See* **mirror, plane.**

**plane, nodal** A plane, perpendicular to the optical axis, which passes through one of the nodal points of an optical system (Fig. P8).
*See* **points, nodal.**

**plane, object** A plane perpendicular to the optical axis at any axial object point of an optical system.

**plane, principal** A plane perpendicular to the optical axis of an optical system at the point where the incident rays parallel to the optical axis intersect the refracted rays converging to the secondary focal point (**secondary principal plane**); or in which the refracted rays parallel to the optical axis intersect the incident rays coming from the primary focal point (**primary principal plane**). Each

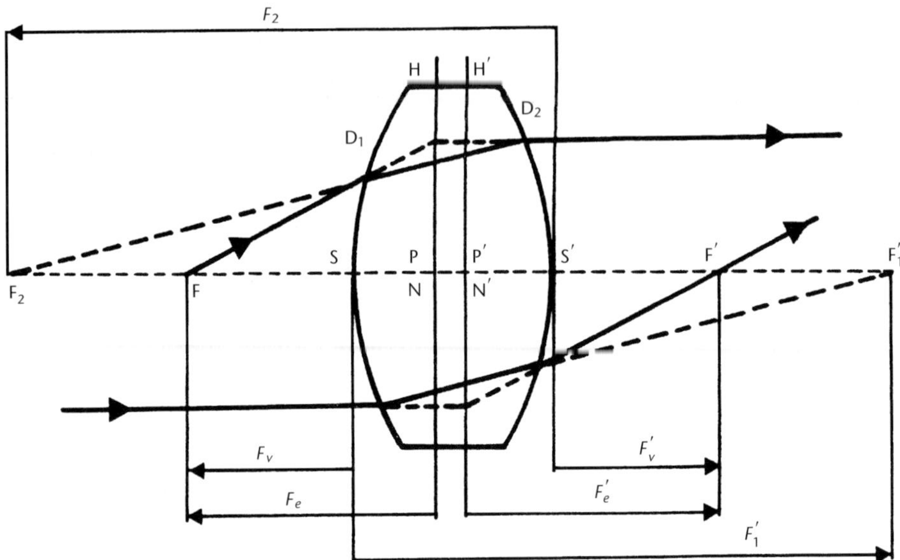


**Fig. P8** Primary and secondary principal planes HP and H′P′ of a thick lens in air (PF, anterior focal length; P′F′, posterior focal length; SF, front vertex focal length; S′F′, back vertex focal length; SF′$_1$, back focal length of the first surface D$_1$; S′F$_2$, front focal length of the second surface D$_2$; N and N′, nodal points)

plane is an erect image of the other, and of the same size. For this reason they are sometimes also referred to as **unit planes** as they are conjugate planes in which the magnification is +1. In a thin lens these planes coincide at the lens. (Fig. P8)
*See* **distance, image; distance, object; length, focal; lens, thin; points, nodal; points, principal; power, equivalent.**

**plane of regard** Plane containing the fixation point, the axes of fixation from the two eyes and the base line. *Syn.* plane of fixation.
*See* **line, base; line, median.**

**plane, sagittal** A vertical plane parallel to the median plane as, for example, the *yz* plane.
*See* **plane, *yz*.**

**plane, spectacle** A plane representing the orientation of the spectacle lenses relative to the eyes and passing through the posterior vertices of the two lenses.
*See* **angle, pantoscopic; angle, retroscopic; vertex; vertex distance.**

**plane, subjective horizontal** Plane fixed with respect to the eye, i.e. horizontal when the eye is in the primary position.
*See* **plane of the eye, horizontal; position, primary.**

**plane of vibration** *See* **light, polarized.**

**plane, visual** The plane containing the two visual axes.

**plane, *xy*** Horizontal plane of the eye containing both the *x*- and *y*-axes.
*See* **axis, anteroposterior; axis, transverse.**

**plane, *yz*** Vertical plane of the eye containing both the *y*- and *z*-axes.
*See* **axis, anteroposterior; axis, vertical.**

**planes, cardinal** Planes, normal to the optical axis, which pass through the cardinal points of a lens or optical system. They are the focal planes, the nodal planes and the principal planes. (Sometimes, this definition also includes the object and image planes.)
*See* **points, cardinal.**

**planes, unit** *See* **plane, principal.**

**plano lens** *See* **lens, afocal.**

**planoconcave lens** *See* **lens, planoconcave.**

**planoconvex lens** *See* **lens, planoconvex.**

**plaques, Hollenhorst's** Orange-yellow spots, usually found at branching sites of retinal arterioles. They are due to necrosis and ulceration of atheromatous, cholesterin-containing emboli in the carotid arteries which discharge into the circulation. They do not usually obstruct the retinal arterioles and as such do not cause visual symptoms. However, they indicate the possible development of larger emboli (**fibrinoplatelets**) that may temporarily obstruct the retinal circulation and cause amaurosis fugax, and may even presage a myocardial infarction or stroke.

*See* **amaurosis fugax; arcus senilis; atheroma; xanthelasma.**

**plastic** Various organic or synthetic materials (e.g. CR-39, HEMA, polymethyl methacrylate, polycarbonate, etc.) which can be transformed into solid shapes to make spectacle frames, contact lenses, ophthalmic lenses, etc. and can be made to have good optical surfaces, high light transmission and refractive indices and dispersions similar to that of crown or flint glass.
*See* **acetone; CR-39; HEMA; index of refraction; polymethyl methacrylate; spectacle frame, plastic.**

**plastic period** *See* **period, critical.**

**plastic spectacle frame** *See* **spectacle frame, plastic.**

**plateau iris** *See* **iris, plateau.**

**Plateau's spiral** *See* **spiral, Plateau's.**

**plates, pseudoisochromatic** Charts for testing colour vision on which are printed dots of various colours, brightness, saturation and sizes, arranged so that the dots of similar colour form a figure (a letter, a numeral, a geometrical shape or winding path) among a background of dots of another colour. The colours of the figure and the background correspond to the confusion colours of the various types of anomalous colour vision. A dichromat or an anomalous trichromat has difficulty in perceiving the pattern because it is distinguishable from the background only by its difference in hue. There are many different sets of such plates, some using figures (circles, crosses or triangles) such as the **AO, HRR** plates, or numbers or lines such as those of **Ishihara** (Fig. P9) and **Dvorine**, or five spots such as the **City University test** (CUT) in which the subject chooses the spot most closely matching the colour of the central spot, etc.

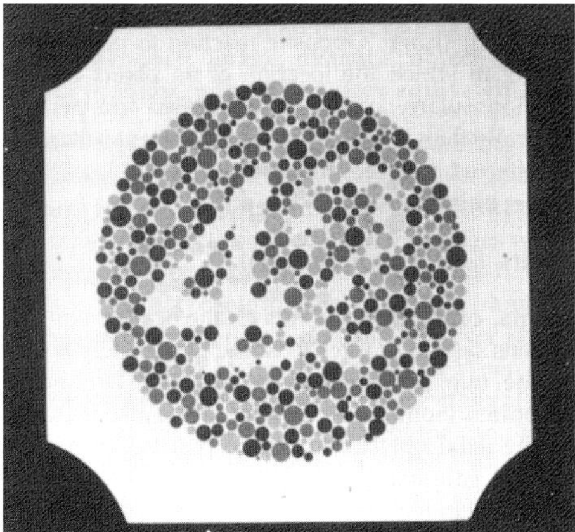

**Fig. P9** One of the Ishihara pseudoisochromatic plates

*See* **colours, confusion; colour vision, defective; lamp, Macbeth.**

**pleochroism** The property of an optically anisotropic medium (that is certain crystals) to exhibit different brightness and/or colour when the light transmitted through it is viewed from different directions. (A particular case of pleochroism is dichroism.) *Syn.* polychroism.
*See* **anisotropic; dichroism.**

**pleomorphism, endothelial** *See* **polymorphism, endothelial.**

**pleoptics** A method of treating amblyopia with eccentric fixation which consists of dazzling the eccentrically fixating retinal area with high illumination while protecting the fovea with a disc projected onto the fundus and thereby rendering the fovea more responsive to fixation stimuli. There exist several variations of this procedure, but the therapy is very fastidious.
*See* **amblyopia; occlusion treatment; orthoptics; Visuscope.**

**plexiform layer** *See* **retina.**

**plexus, cavernous** A network of nerve fibres derived from the internal carotid nerve and located on the inferotemporal aspect of the internal carotid artery in the cavernous sinus. It supplies sympathetic innervation to almost all of the orbit, including fibres to the dilator pupillae muscle, Müller's superior palpebral muscle, the ciliary muscle and vasoconstrictor fibres for the blood vessels of the eye.
*See* **syndrome, Horner's.**

**plexus, deep episcleral** *See* **plexus, pericorneal.**

**plexus, episcleral venous** A network of vessels near the limbus which receives blood from the intrascleral plexus and canal of Schlemm via collector channels and drains into the anterior ciliary veins. It also receives blood from the conjunctival veins and drains the perilimbal conjunctiva.

**plexus, internal carotid** A network of nerve fibres derived from the internal carotid nerve and located on the lateral side of the internal carotid artery near the apex of the petrous bone. It sends sympathetic axons to the abducens, ophthalmic and nasociliary nerves, the deep petrosal nerve, the caroticotympanic nerve and the ophthalmic and lacrimal arteries.
*See* **ganglion, superior cervical.**

**plexus, intrascleral venous** A network of vessels situated in the deep layers of the sclera near the limbus. It is made up of the deep and mid scleral plexuses. It receives aqueous humour from the canal of Schlemm via collector channels,

a high magnification slit-lamp. If the condition is caused by contact lens wear, management consists of refitting the patient with daily wear contact lenses of higher oxygen transmissibility.
*See* **corneal endothelium; microscope, specular; polymorphism, endothelial.**

**polymethyl methacrylate (PMMA)** Polymerized methyl methacrylate forming a light transparent thermoplastic material used in the manufacture of hard contact lenses and some spectacle lenses.
*See* **index of refraction; modulus of elasticity; plastic; siloxane; spectacle frame, plastic.**

**polymorphism, endothelial** The presence of many cell shapes which accompanies polymegethism. *Syn.* endothelial pleomorphism.
*See* **polymegethism, endothelial.**

**polymyxin B** An antibiotic solution effective against many gram-negative organisms and particularly *Pseudomonas aeruginosa*, but not *Proteus*. It is used topically in combination with either bacitracin as an ointment, or trimethoprim as drops or ointment or neomycin plus gramicidin as drops. These combinations render polymyxin B active against a wide range of bacteria.
*See* **antibiotic.**

**polyopia** A condition in which more than one image of a single object is perceived. It may be double vision but more commonly it is multiple vision. Irregular ocular refraction as in some cataracts may sometimes be the cause. *Syn.* multiple vision.
*See* **diplopia; triplopia.**

**polystichia** A condition in which there are two or more rows of eyelashes in a single eyelid.
*See* **distichiasis; eyelashes.**

**polyvinyl alcohol** *See* **wetting solution.**

**Ponzo visual illusion** *See* **illusion, Ponzo visual.**

**porphyropsin** Visual pigment found in the retinas of freshwater fish. It differs from rhodopsin in having its maximum absorption at about 522 nm.
*See* **pigment, visual.**

**port-wine stain** *See* **syndrome, Sturge–Weber.**

**portion** *See* **lens, bifocal; segment of a bifocal lens.**

**portion, intermediate** That portion of a trifocal lens which has the correction for vision of an area situated between distance and near.
*See* **lens, trifocal.**

**position, active** Position of the eyes characterized by foveal fixation of an object by both eyes. Thus, they are under the control of postural, fixation and fusion reflexes.
*See* **esophoria; exophoria; position, passive; reflex.**

**position, dissociated** *See* **dissociation.**

**position, passive** Position of the eyes when they are only under the control of the postural and fixation reflexes, but not the fusion reflex, as, for example, when one eye is covered and the other is fixating an object.
*See* **heterophoria.**

**position, primary** The position of an eye in relation to the head, from which a pure vertical and a pure horizontal movement is not associated with any degree of torsion. The eye is usually, but not necessarily, in the **straight ahead** (or **straightforward**) position.
*See* **centre of rotation of the eye; torsion.**

**position of rest, anatomical** Position of the eyes when they are completely devoid of tonus, as in death.
*See* **tonus.**

**position of rest, physiological** Position of the eyes when they are only under the control of the postural reflexes, but completely free from any visual stimuli.
*See* **accommodation, resting state of; convergence, initial; tonus; vergence, tonic.**

**position, secondary** Movement of an eye represented by a horizontal or vertical rotation away from the primary position.
*See* **version.**

**position, straight ahead; straightforward** *See* **centre of rotation of the eye; position, primary.**

**position, tertiary** Movement of an eye to an oblique position, as, for example, 'up and in'.
*See* **version.**

**positions of gaze, cardinal** *See* **cardinal positions of gaze.**

**positions of gaze, diagnostic** Method of evaluating the integrity of the extraocular muscles by testing the primary, the four secondary and the four tertiary positions of gaze, monocularly or binocularly.
*See* **test, motility; version.**

**positive eyepiece** *See* **eyepiece, positive.**

**positive lens** *See* **lens, converging.**

**positive spherical aberration** *See* **aberration, spherical.**

**Posner–Schlossman syndrome** *See* **syndrome, Posner–Schlossman.**

**posterior chamber** *See* **chamber, posterior.**

**posterior embryotoxon** *See* **ring of Schwalbe, anterior limiting.**

**posterior pole** *See* **poles of the eyeball.**

**posterior polymorphous dystrophy** *See* **dystrophy, posterior polymorphous.**

**posterior segment of the eye** Posterior portion of the eye comprising the vitreous humour, the retina, the optic disc, the choroid and most of the sclera.
*See* **anterior segment of the eye.**

**posterior synechia; uveitis** *See* under the nouns.

**postlenticular space, Berger's** A space between the posterior surface of the crystalline lens and the hyaloid fossa of the vitreous. The space is believed to be filled with aqueous humour. *Syn.* retrolental space of Berger.
*See* **fossa, hyaloid.**

**post-operative overcorrection** *See* **strabismus, consecutive.**

**potential, action** The electric current generated in an axon of a nerve cell in response to a stimulus. The stimulus must be above a certain threshold value to have an effect. The **sodium pump** (or **sodium/potassium pump**) which transports most sodium ions outside the cell and potassium ions inside the cell ceases to function and the sodium ions rush in making the interior of the axon a positive voltage with respect to the outside. The voltage changes from about −70 mV to +40 mV and then falls rapidly back to the resting membrane potential as the sodium pump regains its effect. The whole process takes less than one millisecond and its amplitude is always the same (all or none law) for a given axon, whatever the magnitude of the stimulus. The action potential is followed by an inexcitable period called the **refractory period** which usually lasts one or two milliseconds. The action potential travels as a wave in both directions from the point of stimulation and the speed is faster in myelinated than in unmyelinated nerve fibres. *Syn.* nerve impulse.
*See* **adaptation; law, all or none; neuron; potential, receptor; potential, resting membrane; synapse.**

**Potential Acuity Meter** *See* **maxwellian view system, clinical.**

**potential, early receptor (ERP)** This is an early rapid response that can be detected when the retina is stimulated with an intense flash of light, approximately $10^6$ times brighter than that required to elicit the ERG. It is completed within 1.5 ms and is followed by the a-wave of the ERG. It is primarily, in man, a cone-generated potential.
*See* **electroretinogram.**

**potential of the eye, dark** *See* **potential of the eye, resting.**

**potential of the eye, resting** A direct current potential which exists between the anterior and posterior poles of the eye, the cornea being positive relative to the back of the eye. It is of the order of several mV in humans. This potential is used in recording the electro-oculogram. *Syn.* dark potential of the eye; standing potential of the eye.
*See* **electro-oculogram.**

**potential of the eye, standing** *See* **potential of the eye, resting.**

**potential, membrane** *See* **potential, resting membrane.**

**potential, receptor** Difference in potential occurring in a receptor in response to a stimulus. This is a graded type of response with an amplitude proportional to the intensity of the stimulus. The photoreceptors and the bipolar cells produce a receptor potential but, surprisingly, it is a hyperpolarization, i.e. the inside of the membrane becomes more negative with respect to the outside. The ganglion cells respond with action potentials.
*See* **potential, action; rhodopsin.**

**potential, resting membrane** Difference in direct current potential between the inside and outside of a living cell. The inside of the cell is usually about −70 mV compared to the outside, but this value depends on the quantity of potassium (mainly), sodium and chloride ions on both sides of the membrane, and the permeability to these ions of the membrane itself. *Syn.* membrane potential; transmembrane potential.
*See* **depolarization; hyperpolarization; potential, action; tonus.**

**potential, standing** *See* **electro-oculogram.**

**potential, transmembrane** *See* **potential, resting membrane.**

**potential, visual evoked cortical (VECP)** An electrical potential measured at the level of the occipital cortex in response to a light stimulation. Recording requires repetition of the stimulus and a computer synchronized with the onset of that stimulus, to average out the background noise produced by the spontaneous brain potentials (e.g. alpha, beta, delta, theta waves). This potential has clinical application and is used to objectively measure refraction, visual acuity, amblyopia, binocular anomalies and help in the diagnosis of some demyelinating diseases (e.g. multiple sclerosis), etc. Many abbreviations are also used, although they are not strictly correct. They are EP (evoked potential),

P

VEP (visually evoked potential), VER (visual evoked response), and pVER (indicating that this potential is pattern-elicited).
*See* **accommodation, objective; artifact; electrodiagnostic procedures; sclerosis, multiple.**

**potentials, oscillatory (OP)** Subwaves of low amplitude but high frequency (70–140 Hz) superimposed on the b-wave of the electroretinogram. The amplitude of these oscillatory responses is usually enhanced by a filtering technique. These potentials are presumed to originate from the vicinity of the inner plexiform layer of the retina (probably the amacrine cells) and may reflect disturbances of that part of the retina.
*See* **electroretinogram; retina.**

**power** General term which may refer to any power such as effective, equivalent, dioptric, focal, refractive, surface or vergence power.

**power, aligning** *See* **acuity, vernier visual.**

**Table P5** Power (in dioptres) of the surfaces and structures of an average adult Caucasian eye*

| | |
|---|---|
| anterior surface of the cornea | 48.21 |
| posterior surface of the cornea | −5.97 |
| complete corneal system | 42.34 |
| anterior surface of the lens | 7.92 |
| accommodated | 13.77 |
| posterior surface of the lens | 13.54 |
| accommodated | 15.84 |
| complete lens system | 21.19 |
| accommodated | 29.42 |
| complete eye | 59.44 |
| accommodated | 67.56 |
| refraction of the eye | +0.50 |
| ocular accommodation | 8.12 |

*see constants of the eye.

**power, approximate** *See* **power, nominal.**

**power, back vertex (BVP)** The reciprocal of the back vertex focal length. It is equal to

$$F'_v = \frac{n'}{SF'}$$

where $n'$ is the refractive index of the second medium, $S$ is the point on the back surface through which passes the optical axis and $F'$ the second principal focus. *Symbol*: $F'_v$. Other formulae for the back vertex power of a lens (or an optical system) are

$$F'_v = \frac{F_1}{1-(d/n)F_1} + F_2 = \frac{F_e}{1-(d/n)F_1}$$

where $d$ is the thickness of the lens, $n$ the index of refraction of the lens, $F_1$ the power of the front surface, $F_2$ the power of the back surface and $F_e$ the equivalent power. The powers are in dioptres and the length in metres. The back vertex power is the usual measurement made by a focimeter. *Syn.* back power.
*See* **power, effective; power, equivalent; vergence; vertex focal length.**

**power, dioptric** *See* **power, refractive.**

**power, dispersive** *See* **dispersion.**

**power, effective** The power of a lens or surface measured in a plane other than the principal plane and usually remote from the lens or surface. If a thin lens or surface of power $F$ is illuminated by parallel incident light, the effective power $F_x$ of another lens placed at a distance $d$

**Table P6** Powers of the surfaces of contact lenses of thickness $d = 0.20$ mm, in which the radius of curvature of the back optic zone is constant and that of the front optic zone varies to produce various back vertex powers and equivalent powers. The index of refraction of these lenses is assumed to be 1.49

| radius of back optic zone (mm) | back surface power (D) $F_2$ | radius of front optic zone (mm) | front surface power (D) $F_1$ | power of lens (D) considered thin $F_1 + F_2$ | equivalent power (D) $F_e$ | back vertex power (D) $F'_v$ |
|---|---|---|---|---|---|---|
| 7.8 | −62.82 | 7.2 | 68.06 | +5.24 | +5.81 | +5.86 |
| 7.8 | −62.82 | 7.4 | 66.22 | +3.40 | +3.95 | +3.99 |
| 7.8 | −62.82 | 7.6 | 64.47 | +1.65 | +2.20 | +2.22 |
| 7.8 | −62.82 | 7.8 | 62.82 | 0.00 | +0.53 | +0.53 |
| 7.8 | −62.82 | 8.0 | 61.25 | −1.57 | −1.05 | −1.06 |
| 7.8 | −62.82 | 8.2 | 59.76 | −3.06 | −2.56 | −2.58 |
| 7.8 | −62.82 | 8.4 | 58.33 | −4.49 | −4.00 | −4.03 |
| 7.8 | −62.82 | 8.6 | 56.98 | −5.84 | −5.36 | −5.40 |
| 7.8 | −62.82 | 8.8 | 55.68 | −7.14 | −6.67 | −6.72 |
| 7.8 | −62.82 | 9.0 | 54.44 | −8.38 | −7.92 | −7.98 |
| 7.8 | −62.82 | 9.2 | 53.26 | −9.56 | −9.11 | −9.18 |
| 7.8 | −62.82 | 9.4 | 52.13 | −10.69 | −10.25 | −10.33 |

from the original lens and forming an image in the same position, is given by the equation

$$F_x = \frac{F}{1 - dF}$$

where $d$ is in metres and positive when measured from left to right. *Examples*: (1) If a hyperopic eye is corrected by a lens $F = +5\,\text{D}$ placed 12 mm from the cornea, the ocular refraction is

$$F_x = \frac{5}{1 - (0.012 \times 5)} = +5.32\,\text{D}$$

(2) If an eye has an ocular refraction of $-10\,\text{D}$, its spectacle refraction at a vertex distance of 10 mm is

$$F_x = \frac{10}{1 - (-0.01 \times -10)} = -11.11\,\text{D}$$

*See* **plane, principal; refractive error; vertex distance.**

**power, equivalent** The refractive power of a lens or an optical system expressed with reference to the principal points. It corresponds to the refractive power of a thin lens placed in the second principal plane which would form an image of a distant object of the same size as that produced by the system that it replaces. It is equal to

$$F_e = \frac{n'}{f'} = -\frac{n}{f}$$

where $n$ and $n'$ are the indices of refraction of the object and image space, respectively, $f$ and $f'$ the distances (in metres) between the first and second principal points and the first and second principal foci, respectively. The equivalent power (*symbol*: $F_e$) is in dioptres. It is also equal to

$$F_e = F_1 + F_2 - \left(\frac{d}{n}\right) F_1 F_2$$

where $F_1$ and $F_2$ are the powers of the lenses or surfaces comprising the system, $d$ is the distance between the two and $n$ the index of refraction of the intervening medium. *Example*: If the anterior surface power of the cornea is equal to $+48.21\,\text{D}$, the posterior surface power is equal to $-5.97\,\text{D}$, the thickness of the cornea 0.5 mm and the index of refraction 1.376, the equivalent power will be

$$F_e = 48.21 - 5.97 - \frac{0.0005}{1.376} \times 48.21 \times (-5.97)$$
$$= +42.34\,\text{D}$$

*Syn.* true power.
*See* **length, equivalent focal; plane, principal; points, principal; power, nominal.**

**power factor** *See* **magnification, spectacle.**

**power, focal** *See* **paraxial equation, fundamental; power, refractive.**

**Table P7** Contact lens power (or ocular refraction) corresponding to a spectacle lens situated at two vertex distances

| spectacle lens power (D) | contact lens power (D) | |
|---|---|---|
| | 10 mm | 14 mm |
| −16 | −13.79 | −13.07 |
| −14 | −12.28 | −11.71 |
| −12 | −10.71 | −10.27 |
| −10 | −9.09 | −8.77 |
| −9 | −8.26 | −7.99 |
| −8 | −7.41 | −7.19 |
| −7 | −6.54 | −6.38 |
| −6 | −5.66 | −5.53 |
| −5 | −4.76 | −4.67 |
| −4 | −3.85 | −3.79 |
| −3 | −2.91 | −2.88 |
| +3 | +3.09 | +3.13 |
| +4 | +4.17 | +4.24 |
| +5 | +5.26 | +5.38 |
| +6 | +6.38 | +6.55 |
| +7 | +7.53 | +7.76 |
| +8 | +8.70 | +9.01 |
| +9 | +9.89 | +10.30 |
| +10 | +11.11 | +11.63 |
| +12 | +13.64 | +14.42 |

**power, front vertex (FVP)** The reciprocal of the front vertex focal length. It is equal to

$$F_v = \frac{n}{SF}$$

where $n$ is the refractive index of the first medium, $S$ is the point on the front surface through which passes the optical axis and $F$ is the first principal focus. *Symbol*: $F_v$. Other formulae for the front vertex power of a lens (or an optical system) are

$$F_v = \frac{F_2}{1 - (d/n)F_2} + F_1 = \frac{F_e}{1 - (d/n)F_2}$$

where $d$ is the thickness of the lens, $n$ the index of refraction of the lens, $F_1$ the power of the front surface, $F_2$ the power of the back surface and $F_e$ the equivalent power. The powers are in dioptres and the length in metres. *Syn.* front power.
*See* **power, effective; power, equivalent; vergence; vertex focal length.**

**power, magnification** *See* **magnification, spectacle.**

**power, magnifying** *See* **magnification, apparent.**

**power, nominal** An estimate of the power of a lens, calculated as the sum of the front and back surface powers, i.e.

$$F = F_1 + F_2$$

p

*Syn.* approximate power.
*See* **power, equivalent; power, surface.**

**power, prism** The amount of deviation of a ray of light transmitted through a prism or lens (outside its optical centre). It is usually expressed in prism dioptres (Δ) and given by the following approximate formula for small angle prisms (in air)

$$P = 100(n - 1)a$$

where $a$ is the prism angle in radians and $n$ the index of refraction of the prism. *Example*: What is the power of a prism with an apex angle of 6° and a refractive index of 1.50? $P = 100(1.50 - 1)(6/57.3) = 5.24\,\Delta$ which corresponds to the deviation of a ray of light equal to 5.24 cm at 100 cm. *Syn.* prismatic power.
*See* **dioptre, prism; law, Prentice's.**

**power, prismatic** *See* **power, prism.**

**power, refractive** The ability of a lens or an optical system to change the direction of a pencil of rays. It is equal to

$$F = \frac{n'}{f'} = -\frac{n}{f}$$

where $n$ and $n'$ are the refractive indices of the object and image space, respectively, $f$ and $f'$ the first and second focal length, respectively, in metres, and the power $F$ is expressed in dioptres. *Symbol*: $F$. *Syn.* dioptric power; focal power; vergence power.
*See* **dioptre; length, focal; paraxial equation, fundamental; power, equivalent; vergence.**

**power, resolving** *See* **resolution, limit of.**

**power, surface** The dioptric power of a single refracting or reflecting surface. It is equal to

$$F = \frac{n' - n}{r}$$

where $F$ is the power in dioptres, $n$ and $n'$ are the refractive indices of the media on each side of the surface and $r$ is the radius of curvature of the lens or mirror surface, in metres. This equation forms part of the fundamental paraxial equation. For a spectacle lens in air ($n = 1$) the power of the surface becomes

$$F = \frac{n' - 1}{r}$$

*Examples*: Power of the corneal surfaces.
(1) Anterior surface

$$F = \frac{1.376 - 1}{0.0078} = 48.21\ \text{D}$$

where the refractive index of the cornea is 1.376 and the surface has a radius of curvature of 7.8 mm.

(2) Posterior surface

$$F = \frac{1.336 - 1.376}{0.0067} = -5.97\ \text{D}$$

where the refractive indices of the aqueous humour and the cornea are 1.336 and 1.376, respectively, and the surface has a radius of curvature of 6.7 mm.
For a thin spectacle lens in air, the sum of the powers of the two surfaces $F_1 + F_2$ represents the total power of the lens and is equal to

$$F = F_1 + F_2 = (n - 1)\left(\frac{1}{r_1} - \frac{1}{r_2}\right)$$

where $n$ is the index of refraction of the lens and $r_1$ and $r_2$ the radii of curvature of its two surfaces.
*See* **paraxial equation, fundamental.**

**Table P8** Surface power of the anterior surface of the cornea (in dioptres) corresponding to various radii of curvature (in mm). Calculations were made using 1.376 as the index of refraction of the cornea

| radius | power | radius | power |
|---|---|---|---|
| 6.80 | 55.29 | 7.80 | 48.20 |
| 7.00 | 53.71 | 7.85 | 47.90 |
| 7.10 | 52.96 | 7.90 | 47.59 |
| 7.20 | 52.22 | 7.95 | 47.30 |
| 7.30 | 51.51 | 8.00 | 47.00 |
| 7.40 | 50.81 | 8.10 | 46.42 |
| 7.50 | 50.13 | 8.20 | 45.85 |
| 7.55 | 49.80 | 8.30 | 45.30 |
| 7.60 | 49.47 | 8.40 | 44.76 |
| 7.65 | 49.15 | 8.50 | 44.23 |
| 7.70 | 48.83 | 8.60 | 43.72 |
| 7.75 | 48.52 | 8.80 | 42.73 |

**power, true** *See* **power, equivalent.**

**power, vergence** *See* **paraxial equation, fundamental; power, refractive; vergence.**

**power, vertex** *See* **power, back vertex; power, front vertex.**

**precorneal film** *See* **film, precorneal.**

**prednisolone** *See* **antiinflammatory drugs.**

**preferential looking** *See* **method, preferential looking.**

**prelens tear film** *See* **tear film, prelens.**

**prelumirhodopsin** *See* **rhodopsin.**

**Prentice's law; rule** *See* **law, Prentice's.**

**preocular tear film** *See* **film, precorneal.**

**preretinal haemorrhage** *See* **haemorrhage, preretinal.**

**preretinal membrane** *See* **fibrosis, preretinal macular.**

**presbyope** A person who has presbyopia.

**presbyopia** A refractive condition in which the accommodative ability of the eye is insufficient for near vision work, due to ageing. This is due to a hardening of the lens and a reduction of the elasticity of its capsule. The main symptom is blurred vision, or difficulty in sustaining clear vision, at the working distance. It is corrected by positive lenses (called the **addition**). This condition usually occurs when the amplitude of accommodation has decreased to 4 D. This condition generally occurs between the age of 42 and 48 in people living in European and North American countries. People living in hot climates become presbyopic earlier. *Syn.* old sight (colloquial).
*See* **accommodative insufficiency; addition, near; capsule, crystalline lens; distance, reading; lens, bifocal; lens, hyperchromatic; lens, progressive; lens, trifocal; modulus of elasticity; monovision.**

**presbyopia, premature** *See* **accommodative insufficiency.**

**prescription** A written formula for the preparation and administration of any treatment. At a minimum, medication prescriptions should include the name of the medication to be used, instructions for its usage and the amount of medication to be dispensed. A spectacle prescription may include a spherical component (often called the **spherical error** or the **sphere**), a cylindrical component (often called the **cylindrical error**), a prismatic component, an addition for near vision and the interpupillary distance. *Example*: +3.00 D (−1.50 D × 90°) 1.5 ΔBI, OU add: +1.75 D, 64 mm. Prescriptions for contact lenses include very specific information regarding the lenses, besides the refraction adjusted for the corneal plane. The form and terminology nowadays usually conform to the recommendations of the International Standards Organization.
*See* $R_x$.

**preseptal cellulitis** *See* **cellulitis, preseptal.**

**preservative agents** *See* **antiseptic.**

**press-on prism** *See* **prism, Fresnel Press-On.**

**pressure, blood** *See* **sphygmomanometer.**

**pressure, equivalent oxygen** *See* **oxygen pressure, equivalent.**

**pressure, intraocular (IOP)** The pressure within the eyeball occurring as a result of the constant formation and drainage of the aqueous humour. This is measured by means of a manometer. What is actually measured in the human eye is the **ocular tension** by means of a tonometer. This is an indirect measure of the IOP as it depends on the thickness and rigidity of the tunics of the eye besides the IOP. Both terms, intraocular pressure and ocular pressure, are usually

**Table P9** Abbreviations commonly used in prescriptions

| abbreviation | Latin | meaning |
|---|---|---|
| *ac* | ante cibum | before meals |
| *ad lib* | ad libitum | freely, as desired |
| *agit.ante us* | agita ante usum | shake before taking |
| *alt hor* | alternis horis | every other hour |
| *bid* | bis in die | use twice a day |
| *c* | cum | with |
| *gtt* | guttae | drops |
| *od* | omni die | every day |
| *oh* | omni hora | every hour |
| *om* | omni mane | every morning |
| *on* | omni nocte | every night |
| *pc* | post cibum | after eating |
| *po* | per os | by mouth |
| *prn* | pro re nata | use as needed |
| *qd* | quaque in die | use every day |
| *qh* | quaque hora | use every hour |
| *qid* | quater in die | use four times a day |
| *ql* | quantum libet | as much as desired |
| *s* | sine | without |
| *sig* | signa | label |
| *soln* | solutio | solution |
| *tab* | tabella | tablet |
| *tid* | ter in die | use three times a day |
| *ung* | unguentum | ointment |

regarded as synonymous. Normal IOP is usually considered to be between 10 and 22 mmHg. However, there may be cases of glaucoma with lower IOP than 22 mmHg and there are also many normal cases with IOP greater than 22 mmHg. There is a slight increase in IOP with age (about 2 mmHg), in the morning as compared to the evening (about 3–4 mmHg), in the supine position as compared to the sitting position (about 3–4 mmHg), and a decrease during accommodation (about 4 mmHg).
*See* **adrenergic receptors; diurnal variations, in intraocular pressure; glaucoma; hypertension, ocular; hypotonia, ocular; indentation, scleral; iridectomy; law, Imbert–Fick; rigidity, ocular; test, differential intraocular pressure; test, provocative; tonometer.**

**pressure, osmotic** The pressure in a solution by which water is drawn into it through a semipermeable membrane (e.g. corneal endothelium). The more concentrated the solution, the greater the osmotic pressure.
*See* **solution, hypertonic; solution, hypotonic; solution, isotonic.**

**pressure, pulse** *See* **sphygmomanometer.**

**prevalence** The number of people with a disease or condition in a given population at a specific time, either a point in time (**point prevalence**) or over a period of time (**period prevalence**). *Example*: the prevalence of keratoconus in Olmsted County, Minnesota on the third of December 1982 was 54.5 per 100 000 population.
*See* **incidence.**

**primary action** Term referring to the greatest effect of an extraocular muscle in one plane. The other actions are called the **subsidiary** or **secondary** and **tertiary** actions. The primary action of the inferior rectus is depression; of the superior rectus, elevation; of the inferior oblique, extorsion; and of the superior oblique, intorsion. The medial and lateral recti muscles exert their primary action in the primary position, that is pure adduction for the medial rectus and pure abduction for the lateral rectus.
*See* **muscles, extraocular; tertiary action; test, forced duction; test, red glass.**

**primary position** *See* **position, primary.**

**primary visual area** *See* **area, visual.**

**Prince rule** *See* **rule, Prince.**

**principal direction** *See* **line of direction.**

**principal plane; points; ray** *See* under the nouns.

**prism** A transparent body (e.g. plastic, glass) bounded by two inclined plane surfaces which intersect in a straight line called the **apex** and form an angle called the **prism angle**. The face opposite the apex is called the **base**. It is an optical element used to deviate light (towards the base of the prism). The angle of deviation $d$ of a prism in air is given by the following formula

$$d = i + i' - a$$

where $i$ is the angle of incidence, $i'$ the angle of emergence and $a$ the prism angle (Fig. P11).
*See* **adaptation, vergence; angle, prism; base setting; dioptre, prism; law of refraction; power, prism; prism, minimum deviation of a; prism, ophthalmic; spectacles, recumbent; spectroscope.**

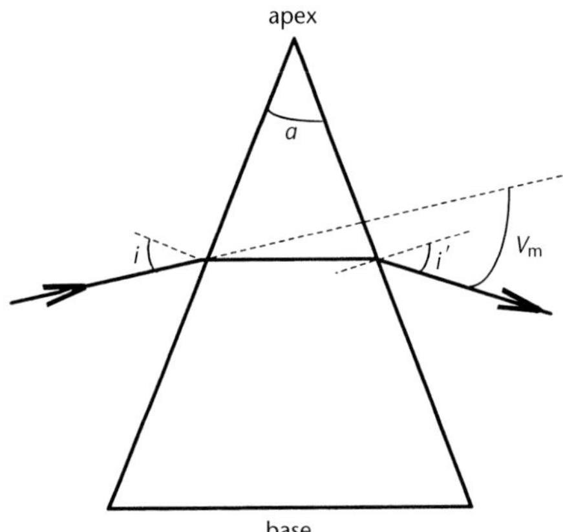


**Fig. P11** Prism ($a$, prism angle; $i$, angle of incidence = $i'$, angle of emergence; $V_m$, angle of minimum deviation)

**prism, achromatic** A prism that deviates light without dispersion. It consists of two prisms, usually one of crown glass and the other of flint, of equal angular dispersions and mounted so that the apex of one is against the base of the other.
*See* **dispersion.**

**prism adaptation** *See* **adaptation, vergence; test, prism adaptation.**

**prism, aligning** *See* **heterophoria, associated.**

**prism ballast lens** *See* **ballast.**

**prism bar** Clinical device consisting of a series of prisms of increasing strengths arranged in a convenient mount for rapid positioning in front of an eye. It can be used with the cover test or even to measure fusional responses when determining the zone of clear, single, binocular vision if rotary prisms are not available.
*See* **prism, rotary; test, cover.**

**prism, base-in; base-out** *See* **base setting.**

**prism, bi-** *See* **bi-prism, Fresnel's.**

**prism binoculars** *See* **binoculars.**

**prism, compensating** *See* **heterophoria, associated; prism, relieving.**

**prism dioptre** *See* **dioptre, prism.**

**prism, dissociating** A prism which, when placed in front of an eye, produces dissociation.
*See* **dissociation.**

**prism, double** *See* **bi-prism; test, double prism.**

**prism, Dove; erecting** *See* **erector.**

**prism, Fresnel Press-On** A tradename for a thin disc of transparent plastic consisting of one flat surface which can adhere to a clean lens surface when pressed in place, and another surface on which are incorporated small prismatic elements laid parallel to one another. Large optical effects can thus be provided in a much thinner and lighter form. These Press-On Fresnel prisms can be cut to any desired shape and are used commonly in orthoptics treatment.
*See* **lens, Fresnel; orthoptics.**

**prism, induced** Prismatic effect created when the patient's visual axis does not pass through the optical centre of an ophthalmic lens. The amount of prism power is given by Prentice's law.
*See* **convergence, correction induced; law, Prentice's.**

**prism, lacrimal** *See* **tear meniscus.**

**prism, minimum deviation of a** The deviation of light rays from their original path is minimum when light passes symmetrically through a prism so that the incident and emergent angles are equal (Fig. P11).
*See* **angle of deviation; prism.**

**prism, Nicol** An optical device for producing a beam of plane polarized light. It is made from a piece of calcite crystal cut diagonally in half with the two halves cemented together. Incident light is split into ordinary and extraordinary linearly polarized rays in the prism: the ordinary ray reaches the interface and is totally reflected, while the extraordinary ray is transmitted (Fig. P12).
*See* **analyser; birefringence; index of refraction; light, polarized; polarizer.**

**prism, ophthalmic** A prism used in the correction or in the measurement of a deviation of the eyes. The power of such a prism is usually only a few prism dioptres. The power of a thin prism in air, represented by the angle of deviation $d$, is given by the approximate formula

$$d = (n - 1)a$$

where $n$ is the index of refraction of the prism and $a$ the prism angle. *Example*: if the prism angle is equal to 10° and the index of refraction

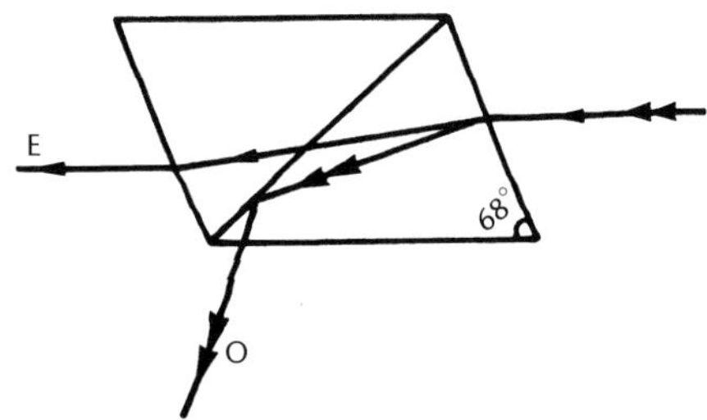


**Fig. P12** Nicol prism (O, ordinary ray; E, extraordinary ray)

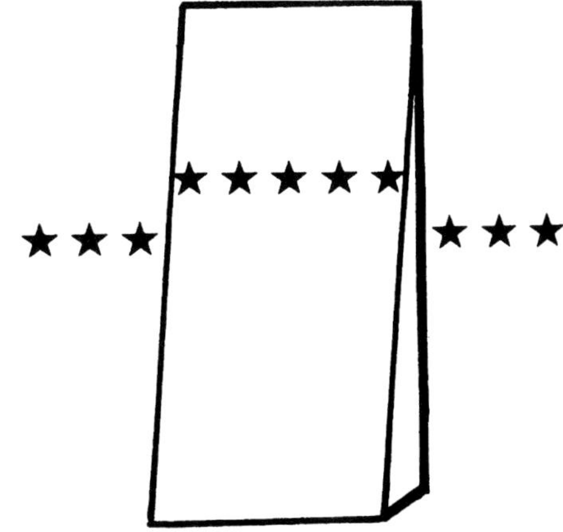

**Fig. P13** A line of stars seen through a prism base down

of the prism is 1.523, the deviation will be equal to 5.23° or 9.12 Δ. (Fig. P13)
*See* **dioptre, prism; power, prism; prism.**

**prism, penta** *See* **Fig. P14.**

**prism, polarizing** A prism made from doubly refracting material. *Example*: quartz.
*See* **analyser; light, polarized; polarizer.**

**prism, Porro** *See* **erector.**

**prism power** *See* **power, prism.**

**prism, reflecting** A prism in which light is internally reflected at one or more of the plane surfaces before emerging. This happens when the angle of incidence at the surface is greater than the critical angle (Fig. P14). *Syn.* total reflecting prism.
*See* **angle, critical; reflection, total.**

**prism reflex test** *See* **method, Krimsky's.**

**prism, relieving** An ophthalmic prism prescribed to relieve symptoms caused by an uncompensated heterophoria. *Syn.* compensating prism.
*See* **heterophoria, uncompensated.**

**Table P10** Approximate deviation of thin ophthalmic prisms of various apical angles and of two different refractive indices

| | deviation | | | |
|---|---|---|---|---|
| | spectacle crown glass ($n$ = 1.523) | | extra dense flint glass ($n$ = 1.70) | |
| apical angle in degrees (°) | degrees (°) | Δ | degrees (°) | Δ |
| 1 | 0.52 | 0.91 | 0.70 | 1.22 |
| 2 | 1.05 | 1.84 | 1.40 | 2.45 |
| 3 | 1.57 | 2.75 | 2.10 | 3.67 |
| 4 | 2.09 | 3.66 | 2.80 | 4.90 |
| 5 | 2.61 | 4.57 | 3.50 | 6.12 |
| 6 | 3.14 | 5.49 | 4.20 | 7.35 |
| 7 | 3.66 | 6.40 | 4.90 | 8.57 |
| 8 | 4.18 | 7.31 | 5.60 | 9.80 |
| 9 | 4.71 | 8.24 | 6.30 | 11.02 |
| 10 | 5.23 | 9.15 | 7.00 | 12.25 |
| 11 | 5.75 | 10.06 | 7.70 | 13.47 |
| 12 | 6.28 | 10.99 | 8.40 | 14.70 |

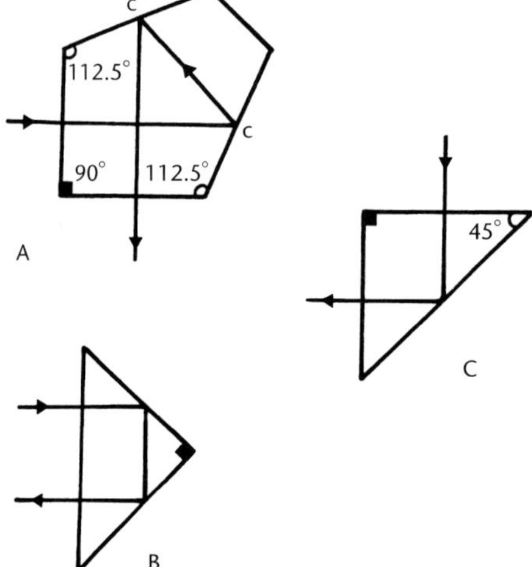


**Fig. P14** Examples of reflecting prisms (A, penta prism, with surfaces C coated with silver or aluminium; B and C, in which the surfaces reflect light by total internal reflection)

**prism, Risley** *See* **prism, rotary.**

**prism, rotary** A pair of identical thin prisms mounted one in front of the other, so that they can be rotated by equal amounts in opposite directions to give a resultant power in a single meridian. The power can vary from zero when the apex of one prism coincides with the base of the other, to the sum of the powers of the two prisms when the apices coincide. The **Risley prism** is a very common type of rotary prism. It is used to determine the limits of the zone of clear, single, binocular vision and also in some stereoscopes (e.g. variable prism stereoscope). *Syn.* variable prism.
*See* **base setting; stereoscope, variable prism.**

**prism, tear** *See* **tear meniscus.**

**prism test, double** *See* **test, double prism.**

**prism, total reflecting** *See* **prism, reflecting.**

**prism, Wollaston** Two right-angled prisms of equal angle made of a double refracting crystal such as quartz or calcite cemented together by their hypotenuse faces to form a rectangular unit. The optical axis of the crystal in one prism is perpendicular to that in the other prism and both axes are also perpendicular to the direction of the incident light. A beam of unpolarized light incident on a Wollaston prism will emerge as two diverging beams which are oppositely polarized and almost free of dispersion. This prism is used in some types of keratometers (e.g. Javal–Schiotz). *Syn.* Wollaston polarizer.
*See* **analyser; keratometer; light, polarized; refraction, double.**

**prisms, version** *See* **prisms, yoke.**

**prisms, yoke** Two prisms, one in front of each eye, of equal deviation and direction. 2 ΔBU, OU. The apparent view moves towards the apex of the prisms. These are sometimes prescribed in the management of nystagmus, in visual training, for the bedridden (BD prisms) and in some cases of physical disability. (Fig. P15) *Note*: also spelt yoked prisms. *Syn.* version prisms.

**prismatic effect, differential** *See* **effect, differential prismatic.**

**prismatic imbalance** *See* **effect, differential prismatic.**

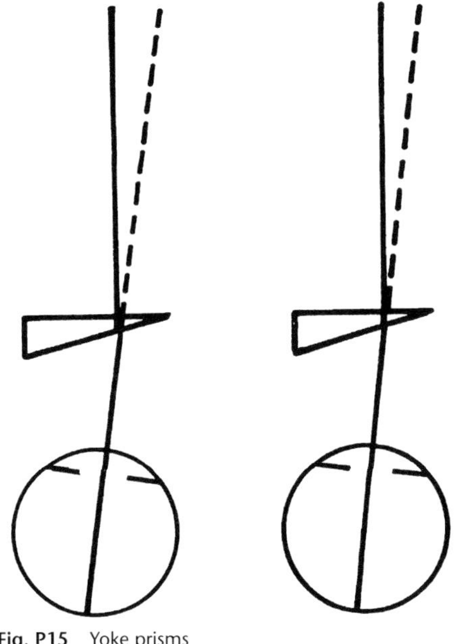

Fig. P15 Yoke prisms

**prismatic jump** *See* **jump.**

**prismatic power** *See* **power, prism.**

**procaine hydrochloride** A local anaesthetic of the amide type used in eye surgery. It is used in 1–10% solution and its action lasts for nearly 1 hour.
*See* **anaesthetics; bupivacaine; lidocaine.**

**prognosis** The prediction of the probable course of a disease or visual anomaly based on all the relevant facts of the case.
*See* **diagnosis; sign.**

**progression** *See* **lens, progressive.**

**progressive myopia** *See* **myopia, pathological.**

**projection 1.** Localization of visual impressions from the eye to the apparent source of the stimulus, such as up and to the left. This is sometimes referred to as mental projection. **2.** A prominence. **3.** The imaging of an object onto a screen or a surface.

**projection, erroneous** *See* **projection, false.**

**projection, false** The false positioning in space of a visual sensation arising from a retinal image formed in an eye with paresis of an extraocular muscle. The visual sensation appears in the direction of normal action of the paretic muscle. *Example*: past-pointing. *Syn.* erroneous projection; malprojection.
*See* **pointing, past-.**

**projector** An optical instrument which forms a magnified image of an object (e.g. a slide) onto a screen.

**prolapse of the iris** *See* **iris, prolapse of the.**

**proliferative retinopathy** *See* **retinopathy, proliferative.**

**prone test** *See* **test, provocative.**

**propamidine isethionate** An antibiotic agent used topically in solution 0.1%, especially in the treatment of acanthamoeba keratitis. It is a member of the diamidine group of antibiotics. Although it may be used alone it is most commonly used with polyhexamethylene biguanide, or with neomycin, or with chlorhexidine.
*See* **keratitis, acanthamoeba.**

**proparacaine hydrochloride** *See* **proxymetacaine.**

**propranolol** *See* **miotics.**

**proprioception** Awareness of posture, balance or position due to the reception of stimuli, produced within the organism, which stimulate receptors (called **proprioceptors**) located within muscles, tendons, joints and the vestibular apparatus of the inner ear. The precise role of proprioception regarding the visual apparatus is uncertain.
*See* **Table N1; reflex, tonic neck.**

**proptosis** *See* **exophthalmos.**

**prosopagnosia** Inability to recognize faces. It may be due to a lesion in one area of the inferotemporal (IT) cortex.
*See* **agnosia.**

**prostaglandin analogues** Drugs used in the treatment of open-angle glaucoma or ocular hypertension. At specific dosages they lower the intraocular pressure, supposedly by increasing the outflow of aqueous humour via the uveoscleral pathway. Common agents include latanoprost, travoprost, bimatoprost and unoprostone isopropyl.

**prosthesis, ocular** An artificial eye or ocular implant. *Note*: also spelt prothesis.
*See* **conjunctivitis, giant papillary; eye, artificial; implant, intraocular lens; ocularist.**

**protan** Person who has either protanopia or protanomaly.

**protanomal** Person who has protanomaly.

**protanomaly** A type of anomalous trichromatism in which an abnormally high proportion of the red primary stimulus is needed when mixing red and green to match a given yellow. This is due to the fact that the luminosity function of a

protanomal is reduced for the red radiations. The condition occurs in less than 1% of the male population. *Syn.* protanomalous trichromatism; protanomalous vision; red-weakness.
*See* **anomaloscope; colour vision, defective; plates, pseudoisochromatic; trichromatism.**

**protanope** Person who has protanopia.

**protanopia** Type of dichromatism in which only two hues are seen: below 493 nm all radiations appear bluish whereas above it they all appear yellowish. Around 493 nm is the neutral point. The luminosity function of protanopes is significantly decreased for red radiations (for which he or she is almost blind). The condition occurs in about 1% of the male population. *Syn.* red blindness.
*See* **dichromatism; plates, pseudoisochromatic; point, neutral.**

**protective lens** *See* **lens, plastic.**

**protein removal** *See* **enzyme.**

**prothesis** *See* **prosthesis, ocular.**

**protractor 1.** Instrument used to measure or set out angles on paper. **2.** A scale containing a circle graduated in degrees and a set of axes emerging from the centre of the circle used to set the axis of an astigmatic ophthalmic lens. It also includes various other scales for positioning the optical centre of lenses.
*See* **lens, astigmatic.**

**provocative test** *See* **test, provocative.**

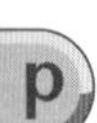

**proximal** Nearest to a central point.
*See* **distal.**

**proximal convergence** *See* **convergence, proximal.**

**proxymetacaine hydrochloride** A topical anaesthetic, commonly used in 0.5% solution. It has a greater potency than tetracaine (amethocaine) and causes less stinging and squeezing of the eyes when instilled. *Syn.* proparacaine hydrochloride.
*See* **anaesthetics; tetracaine.**

**pseudo-** A prefix meaning false or spurious (e.g. pseudochalazion, pseudoglaucoma, pseudopapilloedema, etc.).

**pseudoesotropia** *See* **epicanthus.**

**pseudoexfoliation (PXF)** Deposition of greyish-white, flake-like basement membrane material on the anterior lens capsule, the iris and the ciliary processes with free-floating particles in the anterior chamber. It occurs mainly in the elderly. It often gives rise to open-angle glaucoma (called **capsular glaucoma** or **pseudoexfoliation glaucoma**) which is frequently resistant to medical therapy and requires laser trabeculoplasty. The origin of the pseudoexfoliative material is believed to be secondary to an abnormal basement membrane, produced by ageing epithelial cells in the eye, as well as in the skin and visceral organs. Therefore pseudoexfoliation is thought to be part of a generalized basement membrane disorder and thus also referred to as **exfoliation syndrome** or **pseudoexfoliation syndrome** (PXS). *Syn.* exfoliation syndrome; pseudoexfoliation syndrome.
*See* **exfoliation.**

**pseudo-hemianopia** *See* **phenomenon, extinction.**

**pseudoisochromatic plates** *See* **plates, pseudoisochromatic.**

**pseudomembrane** A type of inflammatory response characterized by the production of mucus which adheres to the adjacent conjunctiva. This differs from a true membrane in that the latter is firmly attached to the conjunctival surface and is composed of dead cells and debris.

**pseudomyopia** *See* **accommodation, spasm of.**

**pseudopapilloedema** A benign condition in which the optic disc is elevated resembling papilloedema. The condition is usually induced by optic disc drusen, hypermetropia greater than 4 D, persistent hyaloid artery or myelinated nerve fibres.
*See* **drusen; fibres, myelinated nerve; hyaloid remnant.**

**pseudophakic eye** *See* **eye, pseudophakic.**

**pseudopterygium** A fold of conjunctiva that has become attached to the cornea as a result of injury or ulcer near the limbus. Hard contact lens wear has occasionally given rise to pseudopterygium: refitting with soft contact lenses may then be indicated. In the case of pseudopterygium a probe can be passed beneath it near the limbus whereas this is impossible in true pterygium.
*See* **pterygium.**

**pseudoptosis** A condition resembling ptosis, due to abnormalities other than those found in the eyelid elevator muscles. Causes include blepharophimosis, dermatochalasis, ipsilateral hypotropia, phthisis bulbi, microphthalmos, anophthalmos, or a decrease in orbital volume as in enophthalmos. *Syn.* apparent ptosis.
*See* **blepharophimosis; dermatochalasis; elevator; ptosis; syndrome, blepharophimosis.**

**pseudosclerosis of Westphal** *See* **disease, Wilson's.**

**pseudoscope** An instrument which, by means of prisms or mirrors, transposes to one eye the image seen normally by the other eye. Thus the sense of depth is reversed and peaks are seen as troughs and vice versa. (Fig. P16)

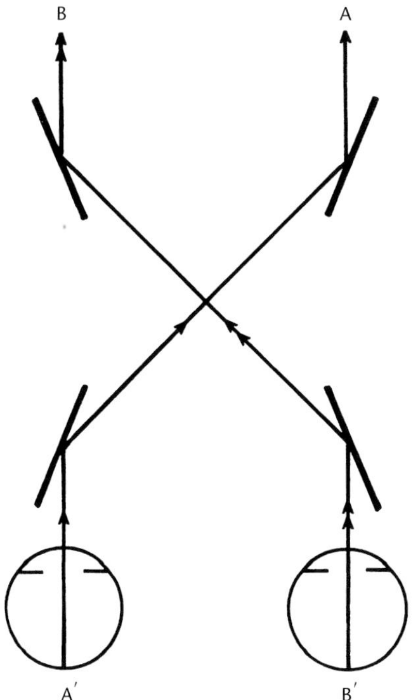


**Fig. P16** Optical principle of a pseudoscope

**pseudostrabismus** *See* **strabismus, apparent.**

**pseudotumour, orbital** *See* **syndrome, orbital inflammatory.**

**pseudoxanthoma elasticum** *See* **angioid streaks.**

**psychophysics** Branch of science which deals with the relationship between the physical stimuli and the sensory response. The measurements of thresholds (e.g. visual acuity, dark adaptation) or matching of stimuli (as in the spectral luminous efficiency curve) are examples of psychophysics.
*See* **optometry, experimental.**

**pterygium** A triangular fold of bulbar conjunctiva, in the interpalpebral fissure, with its apex advancing progressively towards the cornea, usually from the nasal side. A pinguecula often precedes its development. It is considered to be due to a degenerative process caused by recurrent dryness or irritation from wind and dust or prolonged exposure to sunlight, especially UV. It becomes more prevalent with age. Symptoms are usually absent unless the pterygium encroaches on the cornea and vision may then be affected: surgical intervention is then necessary. Some pterygia tend to recur after excision. UV absorptive lenses may help decrease the incidence.
*See* **dellen; dyskeratosis; lens, absorptive; line, Stocker's; pinguecula; pseudopterygium.**

**ptosis** Drooping of the upper eyelid causing a narrowing of the palpebral fissure. It is often divided into two main types: congenital and acquired. The congenital type present at birth is usually the result of interference with the superior division of the oculomotor nerve. The acquired type may result from any affection of the nerve supply of the upper eyelid musculature, from a disease of the muscles themselves or from mechanical interference in elevating the eyelid due to the weight of a tumour, trauma or chronic tissue hypoxia (e.g. diabetes). The correction is usually surgical. Sometimes a **ptosis crutch**, which is attached to the spectacles and elevates the eyelid, may be useful. There are also special contact lenses designed to support the upper eyelid. *Syn.* blepharoptosis.
*See* **ataxia, hereditary spinal; epicanthus inversus; myasthenia gravis; phenomenon, jaw-winking; sign, Cogan's lid twitch; spectacles, orthopaedic; syndrome, Horner's.**

**ptosis, acquired aponeurotic** Ptosis caused by a partial disinsertion, dehiscence or weakness of the aponeurosis of the levator palpebrae superioris muscle. It usually occurs in old age and is bilateral, but disinsertion can result from trauma to one eye (e.g. following eye surgery). Occasionally an abnormal attachment to the superior border of the tarsal plate is present as well. This is the most common form of acquired ptosis. The typical treatment is by resection of the levator palpebrae muscle.
*See* **muscle, levator palpebrae superioris.**

**ptosis adiposa** *See* **dermatochalasis.**

**ptosis, pseudo-** *See* **pseudoptosis.**

**pucker, macular** *See* **fibrosis, preretinal macular.**

**Pulfrich refractometer** *See* **refractometer.**

**Pulfrich stereophenomenon** *See* **stereophenomenon, Pulfrich.**

**Pulsair non-contact tonometer** *See* **tonometer, non-contact.**

**pulvinar** The prominence of the posterior portion of the thalamus overlapping the superior colliculus. It receives projections from the auditory, somatosensory and visual cortex regions. It is involved in visual attention, suppression of irrelevant stimuli and utilizing information to initiate eye movements.

**punctal occlusion** *See* **occlusion, punctal.**

**punctate epithelial keratitis** *See* **keratitis, punctate epithelial.**

**punctum caecum** *See* **blind spot.**

**punctum lacrimale** *See* **lacrimal apparatus.**

**punctum luteum** *See* **macula lutea.**

**punctum proximum** *See* **accommodation.**

**punctum remotum** *See* **accommodation, far point of.**

**pupil** Aperture within the iris, normally circular, through which light penetrates into the eye. It is located slightly nasally to the centre of the iris. Its diameter can vary from about 2 to 8 mm. It is often slightly smaller in old age.
*See* **acorea; anisocoria; corectopia; dicoria; dyscoria; hippus; iridectomy; iris; microcoria; miosis; muscle, dilator pupillae; muscle, sphincter pupillae; mydriasis; nucleus, Edinger–Westphal; polycoria; polyopia; reflex, pupil light.**

**pupil, Adie's** A pupil in which the reactions to light, direct or consensual, are almost abolished, with a reaction occurring only after prolonged exposure to light or dark. The reaction of the pupil to a near target is also delayed and slow. The condition is usually unilateral with the affected pupil being the larger of the two. It may be due to a disease of, or injury to, the ciliary ganglion or to the short ciliary nerves. Other causes include temporal arteritis in elderly patients, syphilis or diabetes. *Syn.* myotonic pupil; pupillotonia; tonic pupil (some authors use this last term when the cause is known and Adie's pupil when the cause is unidentified).
*See* **syndrome, Adie's; reflex, pupil light.**

**pupil, amaurotic** Miotic pupil that does not react to direct and consensual ipsilateral light stimulation, but does react consensually to contralateral stimulation. It is most often noted in cases of severe optic nerve dysfunction or retinal disease.

**pupil, apparent** *See* **pupil of the eye, entrance.**

**pupil, Argyll Robertson** Pupil which reacts when the eye accommodates and converges but fails to react directly and consensually to light. The condition is bilateral, the pupils are small and usually unequal. It is usually a sign of neurosyphilis. *See* **iridoplegia; reflex, pupil light; tabes dorsalis.**

**pupil, artificial 1.** Pupil made by iridectomy. **2.** A circular aperture made in a diaphragm which can be mounted in front of the eye to provide a constant and smaller pupil size. It is used in research but also as a clinical test.
*See* **disc, pinhole; iridectomy.**

**pupil block** *See* **pupillary block.**

**pupil constriction** *See* **miosis; reflex, pupil light.**

**pupil dilatation** *See* **mydriatic; reflex, pupil light.**

**pupil, ectopic** *See* **corectopia.**

**pupil of the eye, entrance** This is the image of the iris aperture formed by the cornea. It is what one sees when one looks at an eye. It is some 13% larger than the real pupil and located slightly in front of it. *Syn.* apparent pupil.

**pupil of the eye, exit** This is the image of the iris aperture formed by the crystalline lens. It is slightly larger than the real pupil and situated slightly behind it.

**pupil, Hutchinson's** A pupil which is dilated and completely inactive to all stimuli. It is associated with lesions of the central nervous system, as may occur in head injury.

**Table P11** Examples of pupil abnormality

| defect | appearance | light response* | consensual light response* | near response |
|---|---|---|---|---|
| Adie's pupil | large | impaired | impaired | slow |
| Argyll Robertson | both pupils small, unequal +irregular | almost abolished | almost abolished | normal |
| blindness in one eye | normal | abolished | abolished | normal |
| Horner's syndrome | small + ptosis | normal | normal | normal |
| Hutchinson's pupil | large | abolished | abolished | abolished |
| optic neuritis | normal/large | impaired | impaired | normal |
| 3rd nerve paralysis† | large + ptosis | abolished | abolished | abolished |

*To stimulation of the affected eye.
†When caused by an aneurysm of the posterior communicating artery.

**pupil, keyhole** A pupil shaped like a keyhole due to iridectomy in which a section of the iris extending from the pupillary margin to the periphery has been excised, or due to coloboma or trauma to the iris.

**pupil light reflex** *See* **reflex, pupil light.**

**pupil, Marcus Gunn** A defect of the pupillary reflex characterized by a smaller constriction of both pupils when the affected eye is stimulated by light as compared to that occurring when the normal eye is stimulated. It is easier, however, to observe this phenomenon when swinging a light from one eye to the other in a darkened room while the subject is fixating a distant object (this is called the **swinging flashlight test**). Stimulation of the normal eye will cause constriction of both pupils whereas rapid stimulation of the affected eye will lead to a small dilatation (a paradoxical reaction, sometimes referred to as **pupillary escape**). This condition is due to a lesion in one of the optic nerves which affects the afferent pupillary pathway. It is often the result of multiple sclerosis or optic neuritis or retrobulbar optic neuritis. *Syn.* relative afferent pupillary defect (RAPD).

**pupil, myotonic** *See* **pupil, Adie's.**

**pupil reflex** *See* **reflex, pupil.**

**pupil, tonic** *See* **pupil, Adie's.**

**pupil, white** *See* **leukocoria.**

**pupillae ectopia** *See* **corectopia.**

**pupillae muscle, dilator** *See* **muscle, dilator pupillae.**

**pupillary axis** *See* **axis, pupillary.**

**pupillary block** A blockage of the normal flow of aqueous humour from the posterior to the anterior chamber of the eye. It may be caused by a posterior annular synechia occurring during anterior uveitis, by luxation of the lens anteriorly occluding the pupil, or by adhesion of the iris to the vitreous or to the posterior capsule following extracapsular cataract extraction (called **aphakic pupillary block**). It may produce an attack of angle-closure glaucoma as the iris may be pushed forward blocking the drainage angle. *Syn.* pupil block.
*See* **glaucoma, angle-closure; iris bombé; luxation of the lens; seclusio pupillae; synechia, annular.**

**pupillary defect; escape** *See* **pupil, Marcus Gunn.**

**pupillary membrane** *See* **membrane, pupillary.**

**pupillary reflex** *See* **reflex, pupil light.**

**pupillometer 1.** An instrument for measuring the diameter of the pupil. There exist several types but the most common is a series of graduated filled circles whose sizes are compared with the pupil (**Haab's pupillometer**). It is also common to measure pupil size by photography or video after appropriate calibration of the method. (Fig. P17) *Syn.* coreometer. **2.** Although incorrectly used, it refers to an instrument for measuring the interpupillary distance (PD). These instruments are based either on using the pupil centres (e.g. Reichert PD gauge) or the corneal reflections (e.g. Essilor Corneal Reflection Pupillometer; Seiko SP-100 Pupillometer), but the latter can be used on the basis of the pupil centres as well. In the instruments using corneal reflections the subject views the image of a small illuminated target surrounding the observation aperture used by the examiner or made to appear as if it came from the observer's eye. That image is formed at infinity by a lens placed in front of the subject's eyes. The examiner moves a hair line to coincide with the centre of the corneal reflections and reads the monocular and total interpupillary distances. *Syn.* interpupillometer (this is the most appropriate term for this instrument); PD gauge; PD meter.
*See* **distance, interpupillary; rule, PD.**

**pupillometer, Broca's** A subjective instrument for measuring the diameter of the pupil. It

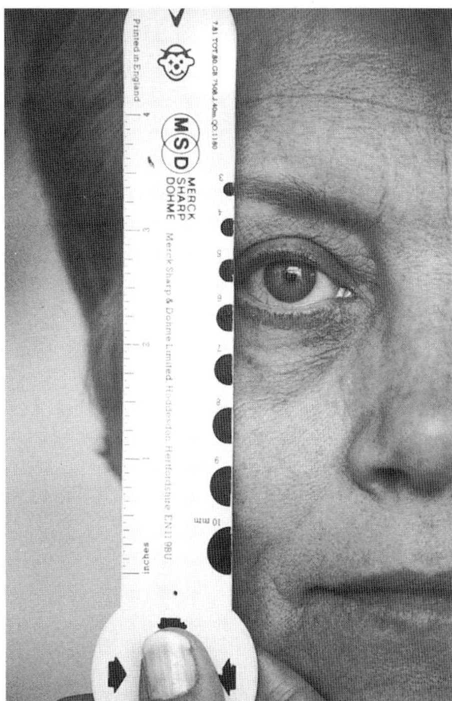

**Fig. P17** Typical pupillometer

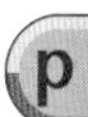

consists of a pair of very small light sources placed at the anterior focal plane of the eye. The two sources are separated until the circular, out of focus images on the retina are seen in juxtaposition. The distance between the two sources represents the diameter of the pupil.

**pupilloscope** Instrument for observing the pupil.

**pupillotonia** *See* **pupil, Adie's.**

**purity** *See* **saturation.**

**Purkinje after-image** *See* **after-image.**

**Purkinje figures; shadows** *See* **angioscotoma.**

**Purkinje shift** Reduction in the luminosity of a red light relative to that of a blue light when the luminances are reduced from photopic to scotopic levels of illumination. This is due to the shift of the spectral sensitivity curve from a maximum at 555 nm to 507 nm when passing from light to dark adaptation. *Syn.* Purkinje's phenomenon.
*See* **interval, photochromatic; theory, duplicity.**

**Purkinje tree** *See* **angioscotoma.**

**Purkinje–Sanson images** *See* **images, Purkinje–Sanson.**

**purple** A mixture, in suitable proportions, of short wave radiations (less than 400 nm) and long wave radiations (greater than 700 nm). It is a complementary colour to yellow-green. Purples are colour stimuli represented on the chromaticity diagram by the straight line joining the ends of the spectrum locus. *Syn.* non-spectral colour; non-spectral purple.
*See* **chromaticity diagram; colour, complementary; spectrum locus.**

**pursuit movement** *See* **movement, pursuit.**

**push-up** *See* **method, push-up; test, push-up.**

# Q

**quadrantanopsia** Visual field loss in a quarter of the visual field of the eye. The defect is usually bilateral as it is caused by a lesion past the optic chiasma. It may be homonymous (binasal, bitemporal, upper or lower), crossed (one upper and the other lower), congruous (equal size of the defects), or incongruous (unequal size of the defects). (Fig. Q1) *Syn.* quadrantic anopsia; quadrantic hemianopsia.
*See* **hemianopsia.**

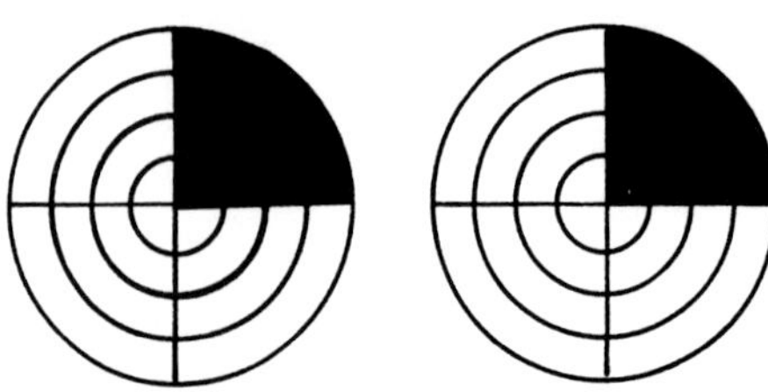

**Fig. Q1** Complete, right, superior homonymous quadrantanopsia due to a lesion of the optic radiations in the left temporal lobe

**quadrantanopsia, superior** A superior, homonymous quadrantanopsia due to a lesion of the most anterior and inferior fibres of the optic radiations that is in Meyer's loop, on the contralateral side of the visual pathway. *Syn.* 'pie in the sky' defect.
*See* **loop, Meyer's; radiations, optic.**

**quadrigemina, corpora** *See* **colliculi.**

**quantity of light** *See* **light, quantity of.**

**quantum** *See* **photon.**

**quantum theory** *See* **theory, quantum.**

**quartz** *See* **prism, Wollaston.**

**quinine amblyopia** *See* **amblyopia.**

**quinolones** A class of broad-spectrum antibacterial drugs of which the main ophthalmic agents are **ciprofloxacin** and **ofloxacin**. They are used topically in 0.3% solution. They are effective against the majority of gram-negative pathogens, including *Haemophilus*, *Neisseria gonorrhoeae*, *Chlamydia trachomatis*, *Pseudomonas aeruginosa* (especially ciprofloxacin), staphylococci and streptococci. They are used in the treatment of conjunctivitis, blepharitis, keratoconjunctivitis and corneal ulcers.
*See* **antibiotic.**

# R

**radial keratotomy** *See* **keratotomy, radial.**

**radiant flux** *See* **flux, radiant.**

**radiation** **1.** Emission or transfer of energy in the form of electromagnetic waves or particles. **2.** A group of nerve fibres that diverge in all directions from a point of origin. *Example*: the optic radiations.
*See* **radiations, optic; spectrum, electromagnetic.**

**radiation, black body** The radiation emitted by a heated black body.
*See* **body, black; colour temperature.**

**radiations, optic** That part of the visual pathway which consists of axons arising in the lateral geniculate body and terminating in a fan-shaped manner in the visual area of the occipital lobe. As they emerge from the lateral geniculate body the inferior fibres loop forward in the temporal lobe before swinging back toward the occipital cortex. These fibres form what is called **Meyer's loop** (or **Archambault's loop**). They receive impulses from the inferior retinal quadrants (corresponding to the superior aspect of the contralateral visual field). They terminate on the inferior lip of the calcarine fissure. *Syn.* optic radiations of Gratiolet; geniculocalcarine tract.
*See* **area, visual; pathway, visual.**

**radiology** A science dealing with techniques that use radiant energy (e.g. X-rays) for diagnosis and therapy.
*See* **angiography, fluorescein; magnetic resonance imaging; tomography, computerized.**

**radiuscope** Instrument used for measuring the radius of curvature of the surfaces of a contact lens. It is based on the Drysdale method. *Syn.* optical microspherometer.
*See* **method, Drysdale's; Toposcope.**

**Raman effect** *See* **effect, Raman.**

**Ramsden eyepiece** *See* **eyepiece, Ramsden.**

**ramus communicans** *See* **ganglion, ciliary; nerve, ophthalmic.**

**random-dot stereogram** *See* **stereogram, random-dot.**

**random-dot E test** *See* **stereogram, random-dot.**

**range of accommodation** *See* **accommodation, range of.**

**raphe, retinal** A horizontal line of demarcation or seam, on the temporal side of the macula, separating the arcuate nerve fibres from the upper and lower retina.
*See* **fibres, arcuate; fibres, papillomacular; scotoma, arcuate; scotoma, Bjerrum's.**

**ratio, AV** The ratio of the diameter of the retinal arteries to that of the retinal veins. It is usually around two-thirds. Deviations from this value may indicate a vascular disease (e.g. hypertension).

**ratio, cup-disc (C/D)** The ratio of the horizontal diameter of the physiological cup to that of the horizontal diameter of the optic disc. It should be less than 0.5. If it exceeds that value, or if there is a difference in ratio between the two eyes, or if there is a progressive enlargement of the cup, glaucoma may be suspected (Fig. R1).
*See* **cup, glaucomatous.**

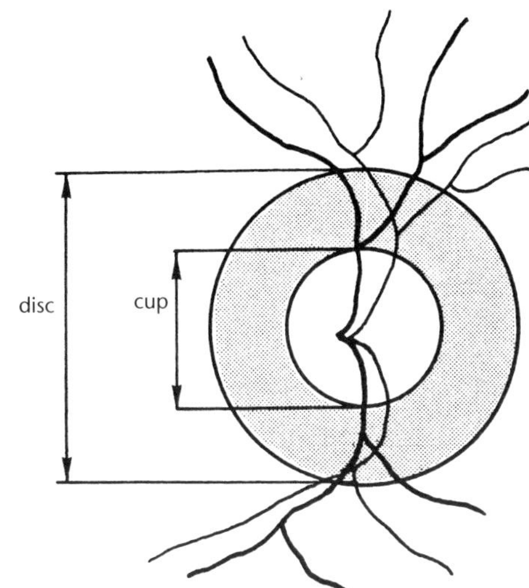


**Fig. R1** Diagram of the physiological cup with a cup–disc ratio of 0.5

**Raubitschek chart** *See* **chart, Raubitschek.**

**ray** In geometrical optics, a straight line representing the direction of propagation of light.

**ray, axial** A ray which is coincident with the axis of an optical system.

**ray, chief** A ray joining an object point to the centre of the entrance pupil of an optical system (Fig. R2).
*See* **light, pencil of.**

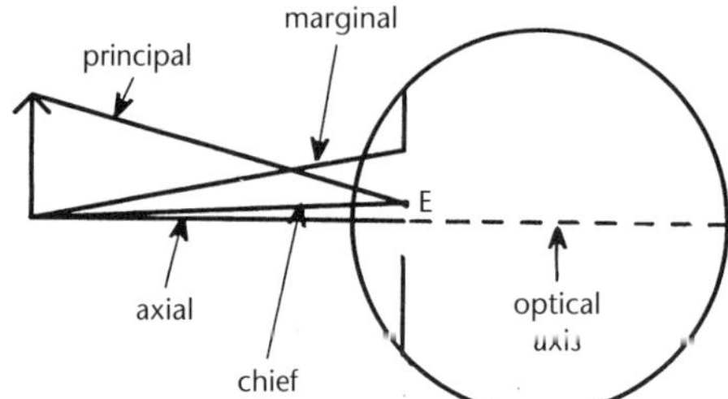


**Fig. R2** Rays of light incident to the eye (E, centre of the entrance pupil of the eye)

**ray, emergent** A ray of light in image space either after reflection (**reflected ray**) or after refraction (**refracted ray**).

**ray, extraordinary** *See* **birefringence.**

**ray, incident** A ray of light in object space which strikes a reflecting or refracting surface.

**ray, marginal** A ray joining the axial point of an object to the edge or margin of an aperture or pupil.

**ray, ordinary** *See* **birefringence.**

**ray, paraxial** A light ray which forms an angle of incidence so small that its value in radians is almost equal to its sine or its tangent. (i.e. $\sin\theta = \theta$ or $\tan\theta = \theta$. These are approximate expressions referred to as the **paraxial approximation** (or the **gaussian approximation.**)
*See* **angle of incidence; optics, paraxial; paraxial region; theory, gaussian.**

**ray, principal** A ray joining the extreme off-axis object point to the centre of the entrance pupil or aperture.

**ray tracing** Technique used in optical computation consisting of tracing the paths of light rays through an optical system by graphical methods or by using formulae. Nowadays, computer methods are used.
*See* **sign convention.**

**Rayleigh criterion** *See* **criterion, Rayleigh.**

**Rayleigh equation** A colour equation representing a match of yellow (usually 589 nm) with a mixture of red (usually 670 nm) and green (usually 535 nm). It is used to differentiate certain types of colour deficiencies. The anomaloscope is built on this principle.
*See* **anomaloscope; colour vision, defective.**

**Rayleigh scattering** *See* **scattering, Rayleigh.**

**reaction time** The time interval between the onset of a stimulus and the response of a subject. Visual stimulations with a flash of light give rise to reaction times varying between 130 and 180 ms.

**reading** The act of viewing and interpreting letters, words, sentences, etc. It consists of a pattern of eye movements. The eyes proceed along a line in a series of step-like saccades, separated by fixation pauses during which information from the text is acquired. The amount of reading matter correctly identified during the fixation pause is called the span of recognition or the perceptual span. Most saccades are made from left to right but some occur in the opposite direction (called regression) to return to text recently

**Table R1** Differences between the sine and the tangent values of various angles (in degrees and radians). The error is calculated between the sine value and the value in radians and between the value in radians and the tangent value

| angle (deg) | angle (rad) | sine value | tangent value | error (%) sine error | error (%) tangent error |
|---|---|---|---|---|---|
| 0.5 | 0.008 727 | 0.008 727 | 0.008 727 | 0.00 | 0.00 |
| 1 | 0.017 453 | 0.017 452 | 0.017 455 | 0.01 | 0.01 |
| 2 | 0.034 907 | 0.034 899 | 0.034 921 | 0.02 | 0.04 |
| 3 | 0.052 360 | 0.052 336 | 0.052 408 | 0.05 | 0.09 |
| 4 | 0.069 813 | 0.069 756 | 0.069 927 | 0.08 | 0.16 |
| 5 | 0.087 266 | 0.087 156 | 0.087 489 | 0.13 | 0.25 |
| 6 | 0.104 720 | 0.104 528 | 0.105 104 | 0.18 | 0.37 |
| 7 | 0.122 173 | 0.121 869 | 0.122 785 | 0.25 | 0.50 |
| 8 | 0.139 626 | 0.139 173 | 0.140 541 | 0.33 | 0.65 |
| 10 | 0.174 533 | 0.173 648 | 0.176 327 | 0.51 | 1.03 |
| 15 | 0.261 799 | 0.258 819 | 0.267 949 | 1.15 | 2.35 |
| 20 | 0.349 066 | 0.342 020 | 0.363 970 | 2.06 | 4.27 |
| 30 | 0.523 599 | 0.500 000 | 0.577 350 | 4.72 | 10.27 |

read but not yet fully perceived. At the end of the line the eyes make a return sweep to the next line of text (Fig. R3).
*See* **movement, saccadic eye; test, developmental eye movement.**

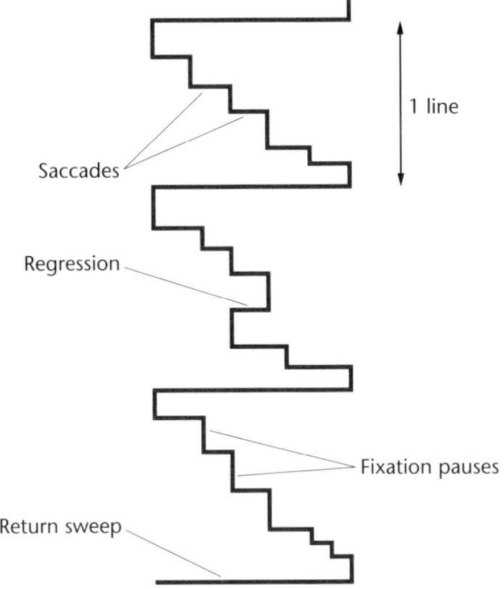


**Fig. R3** Schematic illustration of eye movements during reading. Horizontal lines represent eye movements and vertical lines fixation pauses

**reading addition** *See* **addition, near.**

**reading distance; lens** *See* under the nouns.

**reading portion** *See* **segment of a bifocal lens.**

**reading slit** *See* **typoscope.**

**receptive field** *See* **field, receptive.**

**receptor** *See* **photoreceptor.**

**receptors, adrenergic** *See* **adrenergic receptors.**

**recession** A surgical procedure used in strabismus in which an extraocular muscle is removed from its insertion and repositioned elsewhere on the globe (usually further back).
*See* **resection; strabismus.**

**reciprocal innervation** *See* **law of reciprocal innervation, Sherrington's.**

**reciprocal metre** *See* **curvature of a surface.**

**reciprocity, law of** *See* **law, Bunsen–Roscoe.**

**von Recklinghausen's disease** *See* **disease, von Recklinghausen's.**

**recovery point** The point at which fusion is regained on decreasing the prism or lens power which originally induced diplopia in investigation of relative accommodation and convergence.
*See* **convergence, relative.**

**rectus muscles** *See* **muscles.**

**recumbent spectacles** *See* **spectacles, recumbent.**

**recurrent corneal erosion** *See* **corneal erosion, recurrent.**

**red** One of the hues of the visible spectrum evoked by stimulation of the retina by wavelengths beyond 630 nm. The complementary colours to red are blue-green (between 490.4 and 492.4 nm).
*See* **colour, complementary.**

**red blindness** *See* **protanopia.**

**red glass test** *See* **test, red glass.**

**red reflex** *See* **reflex, fundus.**

**red-green colour deficiency** A general term indicating a colour vision deficiency which is either of the deutan (green colour vision defect) or of the protan (red colour vision defect) type. These defects are mostly hereditary and affect both eyes equally. Most cases are inherited in X-linked recessive manner.
*See* **colour vision, defective; deutan; protan; rule, Kollner's.**

**reduced eye; vergence** *See* under the nouns.

**refixation reflex** *See* **reflex, refixation.**

**reflectance** *See* **factor, reflection.**

**reflecting prism; telescope** *See* under the nouns.

**reflection** Return or bending of light by a surface such that it continues to travel in the same medium.

**reflection, angle of** *See* **angle of reflection.**

**reflection, diffuse** Reflection from a surface which is not polished and light is reflected in many or all directions (Fig. R4). *Syn.* irregular reflection.
*See* **diffusion; glossmeter; matt surface.**

**reflection, direct** *See* **reflection, regular.**

**reflection factor** *See* **factor, reflection.**

**reflection, irregular** *See* **reflection, diffuse.**

**reflection, law of** *See* **law of reflection.**

**reflection, mixed** The simultaneous occurrence of regular and diffuse reflection.
*See* **reflection, diffuse; reflection, regular.**

**reflection, regular** Reflection from a polished surface in which there is no scattering and light travels back in a definite direction (Fig. R4). *Syn.* direct reflection; specular reflection.
*See* **microscope, specular.**

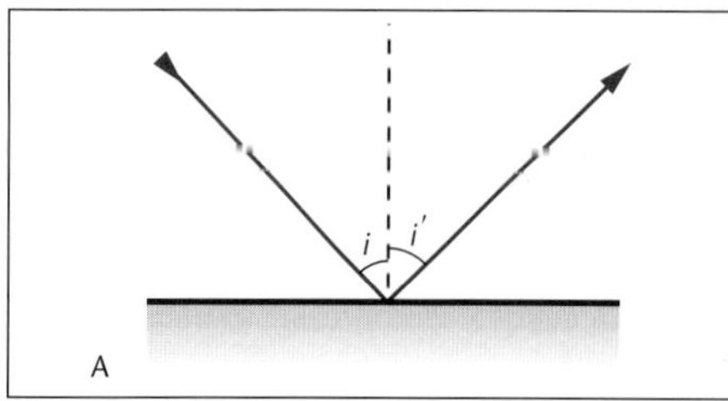


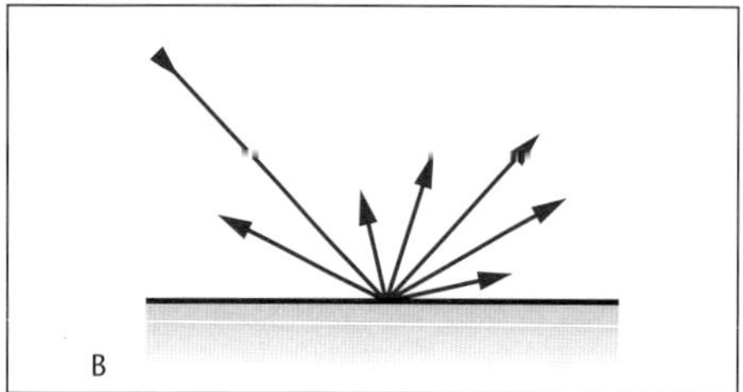


**Fig. R4** A, specular reflection; the angle of incidence *i* is equal to the angle of reflection *i'*. B, diffuse reflection.

**reflection, specular** *See* **reflection, regular.**

**reflection, surface** Light reflected at a surface according to Fresnel's formula.
*See* **Fresnel's formula.**

**reflection, total** Reflection occurring when light is incident at an angle greater than the critical angle. *Syn.* total internal reflection.
*See* **angle, critical; prism, reflecting.**

**reflection, total internal** *See* **reflection, total.**

**reflector** Any device which reflects light (e.g. glass-plate, prism, mirror).

**reflex 1.** Involuntary response to a stimulus. **2.** Reflection or an image formed by reflection (e.g. corneal reflex).

**reflex, accommodative** *See* **reflex, near.**

**reflex arc, pupillary** *See* **reflex, pupil light.**

**reflex, blinking** Blinking in response to various stimulations such as a light source or a mechanical threat.
*See* **pathway, retinotectal.**

**reflex, cat's eye** A whitish, bright reflection observed in the normally black pupil in several conditions, such as leukocoria, retinoblastoma, Coats' disease or persistent hyperplastic primary vitreous. It resembles the reflection from the tapedum lucidum of a cat when a light is shined at night.
*See* **disease, Coats'; leukocoria; retinoblastoma; tapedum lucidum.**

**reflex, consensual light** *See* **reflex, pupil light.**

**reflex, corneal 1.** Blinking in response to a threat, or to tactile stimulation of the cornea, as for example when measuring objectively the corneal touch threshold. **2.** Image formed by reflection of light from the cornea (Fig. R5).
*See* **aesthesiometer; blink; method, Hirschberg's; method, Krimsky's; pupillometer; strabismus, apparent.**

**reflex, direct light** *See* **reflex, pupil light.**

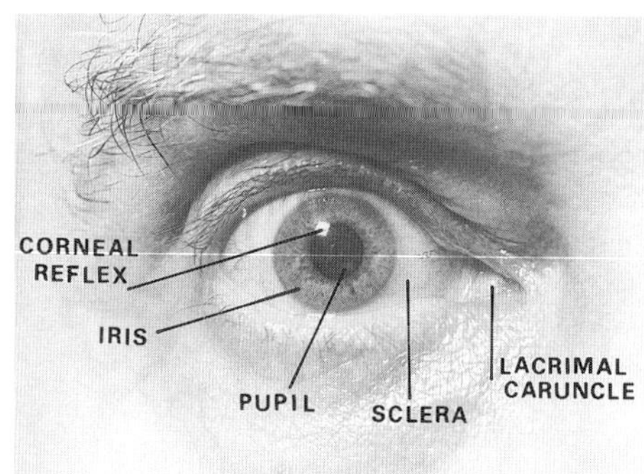


**Fig. R5** Frontal view of the right eye

**reflex, eyeball compression** *See* **reflex, oculocardiac.**

**reflex, fixation** Psycho-optical reflex consisting of an involuntary movement of the eye (or eyes) aimed at placing on the foveola the retinal image of an object which was formed in the retinal periphery.
*See* **reflex, psycho-optical; reflex, re-fixation.**

**reflex, foveal** Tiny reflection from the concave surface of the foveal depression of the retina seen in ophthalmoscopy. It is not usually visible in old eyes.
*See* **fovea centralis.**

**reflex, fundus** Light reflected by the fundus of the eye, as seen in retinoscopy and ophthalmoscopy. It appears as a red glow in the plane of the pupil in retinoscopy. It is absent when the eye has a dense cataract. *Syn.* red reflex.
*See* **fundus, ocular; ophthalmoscope; retinoscope.**

**reflex, fusion** *See* **fusion, motor.**

**reflex, hemianopic pupillary** In hemianopsia, a loss of pupillary constriction when light falls on the blind side of the retina while pupillary constriction is maintained when light stimulates the unaffected side of the retina. *Syn.* Wernicke's hemianopic pupil; Wernicke's pupillary reaction; Wernicke's pupillary reflex; Wernicke's sign.
*See* **hemianopsia.**

**reflex, indirect light** *See* **reflex, pupil light.**

**reflex, lacrimal** Secretion of tears in response to irritation of the cornea or conjunctiva as, for example, when first wearing contact lenses (hard in particular), but it may also be induced by eyestrain, glare, laughing, etc. Physiologically, some believe that reflex tearing acts as a natural defence mechanism to flush or clean the eye of irritants (i.e. foreign bodies, noxious fumes etc.) *Syn.* lacrimation reflex; weeping reflex.
*See* **lacrimal apparatus; lacrimation; reflex, tearing.**

**reflex, lacrimation** *See* **reflex, lacrimal.**

**reflex, light 1.** That light which appears in the pupil in retinoscopy. It is light reflected by the retina. *Syn.* retinoscopic light. **2.** Any reflected light.
*See* **reflex, pupil light; retinoscope.**

**reflex, near** Reflex evoked by a blurred retinal image, as when fixating from far to near. It consists of three responses: (1) increased convexity of the crystalline lens; (2) constriction of the pupils; and (3) convergence of the eyes. This reflex is not a pure reflex since each of the three components can act independently of the other two; convergence by means of prisms, accommodation by means of lenses and miosis by light stimulation. *Syn.* accommodative reflex; near-triad reflex; synkinetic near reflex.
*See* **accommodation, mechanism of; accommodative response; pupil.**

**reflex, near-triad** *See* **reflex, near.**

**reflex, oculocardiac** A decrease in pulse rate following compression of the eyeball or traction on the extraocular muscles. It may produce a systolic cardiac arrest. *Syn.* Ascher's phenomenon; Ascher's reflex; eyeball compression reflex.

**reflex, optokinetic** *See* **reflex, vestibulo-ocular.**

**reflex, postural** A reflex which helps to maintain static or dynamic posture of the body, for example, the **righting reflex**, in which visual stimuli help to maintain a correct position of the head in space by activating the muscles of the neck and limbs.
*See* **reflex, static eye.**

**reflex, psycho-optical** Reflexes involving the eye which are mediated by the occipital cortex such as the accommodative, fixation, fusion, version and vergence reflexes.

**reflex, pupil** Any alteration of the pupil size in response to stimuli other than light (e.g. a sudden noise).
*See* **reflex, pupil light.**

**reflex, pupil light 1.** Constriction of the pupil in response to light stimulation of the retina. The response of an eye to light stimulation can occur either with a light shining on it directly (the **direct light reflex**) or when the other eye is stimulated (the **consensual** or **indirect light reflex**). The **reflex arc** consists of four neurons beyond the ganglion cells. The **first** afferent neuron transmits nervous impulses from the retina to the two pretectal nuclei, located on the lateral side of the superior colliculi, in response to light stimulation of the photoreceptors. The **second** neurons, called the internuncial neurons, connect each pretectal nucleus to both Edinger–Westphal nuclei which form part of the oculomotor nuclei. The **third** efferent neurons connect the latter nuclei, via the third nerve (oculomotor nerve) to the ciliary ganglion where there is a synapse. The **fourth** efferent neurons connect the latter, via the short ciliary nerves, to the sphincter pupillae muscle of each iris and constrict the pupil. The efferent path represents the **parasympathetic** innervation (Fig. R6). **2.** Dilatation of the pupil in response to a reduction of the light stimulation of the retina. It is effected by **sympathetic** innervation which originates in the hypothalamus and descends down the brainstem to the ciliospinal centre, located between C8 and C12. From there fibres pass to the superior cervical ganglion in the neck, then ascend along the internal carotid artery until they join the ophthalmic division of the trigeminal nerve. The fibres reach the dilator pupillae muscle of the iris via the nasociliary and long ciliary nerves which enter the eyeball behind the equator. *Syn.* light reflex.
*See* **fibres, pupillary; ganglion, ciliary; muscle, sphincter pupillae; nerve, oculomotor; nerves, short ciliary; nucleus, Edinger–Westphal; pathway, retinotectal; reflex, accommodative.**

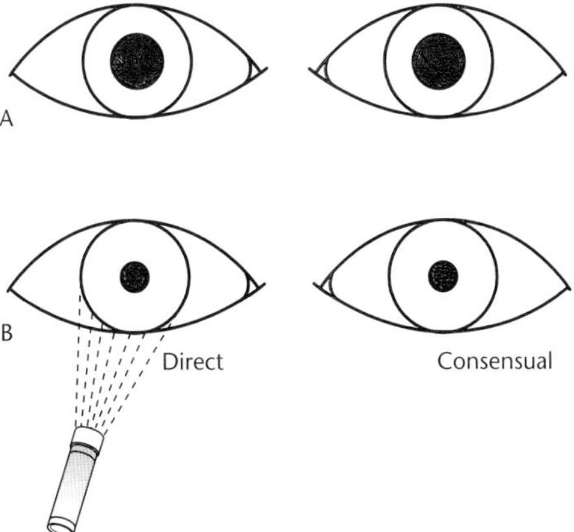


**Fig. R6** A, pupils under low illumination. B, direct pupil light reflex of the right eye in response to light stimulation, accompanied by a consensual light reflex of the left eye

**reflex, red** *See* **reflex, fundus.**

**reflex, re-fixation** This reflex occurs while fixating one object and another in the visual field attracts the attention. The eye then turns to fixate on the new object. This is a special case of the fixation reflex.
*See* **reflex, fixation.**

**reflex, retinoscopic** *See* **reflex, light; retinoscope.**

**reflex, righting** *See* **reflex, postural.**

**reflex, static eye** A higher order postural reflex which helps to maintain the eye static with respect to the visual environment by action on the extraocular muscles (possibly via the utricular receptors of the vestibular system) during head or body movements. *Syn.* compensatory eye movements.

**reflex tearing** Tears produced in response to irritation to the cornea or to the conjunctiva.
*See* **tear secretion; tears; test, Schirmer's.**

**reflex, tonic neck** Orientation of the head, eyes and body in response to proprioceptive information provided by the activity of the muscles of the neck.
*See* **proprioception.**

**reflex, vergence** A disjunctive fixation reflex in response to an object which moves closer or further than the original position of the fixation point.
*See* **movements, disjunctive eye.**

**reflex, version** A conjugate fixation reflex in response to an object moving in the same frontal plane.
*See* **version.**

**reflex, vestibulo-ocular** A conjugate movement of the eyes in the direction opposite to a head movement. This reflex is triggered by stimulation of the semicircular canals. It is aimed at maintaining a stable image on the retina during head movement. This reflex responds best at high velocities and frequencies of the visual stimulus. At low velocities and frequencies the stabilization of the retinal image is attempted by the **optokinetic reflex**, which is triggered only by retinal stimulation. It complements the vestibulo-ocular reflex.
*See* **nystagmus; optokinetic.**

**reflex, weeping** *See* **reflex, lacrimal.**

**reflex, Wernicke's pupillary** *See* **reflex, hemianopic pupillary.**

**reflex, white pupillary** *See* **leukocoria.**

**refract 1.** To bend a ray of light when it passes through a surface separating media of different refractive indices. **2.** To measure the refractive state of the eye.

**refracting angle** *See* **angle, prism.**

**refracting unit** *See* **phoropter.**

**refraction 1.** The change in direction of the path of light as it passes obliquely from one medium to another having a different index of refraction. **2.** The process of measuring and correcting the refractive error of the eyes. *Syn.* refraction of the eye; sight testing (obsolete term). **3.** *See* **refractive error.**
*See* **law of refraction.**

**refraction, angle of** *See* **angle of refraction.**

**refraction, binocular** A clinical procedure in which the subjective measurement of refraction of each eye is performed while both eyes are viewing a test. The visual examination is thus carried out under more natural conditions than when one eye is closed; the sizes of the pupils are similar and the accommodation-convergence relationship is maintained. There are various such methods; using polarized targets (e.g. Vectograph slides; Parallel-testing Infinity Balance test), using a septum (e.g. Turville Infinity Balance test), or fogging (e.g. Humphriss Immediate Contrast test). These methods give better results than refracting monocularly, especially in latent hypermetropia, hypermetropic anisometropia, pseudomyopia, cyclophoria, etc. and no additional step for binocular balancing is necessary.
*See* **method, Humphriss; test, balancing; test, Turville, infinity balance; testing in parallel.**

**refraction, cycloplegic** Assessment of the refractive state of the eye when accommodation has been totally or partially paralysed by a cycloplegic (e.g. cyclopentolate 1% eyedrops, or atropine 0.5 or 1% ointment). This may be carried out in children to reveal the full extent of a hypermetropia or in the initial assessment of accommodative esotropia, but only occasionally in adults as fogging methods usually suffice for them.
*See* **accommodative esotropia; cycloplegia; method, fogging.**

**refraction, double** The splitting of an incident ray into two (ordinary and extraordinary) by a birefringent medium.
*See* **anisotropic; birefringence; prism, Nicol; prism, Wollaston.**

**refraction, dynamic** Determination of the refractive state of the eye when accommodation is stimulated, as distinguished from **static refraction** which is the determination of the refractive state of the eye when accommodation is at rest or paralysed.
*See* **refractive error; retinoscopy, dynamic.**

**refraction, error of** *See* **ametropia**; **refractive error.**

**refraction of the eye** **1.** *See* **refraction. 2.** Refraction of light by the optical media of the eye. **3.** *Syn.* for ametropia.
*See* **ametropia; refractive error.**

**refraction, index of** *See* **index of refraction.**

**refraction, laser** A method of subjective refraction in which the patient observes a slowly rotating drum on the surface of which is perceived a speckle pattern resulting from illumination by a laser. The speckle pattern appears to move only when the eye is not focused for the fixation distance. If the perceived movement of the pattern is opposite to that of the drum, the eye is myopic and if the perceived movement of the pattern is in the same direction as the drum, the eye is hyperopic. Correction can be determined by placing a lens in front of the eye which will neutralize the movement; at that point the eye is focused for the fixation distance. Astigmatism can be measured by rotating the drum in various meridians. The drum can be placed at infinity or at near (an allowance for the radius of curvature of the drum and the distance must then be made). This method can be useful for mass screening, especially children, as accommodation is not stimulated as much as with Snellen letters. It has been very useful as a research tool for accommodation studies where it is arranged as part of a Badal optometer.
*See* **optometer, Badal's; refractive error.**

**refraction, manifest** The refractive error or the process of determining it, when accommodation is at rest (but not paralysed).
*See* **refraction, cycloplegic.**

**refraction, objective** Measurement of the refraction of the eye which is not based on the patient's judgements, as when using an objective optometer.
*See* **optometer; retinoscope.**

**refraction, over-** *See* **over-refraction.**

**refraction, static** *See* **refraction, dynamic**; **refractive error.**

**refraction, subjective** Measurement of the refraction of the eye based on the patient's judgements.
*See* **method, fogging; optometer; test, fan and block; test, plus 1.00 D blur.**

**refractionist** One who measures and corrects the refractive state of the eye.
*See* **optometrist.**

**refractive amblyopia** *See* **amblyopia.**

**refractive correction** *See* **correction.**

**refractive error** The dioptric power of the ametropia of the eye. It is equal to $1/k$ in dioptres, where $k$ is the distance between the far point and either the spectacle plane (**spectacle refraction**), or the principal point of the eye, or the refracting surface of the reduced eye (**ocular refraction**), in metres. $K$, thus

$$K = \frac{1}{k}$$

when the eye is situated in air *Syn.* ametropia (although this is not strictly so as ametropia is the anomaly); refraction of the eye; refractive status; static refraction.
*See* **accommodation, far point of; ametropia; correction; cycloplegia; experiment, Scheiner's; method, fogging; optometer; photorefraction; potential, visual evoked; Simultantest; test, duochrome; velonoskiascopy.**

**refractive index** *See* **index of refraction.**

**refractive keratoplasty** *See* **epikeratoplasty; keratomileusis; keratophakia; keratotomy, radial; LASIK.**

**refractive power** *See* **power, refractive.**

**refractivity** *See* **dispersion.**

**refractometer** **1.** An instrument for measuring the refractive index of transparent objects. There exist several types: **Abbé's refractometer** which is based on the measurement of the critical angle at the interface between a sample and a prism of known index of refraction and uses white light whereas that of **Pulfrich**, which is based on the same principle as Abbé's, uses monochromatic light. As the refractive index of some materials is related to their water content, the hand-held **Atago CL-1 Soft lens Refractometer** has been calibrated to provide a reading of the percentage of water content of soft contact lenses. **2.** *See* optometer.
*See* **angle, critical; index of refraction; optometer; oxygen permeability; water content.**

**refractometry** **1.** Measurement of the refractive error of the eye with a refractometer or optometer. **2.** Measurement of the index of refraction of a medium with a refractometer (e.g. Abbé's refractometer).
*See* **refractometer.**

**refractor** *See* **phoropter.**

**refractory period** *See* **potential, action.**

**Rieger's syndrome** *See* **syndrome, Rieger's.**

**Reis–Buckler dystrophy** *See* **dystrophy, Reis–Buckler.**

**Reiter's disease** *See* **disease, Reiter's.**

**relative afferent pupillary defect** *See* **pupil, Marcus Gunn.**

**relative amplitude of accommodation; convergence; scotoma** *See* under the nouns.

r

**relative scotoma** *See* **scotoma, relative.**

**reliability** The extent to which multiple measurements of the same thing, made on separate occasions, yield approximately the same results. The reliability between two sets of scores can be assessed by determining the correlation coefficient (**test-retest reliability** coefficient).
*See* **validity.**

**relief 1.** Quality of an object or of different parts of a surface to stick out from the background or general plane in which it is situated. The perception of relief is a special case of depth perception. **2.** A feeling of gladness that something unpleasant or painful has not occurred or has ceased.
*See* **perception, depth; stereopsis.**

**relieving prism** *See* **prism, relieving.**

**remotum, punctum** *See* **accommodation, far point of.**

**Remy separator** A simple, hand-held instrument for separating the vision of both eyes and commonly used for anti-suppression or divergence training. It consists of a vertical septum in the median plane, which is attached to, and divides a target holder at one end. The other end of the septum rests against the patient's nose so that a target on either side of the septum is seen by only one eye. (Fig. R7)
*See* **suppression.**

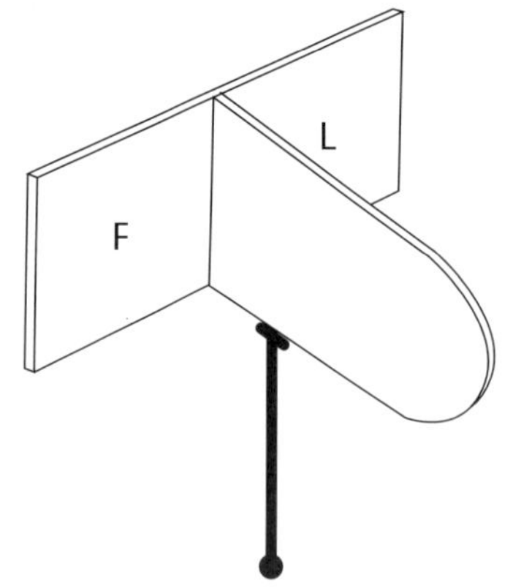


**Fig. R7** Remy separator

**resection** A surgical procedure used in strabismus in which a portion of an extraocular muscle is removed (usually at its insertion) and the muscle is reattached at or near the original site of insertion. This is carried out to shorten the muscle.
*See* **enophthalmos; recession; strabismus.**

**residual astigmatism** *See* **astigmatism, residual.**

**residual error of refraction** *See* **refraction, over.**

**reserve of accommodation** *See* **addition, near.**

**reserve, convergence fusional** *See* **convergence, relative.**

**resolution, limit of** The least separation of two images so that they are seen as separate when viewed through an optical instrument. This is usually evaluated in terms of the separation between the maximum of the intensity distribution curve of the diffraction pattern (or Airy's disc) of the images; it is commonly assumed that two points will be resolved if the centre of one pattern falls on the first dark ring of the other. The limit of resolution is greater the larger the aperture of the system. *Syn.* resolving power; resolution threshold.
*See* **criterion, Rayleigh; diffraction; disc, Airy's; minimum separable.**

**resolution, spurious** If the contrast sensitivity function (CSF) is measured when the eye is not in focus for the grating (e.g. due to a lack of correction or an erroneous correction), the CSF will suffer appreciably and fall much more rapidly with increasing spatial frequency towards zero contrast sensitivity. At this point the grating can no longer be resolved and appears a uniform grey. At spatial frequencies greater than this threshold value there may occur a phenomenon known as spurious resolution in which the CSF rises above zero. Thus, the grating may become visible again at higher spatial frequencies than that at which it first disappeared. *Example*: spurious resolution can be observed when looking at a radial grating (or star sector target) in which the spatial frequencies increase towards its centre. If the grating is held close to the eye with the accommodation relaxed one can see a grey annulus (and sometimes two) separating a zone (or two) of spurious resolution.
*See* **sensitivity, contrast.**

**resolution visual acuity** *See* **acuity, visual.**

**response, SILO** An acronym for small in large out. It refers to the presumed change of the perceived size of a test object that a patient experiences, while maintaining fusion when convergence or divergence is varied. When convergence is increased, with BO prisms, the object may appear to become smaller and nearer. When divergence is increased with BI prisms the object may appear larger and further away. The SILO is not universal; children tend to respond that way, but adults commonly respond in the opposite way, that is, if the test object becomes smaller they report it as moving away from them. The acronym is then given as SOLI. The response is used in visual therapy as a feedback mechanism to patients about their performance.
*See* **biofeedback; fusion, sensory; prism.**

**restriction** An interference in normal eye movement. This is most often due to the development of abnormal tissue that acts to limit free movement of the eye.
*See* **disease, Graves'.**

**ret** *See* **retinoscopy.**

**reticule** *See* **graticule.**

**reticulosis** *See* **syndrome, Mikulicz's.**

**retina** The light-receptive, innermost nervous tunic of the eye. It is a thin transparent membrane (125 μm near the ora serrata and 350 μm near the macula) and which extends over an area of about 266 $mm^2$. It lies between the vitreous body and the choroid, and extends from the optic disc to the ora serrata. Near the posterior pole and temporal to the optic disc is the macula, at the centre of which is the foveola which provides the best visual acuity. The retina contains at least 10 distinct layers, of which there are two synaptic layers. They are from the outermost layer to the innermost: (1) the pigment epithelium; (2) the layer of rods and cones; (3) the external limiting membrane; (4) the outer nuclear layer; (5) the outer molecular (or outer plexiform) layer; (6) the inner nuclear layer (which contains the bipolar, amacrine and horizontal cells and nuclei of the fibres of Mueller); (7) the inner molecular (or inner plexiform) layer; (8) the ganglion cell layer; (9) the nerve fibre layer (or stratum opticum); and (10) the internal limiting membrane. The two synaptic layers where visual signals must synapse as they emerge from the rods and cones on their way to the optic nerve are the two molecular layers (5 and 7). (Fig. R8)
*See* **astrocytes; cell, amacrine; cell, bipolar; cell, cone; cell, ganglion; cell, horizontal; cell, Mueller's; cell, rod; cup, optic; disc, optic; fovea; fundus, ocular; layer of Henle, fibre; macula; membrane of the retina, external limiting; membrane of the retina, internal limiting; retina, neurosensory; retinitis; retinopathy.**

**retina, converse** *See* **retina, inverted.**

**retina, fleck** Term referring to a retina with multiple, small or yellow spots which are seen in various conditions: actinic keratopathy, drusen, fundus albipunctatus, fundus flavimaculatus.
*See* **pisciform lesions.**

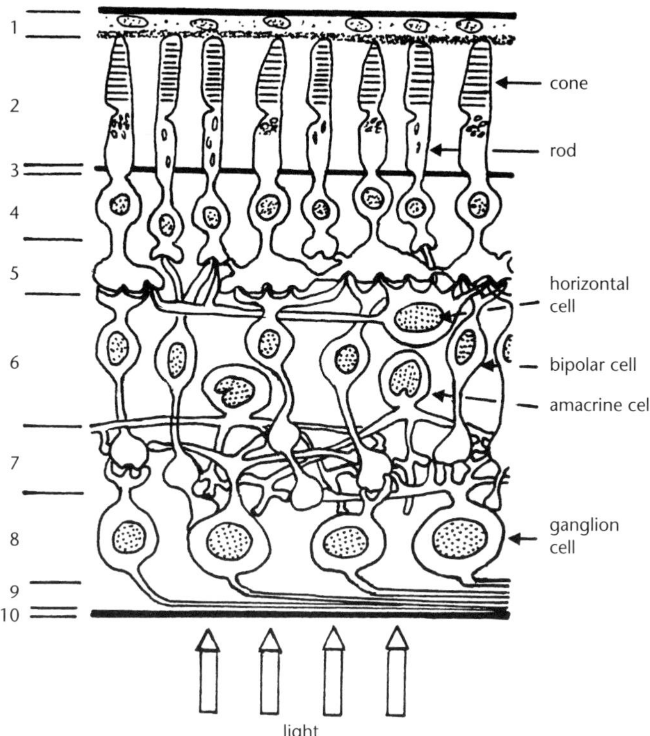


**Fig. R8** Schematic representation of the cells and layers of the central primate retina (1: retinal pigment epithelium; 2: layer of rods and cones; 3: external limiting membrane; 4: outer nuclear layer; 5: outer plexiform layer; 6: inner nuclear layer; 7: inner plexiform layer; 8: ganglion cell layer; 9: nerve fibre layer; 10: internal limiting membrane)

**Table R2** Some approximate retinal dimensions

| structure | diameter mm | degrees | distance from centre of foveola |
|---|---|---|---|
| foveola | 0.4 | 1.3 | |
| fovea centralis | 1.5 | 5.0 | |
| macula lutea | 4.0 | 14 | |
| optic disc* | | | |
| horizontal | 1.8 | 6.0 | |
| vertical | 2.1 | 7.5 | |
| nasal disc margin | | | 5.5 mm or 18.5° |
| temporal disc margin | | | 3.5 mm or 12.5° |
| centre of disc | | | 4.6 mm or 15.5° |

*The figures given for the size of the disc are those corresponding to the blind spot. Anatomically the optic disc is slightly smaller.

**retina, inverted** Term which refers to the fact that the retina of vertebrates is orientated so that the light has to pass through all the neuronal layers before reaching the photoreceptors. However, the retina of invertebrates is normally orientated so that light passes first through the photoreceptors as it traverses the retina: such a retina is called a **verted** or **converse retina.**

**retina, lattice degeneration of the** A vitreoretinal degeneration usually found between the equator and the ora serrata leading to a thinning of the retina and characterized by a lesion made up of fine white lines and some pigmentation. It may result in holes or tears and in retinal detachment by which time the patient usually complains of floaters. The condition is most common in myopes and often found in patients with Marfan's syndrome.
*See* **floaters; retinal tear; retinal detachment; retinoschisis; syndrome, Marfan's.**

**retina, leopard** *See* **fundus, leopard.**

**retina, neurosensory** This is composed of all the layers of the retina, except the outer pigmented layer (called retinal pigment epithelium). It comprises three main groups of neurons: (1) the photoreceptors, (2) the bipolar cells, and (3) the ganglion cells. In addition, there are other connecting neurons: the horizontal and amacrine cells. The neurosensory layer is derived embryologically from the inner layer of the optic cup whereas the pigmented layer is derived from the outer layer of the optic cup and they are separated by a potential space which facilitates their separation, as occurs in detached retina.
*See* **cup, optic; retinal detachment; retinal pigment epithelium.**

**retina, tessellated** *See* **fundus, tessellated.**

**retina, tigroid** *See* **fundus, tessellated.**

**retina, verted** *See* **retina, inverted.**

**retinal 1.** *See* **rhodopsin. 2.** Pertaining to the retina.

**retinal arterial occlusion** Occlusion of the central retinal artery (CRAO) is characterized by a sudden loss of vision and a defective direct pupil light reflex. The retinal arterioles are constricted while the veins are full but a venous pulse is absent. The retina appears white and swollen, especially near the posterior pole, and the choroid is seen through it as a cherry-red spot. If the occlusion persists the cherry-red spot disappears after several weeks, the retinal arterioles remain attenuated, eventually becoming white threads, and the optic disc becomes atrophic.
Occlusion is more frequently limited to one branch of the central retinal artery (BRAO). In this case, the clinical picture is limited to the area supplied by the branch and this is associated with a visual field defect in that region. Causes include retinal emboli due to a cardiovascular disease, systemic hypertension, temporal arteritis, oral contraceptives, syphilis, intravenous drug abuse or trauma. Treatment is urgent as there is an extremely serious risk of blindness.
*See* **amaurosis fugax; angiography, fluorescein; arteritis, temporal; atheroma; cherry-red spot; plaques, Hollenhorst's; reflex, pupil light.**

**retinal break** *See* **retinal tear.**

**retinal correspondence, abnormal (ARC)** A type of retinal correspondence in which the fovea of one eye is associated with an extrafoveal area of the other eye to give rise to a perception of a single object. This phenomenon is common in strabismus, but may also occur as a result of a macular lesion. ARC is often classified in three types: (1) **Harmonious**, in which the angle of anomaly is equal to the objective angle of deviation. This indicates that the ARC fully corresponds to the strabismus. (2) **Unharmonious**, in which the angle of anomaly is less than the

objective angle of deviation. (3) **Paradoxical**, when the angle of anomaly is greater than the objective angle of deviation. ARC can be detected by examination with a major amblyoscope, with the after-image test, or by comparison between the objective and the subjective angles of deviation measured with the alternate cover test and either a Maddox rod or the von Graefe's test, respectively (a difference between the objective and the subjective angles indicates ARC). (Fig. R9) *Syn.* anomalous retinal correspondence; retinal incongruity.
*See* **angle of anomaly; diplopia, incongruous; diplopia, physiological; glass, Bagolini's; movement, phi; test, after-image.**

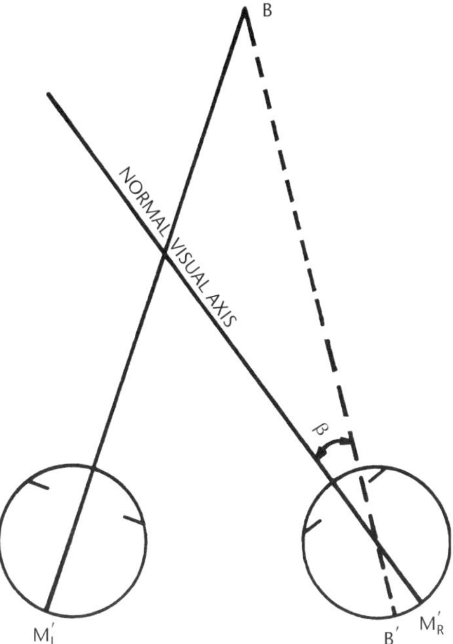


**Fig. R9** Abnormal retinal correspondence between $M'_L$ and B′ in right esotropia ($M'_R$, fovea of the right eye)

**retinal corresponding points** Two points (or small areas), one in each retina, which when simultaneously stimulated give rise to the perception of a single object. These points share a common line of direction and this explains why stimulating them is perceived as arising from the same point in space. *Syn.* normal retinal correspondence (NRC).
*See* **area, Panum's; disparity, retinal; horopter; law of identical visual directions; test, after-image transfer.**

**retinal detachment (RD)** Separation of the neurosensory retina from the pigment epithelium layer. Fluid collects in that potential space (this is called **serous retinal detachment**). It may do so from the vitreous when there is a retinal hole or tear (this is **rhegmatogenous retinal detachment**) or from the choroid when the retinal pigment epithelium is damaged (this is called **exudative** or **secondary retinal detachment**). Retinal detachment may also occur when the vitreoretinal membranes pull the neurosensory retina away from the retinal pigment epithelium (this is called **traction retinal detachment**). It can be observed with the ophthalmoscope as it is raised above the level of the surrounding retina requiring more plus power to focus on it. The detached retina appears dark red to grey and may show some folds. The condition occurs most commonly in eyes with degenerative myopia, and in the elderly. Ocular trauma, tumour, degeneration of the retina, shrinkage of the vitreous or after cataract surgery are other possible causes. Symptoms include a loss of vision in the visual field corresponding to the detached area, photopsia and a sudden shower of floaters. If the lesion is small, retinochoroidal adhesion may be achieved with either laser photocoagulation or cryotherapy. Management may require the patient to rest flat in bed but the typical treatment is surgical and urgent before the macular area becomes detached. It consists of indenting the sclera over the detached area (called **scleral buckling**) and usually draining the subretinal fluid. *Syn.* ablatio retinae.
*See* **disease, Coats'; floaters; macular hole; metamorphopsia; photocoagulation; photopsia; retina, lattice degeneration of the; retinal dialysis; retinal tear; retinopathy, central serous; retinopathy of prematurity; retinoschisis; sign, Shafer's; striae retinae; syndrome, Ehlers–Danlos; ultrasonography; vitrectomy; vitreous detachment.**

**retinal dialysis** A retinal tear at the ora serrata. It usually results from trauma, although some tears occur spontaneously. If the trauma is intense there may also be a retinal tear at the optic disc but the most frequent location is in the lower temporal quadrant. The condition is most typically asymptomatic. However, as it often gives rise to retinal detachment, the patient may report some of the symptoms associated with the latter. Perimetry and binocular indirect ophthalmoscopy are essential in the examination of this condition. In some cases the tear does not progress, but because of the risk of retinal detachment, patients must be referred to a retinal specialist. *Syn.* retinal disinsertion.
*See* **ora serrata; retinal detachment.**

**retinal disinsertion** *See* **retinal dialysis.**

**retinal disparity; embolism** *See* under the nouns.

**retinal glioma** *See* **retinoblastoma.**

**retinal hypoxia** *See* **hypoxia.**

**retinal illuminance** Luminous flux incident on the retina. The simplified formula is

$$T = LS$$

where $L$ is the luminance of the stimulus in $cd/m^2$ and $S$ is the area of the pupil in $mm^2$. The retinal illuminance $T$ is then given in trolands. *Syn.* retinal illumination.
*See* **troland; vignetting.**

**retinal image, stabilized** *See* **stabilized retinal image.**

**retinal incongruity** *See* **retinal correspondence, abnormal.**

**retinal line** *See* **line, retinal.**

**retinal mosaic** *See* **mosaic, retinal.**

**retinal pigment epithelium (RPE)** Brown layer of the retina situated next to the choroid composed of cells filled with pigment (mainly fuscin and melanin). Depending upon the amount of pigment, the fundus will appear dark or light. It is also responsible for supplying metabolites and other needs to the photoreceptors, and helps in retinal adherence and vitamin A metabolism. A dysfunction of this tissue can be detected with the electro-oculogram. This tissue can be transplanted and this may help treat age-related maculopathy.
*See* **electro-oculogram; fuscin; melanin; membrane, Bruch's; syndrome, Usher's.**

**retinal pigment epithelium hyperplasia** An abnormal proliferation of retinal pigment epithelium. This condition is thought to be due to persistent, abnormal traction on the RPE, causing it to proliferate. This finding has been noted along the vitreous base as well as in areas of inflammation and trauma. There is no particular visual significance to this lesion.

**retinal raphe** *See* **raphe, retinal.**

**retinal rivalry** When the two eyes are simultaneously or successively stimulated on corresponding retinal areas by dissimilar images (e.g. a green source to one eye and a red to the other, or lines orientated in one direction to one eye and in the other direction to the other), there results either an alternation of perception (complete or partial) or even a constant dominance of one eye. (Fig. R10) *Syn.* binocular rivalry.
*See* **effect, Cheshire cat; suppression.**

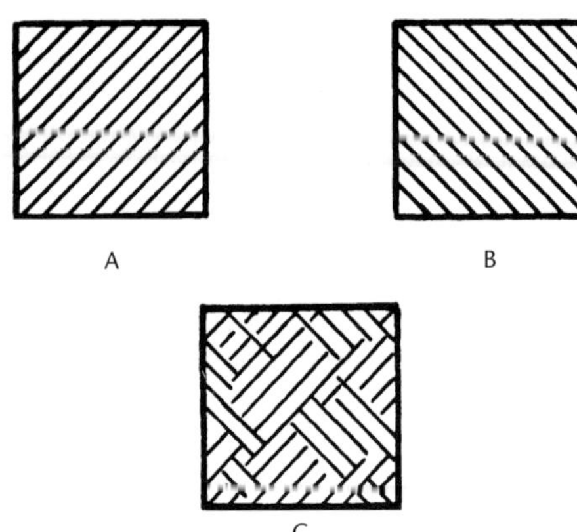


**Fig. R10** Retinal rivalry. Target A is seen by one eye. Target B is seen by the other eye. Target C is seen by both eyes simultaneously

**retinal slip** *See* **disparity, retinal.**

**retinal tear** An opening in the retina that may be caused by trauma, degeneration or most commonly proliferative vitreoretinopathy in which the vitreous adheres to the retina and pulls it from the point of adherence during or just after an abrupt eye movement. The tear appears horseshoe-shaped or round or occasionally slit-like. The patient often complains of photopsia and seeing floaters and they may present with a vitreous haemorrhage. Retinal tears may lead to rhegmatogenous or traction retinal detachment. Management includes laser photocoagulation or cryopexy.
*See* **retinal detachment.**

**retinal vasculitis** *See* **disease, Eales'.**

**retinal vein occlusion** Occlusion of the central retinal vein (CRVO) can be either **non-ischaemic** CRVO (or **venous-stasis retinopathy**) which is the most common type, or **ischaemic** CRVO (or **haemorrhagic retinopathy**). The non-ischaemic type is characterized by some loss of vision, slight impairment of the pupil responses to light and partial or complete central scotoma due to macular oedema. The ophthalmoscopic picture shows retinal haemorrhages, flame-shaped in appearance and distributed throughout the whole fundus, dilated and tortuous veins and a swollen optic disc. In some cases cotton-wool exudates are also noted. When the condition affects young adults it is commonly referred to as **papillophlebitis** (or **optic disc vasculitis**) in which the clinical picture is similar except that the pupillary responses to light are normal and the patient is often asymptomatic. The ischaemic type which usually affects older people is a more severe type and the signs and symptoms are much more marked than in the non-ischaemic type.
Occlusion is more frequently limited to one branch of the central retinal vein (BRVO). In this case the clinical picture is limited to the retinal

area drained by the occluded branch, but most patients will have some loss of vision depending on the extent of the macular oedema. Predisposing causes are cardiovascular disease, systemic hypertension, diabetes or raised intraocular pressure. Treatment depends on the primary cause. Photocoagulation is used in some cases.
*See* **angiography, fluorescein; exudates; haemorrhage, preretinal; rubeosis iridis; vein, central retinal.**

**retinex** A theory proposed to explain colour and brightness perception and constancies. It postulates that the colour of an object is not determined by the spectral composition of the light stimulus coming from an object. It is determined by information obtained from a comparison of three lightnesses generated by the light absorption of the three types of cone cell. The name of the theory 'retinex' reflects the fact that the perception of the image results from the retina and the cortex.

**retinitis** Inflammation of the retina. This usually follows inflammations of the vitreous body, retinal vessels and especially of the choroid. Retinitis leads to an exudation of cells into the vitreous body and, if serious, vision will be affected. If the inflammation affects the macular area there will be a loss of vision. Haemorrhages and oedema (producing a blurring of the margins of the optic disc) are also usually present.

**retinitis, cytomegalovirus** A rare chronic, diffuse infection of the retina caused by the cytomegalovirus (CMV), a member of the herpesvirus group. It affects people with an impaired immune system as a result of either AIDS, organ transplantation or chemotherapy for some malignancies such as leukaemia. The signs are whitish retinal lesions which look granular (not fluffy, cottonwool spots). These lesions progress into retinal necrosis with absolute visual field loss in that area. The lesions are usually accompanied by haemorrhages. Eventually the lesions coalesce and involve the entire fundus, resulting in complete visual loss. In the initial phase of the disease most patients are usually asymptomatic while those with symptoms will complain of floaters, blurred vision, photopsia, scotomas, metamorphopsia, etc. In some cases, retinal detachment follows the disease. Treatment with dihydroxy propoxymethyl guanine and ganciclovir produces some regression of the disease.
*See* **metamorphopsia; necrosis; photopsia; syndrome, acquired immunodeficiency.**

**retinitis exudativa externa** *See* **disease, Coats'.**

**retinitis pigmentosa (RP)** A primary pigmentary dystrophy of the retina followed by migration of pigment. It is an inherited disease characterized by night blindness and constricted visual fields. The condition is usually bilaterally symmetrical. The rod system is damaged but cones are also involved to some degree and the electroretinogram amplitude is subnormal. The disease usually begins in adolescence with night blindness, followed by a ring scotoma in the periphery that spreads until only a small contracted central field remains. Ophthalmoscopic examination reveals a yellowish atrophy of the optic nerve, severe arterial attenuation and conspicuous pigment proliferation which begins in the equatorial region. The areas of pigment have dense centres and irregular processes shaped like bone corpuscles. *Syn.* primary pigmentary retinal dystrophy.
*See* **electroretinogram; fundus, leopard; hemeralopia; keratoconus; tritanopia; vision, tunnel.**

**retinitis proliferans** *See* **retinopathy, proliferative.**

**retinitis, solar** *See* **retinopathy, solar.**

**retinoblastoma** A congenital malignant tumour of the retina usually noted in the first two years of life, although in some cases it may not be until after age 5 years. It is the most common intraocular tumour of childhood. There is a retinoblastoma gene; it was identified on chromosome 13q14. Most individuals who inherit a mutant copy of the retinoblastoma gene sustain a second hit to the remaining normal copy of the gene and develop the disease. The most common ocular manifestations are leukokoria and strabismus and sometimes, red eye, glaucoma and orbital cellulitis. Diagnosis is usually made by the appearance of a greyish reflex of light observed at the pupil, although often by that time the pupil is fixed and the eye is blind. Treatment includes external beam radiotherapy, photocoagulation, cryotherapy and chemotherapy while advanced tumours are managed by enucleation. *Syn.* retinal glioma.
*See* **leukocoria; reflex, cat's eye.**

**retinochoroiditis** Inflammation of both the retina and the choroid.
*See* **toxoplasmosis.**

**retinol** *See* **vitamin A deficiency.**

**retinopathy** A disease of the retina.
*See* **retinitis; tritanopia.**

**retinopathy, arteriosclerotic** *See* **arteriosclerosis.**

**retinopathy, background diabetic** A progressive microangiopathy of the retinal vessels occurring in the early stage of diabetic retinopathy. It is characterized by microaneurysms, dot-blot haemorrhages, flame-shaped haemorrhages, hard exudates and retinal oedema. Retinal veins may also become dilated and tortuous. If the

microvascular occlusion progresses there will be signs of ischaemia and multiple cotton-wool spots will appear, as well as more venous changes and maculopathy, producing the clinical picture of **preproliferative diabetic retinopathy**. If the macular oedema is not clinically significant the patient remains asymptomatic, although a blue-yellow colour vision defect will usually develop. *Syn.* non-proliferative diabetic retinopathy (NPDR).
*See* **retinopathy, diabetic.**

**retinopathy, central serous (CSR)** An accumulation of serous fluid in the subretinal space which leads to a retinal detachment. It usually occurs in the central area of the retina and results in a sudden blurring and/or distortion of vision. The condition typically affects men between the ages of 20 and 45 years. It subsides by itself within a few months in most cases; otherwise photocoagulation may be necessary. *Syn.* central serous chorioretinopathy.
*See* **photocoagulation; retinal detachment.**

**retinopathy, diabetic (DR)** Retinal changes occurring in long standing cases of diabetes mellitus. It is the most common retinal vascular disease. In general, the severity of the retinopathy parallels the duration of the diabetes. The retinopathy is characterized by the presence of new blood vessels (neovascularization) which proliferate on or near the optic disc on the surface of the retina, microaneurysms (small round red spots) and sharply defined white or yellowish waxy exudates. Vitreous detachment is a likely outcome. If the vessels bleed there can be a preretinal haemorrhage with visual loss. Both eyes are usually involved although to different degrees. Visual acuity may be unaffected unless the fovea is involved. After the condition has reached the stage of proliferative retinopathy, the principal treatment is with laser photocoagulation which reduces the risk of further visual loss. Low vision aids may be needed afterward. *Syn.* diabetic retinitis; proliferative diabetic retinopathy (PDR).
*See* **aneurysm; angiography, fluorescein; exudate; microaneurysm; photocoagulation; retinopathy, proliferative.**

**retinopathy, haemorrhagic** *See* **retinal vein occlusion.**

**retinopathy, hypertensive** Retinal changes occurring in malignant hypertension. It is characterized by attenuation and local arteriolar constriction (grades 1 and 2). As the condition progresses, flame-shaped haemorrhages, cotton-wool exudates and oedema appear (grade 3) and at the most advanced stage (grade 4) papilloedema occurs. Arteriosclerotic retinopathy may also accompany this disease.
*See* **arteriosclerosis; exudate; hypertension; macular star; sphygmomanometer.**

**retinopathy, non-proliferative** *See* **retinopathy, background diabetic.**

**retinopathy of prematurity (ROP)** A bilateral retinal disease which commonly affects premature infants exposed to high ambient oxygen concentrations. It is characterized by proliferation and tortuosity of blood vessels, usually with haemorrhages and retinal detachment accompanied by an accumulation of fibrous tissue on the surface of the retina. Some of the infants may develop cicatricial complications which may be innocuous or may progress to cover the central region of the retina and cause blindness. Other complications may be myopia or glaucoma. This condition is less common nowadays. *Syn.* retrolental fibroplasias (RLF).
*See* **leukocoria.**

**retinopathy, proliferative** Neovascularization of the retina extending into the vitreous with connective tissue proliferation surrounding the vessels. The vessels usually arise from a retinal vein near an arteriovenous crossing at the posterior pole and from the surface of the optic disc. It occurs as a result of certain inflammatory conditions and in diabetes. Visual acuity may be affected. *Syn.* retinitis proliferans.
*See* **fibrosis, preretinal macular; hypoxia; retinopathy, diabetic; vitrectomy.**

**retinopathy, solar** Macular damage caused by fixating the sun without adequate protection, usually viewing a solar eclipse, but also in people staring at the sun as part of sun worship or psychosis. The retina presents at first with retinal oedema which may develop into an atrophy of the tissue and produce a circumscribed hole or cyst in the fovea. This latter event results in a permanent central scotoma. There is no specific treatment but the condition can be prevented by wearing very dense light filters or viewing through photographic films. *Syn.* eclipse retinopathy; foveomacular retinitis; solar retinitis.
*See* **actinic; hole, macular.**

**retinopathy, toxaemic of pregnancy** Sudden angiospasm of retinal arterioles, later followed by the typical picture of advanced hypertensive retinopathy. Restitution follows rapidly after the termination of pregnancy.
*See* **retinopathy, hypertensive.**

**retinopathy, venous-stasis** *See* **retinal vein occlusion.**

**retinoschisis** A vitreoretinal degeneration characterized by splitting of the retina into two layers. It occurs either as a hereditary disease or as an acquired condition (70% of these patients are hypermetropic). The X-linked hereditary condition (called **juvenile retinoschisis**) affects only males and usually involves the macula with loss of central vision. The congenital condition is

characterized by a splitting of the nerve fibre layer from the retina whereas the acquired form, which is the most common, results in a splitting at the outer plexiform layer. The latter usually begins in the temporal periphery appearing as a coalescence of microcystoid degenerations with a smooth transparent elevation and associated with an absolute scotoma. The condition may spread to involve the entire peripheral fundus. Holes in the two layers are common and are a sign of progression. The inner layer contains blood vessels and sometimes has small whitish flakes on it which are called 'snowflakes'.
*See* **retinal detachment.**

**retinoschisis, juvenile** *See* **retinoschisis.**

**retinoscope** An instrument for determining objectively the refractive state of the eye. It consists of a light source, a condensing lens and a mirror. The mirror is either semi-transparent or has a hole through which the retinoscopist can view the patient's eye along the retinoscope's beam of light. A patch of light is formed on the patient's retina and by moving that patch in a given direction and observing the direction in which it appears to move after refraction by the patient's eye, the retinoscopist can determine whether the patient's retina is focused in front of, at, or behind the retinoscope's sight hole. If the light reflected from the patient's fundus (called the **retinoscopic reflex** or **light reflex**) and observed in the patient's pupil through the retinoscope moves in the same direction as the movement of the mirror (this is referred to as a **with movement**), the eye is hypermetropic. If the reflex moves in the opposite direction to that of the mirror (**against movement**), the eye is myopic. Sometimes it is impossible to see a clear movement one way or the other but only a bipartite reflex, showing opposite movements in the two sectors of the pupils (this is called a **split reflex** or a **scissors movement**). The refractive error is determined by placing lenses of various powers in front of the patient's eye until no movement is seen, i.e. the whole pupil is either illuminated or dark and the image of the patient's retina is then conjugate with the plane of the retinoscope's sight hole. When this phenomenon occurs the **neutral point** has been reached. The neutral point is measured for each principal meridian of the eye if it is astigmatic. To arrive at the patient's error of refraction the dioptric power corresponding to the distance between patient and retinoscope (called the **working distance**) is subtracted from the total lens power used to obtain neutralization. The amount of dioptric power subtracted is called the **allowance**. (Fig. R11) *Syn.* skiascope.
*See* **band, retinoscopic; chromoretinoscopy; distance, working; point, neutral; reflex, fundus; velonoskiascopy.**

**retinoscope, spot** A retinoscope which projects a circular beam of light upon the patient's retina.

**retinoscope, streak** A retinoscope which projects into the patient's eye an oblong streak which can be adjusted in width and rotated in various meridians. It is more efficient than the spot retinoscope in determining astigmatism.

**retinoscopic artifact** An error encountered in determining the refractive error by retinoscopy. This error is due to the fact that the retinal layer which reflects the retinoscopic light is not situated within the photoreceptors (where an image must be formed to appear in focus) but in front of them. Retinoscopic light is reflected by the vitreous–retina interface due to the difference in their refractive indices (that difference may not exist in some species and in old eyes). Consequently retinoscopic results tend to be more hyperopic or less myopic than is actually the case. The smaller the eye the greater the error because the thickness of the retina is nearly constant across species. This error is equal to about 0.25 D in young human adults, about 1 D in

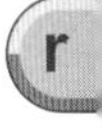


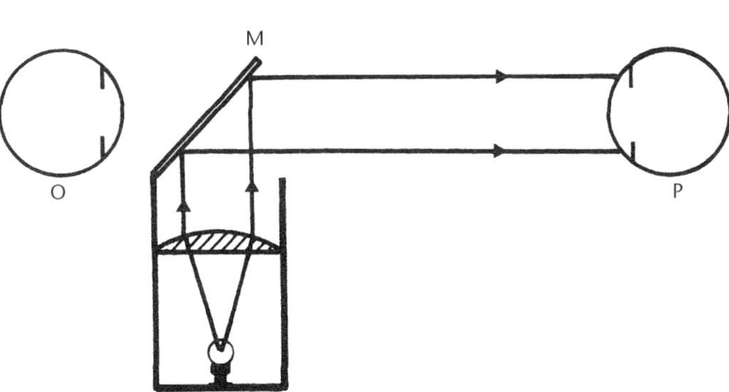


**Fig. R11** Optical principle of a retinoscope (O, observer's eye; P, patient's eye; M, semi-silvered mirror)

infant eyes and can reach some 8 D in very small animals. *Syn.* retinoscopic error; small eye artifact (so called because the effect is much greater for small eyes than for large eyes).

**retinoscopy (ret)** The determination of the refractive state of the eye by means of a retinoscope. *Syn.* skiascopy; shadow test.
*See* **chromoretinoscopy.**

**retinoscopy, dynamic** Retinoscopy performed with the patient fixating binocularly a near object such as a letter, a word, or a picture mounted on, or held close to, the retinoscope and wearing the distance correction. No working distance lens power is subtracted or added to the finding since the plane of regard is at the same distance as the retinoscope. *Syn.* book retinoscopy (this term is restricted to the case when the patient is reading a text); cognitive retinoscopy (when the patient fixates a single letter or reads some words); near point retinoscopy.
*See* **accommodation, lag of; accommodation, objective; retinoscopy, MEM; retinoscopy, near; retinoscopy, static.**

**retinoscopy, MEM** A type of dynamic retinoscopy in which the retinoscope is held in the same plane as the near fixation target and lenses are interposed very briefly in front of one eye, while the other eye fixates the target. The aim of the method is to estimate the fundus reflex motion without disturbing the accommodative stance, that is by leaving each lens in front of one eye for less than one second, until the neutral point is achieved. The results in non-presbyopic subjects generally show a lag of accommodation of 0 to + 0.75 D. *Note*: MEM is an acronym of 'monocular estimate method'.
*See* **retinoscopy, dynamic.**

**retinoscopy, near** Retinoscopy performed in a darkened room at 50 cm (or 20 inches) with the patient fixating the retinoscope light monocularly (the other eye being occluded). Distance retinoscopic refraction is derived by adding − 1.00 D (to take into account the working distance and the state of accommodation in the dark) to the value found by near retinoscopy. The technique is used in paediatric optometry. A better terminology for this term should be **monocular near retinoscopy** to avoid confusion with near point retinoscopy.
*See* **accommodation, resting state of; retinoscopy, dynamic; retinoscopy, MEM; retinoscopy, static.**

**retinoscopy, near point** *See* **retinoscopy, dynamic.**

**retinoscopy, static** Retinoscopy performed with the patient fixating a target at distance or with accommodation paralysed.
*See* **retinoscope.**

**retinotectal pathway** *See* **pathway, retinotectal.**

**retinotopic map** Term referring to the fact that the precise spatial arrangement of the retina is maintained throughout the visual pathway.
*See* **geniculate bodies, lateral; pathway, visual.**

**retraction syndrome, Duane's** *See* **syndrome, Duane's.**

**retrobulbar** Behind the eyeball as, for example, retrobulbar optic neuritis.
*See* **neuritis, optic.**

**retrobulbar optic neuritis** *See* **neuritis, optic.**

**retrography** *See* **mirror writing.**

**retro-illumination** *See* **illumination, retro-.**

**retrolental fibroplasia** *See* **retinopathy of prematurity.**

**retrolental space of Berger** *See* **postlenticular space, Berger's.**

**retroscopic angle** *See* **angle, retroscopic.**

**reversed image** *See* **image, inverted.**

**reversible spectacles** *See* **spectacles, reversible.**

**rhegmatogenous retinal detachment** *See* **retinal detachment.**

**rheumatoid arthritis** A chronic systemic disease of unknown cause characterized by swelling of the joints causing pain and sometimes deformity. It is often accompanied by ocular inflammations which include corneal (keratitis sicca), scleral (scleritis) and uveal (iridocyclitis), as well as scleral thinning (scleromalacia). The juvenile type of the disease (Still's disease) is often accompanied by **band-shaped keratopathy** (in which calcium appears in the superficial layers of the cornea), cataract and iridocyclitis.
*See* **cataract; disease, Reiter's; disease, Still's; iridocyclitis; keratitis sicca; keratopathy; scleritis; scleromalacia; syndrome, Sjögren's; uveitis.**

**rhodopsin** Visual pigment contained in the outer segments of the rod cells of the retina and involved in scotopic vision. When light stimulates the retina, the chromophore of the pigment molecule '11-*cis*' retinal (which is vitamin A aldehyde) isomerizes to 'all-*trans*' retinal. This leads to other chemical transformations which carry on even in the absence of light. The first stage is **prelumirhodopsin**, then **lumirhodopsin** and finally **metarhodopsin** (of which there are two types). This last transformation may lead to the breakdown of the molecule into **retinal** and **opsin**. The molecule is regenerated by recombining retinal and opsin with some enzymes. The absorption spectrum of rhodopsin has a maximum around 498 nm. The isomerization

from '11-*cis*' to 'all-*trans*' also gives rise to the process of **transduction** in which the membrane potential covering the pigment molecules in the outer segment changes towards a hyperpolarization of the cell. This is the first step in the nervous response to a light stimulation of the retina. *Syn.* visual purple (not used any more); erythropsin.
*See* **adaptation, dark; bleaching; cell, rod; pigment, visual; potential, receptor; spectrum, absorption; transduction.**

**rhythm, circadian** The characteristic of some processes to repeat at approximately 24-hour intervals. *Examples*: intraocular pressure is at its lowest every evening and highest every morning; corneal sensitivity is at its lowest every morning and highest every evening. *Syn.* diurnal cycle (provided the variation in activity or behaviour is more or less divided equally between night and day).

**Ricco's law** *See* **law, Ricco's.**

**Riddoch phenomenon** *See* **phenomenon, Riddoch.**

**Rieger's syndrome** *See* **syndrome, Rieger's.**

**rigid lens** *See* **lens, contact.**

**rigidity, ocular** The resistance of the coats of the eye to indentation. This factor is taken into account in the tables used when determining the intraocular pressure by means of an indentation tonometer such as that of Schiötz. The tables are based on an eye of average ocular rigidity but, if the eye has high or low rigidity, an error is introduced into the readings: means of minimizing this effect have been devised.
*See* **tonometer, impression.**

**Riley–Day syndrome** *See* **syndrome, Riley–Day.**

**rim** That part of a spectacle frame which partly or completely surrounds the lens.

**rimexolone** *See* **antiinflammatory drug.**

**rimless fitting** Fitting an edged lens to a rimless mount. The process may include drilling, slotting, strap adjustment, etc. (British Standard).
*See* **lens groove; spectacles, rimless.**

**rimless spectacles** *See* **spectacles, rimless.**

**ring, Coat's white** A small, oval or circular, whitish-grey ring opacity in the cornea found at the level of Bowman's membrane, usually near the periphery. It is composed of a deposition of iron, possibly located at the site of a previous foreign body injury. No treatment is necessary.
*See* **line, iron.**

**ring, Fleischer's** A narrow ring of brownish or greenish pigment containing iron, deposited in the epithelium of the cornea and surrounding (completely or partially) the base of the cone in keratoconus. It is not always present in that disease. *Syn.* Fleischer's line.
*See* **keratoconus; line, iron.**

**ring, Kayser–Fleischer** A ring of pigment granules containing copper located in Descemet's membrane around the periphery of the cornea. It has a brown or greyish-green colour to the unaided eye or golden brown to reddish colour when viewed through the slit-lamp and appears in nearly all cases of Wilson's disease.
*See* **disease, Wilson's.**

**ring, Landolt** *See* **Landolt ring.**

**ring of Schwalbe, anterior limiting** A bundle of connective tissue and elastic fibres forming the junction between the anterior termination of the trabecular meshwork and Descemet's membrane of the cornea. If it is unusually thickened or prominent, it is called **posterior embryotoxon**. *Syn.* line of Schwalbe.
*See* **gonioscopy, direct; meshwork, trabecular; syndrome, Axenfeld's; syndrome, Rieger's.**

**ring, scleral** The appearance of a white patch of sclera adjacent to the optic disc when the retinal pigment epithelium and the choroid do not extend to the optic disc.

**ring scotoma** *See* **scotoma, ring.**

**ring, Soemmering's** Lens remnants found within the periphery of the capsular bag. It may occur following trauma to the lens in which the nucleus and cortex are destroyed, but most commonly following extracapsular cataract extraction. The pupillary area is usually left relatively free.
*See* **after-cataract; cataract extraction, extracapsular.**

**ring, Wessley** A disc-shaped greyish opacity made up of inflammatory cells consisting of antigen-antibody complexes located in the corneal stroma. It is seen in stromal interstitial keratitis resulting from a herpes simplex virus or disciform keratitis. The ring may attract neovascularization. *Syn.* immune ring of Wessley.
*See* **keratitis, disciform; keratitis, interstitial.**

**rings, Newton's** *See* **Newton's rings.**

**Riolan muscle** *See* **muscle of Riolan.**

**Risley prism** *See* **prism, rotary.**

**river blindness** *See* **onchocerciasis.**

**Rizzuti's sign** *See* **sign, Rizzuti's.**

**rod cell** *See* **cell, rod.**

**rod-free area** *See* **foveola.**

**rod monochromat** *See* **monochromat.**

**Roenne nasal step** When scotomata occur above and below the fixation point they meet in the nasal field and form a horizontal step-like defect. It is one of the signs of glaucoma.
*See* **glaucoma, open-angle; scotoma, Bjerrum's.**

**room, Ames** A specially constructed room in which all the visible features have been distorted to make the room appear rectangular from one specific point of observation. In particular, the back wall of the room appears perpendicular to the line of sight, with left and right corners appearing equidistant to the observer, although in reality one corner is much further away. To an observer looking into the room, people of identical heights standing one in each corner of the room appear of clearly different height. The person standing in the far away corner does indeed produce a smaller retinal image, but since the observer believes that they are at the same distance, the person standing closer 'must be larger'. The Ames room demonstrates how perceived distance influences perceived size. *Syn.* Ames distorted room.
*See* **illusion, moon; perception, depth.**

**room, leaf** A cubical box, about 2 metres square with its walls vertical and one open side. The interior surfaces are covered with artificial leaves of various sizes which stick out in a random manner. An observer looking binocularly into the room from the centre of the open side will see its cubical shape due to stereopsis. However, monocularly the room appears almost flat as the monocular cues to depth perception are almost completely eliminated in this room. The leaf room is used to detect and measure spatial distortions resulting from aniseikonia. It can also be used to demonstrate spatial distortion using meridional size lenses.
*See* **aniseikonia; lens, aniseikonic; perception, depth; stereopsis.**

**rosacea, acne** *See* **acne rosacea.**

**rosacea keratitis** *See* **keratitis, rosacea.**

**rose bengal** An iodine derivative of fluorescein having vital staining properties but unlike fluorescein it is a true histological stain which binds strongly and selectively to cellular components. The colour of this stain is red. It has the disadvantage of causing some pain in a good percentage of eyes. It stains dead or degenerated epithelial cells but not normal cells and is used to help in the diagnosis of corneal abrasion, keratitis, keratitis sicca, lagophthalmos, etc.
*See* **fluorescein; lissamine green.**

**Rosenmuller, valve of** *See* **valve of Rosenmuller.**

**rotary prism** *See* **prism, rotary.**

**rouge** A powder consisting of iron oxide, used to polish lenses, metals, etc.
*See* **polishing; surfacing.**

**rubeosis iridis** Neovascularization of the iris characterized by numerous coarse and irregular vessels on the surface and stroma of the iris. The new blood vessels may cover the trabecular meshwork, cause peripheral anterior synechia and give rise to secondary glaucoma. The most frequent causes are diabetes mellitus and central retinal vein occlusion.
*See* **diabetes; glaucoma, neovascular; glaucoma, secondary; iritis; retinal vein occlusion; synechia.**

**Rubin's vase** *See* **vase, Rubin's.**

**rule, Javal's** *See* **Javal's rule.**

**rule, Kestenbaum's** A procedure designed to estimate the power of the addition needed to read ordinary newsprint (about Jaeger 5 or N7–8) in low vision patients. It consists of dividing the denominator of the Snellen visual acuity fraction by its numerator (i.e. 1/Snellen visual acuity). *Example*: if the Snellen visual acuity is 6/60 (or 20/200) the power of the add will be +10 D, which corresponds to a magnification of 10/4 = 2.5 ×. *Syn.* Kestenbaum's formula.
*See* **vision, low.**

**rule, Knapp's** *See* **law, Knapp's.**

**rule, Kollner's** Lesions of the outer retinal layers and changes in the ocular media produce a blue-yellow colour vision defect, whereas lesions of the inner retinal layers, the optic nerve and the visual pathway produce a red-green defect. *Examples*: age-related maculopathy causes a blue-yellow defect; optic neuritis causes a red-green defect. There are exceptions to this rule, particularly during the evolution of a disease. *Syn.* Kollner's law.

**rule, near point** A device for measuring the near points of accommodation and convergence. The RAF rule consists of a graduated four-sided bar on which is mounted a movable target holder which can be moved in the median plane of the head. The bar is calibrated in centimetres and dioptres (Fig. R12).
*See* **accommodation, near point of; method, push-up.**

**rule, PD** A ruler calibrated in millimetres used for measuring the interpupillary distance. Some

**Table R3** Power of the addition required (and corresponding focal length) to read ordinary newsprint (about J5 or N8) in low vision patients, for various acuities. The add is calculated according to Kestenbaum's rule and is an estimate

| acuity at 40 cm | Snellen equivalent at 40 cm (m) | (ft) | power of add (D) | focal distance of add (cm) |
|---|---|---|---|---|
| 40/80 | 6/12 | 20/40 | +2 | 50 |
| 40/100 | 6/15 | 20/50 | +2.5 | 40 |
| 40/120 | 6/18 | 20/60 | +3 | 33 |
| 40/140 | 6/21 | 20/70 | +3.5 | 29 |
| 40/160 | 6/24 | 20/80 | +4 | 25 |
| 40/200 | 6/30 | 20/100 | +5 | 20 |
| 40/250 | 6/38 | 20/125 | +6.25 | 16 |
| 40/320 | 6/48 | 20/160 | +8 | 12.5 |
| 40/400 | 6/60 | 20/200 | +10 | 10 |
| 40/500 | 6/75 | 20/250 | +12.5 | 8 |
| 40/600 | 6/90 | 20/300 | +15 | 6.7 |
| 40/800 | 6/120 | 20/400 | +20 | 5 |
| 40/1200 | 6/180 | 20/600 | +30 | 3.3 |
| 40/1600 | 6/240 | 20/800 | +40 | 2.5 |

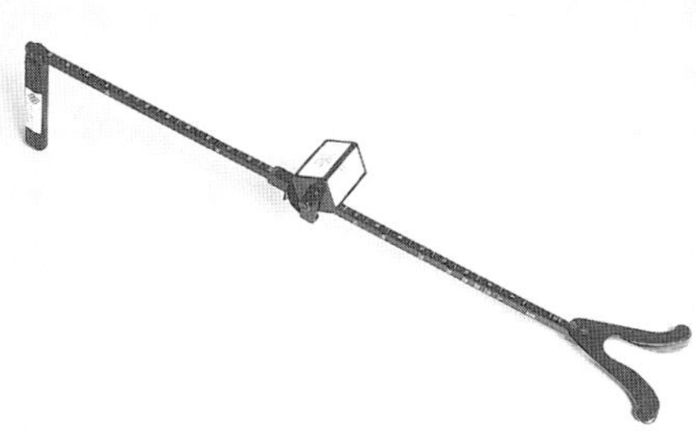

**Fig. R12** The RAF near point rule

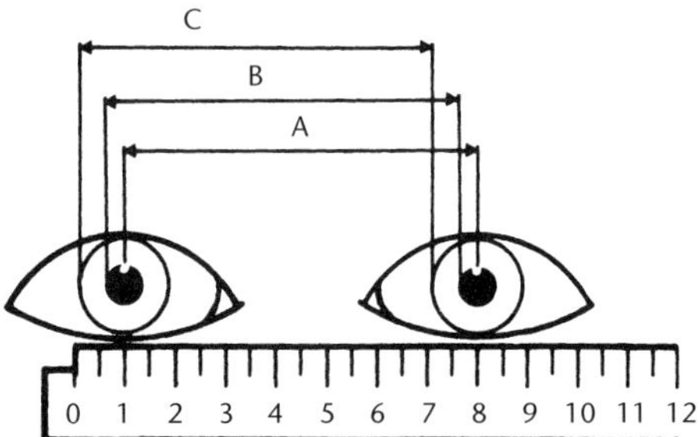


**Fig. R13** PD rule. Measurement of the interpupillary distance is made by measuring the distance A between the two corneal images, or B between the edges of the pupils (if both pupils are of the same size), or C between the edges of the limbus. In normal use, the PD rule is typically placed along the horizontal diameter of the cornea

have the zero point in the middle and the gradations on each side to measure two half-distances thus taking into account facial asymmetry. Many PD rules also have facilities for measuring frames. (Fig. R13) *Syn.* pupillometer (although it is an incorrect use of this term, it is frequently used as a synonym).
*See* **distance, interpupillary; pupillometer.**

**rule, Prentice's** *See* **law, Prentice's.**

**rule, Prince** A device for determining the location of the near point of accommodation and the amplitude of accommodation. It consists of a ruler scaled in dioptres on one side and in millimetres on the other. One end of the ruler is held against the face and a test card is moved along the ruler towards the eye until a blur is noticed. The amplitude of accommodation in dioptres represents either the ocular accommodation (if the reference point is the cornea) or the spectacle accommodation (if the reference point is the spectacle plane).
*See* **accommodation, amplitude of; accommodation, near point of; method, push-up; rule, near point.**

**$R_x$** Traditionally this symbol, which is an abbreviated form of the Latin word recipe meaning take, appears before the main part of a prescription. It is nowadays commonly used as a synonym for prescription.
*See* **prescription.**

# S

**saccade** *See* **movements, fixation.**

**saccadic eye movement** *See* **movement, saccadic eye.**

**saddle bridge** *See* **bridge, saddle.**

**safety glass** *See* **glass, safety**

**sag** Abbreviation for sagitta or sagittal depth; the height of a segment of a circle or sphere.
*See* **lens measure; vertex depth.**

**sagittal depth** *See* **sag; vertex depth.**

**sagittal focus** *See* **astigmatism, oblique.**

**sagittal plane** *See* **plane, sagittal.**

**saline, physiological** A 0.9% sterile solution of sodium chloride in water. This concentration of sodium chloride is considered approximately isotonic with the tears. It is used to store and rinse soft contact lenses, to irrigate the eye, etc. *Syn.* normal saline; NaCl 0.9%.
*See* **eyewash; irrigation; solution, hypertonic; solution, isotonic.**

**'salt and pepper' fundus** *See* **fundus, salt and pepper.**

**sample** *See* **sampling.**

**sampling** The selection of a group of subjects from a population. This is usually done for the purpose of experimentation. The part of the population selected is called the **sample**: it is usually considered to be representative of a given population. A good sample must be **random**, i.e. every possible member of that population has an equal chance of being selected. Otherwise, it is said to be **biased**. Sampling can extend either across geographical areas (**spatial sampling**) or over a period of time (**temporal sampling**).

**Sandhoff's disease** *See* **disease, Sandhoff's.**

**sarcoidosis** *See* **dacryoadenitis; iridocyclitis; keratitis sicca; syndrome, Mikulicz's; uveitis.**

**sarcoma** Malignant tumour formed by proliferation of mesodermal cells.

**Sattler's layer** *See* **choroid.**

**Sattler's veil** Clouding of vision accompanied by seeing coloured haloes around lights caused by corneal oedema resulting from contact lens wear, more frequently the hard lens type (PMMA). The cause has recently been shown to be due to a circular diffraction pattern formed by the basal epithelial cells and the extracellular spaces.
*See* **clouding, central corneal; halo.**

**saturation** Attribute of a visual sensation which permits a judgement to be made of the proportion of pure chromatic colour in the total sensation. *Note*: This attribute is the psychosensorial correlate, or nearly so, of the colorimetric quantity **purity** (CIE).

**scale, Snell–Sterling visual efficiency** *See* **visual efficiency scale, Snell–Sterling.**

**scatter illumination, sclerotic** *See* **illumination, sclerotic scatter.**

**scatter, Tyndall** *See* **effect, Tyndall.**

**scattering, Rayleigh** Diffusion of radiation in the course of its passage through a medium containing particles the size of which is small compared with the wavelength of the radiation (CIE).

**Scheiner's disc; experiment; test** *See* under the nouns.

**schematic eye** *See* **eye, schematic.**

**Schiötz tonometer** *See* **tonometer, impression.**

**Schirmer's test** *See* **test, Schirmer's.**

**Schlemm's canal** *See* **canal, Schlemm's.**

**Schroeder's staircase** This is an ambiguous figure which gives rise to two different perceptions. It consists of a drawing of parallel step-like lines extending from the upper corner of a parallelogram to the lower opposite corner. One either sees a staircase from underneath or a staircase from above and, upon continuous viewing, the impression alternates (Fig. S1). *Syn.* Schroeder's staircase visual illusion.
*See* **figure, Blivet; Necker cube; vase, Rubin's.**

**Schwalbe, anterior limiting ring of; line** *See* **ring of Schwalbe, anterior limiting.**

**science of vision** *See* **vision science.**

**scimitar scotoma** *See* **scotoma, arcuate.**

**scintillans, synchisis** *See* **synchisis scintillans.**

**scintillating scotoma** *See* **scotoma, scintillating.**

**scissors movement** *See* **movement, scissors.**

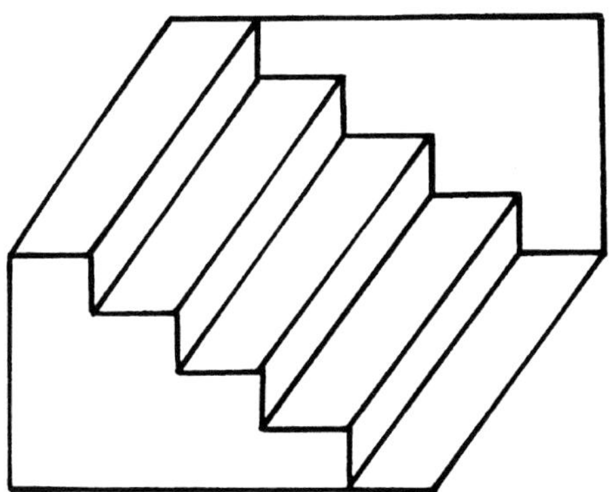

**Fig. S1** Schroeder's staircase

**sclera** The tough, white, opaque, fibrous outer tunic of the eyeball covering most of its surface (the cornea contributes 7% of, and completes, the outer tunic). Its anterior portion is visible and constitutes the 'white' of the eye. In childhood (or in pathological conditions) when the sclera is thin, it appears bluish, while in old age it may become yellowish, due to a deposition of fat. The sclera is thickest posteriorly (about 1 mm) and gradually becomes thinner towards the front of the eyeball. It is a sieve-like membrane at the lamina cribrosa. The sclera is pierced by three sets of apertures: (1) the posterior apertures round the optic nerve and through which pass the long and short posterior ciliary vessels and nerves; (2) the middle apertures, 4 mm behind the equator which give exit to the vortex veins; and (3) the anterior apertures through which pass the anterior ciliary vessels. The tendons of insertion of the extraocular muscles run into the sclera as parallel fibres and then spread out in a fan-shaped manner. The sclera is commonly considered to be divided into three layers from without inward: (1) the episclera, (2) the scleral stroma and (3) the lamina fusca (or suprachoroid) which is interposed between choroid and sclera. *Syn.* sclerotic.
*See* **circle of Zinn; cribriform plate; episclera; evisceration; nerve, optic.**

**sclera, blue** A hereditary defect in which the sclera has a bluish appearance. The sclera is thinner than normal and is susceptible to rupture if the person engages in contact sports. It is often associated with fragility of the bones and deafness as part of a condition called **osteogenesis imperfecta** or (**fragilitas ossium** or **van der Hoeve's syndrome**) and with keratoconus. *Syn.* blue sclerotic.
*See* **keratoconus; syndrome, Ehlers–Danlos; syndrome, Marfan's.**

**scleral buckling** *See* **retinal detachment.**

**scleral crescent** *See* **crescent, myopic.**

**scleral contact lens; ectasia; indentation; rigidity; ring** *See* under the nouns.

**scleral size, back** Maximum internal diameter of the back surface of a scleral contact lens before the outer sharp edge has been rounded. *Syn.* back haptic size.

**scleral spur** A ridge of the sclera at the level of the limbus interposed between the posterior portion of Schlemm's canal and the anterior part of the ciliary body. The scleral spur is the structure from which some of the ciliary muscle fibres originate. *See* **canal, Schlemm's; ciliary body; gonioscopy; muscle, ciliary; sulcus, internal scleral.**

**scleral zone** The portion of a scleral contact lens designed to lie in front of the sclera. *Syn.* haptic. *See* **lens, scleral contact.**

**sclerectasia** *See* **ectasia, scleral.**

**scleritis** Inflammation of the sclera which, in its severe necrotizing or in the posterior type may cause sight-threatening complications such as keratitis, uveitis, angle-closure glaucoma or optic neuropathy. It affects females more commonly than males in the fourth to sixth decades of life. Like episcleritis it has a tendency to recur. It is characterized by pain which can be severe and redness and some patients may develop nodules (**nodular scleritis**). It is often associated with a systemic disease. Common causes are rheumatoid arthritis, herpes zoster, ankylosing spondylitis, syphilis and lupus erythematosus. It can involve part of the sclera, e.g. **anterior scleritis** (that is the most common, and it is classified as diffuse, nodular and necrotizing, with or without inflammation) or **posterior scleritis**. Treatment includes topical and systemic steroids and immunosuppressive drugs for very severe cases. *See* **episcleritis; rheumatoid arthritis; keratitis, acute stromal.**

**scleritis, necrotizing** The most severe form of scleritis, much less common than the other types. About half the patients have one of the following diseases: rheumatoid arthritis, Wegener's granulomatosis, polyarteritis nodosa, systemic lupus erythematosus, or herpes zoster. It is characterized by pain, and white, avascular areas next to damaged areas through which one can see the brown colour of the underlying uveal tissue, and to congested areas of the sclera. In most cases visual acuity is decreased. The necrosis gradually spreads around the globe. Treatment typically consists of topical steroids, immunossuppressive agents and occasionally surgery to repair scleral or corneal perforation.
*See* **scleromalacia.**

**scleritis necroticans** *See* **scleromalacia.**

**scleritis, posterior** Inflammation of the sclera involving the posterior segment of the eye. The condition is often associated with a systemic disease (e.g. rheumatoid arthritis). It is characterized by pain and reduced visual acuity. The severity of the visual impairment depends on the involved tissue and its location. Signs include eyelid oedema, proptosis, limitation of ocular movements and if anterior scleritis is present, redness. The ocular fundus may present disc swelling, choroidal folds, macular oedema and serous retinal detachment. Treatment mainly consists of systemic steroids and immunosuppressive agents.

**sclerokeratitis** Inflammation of both the sclera and the cornea.

**scleromalacia** A bilateral and painless degenerative thinning of the sclera occurring in people with rheumatoid arthritis. In this condition rheumatoid nodules may develop in the sclera and cause perforation (**scleromalacia perforans**). *Syn.* necrotizing scleritis without inflammation; scleritis necroticans.
*See* **rheumatoid arthritis.**

**sclerosis, central areolar choroidal** *See* **dystrophy, central areolar choroidal.**

**sclerosis, multiple (MS)** A disease in which there are disseminated patches of demyelination and sclerosis (or hardening) of the brain, spinal cord and peripheral and optic nerves causing paralysis, tremor, disturbance of speech, nystagmus, diplopia due to involvement of the extraocular muscles and frequently retrobulbar optic neuritis.
*See* **myokymia; neuritis, optic; oscillopsia; potential, visual evoked cortical; pupil, Marcus Gunn; Uhthoff's symptom.**

**sclerotic** *See* **sclera.**

**sclerotic scatter illumination** *See* **illumination, sclerotic scatter.**

**scopolamine hydrobromide** *See* **hyoscine hydrobromide.**

**scotoma** An area of partial or complete blindness surrounded by normal or relatively normal visual field.
*See* **angioscotoma; hemianopsia; quadrantanopsia.**

**scotoma, absolute** A scotoma in which vision is entirely absent in the affected area.
*See* **glaucoma, open-angle; retinoschisis; scotoma, relative.**

**scotoma, annular** *See* **scotoma, arcuate; scotoma, ring.**

**scotoma, arcuate** Scotoma running from the blind spot into the nasal visual field and following the course of the retinal nerve fibres. A double arcuate scotoma extending both in the upper and lower part of the field may join to make an **annular scotoma** or **ring scotoma**. *Syn.* comet scotoma; scimitar scotoma.
*See* **fibres, arcuate; raphe, retinal; scotoma, Bjerrum's; scotoma, ring.**

**scotoma, Bjerrum's** An arcuate scotoma extending around the fixation point (usually located between the 10° and 20° circles) which occurs in open-angle glaucoma. It often extends from the horizontal midline to the optic disc. (Fig. S2)
*Syn.* Bjerrum's sign.
*See* **glaucoma, open-angle; Roenne nasal step; scotoma, Seidel's.**

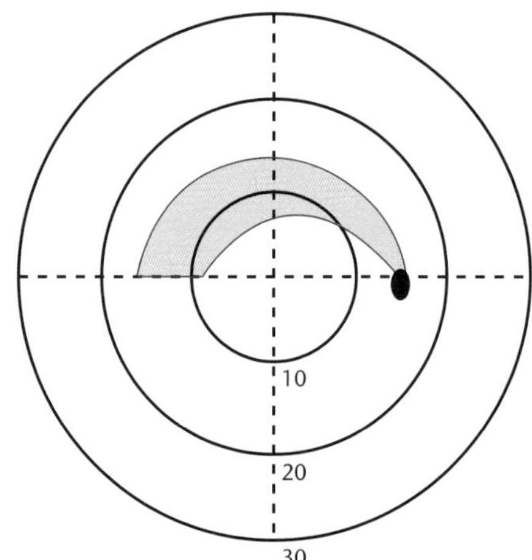


**Fig. S2** Bjerrum's scotoma

**scotoma, central** A scotoma involving the fixation area.

**scotoma, comet** *See* **scotoma, arcuate.**

**scotoma, flittering** *See* **scotoma, scintillating.**

**scotoma, junction** A visual defect due to a lesion (e.g. a pituitary tumour) at the junction of one optic nerve with the chiasma where it is believed that the inferior nasal fibres of the contralateral optic nerve loop before passing backward to the optic tract. The visual defects typically consist of an upper temporal quadrantanopsia in the field of the contralateral eye with, usually, a temporal hemicentral scotoma in the ipsilateral eye. Some authors attribute these visual defects to prechiasmal compression of one optic nerve plus compression of the whole chiasma.
*See* **Wilbrand's knee.**

**scotoma, negative** A scotoma of which the person is unaware. The physiological blind spot is an example of a negative scotoma but it is usually referred to as a **physiological scotoma.** *See* **blind spot.**

**scotoma, paracentral** A scotoma involving the area adjacent to the fixation area.

**scotoma, physiological** *See* **scotoma, negative.**

**scotoma, positive** A scotoma of which the person is aware.

**scotoma, relative** A scotoma in which there is some vision left or in which there is blindness to some stimuli, but not to others. *See* **scotoma, absolute.**

**scotoma, ring 1.** An annular scotoma surrounding the fixation point. It may be formed by the development of two arcuate scotomas. *Syn.* annular scotoma. **2.** A circular area in the peripheral field of view at the edge of a strong convex spectacle lens which is not seen (Fig. S3). This scotoma is due to the prismatic effect at the edge of the lens and unlike other scotomas, not from a pathological condition. When the head turns the ring scotoma also turns and it is then called a **roving ring scotoma**. *See* **phenomenon, jack-in-the-box; scotoma, arcuate.**

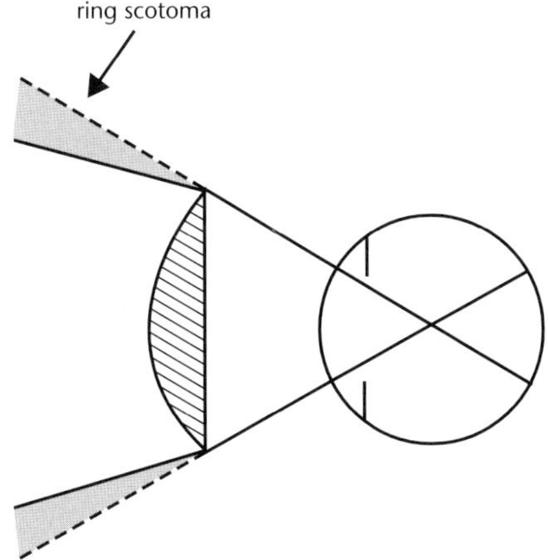


**Fig. S3** Ring scotoma produced by a strong convex spectacle lens (shaded area)

**scotoma, roving ring** *See* **phenomenon, jack-in-the-box; scotoma, ring.**

**scotoma, scimitar** *See* **scotoma, arcuate.**

**scotoma, scintillating** The sudden appearance of a transient, shimmering scotoma with a zigzag outline of bright-coloured lights (also called a **fortification spectrum** or **fortification figures**). It usually occurs as one of the first symptoms of a migraine attack. *Syn.* flittering scotoma. *See* **migraine; teichopsia.**

**scotoma, Seidel's** An arcuate scotoma extending above and below the blind spot found in glaucoma. *Syn.* Seidel's sign. *See* **glaucoma; scotoma, Bjerrum's.**

**scotomas, congruous** Scotomas in the two visual fields which are identical. They form a single defect in the binocular visual field. Such scotomas are often the result of lesions in the visual cortex.

**scotomas, incongruous** Scotomas in the two visual fields which differ in one or more ways. Such scotomas are often the result of lesions in the optic tract.

**scotometer** An instrument such as a campimeter or a perimeter for detecting and plotting the position and magnitude of a scotoma. *See* **campimeter; perimeter.**

**scotopia** *See* **vision, scotopic.**

**scotopic eye** *See* **eye, dark-adapted.**

**scotopic sensitivity syndrome** *See* **syndrome, Meares–Irlen.**

**scotopic vision** *See* **vision, scotopic.**

**screen, Bjerrum's** *See* **screen, tangent.**

**screen, Hess** A black tangent screen for measuring and classifying strabismus. It consists of a chart divided by red lines into small sections of 5° separations. As the screen is flat, the lines are curved in a pincushion pattern (i.e. the middle of the lines is closer to the centre of the screen than the ends of the lines). At the respective positions on the lines in the eight major meridians are small red dots indicating positions 15° and 30° from the fixation point. Two green threads extend from the upper corners of the screen and meet a third green thread which originates on the end of a pointer. The three threads form a figure Y. The patient, wearing a red lens in front of one eye and a green lens in front of the other, moves the pointer until the common origin of the green threads is superimposed on each of the red dots. The discrepancy between the two on the screen indicates the extent of the deviation.

**screen, Lees** An instrument similar to the Hess screen. It consists of two internally illuminated screens placed at right angles. One eye views one screen directly, the other views the second screen via a mirror; hence, the eyes are dissociated. When one eye fixates a point on one illuminated

S

screen, its position as seen by the second eye is indicated with a wand on the second, non-illuminated screen. When this is illuminated, the position of the wand relative to the screen markings indicates whether a muscle or set of muscles is paretic or not.

**screen, tangent** A large plane surface for detecting and plotting the central visual field (about 50° in diameter) by moving the position of a stimulus (e.g. a white 1 mm pinhead). It consists of dull black cloth or other material perpendicular to the line of sight and placed usually 1 m away from the subject (2 m gives more accuracy). In the centre of the screen is a white spot that provides a fixation point and a series of radial and circumferential lines are sewn or drawn to facilitate the localization of the stimulus. *Syn.* Bjerrum's screen.
*See* **campimeter; perimeter.**

**screen test** *See* **test, cover.**

**screener, Harrington–Flocks visual field** A visual field screening instrument consisting of a chin rest, an ultraviolet lamp and a series of 20 cards (10 for each eye). Upon each card is printed a multiple patterned stimulus in fluorescent sulfide ink which fluoresces when illuminated by ultraviolet light. The subjects are instructed to report the number of stimuli (2–4) seen on each card during 0.25 s flash exposure of the ultraviolet source. The serial presentation of all the card patterns is aimed at detecting a scotoma within a central area of 50° in diameter. Once a defect has been detected, it is necessary to use another instrument (e.g. perimeter, tangent screen) to determine the depth and extent of the scotoma. The **Fincham–Sutcliffe screener** is a similar type of instrument but the stimuli are small holes drilled in a grey tangent screen and illuminated by tungsten filament sources. Each pattern can be presented either continuously or for time-limited periods. Each of the 18 patterns consists of 2–4 stimuli. Both instruments lack calibration for either the stimuli or the background.
*See* **analyser, Friedmann visual field; field, visual; perimeter, automated.**

**screener, Fincham–Sutcliffe** *See* **screener, Harrington–Flocks visual field.**

**SEAL** *See* **staining, fluoresecein.**

**sebaceous gland carcinoma** *See* **carcinoma, sebaceous gland.**

**sebum** *See* **glands, meibomian.**

**seclusio pupillae** A complete blocking of the anterior chamber from the posterior chamber by a posterior annular synechia.
*See* **pupillary block; synechia, annular.**

**second degree fusion** *See* **vision, Worth's classification of binocular.**

**secondary cataract; deviation; glaucoma; position** *See* under the nouns.

**see 1.** To perceive by the eye. **2.** To discern. **3.** To note: to understand.

**see-saw nystagmus** *See* **nystagmus.**

**seg height** *See* **segment height.**

**segment height** The vertically measured distance from the lowest point on the lens to the top of the segment of a bifocal (or trifocal) ophthalmic lens. *Syn.* seg height.

**segment of a bifocal lens (seg)** An area of a bifocal lens of a power different to that of the main portion. *Syn.* portion. There is the **distance portion** which has the correction for distance vision, and the **near** or **reading portion** which has the correction for near vision.
*See* **lens, bifocal; portion, intermediate.**

**segment of the eye, anterior** *See* **anterior segment of the eye.**

**segment of the eye, posterior** *See* **posterior segment of the eye.**

**Seidel aberration** *See* **aberration, monochromatic.**

**Seidel's scotoma** *See* **scotoma, Seidel's.**

**semidecussation** *See* **hemidecussation.**

**semi-finished lens** *See* **lens, semi-finished.**

**semilunar fold** *See* **plica semilunaris.**

**senescent cataract** *See* **cataract, senescent.**

**senile macular degeneration** *See* **maculopathy, age-related.**

**senilis, arcus** *See* **arcus, corneal.**

**sensation** The conscious response to the effect of a stimulus exciting any sense organ.
*See* **perception.**

**sensation, visual** A sensation produced by the sense of sight.

**sense** Any faculty (or ability) by which some aspect of the environment is perceived. The five main senses are those of sight, hearing, smell, taste and touch. The sense of sight may be further divided into the colour sense, the form sense, the light sense, the space sense, etc.

**sense organ** A structure especially adapted for the reception of stimuli and the transmission of the relevant information to the brain. The organ of sight is the eye in which light is transduced into nerve signals in the photoreceptors of the retina.

**sensitive period** *See* **period, critical.**

**sensitivity 1.** The capability of responding to or transmitting a stimulus. **2.** The reciprocal of the threshold. **3.** The extent to which a test gives results which are free from **false negatives** (i.e. people found not to have the defect when they actually have it). The fewer the number of false negatives, the greater is the sensitivity of the test. It is usually presented as a percentage of the number of people truly identified as defectives, referred to as **true positives**, A (or hit), divided by the total number of defective people tested. The total number includes all the true positives, A, plus the false negatives, C (or **miss**). Hence,

$$\text{sensitivity (in \%)} = \frac{A}{A + C} \times 100$$

*See* **specificity.**

**sensitivity, contrast** The ability to detect luminance contrast. In psychophysical terms it is the reciprocal of the minimum perceptible contrast. The measurement of the contrast sensitivity of the eye is a more complete assessment of vision than standard visual acuity measurement. It provides an evaluation of the detection of objects (usually sinusoidal gratings on a chart or generated on an oscilloscope display) of varying spatial frequencies and of variable contrast. For each frequency a contrast threshold is obtained and serial measurements yield a **contrast sensitivity function** (CSF). The point where the CSF intercepts the spatial frequency axis represents the standard visual acuity of the subject at 100% contrast. This point is usually referred to as the **cut-off frequency** (Fig. S4). *Example*: following amblyopia treatment, some cases still have the same visual acuity while the CSF is improved.
*See* **acuity, visual; chart, contrast sensitivity; contrast; cycle per degree; function, modulation transfer; glare; grating; resolution, spurious; test, Arden grating; Vistech.**

**sensitivity, corneal** The capability of the cornea to respond to stimulation. Corneal sensitivity to touch is assessed by an aesthesiometer that measures the **corneal touch threshold** (CTT) which is the reciprocal of corneal sensitivity. Sensitivity varies across the cornea, with the centre being the most sensitive. Diseases and rigid contact lens wear greatly reduce the sensitivity of the cornea.
*See* **aesthesiometer; corneal touch threshold; hyperaesthesia, corneal.**

**sensory fusion** *See* **fusion, sensory.**

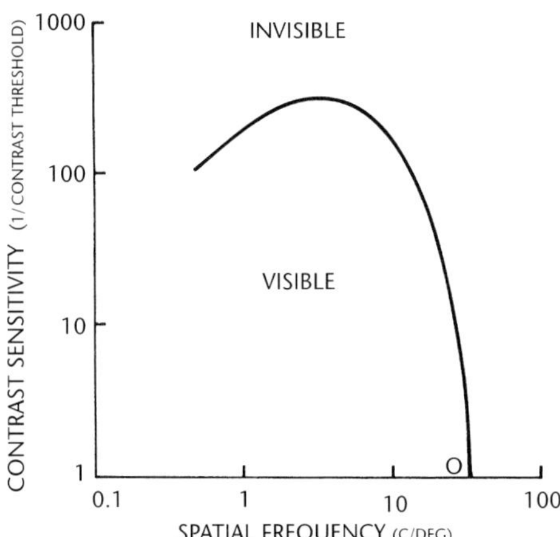


**Fig. S4** Typical contrast sensitivity function of an adult human eye (O, cut-off frequency) (both scales are logarithmic)

**Table S1** Relationship between contrast sensitivity and contrast threshold (contrast sensitivity = 1/contrast threshold). Neither values have units

| contrast sensitivity | $\log_{10}$ contrast sensitivity | contrast threshold decimal | contrast threshold % |
|---|---|---|---|
| 1000 | 3.00 | 0.001 | 0.1 |
| 100 | 2.00 | 0.01 | 1 |
| 20 | 1.30 | 0.05 | 5 |
| 10.00 | 1.00 | 0.1 | 10 |
| 5.00 | 0.70 | 0.2 | 20 |
| 3.33 | 0.52 | 0.3 | 30 |
| 2.50 | 0.40 | 0.4 | 40 |
| 2.00 | 0.30 | 0.5 | 50 |
| 1.67 | 0.22 | 0.6 | 60 |
| 1.43 | 0.15 | 0.7 | 70 |
| 1.25 | 0.10 | 0.8 | 80 |
| 1.11 | 0.05 | 0.9 | 90 |
| 1.00 | 0.00 | 1 | 100 |

**septum orbitale** *See* **orbital septum.**

**serous chorioretinopathy** *See* **retinopathy, central serous.**

**sessile drop test** *See* **test, sessile drop.**

**sex-linked recessive inheritance** *See* **inheritance.**

**shadow** A darkened area from which rays from a source of light are excluded. The shadow patterns cast by light (e.g. sunlight, ceiling fixtures) is such a common sight that if light shines from the opposite direction (e.g. from the ground upward) the normal shadow pattern will be reversed and so will perception; depressions will appear as mounds or vice versa. Shadows

offer a cue to depth perception, as when trying to judge the shape of objects.
*See* **penumbra; perception, depth; stereopsis.**

**shadow test** *See* **test, shadow.**

**Shafer's sign** *See* **sign, Shafer's.**

**Shaffer system** *See* **method, van Herick, Shaffer and Schwartz.**

**shagreen, crocodile** Polygonal greyish-white corneal opacities separated by relatively clear spaces and located in the stroma, either near Bowman's membrane (**anterior crocodile shagreen**) or occasionally near Descemet's membrane (**posterior crocodile shagreen**). They are the result of an irregularity of the stromal collagen lamellae. The condition occurs in old people who are asymptomatic, with little or no effect on vision. *Syn.* crocodile shagreen of Vogt.

**shagreen of the crystalline lens** The slightly irregular or granular appearance of the surfaces of the crystalline lens when viewed with the slit-lamp with specular reflection illumination. The posterior lens shagreen has a slightly yellower tint and is less coarse than the anterior. It is believed to represent variations in the refraction of light within the lens capsule.
*See* **capsule; illumination, specular reflection; lens, crystalline; sign, Vogt's.**

**shape constancy** *See* **constancy, shape.**

**shape factor; magnification** *See* **magnification, shape; magnification, spectacle.**

**Sheard criterion** *See* **criterion, Sheard.**

**sheath syndrome** *See* **syndrome, Brown's superior oblique tendon sheath.**

**shell** *See* **impression, eye.**

**Sheridan–Gardner test** *See* **test, Sheridan–Gardner.**

**Sherrington's law of reciprocal innervation** *See* **law of reciprocal innervation, Sherrington's.**

**shield, eye** 1. *See* **occluder.** 2. A protecting screen against injury or light (Fig. S5).
*See* **goggles; spectacles, industrial.**

**shield ulcer** *See* **ulcer, shield.**

**shingles** *See* **herpes zoster.**

**short-pointing** *See* **pointing, short-.**

**short sight** *See* **myopia.**

**shutter** A device which provides a means (mechanical or electro-optical) for letting a beam of light pass during a given length of time.

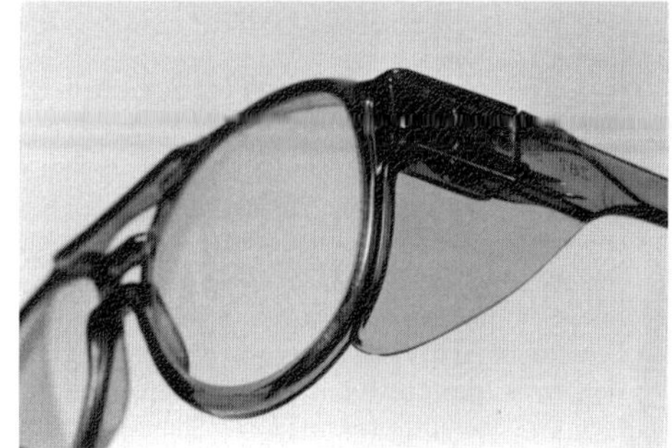

**Fig. S5** Spectacles with protective shield

**SI unit** Abbreviation of **Système International** d'unités (or International System of Units). It is derived from the metric system of physical units. There are seven base units, two supplementary units and many derived units.
*See* **candela per square metre; lumen; lux; micrometre (micron); nanometre.**

**sickle-cell disease** *See* **disease, sickle-cell.**

**Table S2** Base and supplementary SI units, and some derived units

| physical quantity | name | symbol |
|---|---|---|
| **Base units** | | |
| length | metre | m |
| mass | kilogram | kg |
| time | second | s |
| electric current | ampere | A |
| thermodynamic temperature | kelvin | K |
| luminous intensity | candela | cd |
| amount of substance | mole | mol |
| **Supplementary units** | | |
| plane angle | radian | rad |
| solid angle | steradian | sr |
| **Some derived units** | | |
| area | square metre | $m^2$ |
| electric potential difference | volt | V |
| electric resistance | ohm | Ω |
| energy | joule | J |
| force | newton | N |
| frequency | hertz | Hz |
| illuminance | lux | lx |
| luminance | candela per square metre | $cd/m^2$ |
| luminous flux | lumen | lm |
| power | watt | W |
| velocity | metre per second | m/s |
| volume | cubic metre | $m^3$ |

**side** An attachment to the front of a spectacle frame passing towards or over the ear for the purpose of holding the frame in position. *Syn.* temple.
*See* **spectacle frame markings; spectacles; temple, library.**

**side, curl** The end of the side of a spectacle frame which lies along the greater part of the groove behind the ear. It contributes to the stability of the frame and it is particularly useful to children and to people engaged in sports. *Syn.* earpiece.

**siderosis bulbi** Deposit of iron produced by an iron foreign body in the ocular tissues. It is characterized by a reddish-brown discoloration of the surrounding tissue.
*See* **heterochromia; line, iron.**

**sight** The special sense by which the colour, form, position, shape, etc. of objects is perceived when light from these objects impinges upon the retina of the eye.

**sight, line of** *See* **line of sight.**

**sight, night** *See* **hemeralopia.**

**sight, old** *See* **presbyopia.**

**sight, partial** *See* **vision, low.**

**sight, second** Improvement of near vision in the elderly resulting from increased refraction of the nucleus of the crystalline lens. It often occurs in people with incipient cataract. *Syn.* gerontopia; senile lenticular myopia.

**sight, sense of** *See* **sense.**

**sight-testing** *See* **refraction.**

**sign** Objective evidence of a disease as distinguished from **symptom** which is a subjective complaint of a patient.
*See* **diagnosis; prognosis.**

**sign, Argyll Robertson** *See* **pupil, Argyll Robertson.**

**sign, Bell's** Bell's phenomenon occurring on the affected side in Bell's palsy.
*See* **palsy, Bell's; phenomenon, Bell's.**

**sign, Bjerrum's** *See* **scotoma, Bjerrum's.**

**sign, Cogan's lid twitch** A twitch of the upper eyelid in an eye with ptosis when the patient is asked to look in the primary position following a downward look. The eyelid then returns to its ptosis position. This condition occurs in myasthenia gravis.
*See* **myasthenia gravis; ptosis.**

**sign, Collier's** Unilateral, or more commonly bilateral, eyelid retraction that exposes an unusual amount of the sclera of the eye above and below the iris; it gives the person a frightened or startled expression. It is due to a midbrain lesion.
*See* **syndrome, Parinaud's.**

**sign convention** A set of conventions regulating the direction of distances, lengths, and angles measured in geometrical optics. The most common is the **New Cartesian Sign Convention**. It stipulates: (1) All distances are measured from the lens, refracting surface or mirror. Those in the same direction as the incident light, which is drawn travelling from left to right, are positive. Those in the opposite direction are negative. (2) All distances are measured from the axis. Those above are positive. Those below are negative. (3) Angles are measured from the incident ray to the axis, with anti-clockwise angles positive and clockwise angles negative. (4) The power of a converging lens is positive and that of a diverging lens is negative (Fig. S6).
*See* **focal length; law, Lagrange's; law of refraction; Newton's formula; paraxial equation, fundamental.**

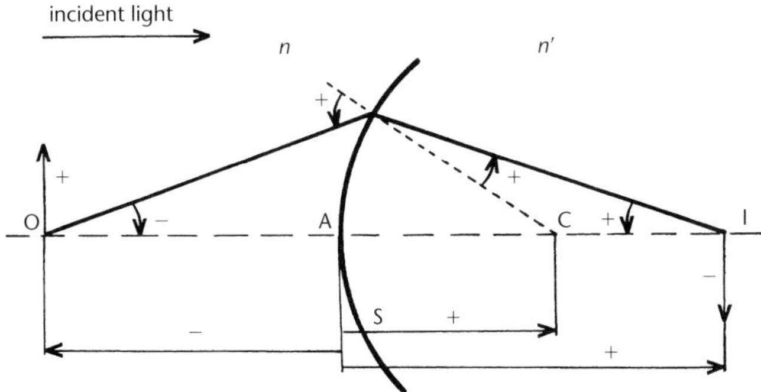


**Fig. S6** Sign convention at a spherical refracting surface S (O, object; A, vertex; C, centre of curvature; I, image; $n$, $n'$, refractive indices)

**sign, Dalrymple's** Retraction of the eyelids causing an abnormally widened palpebral fissure, in primary gaze. This is a sign of Graves' disease. The patient appears to stare and to be frightened as some white sclera may be seen above the upper limbus.
*See* **disease, Graves'.**

**sign, doll's eye** *See* **phenomenon, doll's head.**

**sign, von Graefe's** Immobility or lagging of the upper eyelid when looking downward. This is a sign of Graves' disease.
*See* **disease, Graves'.**

**sign, Hutchinson's** A triad of signs present in congenital syphilis. They are interstitial keratitis, notched teeth and deafness.
*See* **keratitis, interstitial.**

**sign, local** *See* **direction, oculocentric.**

**sign, Moebius'** Convergence weakness occurring in Graves' disease.
*See* **disease, Graves'.**

**sign, Mizuo's** *See* **phenomenon, Mizuo's.**

**sign, Munson's** A sign observed in keratoconus in which the lower lid is bulging as a cone when the patient looks downward.
*See* **keratoconus.**

**sign, Rizzuti's** An arrowhead pattern near the nasal part of the corneoscleral limbus, sometimes seen in advanced keratoconus.
*See* **keratoconus.**

**sign, Seidel's** *See* **scotoma, Seidel's.**

**sign, Shafer's** The presence of pigment granules of various sizes floating in the anterior vitreous. They usually result from a retinal break/s which may progress into retinal detachment. They can easily be seen with a slit-lamp.
*See* **retinal detachment.**

**sign, Vogt's** Loss of the normal shagreen of the front surface of the crystalline lens indicating anterior capsular cataract.
*See* **cataract, anterior capsular; shagreen, crocodile.**

**sign, Uhthoff's** *See* **Uhthoff's symptom.**

**silicone hydrogel lens** *See* **lens, silicone hydrogel.**

**silicone rubber** A polymeric elastomeric, transparent material which is used in the manufacture of silicone rubber contact lenses. It has very high oxygen permeability but it is also very hydrophobic (wetting angle greater than 90°). The surfaces must be specially treated to render them wettable. *Syn.* poly(dimethyl siloxane).
*See* **angle, contact; index of refraction; lens, silicone hydrogel; siloxane.**

**simultanagnosia** Inability to comprehend a whole picture or sustain visual attention across simultaneous elements, although its constituent elements may be recognized. Objects may look fragmented or even sometimes disappear hence the patient may have difficulty recognizing a face as only one part is seen, or difficulty reading. Visual acuity and visual fields are normal. This is often a symptom of Balint's syndrome or the result of a lesion, usually, in both parietal visual cortices, although temporal lobes may also be involved. *Syn.* simultagnosia; visual disorientation.
*See* **syndrome, Balint's.**

**SILO response** *See* **response, SILO.**

**siloxane** A polymeric, transparent material which is used as a component in the manufacture of gas permeable contact lenses. This polymer consists of alternating silicon and oxygen atoms and two organic side groups such as methyl, propyl, phenyl, vinyl or chloropropyl attached to each silicon. Siloxane is very permeable to oxygen and carbon dioxide. Many gas permeable contact lenses are made with a combination of siloxane and polymethyl methacrylate.
*See* **modulus of elasticity; polymethyl methacrylate; silicone rubber.**

**silver wire artery** *See* **arteriosclerosis.**

**simple astigmatism** *See* **astigmatism, simple.**

**simple cell** *See* **cell, simple.**

**simultaneous binocular vision** *See* **vision, Worth's classification of binocular.**

**simultaneous vision** *See* **lens, contact.**

**Simultantest** Tradename for an accessory to be inserted in a lens aperture of a phoropter or trial frame used to refine both the sphere and cylindrical components of a refraction. It provides simultaneous viewing of a distant test object through either a plus and minus sphere lens (+ 0.25 and −0.25 D) or through two + 0.25 sphere, − 0.50 cylinder lens systems with their cylindrical axes perpendicular to each other. Either mode of viewing is obtained by turning a knob which actually rotates one of the lenses in the system.
*See* **phoropter; trial frame.**

**sine condition** The elimination of distortion and coma in an image is met when

$$M = \frac{n \sin u}{n' \sin u'}$$

where $M$ is the lateral magnification, $n$ and $n'$ the refractive indices of the media in the object and image space, and $u$ and $u'$ are the angular apertures on the object and image sides, respectively. *Syn.* Abbé's condition.
*See* **aperture, angular; coma; correction; distortion; magnification, lateral.**

**single binocular vision** *See* **vision, binocular single.**

**single-vision lens** *See* **lens, single-vision.**

**sinus** A hollow space in bone or other tissue.

**sinus, cavernous** One of the two venous sinuses in the dura mater of the brain extending on each side of the pituitary body, behind the orbit. It receives blood from the superior and the inferior ophthalmic veins and the central retinal veins. The third, fourth, fifth and sixth nerves pass through as well as the internal carotid artery. The cavernous plexus is located within this sinus.
*See* **plexus, cavernous.**

**sinus circularis iridis** *See* **canal, Schlemm's.**

**sinus, ethmoidal** Mucus-lined air cavities within the ethmoid bone, between the nose and the orbit. They drain into the nasal cavity. They contain the anterior and posterior ethmoidal nerves and blood vessels and are filled with air. They are separated from adjacent areas by very thin plates through which infection can pass easily and in particular ethmoiditis, which is the most common cause of orbital cellulitis.
*See* **cellulitis, orbital.**

**sinus of Maier** *See* **lacrimal apparatus.**

**sinus, scleral** *See* **canal, Schlemm's.**

**sinus venosus sclerae** *See* **canal, Schlemm's.**

**situs inversus of the disc** *See* **crescent, congenital scleral.**

**sixth cranial nerve** *See* **nerve, abducens.**

**sixth nerve paralysis** *See* **paralysis of the sixth nerve.**

**size, angular** The size of an object measured in terms of the angle it subtends. The point of reference for the eye can be either the nodal point or the centre of the entrance pupil.
*See* **object, extended; size, apparent.**

**size, apparent** **1.** The size of an object represented by the angular size. **2.** The perceived size of an object as distinguished from the actual size.
*See* **size, angular.**

**size constancy** *See* **constancy, size.**

**size lens** *See* **lens, aniseikonic.**

**Sjögren's syndrome** *See* **syndrome, Sjögren's.**

**skiascope** *See* **retinoscope.**

**skiascopy** *See* **retinoscopy.**

**slab-off lens** *See* **lens, slab-off.**

**slit-lamp** Instrument producing a bright focal source of light with a slit of variable width and height. It may be used to examine the tissues of the anterior segment of the eye in conjunction with a microscope (usually binocular) of variable magnification. To examine the internal structures of the eye including the retina an auxiliary lens is required. Many such lenses exist, some which do not make contact with the eye (e.g. Hruby lens, Volk lens) and others which come in contact with the eye, usually like a scleral type of lens (e.g. Goldmann lens, Thorpe four mirror fundus lens, Wilson three mirror fundus lens). A slit-lamp is essential in contact lens practice. This instrument is also commonly called a **biomicroscope**. (Fig. S7)
*See* **biomicroscope; gonioscope; illumination; lens, Hruby; method, van Herick, Shaffer and Schwartz; microscope, slit-lamp; pachometer; polymegethism, endothelial.**

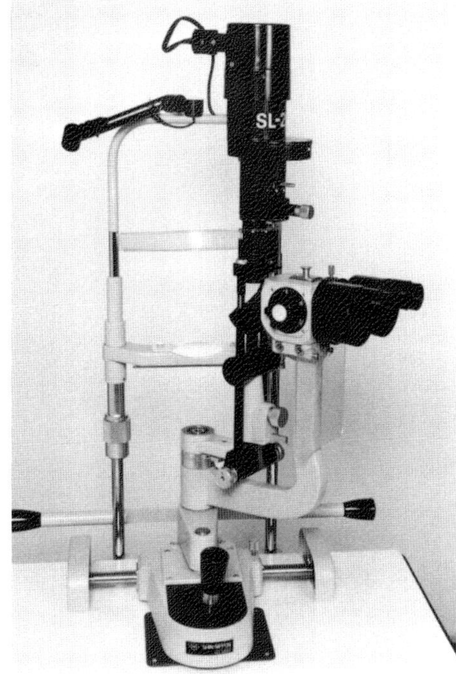

Fig. S7 Slit-lamp (Shin Nippon)

**small angle strabismus** *See* **microtropia.**

**small eye artifact** *See* **retinoscopic artifact.**

**smooth pursuit** *See* **movement, pursuit.**

**Snell's law** *See* **law of refraction.**

**Snellen acuity** *See* **acuity, Snellen.**

**Snellen chart** *See* **chart, Snellen.**

**Snellen equivalent** *See* **acuity, near visual.**

**Snellen fraction** A representation of visual acuity in the form of a fraction (e.g. 6/6 (20/20), 6/24 (20/80), etc.) in which the numerator is the testing distance, usually expressed in metres (or in feet), and the denominator is the distance at which the smallest Snellen letter read by the eye has an angular size of 5 minutes.
*See* **acuity, near visual; acuity, visual; acuity, decimal visual.**

**Table 53** Relationship between Snellen fractions in metres and feet, and for two testing distances (4 and 6 metres)

| (6m) | (20ft) | (4m) |
|---|---|---|
| 6/3 | 20/10 | 4/2 |
| 6/4.8 | 20/16 | 4/3.2 |
| 6/6 | 20/20 | 4/4 |
| 6/7.5 | 20/25 | 4/5 |
| 6/9.5 | 20/32 | 4/6.3 |
| 6/12 | 20/40 | 4/8 |
| 6/15 | 20/50 | 4/10 |
| 6/18 | 20/60 | 4/12 |
| 6/21 | 20/70 | 4/14 |
| 6/24 | 20/80 | 4/16 |
| 6/30 | 20/100 | 4/20 |
| 6/38 | 20/125 | 4/25 |
| 6/48 | 20/160 | 4/32 |
| 6/60 | 20/200 | 4/40 |
| 6/90 | 20/300 | 4/60 |
| 6/120 | 20/400 | 4/80 |
| 6/150 | 20/500 | 4/100 |
| 6/180 | 20/600 | 4/120 |
| 6/240 | 20/800 | 4/160 |
| 6/300 | 20/1000 | 4/200 |

**Snellen test type** *See* **chart, Snellen.**

**Snell–Sterling visual efficiency scale** *See* **visual efficiency scale, Snell–Sterling.**

**snowflake cataract** *See* **cataract, snowflake.**

**snow blindness** *See* **keratoconjunctivitis, actinic.**

**sodium chloride** *See* **saline, physiological.**

**sodium cromoglycate** *See* **conjunctivitis, giant papillary; conjunctivitis, vernal; keratoconjunctivitis, superior limbic; mast cell stabilizers.**

**sodium fluorescein** *See* **fluorescein.**

**sodium pump** *See* **potential, action.**

**sodium/potassium pump** *See* **potential, action; transport, active.**

**soft drusen; exudate** *See* under the nouns.

**solar retinopathy; spectrum** *See* under the nouns.

**solution, hypertonic** A solution with an osmotic pressure greater than that of an isotonic solution. Hypertonic ophthalmic solutions cause some stinging when instilled. *Examples*: sodium chloride 5%: when applied to an oedematous cornea this solution reduces oedema by drawing water from it; sulfacetamide sodium 30%; glycerol (or glycerin), at a dose of 1–1.5 g/kg body weight given as a solution with water or other liquid, which draws water from the eye into the blood and thereby reduces the intraocular pressure. *Syn.* hyperosmotic agent.
*See* **pressure, osmotic; saline, physiological.**

**solution, hypotonic** A solution with an osmotic pressure lower than that of an isotonic solution. Hypotonic ophthalmic solutions generally cause less irritation than hypertonic ones.
*See* **pressure, osmotic.**

**solution, isotonic** A solution with an osmotic pressure equal to that on the other side of a semipermeable membrane. *Example*: sodium chloride 0.9% is considered to be approximately isotonic with the tears.
*See* **pressure, osmotic; saline, physiological.**

**source, coherent** *See* **coherent sources.**

**source, extended** A source consisting of many point sources separated laterally and such that it has a very low degree of coherence. Thus, an extended source has a given size and subtends a given angle.
*See* **coherent sources; light, beam of; light, diffuse; light source.**

**source, point** A source whose dimensions are sufficiently small to cause a radiation with a high degree of coherence. If the point source is situated on the axis of an optical system it gives rise to an axial ray and it is referred to as an **axial point source**.
*See* **coherent sources; ray, axial.**

**space of Berger, postlenticular** *See* **postlenticular space, Berger's.**

**space, gaussian** *See* **paraxial region.**

**space horopter** *See* **horopter, space.**

**spaces, intertrabecular** *See* **meshwork, trabecular.**

**span of recognition** The amount of reading matter which can be correctly identified or perceived during a brief exposure. It is often evaluated in testing and training reading ability.
*See* **reading.**

**sparing of the macula** *See* **macula, sparing of the.**

**spasm of accommodation** *See* **accommodation, spasm of.**

**spasm of the lid** *See* **blepharospasm.**

**spatial frequency; induction; summation** *See* under the nouns.

**spatial vision** *See* **perception, depth.**

**specificity** The extent to which a test gives results which are free from **false positives** (i.e. people found to have the defect when they are actually free of it). The fewer the number of false positives, the greater is the specificity of the test. It is usually presented as the percentage of people truly identified as not defectives, or normal, referred to as **true negatives**, D (or correct reject), divided by the total number of not defectives or normal people tested. The total number includes all the true negatives, D, plus the false positives, B (or **false alarm**). Hence,

$$\text{specificity (in \%)} = \frac{D}{B + D} \times 100$$

*See* **sensitivity.**

**spectacle blur** *See* **blur, spectacle.**

**spectacle crown** *See* **glass, crown.**

**spectacle frame** *See* **spectacles.**

**spectacle frame markings** Numbers shown on a spectacle frame. They are usually the eyesize, the distance between lenses and the side length. Metal frames may also indicate the amount of gold (if any) found in the frame (e.g. 12 k meaning that the material is one-half gold and one-half of another metal). *Example*: 52/22 on the front of the frame means that the eyesize is 52 mm and the DBL is 22 mm, and 140 on the side means that the total length of the side is 140 mm.
*See* **distance between lenses; eyesize; side.**

**spectacle frame, metal** A structure in metal for enclosing or supporting ophthalmic lenses. Common materials include nickel/silver, Hi-nickel alloy, bronze, stainless steel, gold, gold plated, gold coating (commonly referred to as gold filled in which the base metal is most often nickel silver and for better quality frames, monel), copper, beryllium, titanium and sometimes aluminium. Metal spectacle frames are usually more rigid and maintain their shape better than plastic spectacle frames. However, the contacts with the skin of the nose and ears are done with plastic (or silicone) nose pads and temple covers.

**spectacle frame, plastic** A structure in plastic for enclosing or supporting ophthalmic lenses. Common materials include carbon fibre composite materials which are a mixture of principally carbon and nylon in different percentages, cellulose acetate, cellulose propionate, nylon, epoxy resin (tradename Optyl), and Perspex and Plexiglass (which are both tradenames for acrylic plastics containing mainly polymethyl methacrylate). Most of the plastics used are thermoplastic, i.e. a material which softens with heat and can thus be manipulated to fit the patient's head and to insert and remove the lenses.
*See* **frame heater; polymethyl methacrylate.**

**spectacle lens** *See* **lens, spectacle.**

**spectacle magnification** *See* **magnification, spectacle.**

**spectacle refraction** *See* **refractive error.**

**spectacles** An optical appliance consisting of a pair of ophthalmic lenses mounted in a frame or rimless mount, resting on the nose and held in place by sides extending towards or over the ears. *Syn.* eyeglass frame; eyeglasses; eyewear (colloquial); glasses; spectacle frame.
*See* **acetone; angle, pantoscopic; angle, retroscopic; angling; bridge; clipover; eczema; eyesize; front; lorgnette; pad; plastic; rim; side; spectacle frame markings; sunglasses; temple; tortoiseshell.**

**spectacles, aphakic** Spectacles mounted with aphakic lenses used to compensate the loss of optical power resulting from a cataract extraction when no intraocular lens implant has been inserted. *Syn.* cataract glasses.
*See* **cataract extraction; lens, aphakic.**

**spectacles, billiards** Spectacles incorporating joints which enable the wearer to adjust the angle of the sides (British Standard).

**spectacles, folding** Spectacles that are hinged at the bridge and in the sides, so as to fold with the two lenses in apposition.

**spectacles, half-eye** A pair of spectacles designed so that the lenses cover only half of the field of view, usually the lower half (Fig. S8). *Syn.* half-eyes.

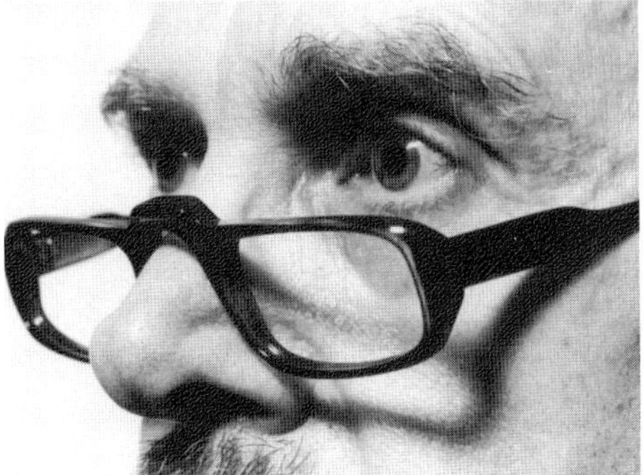

**Fig. S8** Half-eyes spectacles

**spectacles, hemianopsia** Spectacles incorporating a device which provides a lateral displacement of one or both fields of view.

**spectacles, industrial** Spectacles made with plastic or safety glass and solid frame, sometimes with side shields. They are used in industrial occupations where there are possible hazards to the eye. *See* **Fig. S5; glass, safety; goggles; lens, safety.**

**spectacles, library** A plastic spectacle frame with heavyweight front and sides. *Syn.* library frame. *See* **temple, library.**

**spectacles, magnifying** Spectacles containing lenses of high convex power (+10 D or higher) used for near vision.
*See* **vision, low.**

**spectacles, orthopaedic** Spectacles with attachments designed to relieve certain anatomical deformities such as entropion, ptosis, etc.
*See* **entropion; ptosis; syndrome, Horner's.**

**spectacles, pinhole** Spectacles fitted with opaque discs having one or more small apertures. They are used as an aid in certain types of low vision (e.g. corneal scar).
*See* **spectacles, stenopaeic; vision, low.**

**spectacles, recumbent** Spectacles intended to be used while recumbent. They usually incorporate a prism which deflects a beam of light through approximately 90° while keeping the image erect. *Example*: NAP glasses.
*See* **prisms, yoke.**

**spectacles, reversible** Spectacles which are designed to be worn with either lens before either eye.

**spectacles, rimless** Spectacles without rims, the lenses being fastened to the frame by screws, clamps or similar devices.
*See* **lens groove; rim.**

**spectacles, stenopaeic** Spectacles fitted with opaque discs having a slit. They are used as an aid in certain types of low vision.
*See* **disc, stenopaeic; spectacles, pinhole; vision, low.**

**spectacles, supra** Spectacles in which the lenses are held in position by thin nylon threads attached to the rims.
*See* **lens groove; rim.**

**spectacles, telescopic** *See* **lens, telescopic.**

**spectral 1.** Related or belonging to a spectrum. **2.** Related to wavelength.
*See* **wavelength.**

**spectral luminous efficiency** *See* **efficiency, spectral luminous.**

**spectral transmission factor** *See* **spectrophotometer.**

**spectrometer** An instrument for making measurements of the angle of a prism and the index of refraction. It consists of a collimator, an astronomical telescope, a table for carrying a prism and a graduated circle.

**spectrophotometer** An instrument for measuring the relative intensities of the spectrum, wavelength by wavelength. Specifically it measures the spectral **transmission factor** (i.e. the ratio of radiant flux transmitted through a medium to that incident on it) of a medium for a given wavelength. This factor is usually plotted as a graph against many wavelengths providing a spectral transmission curve. Ophthalmic lenses, contact lenses and any other substances (e.g. tear lipids) through which light may be passed can thus be analysed.
*See* **density.**

**spectroscope** An instrument for producing and observing spectra. It consists of a slit, a diffraction grating or a prism to disperse the radiations, achromatic lenses, and an eyepiece to observe them.
*See* **monochromator; spectrum.**

**spectrum 1.** Spatial display of a complex radiation produced by separation of its monochromatic components. **2.** Composition of a complex radiation, e.g. continuous spectrum, line spectrum (CIE). *Plural*: spectra.
*See* **light.**

**spectrum, absorption** The curve representing the relative absorption of a pigment or chemical substance as a function of the wavelength of light. *Example*: the absorption spectrum of rhodopsin. *Syn.* absorbance spectrum.
*See* **pigment, visual; rhodopsin.**

**spectrum, action** A graphical representation of the relative energy necessary to produce a constant biological effect. *Example*: frequency of action potentials in a ganglion cell as a function of wavelength.

**spectrum, continuous** A spectrum in which, over a considerable range, all wavelengths exist without any abrupt variation in intensity. *Example*: the spectrum of hot solids.
*See* **lamp, filament.**

**spectrum, electromagnetic** The total range of all electromagnetic waves. It extends from the longest radio waves of some thousands of metres in wavelength through radar, microwave, infrared rays, visible rays (between wavelengths 780 nm and 380 nm) to ultraviolet rays, X-rays, gamma rays and cosmic rays with

**Table S4** Approximate values of the velocity, frequency and wavelength of electromagnetic radiations in a vacuum (the values represent a point within a range of radiations)

| radiation | velocity (m/s) | frequency (Hz) | wavelength (m) | wavelength (nm) |
|---|---|---|---|---|
| AM radio | $3 \times 10^8$ | $1 \times 10^6$ | $3 \times 10^2$ | $3 \times 10^{11}$ |
| television | $3 \times 10^8$ | $1 \times 10^8$ | 3 | $3 \times 10^9$ |
| radar | $3 \times 10^8$ | $1 \times 10^9$ | $3 \times 10^{-1}$ | $3 \times 10^8$ |
| microwave | $3 \times 10^8$ | $1 \times 10^{10}$ | $3 \times 10^{-2}$ | $3 \times 10^7$ |
| thermal infrared | $3 \times 10^8$ | $1 \times 10^{13}$ | $3 \times 10^{-5}$ | $3 \times 10^4$ |
| near infrared | $3 \times 10^8$ | $1 \times 10^{14}$ | $3 \times 10^{-6}$ | 3000 |
| **light** | | | | |
| red | $3 \times 10^8$ | $3.94 \times 10^{14}$ | $7.6 \times 10^{-7}$ | 760 |
| yellow | $3 \times 10^8$ | $5.45 \times 10^{14}$ | $5.5 \times 10^{-7}$ | 550 |
| violet | $3 \times 10^8$ | $7.50 \times 10^{14}$ | $4.0 \times 10^{-7}$ | 400 |
| ultraviolet | $3 \times 10^8$ | $1 \times 10^{16}$ | $3 \times 10^{-8}$ | 30 |
| X-rays | $3 \times 10^8$ | $1 \times 10^{18}$ | $3 \times 10^{-10}$ | 0.3 |
| gamma rays | $3 \times 10^8$ | $1 \times 10^{21}$ | $3 \times 10^{-13}$ | 0.0003 |

wavelengths as short as $8 \times 10^{-12}$mm. All these electromagnetic waves differ only in frequency (and wavelength) but have the same speed as light in a vacuum.
*See* **infrared; ultraviolet; wavelength.**

**spectrum, equal energy** Spectrum in which all wavelengths have about the same amount of energy.
*See* **achromatic; light, white.**

**spectrum, fortification** *See* **scotoma, scintillating.**

**spectrum, invisible** The portions of the entire electromagnetic spectrum which are made up of radiations other than those of the visible spectrum.

**spectrum, line** Spectrum consisting of a series of discrete monochromatic lines (or narrow bands of monochromatic light) with large intensity differences and separated by intervals without radiations. *Example*: the spectrum emitted by an electric discharge through a gas or vapour under low pressure.

**spectrum locus** The representation of the spectral colour stimuli on a chromaticity diagram.
*See* **chromaticity diagram.**

**spectrum, solar** The spectrum formed by sunlight. It is crossed at intervals by Fraunhofer's lines.
*See* **lines, Fraunhofer's.**

**spectrum, visible** *See* **light.**

**specular microscope** *See* **microscope, specular.**

**specular reflection** *See* **reflection, regular.**

**speed of light** *See* **light, speed of.**

**sphenoid bone** *See* **orbit.**

**sphere** A term commonly used to denote the spherical component of a prescription or of the power of a lens, or even a spherical lens.
*See* **lens, spherical; prescription.**

**sphere, far point** The imaginary spherical surface on which lie the far points of accommodation for all directions of gaze.
*See* **accommodation, far point of.**

**sphere, near point** The imaginary spherical surface on which lie the near points of accommodation for all directions of gaze.
*See* **accommodation, near point of.**

**spherical aberration; equivalent** *See* under the nouns.

**spherical error** *See* **prescription.**

**spherical lens** *See* **lens, spherical.**

**spherometer** *See* **lens measure.**

**sphero-cylindrical lens** *See* **lens, sphero-cylindrical.**

**spherophakia** A congenital, bilateral defect in which the crystalline lens is smaller and more spherical than normal. The zonule of Zinn may also be defective or absent.
*See* **syndrome, Weill–Marchesani.**

**spherule, rod** The foot of a rod located in the outer molecular (or plexiform) layer of the retina.
*See* **cell, rod; retina.**

**sphincter oculi muscle** *See* **muscle, orbicularis.**

**sphincter pupillae muscle** *See* **muscle, sphincter pupillae.**

**sphingomyelin lipidosis** *See* **disease, Niemann–Pick.**

**sphygmomanometer** An instrument for measuring the arterial blood pressure. There are various types, the most common consisting of an inflatable cuff which is placed around the upper arm (usually the left) and air pressure within the cuff is balanced against the pressure of the blood in the brachial artery. The pressure is estimated by means of a mercury or an aneroid manometer. A stethoscope is normally used in conjunction with the instrument to listen to the blood pressure sounds (a stethoscope is not needed with an electronic sphygmomanometer). Normal systolic and diastolic blood pressures in a young adult are about 120/80, respectively. The difference between the two pressures is called the **pulse pressure**. Blood pressure varies with age, gender, altitude, disease, stress, fear, excitement, exercise, etc. A normal range of systolic pressure is usually considered to be 100–140 mmHg and of diastolic pressure below 90 mmHg.
*See* **arteriosclerosis; hypertension; retinopathy, hypertensive.**

**Spielmeyer–Stock disease** *See* **disease, Batten—Mayou.**

**spin-cast contact lens** *See* **lens, spin-cast contact.**

**spindle, Krukenberg's** *See* **Krukenberg's spindle.**

**spindle, muscle** *See* **muscles, extraocular.**

**spiral, Plateau's** A white disc on which there is a black band which winds round and round with each curve outside the previous one and with its origin at the centre of the disc. When the spiral is rotated and fixated at its centre, the circular bands appear to move in and out. When rotation is stopped a **motion after-effect** (or **motion after-image**) appears, i.e. the circular bands now seem to move in the opposite direction, and if another stationary object is fixated it will appear to swell or shrink in size in a direction opposite to that seen when fixating the rotating disc.
*See* **after-effect, waterfall.**

**spots, Elschnig's** Small, yellowish spots found in the fundus in advanced hypertensive retinopathy. They are choroidal infarcts caused by insufficient blood supply.
*See* **retinopathy, hypertensive.**

**spring catarrh** *See* **conjunctivitis, vernal.**

**squamous cell carcinoma** *See* **carcinoma, squamous cell.**

**squint** *See* **strabismus.**

**squinting eye** *See* **eye, deviating.**

**SRK formula** An approximate formula established by Sanders, Retzlaff and Kraft to determine the power of an intraocular lens implant *P*, in aqueous, to render the eye emmetropic (and ignoring the lens thickness)

$$P = A - 2.5X - 0.9K$$

where *A* is a numerical term specific to the implant and to the manufacturer. It is equal, on average, to 115 for anterior chamber implants and 116.8 for posterior chamber implants. *X* is the axial length of the eye (in mm) and *K* is the average keratometer reading (in dioptres). The formula gives satisfactory results for eyes of average length. *Example*: $A = 116.8$, $X = 23$ mm and $K = 43$ D, $P = 116.8 - 57.5 - 38.7 = 20.6$ D. There are several formulae used to predict the power of an intraocular lens implant but the SRK formula is the one most frequently used.
The power of the intraocular lens implant differs in air and is given by the following formula

$$P_{\text{air}} = \frac{n\text{I} - n\text{air}}{n\text{I} - n\text{aqueous}} \times P$$

where $n$I is the index of refraction of the implant and *P* its power in aqueous.
*Example*: assuming $n$I is equal to 1.523 and the power is 20.6 D, $P\text{air} = (1.523 - 1.0)/(1.523 - 1.333) \times 20.6 = 56.70$ D.
*See* **implant, intraocular lens.**

**stabilized retinal image** Image formed on the retina when neutralizing the fixation movements of the eye. The effect of these movements is thus eliminated and the image usually disappears after a few seconds. The methods used for stabilizing a retinal image are: (1) The target is placed at the end of a tube mounted on a tightly fitted contact lens. The whole device moves with every movement of the eyeball and the retinal image remains on the same retinal spot. (2) The subject is also fitted with a tight contact lens on the side of which is attached a small mirror. A test projected on the mirror is reflected onto a screen. The subject views the test through a compensating system of four mirrors and therefore as the eye moves the retinal image moves along with it and stimulates the same retinal spot. (3) Presentation of a target for a length of time smaller than the time necessary for the eye to perform a small eye movement. Presentations of less than 0.01 s usually fulfil this requirement.
*See* **movements, fixation; phenomenon, Troxler's.**

**stage** The platform, at right angles to the optical axis of a microscope, on which the object to be examined is mounted.
*See* **microscope.**

**staining, fluorescein** The artificial coloration of tissue by fluorescein. Under ultraviolet illumination, it stains dead or degenerated corneal epithelial cells due to abrasions, old age or following inadequate contact lens fit, a yellowish-green colour. It also stains the tears, thus facilitating the evaluation of tear drainage or the blood flow through the retina and choroid when injected intravenously. Corneal staining resulting from contact lens wear may present in various shapes, locations, depths or severity. A very common form is punctate staining as appears in punctate epithelial keratitis. There may be arcuate stains located in different parts of the cornea, some inferiorly (called **inferior epithelial arcuate lesions**) or superiorly (called **superior epithelial arcuate lesions**, *acronym*: **SEAL**, or **epithelial splitting**), which usually do not give rise to symptoms and appear mainly with soft or silicone hydrogel lenses. A very severe form of staining is called **epithelial plug**. It is typically round in shape and represents a loss of the full thickness of the epithelium. Corneal staining resulting from contact lens wear typically disappears after cessation of contact lens wear. *See* **angiography, fluorescein; fluorescein; test, dye dilution; test, fluorescein.**

**staining, 3 and 9 o'clock** Punctate corneal staining located just inside the limbus usually on the horizontal meridian on both sides, hence called 3 and 9 o'clock staining (or 4 and 8 o'clock). It may appear only on one side. It is observed with the biomicroscope after instillation of fluorescein. It is very useful to have the patient look nasally to inspect the temporal cornea and then temporally for the nasal portion. This staining is associated with corneal contact lens wear, although in some rare cases mild staining is observed without contact lens wear. It is due to inadequate spreading of the tear film over these areas of the cornea as a result of incomplete and/or infrequent blinking. Another cause for this type of staining is a small contact lens that is too thick. This condition is a mild form of exposure keratitis. *See* **fluorescein; keratitis, exposure; lamp, Burton; test, fluorescein.**

**standard axis notation** *See* **axis notation, standard.**

**standard illuminants** *See* **illuminants.**

**staphyloma** A bulging of the cornea or sclera due to injury, inflammation, glaucoma or pathological myopia, and containing adherent uveal tissue. If only the cornea or sclera stretches without uveal tissue, the condition is called **ectasia**. *See* **ectasia, corneal; myopia, pathological.**

**Stargardt's disease** *See* **disease, Stargardt's.**

**static eye reflex; perimetry; visual acuity** *See* under the nouns.

**stenopaeic disc; slit** *See* **disc, stenopaeic.**

**stenopaeic spectacles** *See* **spectacles, stenopaeic.**

**stereo-acuity** *See* **acuity, stereoscopic visual.**

**stereo-blindness** Complete lack of perception of stereopsis. It may result from blindness in one eye or strabismus, but also from some unknown cause in people with otherwise normal vision in both eyes. Stereo-blindness in some parts of the visual field also occurs in people who have had their corpus callosum or optic chiasma cut or destroyed. However, some depth perception may still exist thanks to monocular cues (e.g. aerial perspective, light and shadow, overlap, relative size).

**stereo-threshold** *See* **acuity, stereoscopic visual.**

**stereogram** Paired similar photographs or drawings which when viewed in a stereoscope give the sensation of stereopsis. Some stereograms are used only to explore fusion. *Syn.* stereoslide. *See* **stereoscope.**

**stereogram, random-dot (RDS)** A stereogram in which the eye sees an array of little characters or dots of a roughly uniform texture and containing no recognizable shape or contours. The only difference is that a certain region in one target has been laterally displaced with respect to the other, to produce some retinal disparity. When they are viewed in a stereoscope, that region is seen in stereoscopic relief. The shape in that region can be any pattern. The effect is remarkable as the shape usually appears to float out from the surround. *Syn.* Julesz random-dot stereogram.
The **random-dot E test** uses a polarized random test pattern and requires the use of Polaroid spectacles to detect whether a subject has stereopsis. The subject will see a raised letter E in the random-dot pattern of one of the test plates. At 50 cm, the retinal disparity induced by the E is 500 seconds of arc. The **TNO test** for stereoscopic vision also uses random-dot stereograms in which the half-images have been superimposed and printed in complementary colours, like anaglyphs. The test plates, when viewed with red and green spectacles, elicit stereopsis. There is a series of plates inducing retinal disparities ranging from 15 to 480 seconds of arc. *See* **acuity, stereoscopic visual; anaglyph; disparity, retinal; stereotest, Frisby; stereotest, Lang; test, two-dimensional; vectogram.**

**stereophenomenon, Pulfrich** If an object swings in the frontal plane and the observer places in front of one eye a light-absorbing filter (any value between 5% and 40%), that object will appear to move along an ellipse. This elliptical movement is virtually horizontal, with one part in front and the other behind the frontal plane. If the filter is placed in front of the other eye, the object will appear to swing along an ellipse but in the opposite direction. *Syn.* Pulfrich effect; Pulfrich phenomenon.

**stereophotography** Photography to produce pictures which give rise to the perception of stereopsis when viewed in a stereoscope. It has been used for determining corneal and optic disc topography.
*See* **photokeratoscopy.**

**stereopsis** Awareness of the relative distances of objects from the observer, by means of binocular vision only and based on retinal disparity. *Syn.* stereoscopic vision; third degree fusion.
*See* **acuity, stereoscopic visual; anaglyph; angle of stereopsis; chromostereopsis; disparity, retinal; perception, depth; room, leaf; stereo-blindness; stereogram, random-dot; stereoscopy; test, Howard–Dolman; test, three needle; test, two-dimensional.**

**stereopsis, chromatic** *See* **chromostereopsis.**

**stereoscope** An instrument which allows targets to be presented independently to the two eyes. The separation of the targets is produced either by tubes, a septum, or an arrangement of mirrors. Stereograms are the targets used with a stereoscope. Stereoscopes are used to test and train binocular fusion and stereopsis, evaluate suppression and view images in three dimensions.
*See* **stereogram.**

**stereoscope, Brewster's** Stereoscope consisting of two tubes separating the two fields of view and convex lenses. The distance between the tubes can be adjusted to suit the viewer's PD. *Syn.* lenticular stereoscope; Brewster–Holmes stereoscope (although this instrument uses a septum to separate the two visual fields, a sliding stereogram holder and decentred convex lenses, usually +5.25 D, to produce BO prisms) (Fig. S9).
*See* **Telebinocular.**

**stereoscope, Brewster–Holmes** *See* **stereoscope, Brewster's.**

**stereoscope, lenticular** *See* **stereoscope, Brewster's.**

**stereoscope, Pigeon–Cantonnet** A stereoscope consisting of three black cardboard leaves attached together as in a book, with a plane mirror placed on one face of the middle leaf and targets on the other two leaves. The subject places the central leaf as a septum and one eye sees one target directly while the other eye sees the other by reflection in the mirror. The angle of convergence may be controlled by the angle between the leaves. This instrument is often used in visual training as well as in orthoptics.
*See* **orthoptics; training, visual.**

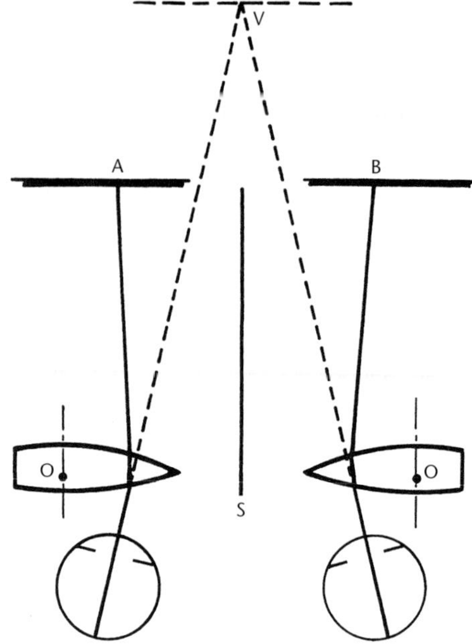


**Fig. S9** Principle of the Brewster–Holmes stereoscope (S, septum; A and B, stereograms; O, optical centre of the convex lenses decentred to produce BO prisms; V, fused images formed by the lenses)

**stereoscope, variable prism** A stereoscope incorporating two Risley prisms and a septum positioned so that each eye sees one half of a stereogram card which can be moved to and fro from the eyes in the median plane of the head. To maintain the normal relationship between accommodation and convergence at a given fixation distance, BO prisms are adjusted before each eye. This instrument is particularly well suited to measure and train fusional reserves of convergence and divergence.
*See* **prism, rotary.**

**stereoscope, Wheatstone** *See* **amblyoscope, Wheatstone.**

**stereoscopic vision** *See* **stereopsis.**

**stereoscopic visual acuity** *See* **acuity, stereoscopic visual.**

**stereoscopy** The science dealing with the perception of three-dimensional effects and of producing them.
*See* **stereopsis.**

**stereoscopy, colour** *See* **chromostereopsis.**

**stereotest, Frisby** A stereoacuity test consisting of a square transparent plate on which four similar patterns (resembling a random-dot stereogram) are printed on one side. In the central part of one of the four patterns is a circular area which is printed on the other side of the plate and can appear in depth. The plate (made of plastic or glass) comes in three thicknesses: 6, 3 and 1 mm. By using the three plates and presenting them at different distances the test can produce a retinal disparity of the circular area between 600 and 7 seconds of arc. In this test the patient's head must be kept still to avoid monocular cues. The plate can be turned upside down or rotated to alter the position of the pattern with relief. *Syn.* Frisby test. *See* **stereogram, random-test.**

**stereotest-housefly** *See* **vectogram.**

**stereotest, Lang** A random-dot stereogram upon which is imprinted a series of parallel strips of cylindrical lenses which act to separate the views seen by each eye. There are three stereoscopic shapes which the patient has to identify: a cat (inducing 1200 seconds of arc of retinal disparity), a star (600 seconds of arc) and a car (550 seconds of arc). The test is administered at 40 cm and exactly in the frontoparallel plane. As there is no need to use special spectacles it is a very useful test for young children. *Syn.* Lang test. *See* **stereogram, random-dot.**

**stereotest, Titmus** *See* **vectogram.**

**stereothreshold** *See* **acuity, stereoscopic visual.**

**sterile infiltrates** A condition often noted in the cornea of contact lens wearers. These lesions differ from infectious infiltrates in so much that the overlying epithelium is usually intact, there is typically little or no pain, and the lesions tend to be small (less than 1.5 mm). The lesions consist of subepithelial infiltrates of leukocytes. It is postulated that these lesions are an immune response to a specific antigen (likely contact lens or solution-related), and not related to a bacterial infection. Treatment is often supportive with cessation of contact lens wear. *See* **corneal infiltrates.**

**sterilization** The process of killing microorganisms in or on materials. It is achieved by heat (dry or moist), ultraviolet light, supersonic waves, etc. or by antiseptic solutions. *See* **antiseptic; disinfection by boiling.**

**steroid** One of a group of hormonal substances produced mainly by the adrenal cortex. They fall into three main groups: glucocorticoids (or glucocorticosteroids), mineralocorticoids and sex hormones. The glucocorticoids have antiinflammatory properties reducing vasodilatation, stabilizing mast cells thus decreasing the release of histamine and maintaining the normal permeability of blood thus preventing oedema. They also inhibit the production of prostaglandins, which mediate some of the effects of inflammation. They are widely used in the treatment of a variety of inflammatory diseases of various organs including the eye (e.g. allergic and vernal conjunctivitis, corneal diseases, iritis, uveitis and sympathetic ophthalmia). The natural glucocorticoids, such as cortisone and hydrocortisone, are effective only at high doses. Synthetic and more potent steroids are used in ophthalmic treatment (when used as ophthalmic preparations they are called **corticosteroids**). They include, betamethasone, dexamethasone, fluorometholone, prednisolone and triamcinolone. *See* **antiinflammatory drug.**

**Stevens–Johnson syndrome** *See* **syndrome, Stevens–Johnson.**

**Stevens' law** *See* **law, Fechner's.**

**stigmatic lens** *See* **lens, anastigmatic.**

**stigmatism** The condition of an optical system in which light from a point source forms an image which is also a point, as distinguished from astigmatism. *See* **astigmatism.**

**stigmatoscope** An instrument for observing or measuring the refractive state of the eye based on the position of best focus of a very small point source. *See* **stigmatoscopy.**

**stigmatoscopy** A method of determining the refractive state of the eye based on the criterion of sharpness of an image. The observer determines the position at which a point source appears in the best focus, while the eye is unaccommodated: this indicates the far point of the eye. If the eye is astigmatic the point source will appear as a line or streak when at the far point of each principal meridian. The distance between the two foci corresponds to the cylinder correction and the slant of the streaks from the horizontal or vertical indicates the axis of the astigmatism. *See* **refractive error; stigmatoscope.**

**Stiles–Crawford effect** *See* **effect, Stiles–Crawford.**

**Stilling canal** *See* **canal, hyaloid.**

**Still's disease** *See* **disease, Still's.**

**Stilling–Turk–Duane syndrome** *See* **syndrome, Duane's.**

**stimuli, heterochromatic** *See* **heterochromatic stimuli.**

**stimulus** Any agent or environmental change which provokes a response. *Plural*: stimuli. *See* **potential, action.**

**stimulus, adequate** A stimulus of sufficient intensity and of appropriate nature to provoke a response in a given receptor. Visible light is the adequate stimulus for the eye, but pressure on the eye which may nevertheless produce a response (called a phosphene) is an **inadequate stimulus.** *See* **phosphene.**

**stimulus, inadequate** *See* **stimulus, adequate.**

**stimulus, liminal** A stimulus of an intensity such that it just provokes a response that is at threshold. *Syn.* threshold stimulus.

**stimulus, threshold** *See* **stimulus, liminal.**

**Stocker's line** *See* **line, Stocker's.**

**Stokes lens** *See* **lens, Stokes.**

**stop** *See* **diaphragm.**

**strabismometer** An instrument for measuring the angle of strabismus.

**strabismus** The condition in which the lines of sight of the two eyes are not directed towards the same fixation point when the subject is actively fixating an object. Thus the image of the fixation point is not formed on the fovea of the deviated eye and there may be diplopia, although in most cases the diplopic image is suppressed and vision is essentially monocular. The prevalence of concomitant strabismus in the population is about 5% and is far more common than paretic strabismus. Management depends on the type of strabismus. However, in all cases the refractive errors must be accurately corrected. If the deviation still prevails, orthoptics and, sometimes, pharmacological (e.g. miotics in accommodative esotropia) treatment is attempted but in many cases surgery is necessary (except where accommodation is faulty or when the deviation is small), usually followed by some orthoptics treatment aimed at developing fusion and stereopsis. *Syn.* heterotropia; squint (this term is commonly used by the general public); tropia.
*See* **angle of anomaly; angle of strabismus; botulinum toxin; chemodenervation; diplopia; eye, deviating; eye, fixating; heterotropia, cyclic; hypertropia, alternating; method, Bruckner's; method, Hirschberg's; method, Javal's; method, Krimsky's; microtropia; movement, phi; myectomy; myotomy; pointing, past-; recession; resection; retinal correspondence, abnormal; suppression; syndrome, Brown's superior oblique tendon sheath; syndrome, Duane's; syndrome, Marfan's; test, cover; test, three-step; theories of strabismus.**

**strabismus, acquired** An abnormal alignment of the visual axes that occurs after the age of six months.

**strabismus, alternating** Strabismus in which either eye may deviate.
*See* **strabismus, unilateral.**

**strabismus, angle of** *See* **angle of deviation.**

**strabismus, apparent** Condition simulating the appearance of strabismus. It may be due to epicanthus, to an abnormally large angle lambda, or to the breadth of the nose, etc. It can be distinguished from a real strabismus by noting that the corneal light reflexes are centrally located in relation to the pupils, or by means of the cover test. *Syn.* pseudostrabismus.
*See* **angle lambda; epicanthus.**

**strabismus, comitant** *See* **strabismus, concomitant.**

**strabismus, concomitant** Strabismus in which the angle of deviation remains the same whichever eye is fixating and in whichever direction the eyes are looking. *Syn.* comitant strabismus.
*See* **concomitance; strabismus, incomitant.**

**strabismus, congenital** *See* **strabismus, infantile.**

**strabismus, consecutive** A deviation of the eye in the opposite direction to what it was previously. This condition may follow surgery although it may occur spontaneously. There are two types: **consecutive exotropia** in a patient who previously had esotropia or esophoria and **consecutive esotropia** in a patient who previously had exotropia or exophoria. *Syn.* post-operative over-correction.

**strabismus, convergent** Strabismus in which the deviating eye turns inward. This is the most common type of strabismus in children. (Fig. S10) *Syn.* crossed eyes (colloquial); esotropia (SOT, ET, esoT).
*See* **pattern, A; pattern, V; syndrome, Swann's; test, prism adaptation.**

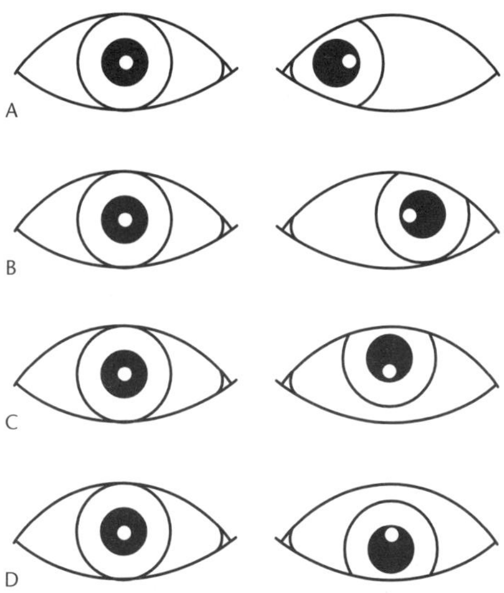


**Fig. S10** A, left convergent strabismus; B, left divergent strabismus; C, left hypertropia; D, left hypotropia

**strabismus, cyclic** *See* **heterotropia, cyclic.**

**strabismus, deorsumvergens** *See* **hypertropia.**

**strabismus, divergent** Strabismus in which the deviating eye turns outward (Fig. S10). *Syn.* exotropia (XOT; XT; exoT).
*See* **pattern, A; pattern, V.**

**strabismus fixus** A congenital condition in which one eye or both eyes are held in a fixed position due to a fibrous and inelastic extraocular muscle (usually the medial or lateral rectus muscle).

**strabismus, incomitant** Strabismus in which the angle of deviation varies with the direction of gaze and with the eye used for fixation. It may be congenital or acquired. The congenital type is due to some developmental anomaly of one or more of the extraocular muscles or of the neural component that serves them. The acquired type may be due to head injury or disease of the oculomotor system. The main symptom of incomitant strabismus is diplopia and it suddenly appears in the acquired type. Abnormal head posture and past-pointing may be present. The affected muscle(s) may be detected by the motility test. Treatment is aimed first at the primary cause but, in general, this type of strabismus does not respond well to orthoptic procedures. In large deviation, surgery is usually the only remedy. *Syn.* nonconcomitant strabismus.
*See* **head posture, abnormal; incomitance; pointing past-; strabismus, paralytic; test, motility.**

**strabismus, infantile** Strabismus which becomes manifest within the first year of life. It is almost always esotropic in nature: exotropia, which is very rare, is usually associated with some neurological condition. Infantile strabismus is characterized by a large angle of squint, hyperopia, alternate fixation which may become unilateral if amblyopia develops, and nystagmus. Management is essentially surgical after correction of the refractive error. A complication following surgery may be dissociated vertical deviation. *Syn.* congenital strabismus; infantile esotropia syndrome.

**strabismus, intermittent** Strabismus which is not present at all times.

**strabismus, monocular** *See* **strabismus, unilateral.**

**strabismus, nonconcomitant** *See* **strabismus, incomitant.**

**strabismus, paralytic** Strabismus due to a paralysis of the extraocular muscles. It usually gives rise to incomitance. The paralysis is usually due to a disorder of the third, fourth or sixth cranial nerve. Diplopia is noticed if the paralysis is recent and it is usually accompanied by an abnormal head posture. In most cases there is not a complete loss of action of a muscle but a partial loss and the condition is referred to as **paretic strabismus**, whether it is congenital or acquired. Orthoptic treatment is very limited in these cases and is not normally appropriate if the deviation was caused by injury or a recent disease. Cosmetic surgery is often necessary.
*See* **head posture, abnormal; incomitance; paralysis of the fourth nerve; paralysis of the sixth nerve; paralysis of the third nerve; test, motility.**

**strabismus, periodic** Strabismus in which the deviation occurs only at certain distances or in certain directions of fixation. *Syn.* relative strabismus.

**strabismus, relative** *See* **strabismus, periodic.**

**strabismus, small angle** *See* **microtropia.**

**strabismus, sursumvergens** *See* **hypertropia.**

**strabismus, unilateral** Strabismus in which the deviating eye is always the same, as distinguished from alternating strabismus. *Syn.* monocular strabismus.
*See* **strabismus, alternating.**

**strain 1.** Internal tension in a lens due to poor annealing, or to glass of a non-uniform coefficient of expansion, or from external pressure on the edge of a glass spectacle lens. It results in birefringence which is observed with a polariscope. **2.** To overwork a faculty (e.g. eyestrain caused by sustained vision of near point objects); or a part of the body (e.g. muscles); or a system (e.g. the effect on corneal metabolism of a closed eye wearing a PMMA lens. This is often referred to as **hypoxic stress**). *Note*: the strain can be either the cause or the effect. *Syn.* stress.
*See* **asthenopia; hypoxia; polariscope.**

**stratum opticum** *See* **retina.**

**stray light** *See* **light, stray.**

**streak retinoscope** *See* **retinoscope, streak.**

**stress** *See* **polariscope.**

**stress, hypoxic** *See* **strain.**

**stress, near point** *See* **asthenopia.**

**stria 1.** Slight dark ridges in the pars plana of the ciliary body, which run parallel with each other from the teeth of the ora serrata to the valleys between the ciliary processes. *Syn.* striae ciliares. **2.** A line in the posterior corneal stroma associated with corneal oedema and sometimes keratoconus. **3.** A vein or streak seen in optical glass which has been contaminated during

manufacture or in which the ingredients have been imperfectly mixed.
*See* **ciliary body; ciliary processes; glass; oedema; ora serrata.**

**striae ciliares** *See* **stria.**

**striae retinae** Concentric lines on the surface of the retina which appear after spontaneous or surgical retinal reattachment.
*See* **retinal detachment.**

**striae, Vogt's** Thin vertical streaks located in the posterior corneal stroma. These folds disappear with external pressure on the globe. They are often present in patients with keratoconus. *Syn.* Vogt's line.
*See* **keratoconus.**

**striate area; cortex** *See* **area, visual.**

**stroboscope** An instrument which produces brief flashes of illumination at a variable frequency. If a moving object is rotating at $x$ rotations per second when the frequency is a full multiple of $x$, one sees the object motionless. If the frequency is decreased the object appears to rotate slowly, but if the frequency is increased the object appears to rotate slowly in the opposite direction to its real rotation. This apparent change of motion or immobilization of an object, when the object is illuminated by a periodically varying light of appropriate frequency, is called a **stroboscopic effect.**

**stroke** *See* **blindness, cortical; hemianopsia, homonymous; ophthalmodynamometer.**

**stroma, corneal** *See* **corneal stroma.**

**Sturge–Weber syndrome** *See* **syndrome, Sturge–Weber.**

**Sturm, conoid of** The bundle of rays formed by an astigmatic optical system consisting of a primary focal line (called **Sturm's line**), a circle of least confusion and a secondary focal line (or Sturm's line) perpendicular to the first.
*See* **astigmatism; circle of least confusion.**

**Sturm, interval of** The linear distance between the two focal lines of an astigmatic optical system. *Syn.* astigmatic interval; focal interval.
*See* **astigmatism; astigmatism, oblique; line, focal.**

**Sturm's line** *See* **line, focal; Sturm, conoid of.**

**stye** *See* **hordeolum.**

**subconjunctival haemorrhage** *See* **haemorrhage, subconjunctival.**

**subhyaloid haemorrhage** *See* **haemorrhage, preretinal.**

**subjective refraction** *See* **refraction, subjective.**

**subliminal perception** *See* **perception, subliminal.**

**subluxation of the lens** *See* **luxation.**

**subnormal vision** *See* **vision, low.**

**substantia propria** *See* **corneal stroma.**

**subtarsal sulcus** *See* **sulcus, subtarsal.**

**successive contrast** *See* **contrast.**

**sulcus, calcarine** *See* **fissure, calcarine.**

**sulcus, ciliary** A groove situated between the posterior root of the iris and the ciliary body. It may be used, sometimes, as a site of fixation of an intraocular lens implant.

**sulcus, inferior palpebral** A furrow in the skin of the lower eyelid. It separates the tarsal from the orbital portion of the lid. It is often not very distinct although it becomes more so with age.

**sulcus, internal scleral** A slight, circular groove situated at the margin between the posterior surface of the cornea and the sclera. It contains the trabecular meshwork and the canal of Schlemm. The posterior lip of the sulcus forms a projecting ridge called the scleral spur.
*See* **scleral spur.**

**sulcus, optic** *See* **pit, optic.**

**sulcus, subtarsal** A groove on the inner surface of the eyelid, near the eyelid margin and parallel to it, which forms the border separating the marginal from the tarsal conjunctiva. Foreign bodies are commonly lodged in this groove.
*See* **eversion, lid; irrigation.**

**sulcus, superior palpebral** A furrow in the skin of the upper eyelid. It separates the tarsal portion which is closest to the lid margin from the orbital portion which extends from the tarsus to the eyebrow. This furrow becomes more prominent with age.
*See* **aperture, palpebral.**

**sulfacetamide sodium** An anti-infective, bacteriostatic drug of the sulfonamide family, used topically against infections and injuries, as well as minor abrasions, of the conjunctiva and cornea. It should not be used immediately following a local anaesthetic. However, **antibiotics** (e.g. bacitracin, chloramphenicol, erythromycin, gentamicin, neomycin, norfloxacin, polymyxin B, tetracycline, tobramycin) which inhibit or destroy a wide range of microorganisms are used more commonly than local sulfonamides.
*See* **antibiotic; antifungal agent; antiinflammatory drug; bacteriostatic; sulfonamide.**

**sulfonamide** Denotes a group of organic derivatives containing $SO_2NH_2$. *Example*: sulfacetamide sodium.

S

**summation** Increased effect produced by a series of stimuli applied either simultaneously or successively (provided the intervals are greater than the latent period). **Binocular summation** usually occurs when the two eyes are stimulated; thus binocular brightness is greater than monocular, except in the unusual Fechner's paradox. Two or more stimuli falling within the excitatory region of a receptive field will increase the excitatory response and similarly two or more stimuli falling within the inhibitory region of a receptive field will increase the inhibition: this is called **spatial summation**. The summation may also occur if successive stimulations are received by the same retinal region: this is called **temporal summation**.
*See* **cell, complex; cell, simple; Fechner's paradox; field, receptive; inhibition, lateral.**

**sun gazing** *See* **retinopathy, solar.**

**sunflower cataract** *See* **chalcosis lentis.**

**sunglasses** Spectacles which have tinted lenses. They are used to protect the eyes from bright sunlight, for special cases (e.g. fear of light) or for cosmetic reasons.
*See* **cataract; lens, tinted; photophobia; pterygium; ultraviolet.**

**sunlight** *See* **light, solar.**

**supercilium** *See* **eyebrow.**

**superimposition** The ability to see two similar images superimposed but not mentally fused. *Examples*: seeing a bird in a cage with both eyes in a synoptophore when one eye is presented with a bird and the other with a cage; seeing the letter E in a synoptophore when one eye is presented with the letter F and the other with the letter L.
*See* **vision, Worth's classification of binocular.**

**superior colliculus; limbic keratoconjunctivitis; oblique muscle; oblique sheath syndrome; ophthalmic vein; orbital fissure; quadrantanopsia; rectus muscle** *See* under the nouns.

**suppression** The process by which the brain inhibits the retinal image (or part of it) of one eye, when both eyes are simultaneously stimulated. This occurs to avoid diplopia as in strabismus, in uncorrected anisometropia, in retinal rivalry, etc. *Syn.* suspenopsia (this term actually refers to voluntary suppression as occurs, for example, when using a monocular microscope with one eye); suspension (most often used when referring to partial suppression).
*See* **cheiroscope; diplopia, physiological; grid, Javal's; Mallett fixation disparity unit; Remy separator; retinal rivalry; test, four prism dioptre base out; test, FRIEND; test, Turville infinity balance; test, Worth's four dot; vectogram.**

**supra** *See* **spectacles, supra.**

**suprachoroid** *See* **sclera.**

**suprachoroidal space** A potential space located between the lamina fusca (or suprachoroid) layer of the sclera and the choroid. In this space are thin, pigmented strands of collagen fibres and it is traversed by the long and short posterior ciliary arteries and nerves.

**supraduction** *See* **elevation of the eye.**

**supranuclear gaze palsy** *See* **palsy, supranuclear gaze.**

**supraorbital artery** *See* **artery, supraorbital.**

**supraorbital nerve** *See* **nerve, ophthalmic.**

**supraorbital notch** An indentation in the orbital margin of the frontal bone, one-third of the way from the nose. The supraorbital nerve and vessels pass through that indentation. Occasionally it is converted into a foramen by ossification.

**supravergence** Movement of one eye upward relative to the other. *Syn.* sursumvergence.
*See* **infravergence; vergence.**

**supraversion** *See* **version.**

**surface, diffusing; matt** *See* **matt surface.**

**surface, optical** *See* **optical surface.**

**surface power** *See* **power, surface.**

**surface, toroidal** *See* **lens, toric.**

**surfacing** The combined processes of roughing, smoothing and polishing of a lens surface to a given curvature.
*See* **glass, ground; lens blank; lens, finished; lens, frosted; moulding; polishing.**

**surfactant** An agent which reduces the surface tension of oil or solid–water interfaces and therefore has cleaning properties. *Note*: the term is an acronym made from the following italic letters; *surf*ace *act*ive *a*ge*nt*.
*See* **deposits, contact lens; disinfection by boiling; enzyme; wetting solution.**

**surrounding field** *See* **field, surrounding.**

**sursumduction** *See* **elevation.**

**sursumvergence** *See* **supravergence.**

**sursumversion** *See* **version.**

**suspenopsia** *See* **suppression.**

**suspension** *See* **suppression.**

**suspensory apparatus of the lens; ligament** *See* **Zinn, zonule of.**

**suture, lens** One of the many radiating lines in the crystalline lens formed by the meeting of lens fibres. Some of these systems of lens fibres form in the fetus or infant a Y, the arms of which are separated by angles of 120°. The anterior Y is upright and the posterior one is inverted. In the adult eye the systems of lens fibres make up more complicated figures, but the Ys present at birth usually persist throughout life (Fig. S11). *See* **fibres, lens; lens, crystalline.**

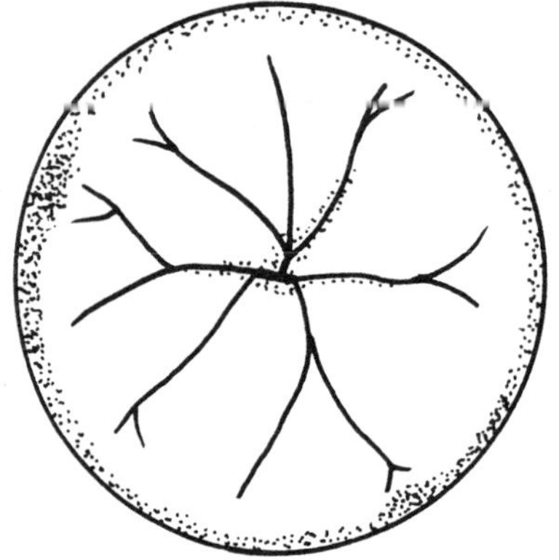

**Fig. S11** Diagram of the anterior aspect of an adult lens sutures showing a 9-point star

**Swann's syndrome** *See* **syndrome, Swann's.**

**swinging flashlight test** *See* **pupil, Marcus Gunn.**

**symblepharon** Adhesion, partial or complete, of the palpebral conjunctiva of the eyelid to the bulbar conjunctiva of the eyeball. It results from disease (e.g. erythema multiforme) or trauma, but is rarely congenital.
*See* **erythema multiforme; syndrome, Stevens–Johnson.**

**sympathetic eye** *See* **eye, sympathetic.**

**sympathetic ophthalmia** *See* **ophthalmia, sympathetic.**

**sympatholytic drugs** Drugs that inhibit nerve impulses in the sympathetic nervous system. They may block the effect of alpha-adrenergic receptors (e.g. thymoxamine which is used to reverse pupillary blockage caused by a mydriatic) or the effect of beta-adrenergic receptors (e.g. betaxolol which block beta 1 receptors; timolol, levobunolol, metipranolol and carteolol which block beta 1 and beta 2 receptors). Beta-blockers are used in the treatment of glaucoma. *Syn.* adrenergic blocking agents.
*See* **alpha-adrenergic antagonist; beta-blocker.**

**sympathomimetic drugs** Drugs that produce an effect similar to that obtained by stimulation of the sympathetic nervous system. Some of these predominantly act on the adrenergic alpha-receptors (e.g. noradrenaline (norepinephrine)), while others act on the adrenergic beta-receptors (e.g. isoproterenol). Others have little direct effect on the adrenergic receptors but enhance the release of natural catecholamine from the sympathetic nerve terminals (e.g. amphetamine, phenylpropanolamine). Sympathomimetic drugs are used (1) in the treatment of open-angle glaucoma by decreasing aqueous humour secretion and increase the outflow through the trabecular meshwork thus reducing the intraocular pressure (e.g. adrenaline (epinephrine), dipivefrin, brimonidine), (2) dilate the pupil without affecting accommodation (e.g. phenylephrine) and (3) constrict conjunctival blood vessels (e.g. naphazoline, tetrahydrozoline). *Syn.* adrenergic stimulating agent.
*See* **alpha-adrenergic agonist; mydriatic.**

**symptom** *See* **sign.**

**synapse** The place where a nerve impulse is transmitted from one neuron to another. That transmission is usually mediated by secretion of neurotransmitters that are released by the axon in the synaptic space (about 20–40 nm wide) and react with the cell membrane of the next dendrites: this leads to a change in electrical potential across the membrane. The main neurotransmitters are **acetylcholine** and **noradrenaline** (norepinephrine), and the action may be either excitation or inhibition. It is estimated that a cortical neuron, for example, makes some 5000–10 000 synapses with surrounding neurons.
*See* **acetylcholine; neuron; neurotransmitter; potential, action.**

**synchisis scintillans** Degenerative condition occurring in older eyes, in myopia, or after injuries and inflammation of the eye (e.g. posterior uveitis) and characterized by the presence of bright, shiny particles floating in a fluid vitreous body. The particles are believed to be composed of cholesterol. Vision may be impaired if the particles float across the visual axis but is restored when the eye is immobile, as they settle at the bottom of the vitreous.
*See* **asteroid hyalosis; floaters; humour, vitreous; uveitis.**

**syndrome** The aggregate of signs and symptoms associated with a disease, lesion, anomaly, etc.

**syndrome A** *See* **pattern, A.**

**syndrome, acquired immunodeficiency (AIDS)** A viral disease characterized by a relentless transition from asymptomatic lymphadenopathy to a wasting condition with infections

(e.g. pneumonia, toxoplasmosis) and malignancies (e.g. Kaposi's sarcoma). It has a long incubation period and a poor prognosis. It is caused by the human immunodeficiency virus (HIV) which breaks down the immune response and is transmitted by exchange of body fluids (e.g. blood, semen) or transfused blood products. In the eye the disease may be accompanied by cotton-wool spots in the retina (the most frequent of the ocular complications), retinal haemorrhages, cytomegalovirus retinitis which is the major cause of visual loss, toxoplasmosis chorioretinitis, herpes zoster ophthalmicus, papilloedema, central retinal vein occlusion (the rarest of ocular complications); limitations of eye movements and pupil abnormalities, reddish-purple nodular tumours in the eyelids and conjunctiva as part of Kaposi's sarcoma.
*See* **retinitis, cytomegalovirus.**

**syndrome, Adie's** A dilated pupil in which all reactions to light are barely existent, together with the absence of tendon reflexes. It typically affects adult women. *Syn.* Holmes–Adie syndrome.
*See* **aniscoria; pupil, Adie's; reflex, pupil light.**

**syndrome, Aicardi's** An inherited disorder that is seen in females consisting of retinal, optic nerve as well as central nervous system abnormalities. Retinal findings consist of multiple, round, chorioretinal depigmented lesions. Additional abnormalities include optic nerve head colobomas, microphthalmos, agenesis of the corpus callosum, seizures and retardation.

**syndrome, Alagille** An autosomal dominant pigmentary retinopathy that includes ophthalmic as well as systemic abnormalities. Systemic abnormalities include heart disease and flattened facial features. Ocular findings include myopia, posterior embryotoxon and Axenfeld's anomaly.
*See* **ring of Schwalbe, anterior limiting; syndrome, Axenfeld's.**

**syndrome, Albright's** A disorder characterized by a host of findings including cutaneous pigmentation, precocious puberty in females, and fibrous dysplasia of the orbital bone/s which may lead to proptosis and optic atrophy.

**syndrome, anterior chamber cleavage** *See* **Peter's anomaly.**

**syndrome, Anton's** Bilateral blindness characterized by a lack of awareness of being blind and near normal pupil reflexes. It is due to a destruction of the cortical visual area.
*See* **blindness, cortical.**

**syndrome, Axenfeld's** A rare, inherited disease characterized by the adhesion of strands of peripheral iris tissue to a prominent Schwalbe's line. It is occasionally associated with glaucoma. *Syn.* Axenfeld's anomaly.
*See* **Peter's anomaly; ring of Schwalbe, anterior limiting; syndrome, Rieger's.**

**syndrome, Balint's** An entity characterized by an inability to fixate voluntarily in different parts of the visual field, to see two objects simultaneously (simultanagnosia) and to mislocate when reaching for, or pointing to, an object (ocular apraxia). Patient has normal visual acuity. This is usually due to a bilateral lesion of an area within the parieto-occipital region of the brain. *Syn.* Balint–Holmes syndrome.
*See* **apraxia, ocular motor; simultanagnosia.**

**syndrome, Bardet–Biedl** *See* **syndrome, Laurence–Moon–Bardet–Biedl.**

**syndrome, Bassen–Kornzweig** An autosomal recessive hereditary disorder characterized by a congenital inability to absorb fats. By the end of the first decade of life the patient develops pigmentary retinopathy which resembles retinitis pigmentosa, although the pigment clumps are scattered throughout the fundus and not confined to the periphery, and night blindness. Treatment with large doses of vitamin A may retard the progression of the condition. *Syn.* abetalipoproteinaemia; acanthocytosis.

**syndrome, Behçet's** *See* **disease, Behçet's.**

**syndrome, Benedikt's** A syndrome caused by a lesion (usually vascular) within the midbrain. It is characterized by an ipsilateral third nerve paralysis and ataxia and tremor of the limbs on the other side of the body.
*See* **paralysis of the third nerve; syndrome, Weber's.**

**syndrome, Bernard–Horner** *See* **syndrome, Horner's.**

**syndrome, blepharophimosis** A rare, autosomal dominant inherited disorder characterized by ptosis, poor levator function, shorter than normal width of the palpebral aperture, telecanthus, epicanthus, partial ectropion of the lower lid, flattening of the supraorbital ridges and amblyopia and strabismus in about half of the cases. Treatment usually begins with surgical correction of the epicanthus and telecanthus, before ptosis surgery.
*See* **blepharophimosis; ectropion, congenital; epicanthus.**

**syndrome, blind spot** *See* **syndrome, Swann's.**

**syndrome, Brown's superior oblique tendon sheath** This syndrome is characterized by limitation of elevation of the eye in adduction, but normal or near normal elevation when the eye is

in abduction. There is limitation of movement of the affected eye in the **forced duction test** when attempting to elevate the eye from the adducted position. The eyes are usually straight in the primary position. The condition seems to be due to a short tendon sheath of the superior oblique muscle and an apparent anomaly of the inferior oblique muscle. *Syn.* Brown's syndrome; sheath syndrome; superior oblique sheath syndrome.
*See* **test, forced duction.**

**syndrome, cat's eye** A condition caused by an extra fragment of a copy of chromosome 22. It is characterized by partial iris coloboma (usually a vertical portion) which makes the patient's eye look like a cat's eye. There are also optic disc coloboma, optic nerve degeneration and microphthalmos. The systemic manifestations include mental and growth retardation and low-set or malformed ears.

**syndrome, Chandler's** A syndrome characterized by a severe corneal endothelial degeneration resulting in corneal oedema and blurred vision. There is also mild iris atrophy and secondary glaucoma. It tends to affect mainly women between 20 and 40 years of age. The therapy is aimed at treating the glaucoma. *Syn.* iridocorneal syndrome.
*See* **syndrome, ICE.**

**syndrome, Cogan's** *See* **keratitis, interstitial.**

**syndrome, Cogan–Reese** *See* **syndrome, ICE.**

**syndrome, computer vision (CVS)** A condition resulting from extensive viewing of computer screens or video display terminals (VDT) or visual display units (VDU). The patient may complain of eyestrain, dry red eyes, headaches, transient blurred vision or diplopia, as well as neckache or backache. The ocular symptoms are caused by continuous accommodative demands produced by the pixels or tiny dots of the computer screen that are difficult to keep in focus, unlike print on a page. Other causes are frequent saccadic eye movements, convergence demands and position of the screen. Management includes exact correction for the distance at which the VDT appears, viewing it about 10°–20° below the straight-ahead position and special dispensing.

**syndrome, corneal exhaustion** An intolerance to continue wearing contact lenses after many years of wear, probably due to endothelial dysfunction as a result of chronic hypoxia and acidosis. It occurs primarily with PMMA lenses but also with other lenses with low oxygen transmissibility. Some of the signs associated with this syndrome are: endothelial polymegethism, corneal oedema, loss of corneal sensitivity, variations in corneal curvature and refractive error, blurred vision, lacrimation, hyperaemia and discomfort. Management usually consists in discontinuing contact lens wear. Refitting with lenses with high oxygen transmissibility is often successful. *Syn.* corneal fatigue syndrome; corneal exhaustion phenomenon.
*See* **hypoxia; syndrome, overwear.**

**syndrome, corneal fatigue** *See* **syndrome, corneal exhaustion.**

**syndrome, Cornelia de Lange** A congenital anomaly characterized by growth and mental retardation, limb malformation, syndactyly, bushy eyebrows meeting in the midline, hairline down on the forehead, depressed bridge of the nose and low-set ears. Ocular manifestations may include ptosis, nystagmus, microcornea and most commonly high myopia. The pathogenesis of the condition is unknown.

**syndrome, dorsal midbrain** *See* **syndrome, Parinaud's.**

**syndrome, Down's** Mental (IQ between 20 and 50) and physical handicap with small stature, obesity, epicanthus, etc. associated with widespread systemic and ocular defects, such as cataract, keratoconus and nystagmus. Cases of high myopia are noted but most subjects tend to have hypermetropia and there is a high prevalence of strabismus. Visual acuity is also reduced, even after correction of the ametropia. *Syn.* trisomy 21 syndrome.

**syndrome, Duane's** A complex disorder found in about 1% of patients with strabismus, it occurs in three different types. All three types are characterized by retraction of the globe into the orbit and by narrowing of the palpebral fissure on attempted adduction. The left eye is affected more often than the right eye and the condition is bilateral in about 20% of patients. In addition, each type presents an abnormal pattern of ocular motility. Type I, the most common affecting over three-quarters of all cases, presents limited or absent abduction and slight esotropia in the primary position, and typically a head turn towards the involved side. Type II presents limited adduction, slight exotropia and relatively normal or slightly limited abduction, and usually a head turn away from the involved side. Type III, the rarest (about 1% of all cases), presents limited abduction and adduction. The aetiology is believed to be a congenital absence of the sixth cranial nerve and its nucleus (partial absence in type II) and fibres from the third cranial nerve innervate the lateral rectus so that innervation results in contraction of both the lateral and medial recti muscles (co-contraction) and the degree of this paradoxical innervation determines the severity of the disorder.

S

Management is frequently surgical especially in types II and III, but prismatic corrections have been found to be beneficial in selected cases. *Syn.* Duane retraction syndrome (DRS); Duane's phenomenon; retraction syndrome; Stilling–Turk–Duane syndrome; Turk's disease.

**syndrome, Ehlers–Danlos** Syndrome characterized by hyperelasticity of the skin, hyperextensibility of the joints and fragile blood vessels. It is inherited as an autosomal dominant disorder of connective tissue with an increase in dermal elastic tissue and a decrease in collagen. The ocular signs include blue sclera, eye elongation and myopia, angioid streaks, ectopia lentis, keratoconus and retinal detachment.

**syndrome, exfoliation** *See* **pseudoexfoliation.**

**syndrome, fallen eye** A condition occurring after a prolonged paresis of the superior oblique muscle of one eye, in which the other eye may not elevate completely, if the paretic eye was always the fixating eye.

**syndrome, floppy eyelid** A condition often occurring in very obese middle-aged males, characterized by a very loose upper eyelid allowing it to be very easily everted and sometimes injured during sleep resulting in papillary conjunctivitis. If severe, treatment is by lid shortening.

**syndrome, Foster Kennedy** A syndrome in which there is optic atrophy in one eye and papilloedema in the other. This is due to direct pressure by a tumour on one optic nerve giving rise to optic atrophy, and as a result of raised intracranial pressure papilloedema develops in the other eye. It is often caused by a tumour at the base of the frontal lobe or an olfactory meningioma. In some cases the patient also reports a loss of smell. *Syn.* Kennedy syndrome. *See* **atrophy, optic; papilloedema.**

**syndrome, Foville's** A disorder of the inferior cerebellar artery which causes a pontine lesion involving the abducens and the facial (or seventh) nucleus or its fasciculus as it leaves the brainstem at the pontine paramedian reticular formation. It is characterized by a paralysis of the conjugate eye movements towards the affected side (horizontal gaze palsy), ipsilateral facial paralysis, hemianaesthesia of the face, contralateral paralysis of the limbs, Horner's syndrome and deafness.

**syndrome, fragile X** An inherited syndrome caused by a constriction and nearly broken long arm of an X chromosome at q27.3. Although males are mainly affected, females are also affected to a lesser extent and carry the genetic defect. Systemic manifestations are mental retardation (the second most common cause after Down's syndrome), enlarged testes, high forehead and large jaws and long ears. The ocular manifestations are strabismus, large refractive errors and poor eye contact.

**syndrome, Fuchs'** Changes in the colour of the iris of one eye associated with a mild inflammation of the iris as well as the ciliary body, often complicated with cataract and sometimes glaucoma. *See* **heterochromia.**

**syndrome, Gerstmann** A disorder believed to result from a lesion at the occipitoparietal border, the angular gyrus and the interparietal sulcus. It is characterized by finger agnosia, agraphia, acalculia and right-left disorientation. Ocular findings are homonymous hemianopsia and visual agnosia for colours.

**syndrome, Gradenigo's** An inflammation of the middle ear (**otitis media**) and mastoid bone (**mastoiditis**) extending to the apex of the petrous temporal bone. It results in ipsilateral deafness, pain in or near the eye on the side of the face (fifth nerve involvement), paralysis of the external rectus muscle (sixth nerve involvement), facial paralysis, reduced corneal sensitivity (fifth nerve involvement) and some increase in body temperature. The condition responds well to antibiotics.

**syndrome, Gregg** *See* **syndrome, rubella.**

**syndrome, Holmes–Adie** *See* **syndrome, Adie's.**

**syndrome, Horner's** Interruption of the sympathetic nerve supply to the dilatator pupillae muscle resulting in miosis, slight ptosis (1 or 2 mm), slight elevation of the lower lid, enophthalmos, heterochromia (mainly in the congenital type), anhidrosis and flushing of the face. *Syn.* Bernard–Horner syndrome.
*See* **anisocoria; enophthalmos; heterochromia; miosis;** Table P11; **ptosis.**

**syndrome, ICE** A syndrome involving the proliferation of corneal endothelium, iris nodules, atrophy of the iris and synechia resulting in secondary glaucoma. ICE is an abbreviation of iridocorneal endothelial. *Syn.* Cogan–Reese syndrome; iridocorneal endothelial syndrome; iris naevus syndrome.
*See* **naevus, iris; syndrome, Chandler's.**

**syndrome, immobile lens** *See* **contact lens acute red eye.**

**syndrome, iridocorneal endothelial** *See* **syndrome, ICE.**

**syndrome, iris naevus** *See* **syndrome, ICE.**

**syndrome, Irlen's** *See* **syndrome, Meares–Irlen.**

**syndrome, Irvine–Gass** *See* **oedema, cystoid macular.**

**syndrome, ischaemic ocular** A syndrome occurring in individuals over the age of 50 with a history of cardiovascular disorders. It is characterized by, usually, unilateral loss of vision which may be acute or may develop over days or months, rubeosis iridis and there may be fadeouts of vision and pain. The fundus may have dilated congested veins with some haemorrhages and macular oedema. Management is directed at the cardiovascular disorder.
*See* **rubeosis iridis.**

**syndrome, Kennedy** *See* **syndrome, Foster Kennedy.**

**syndrome, Laurence–Moon–Bardet–Biedl** An apparently hereditary disorder characterized by mental handicap, dystrophia adiposogenitalis, polydactylism and obesity. The associated ocular abnormalities are retinitis pigmentosa, optic nerve atrophy with reduced visual acuity, night blindness and myopia. *Syn.* Bardet–Biedl syndrome; Moon–Bardet–Biedl syndrome.

**syndrome, Marcus Gunn jaw-winking** *See* **phenomenon, jaw-winking.**

**syndrome, Marfan's** A widespread inherited disorder of connective tissue which affects many organs, including the skeleton, lungs, heart and blood vessels. The ocular signs are subluxation or dislocation of the lens which results from a defective suspensory ligament, myopia due to increased axial length, retinal detachment as well as heterochromia, keratoconus, blue sclerotic, strabismus and glaucoma due to developmental anomalies of the angle of the anterior chamber.
*See* **heterochromia; keratoconus; luxation of the lens; retina, lattice degeneration of the; sclera, blue.**

**syndrome, Meares–Irlen** A visual disorder characterized by difficulties with reading which are mitigated by wearing coloured filters of a specific tint (called **Irlens lens**). The patient often complains of headaches and eye strain and observes illusions of motion, colour and shape distortion of a stationary striped pattern (e.g. grating or text). The patient may also have low amplitude of accommodation and reduced stereoscopic visual acuity. Coloured filters individually selected have been found to help in the management of this condition. *Syn.* Irlen's syndrome; scotopic sensitivity syndrome.
*See* **dyslexia.**

**syndrome, Mikulicz's** A bilateral, painless, symmetrical enlargement of the lacrimal and salivary glands, causing hyposecretion of tears and saliva. It is usually associated with reticulosis, sarcoidosis, tuberculosis or syphilis.
*See* **dacryoadenitis; keratitis sicca; syndrome, Sjögren's.**

**syndrome, Mobius' (or Moebius)** A congenital condition due to a deletion on the long arm of chromosome 13. It is characterized by varying abnormalities of the fifth to the twelfth cranial nerves. The patient may exhibit an expressionless facial appearance, webbed fingers or toes, limb defects, deafness, feeding difficulties and mild mental handicap. The ocular signs include unilateral or bilateral esotropia with inability to abduct the eyes, horizontal gaze palsy and sagging of the lower lids.

**syndrome, monofixation** A condition in which there is an inability in binocular fixation, to fuse images formed on the fovea of each eye while peripheral fusion remains normal. There is limited stereopsis in most cases. One eye is usually amblyopic with a small central scotoma, which accounts for the absence of diplopia. There are cases in which there is no strabismus, although anisometropia is present. When there is strabismus (most commonly esotropia) the angle of deviation is small (less than 8 $\Delta$) and the condition is frequently regarded as a type of microtropia. Management usually consists in correcting the refractive error and often occlusion treatment.
*See* **fusion, sensory; microtropia; occlusion treatment.**

**syndrome, Moon–Bardet–Biedl** *See* **syndrome, Laurence–Moon–Bardet–Biedl.**

**syndrome, nystagmus blockage** A condition in which convergence or adduction of one eye reduces nystagmus.

**syndrome, 'one and one half'** An eye movement disorder resulting from a brainstem lesion of the medial longitudinal fasciculus and the paramedian pontine reticular formation on the same side of the body. It is characterized by a horizontal palsy when the eye looks towards the same side as the lesion and an internuclear ophthalmoplegia (i.e. limited adduction of the eye on the same side and jerk nystagmus of the other eye, when the eyes look to the side of the body opposite to that of the lesion). It is thus named because there is a complete ipsilateral gaze palsy and a contralateral half gaze palsy. *Syn.* paralytic pontine exotropia.
*See* **ophthalmoplegia, internuclear.**

**syndrome, orbital inflammatory** An idiopathic inflammation of orbital tissues causing sudden pain, restricted ocular motility (including diplopia), proptosis, lid oedema and decreased vision. It may occur in children or adults. The abnormality is thought to be due to an inflammation of the orbital structures including the extraocular muscles (myositis) and tendons, vascular system, sclera, and optic nerve sheath.

Lesions may be noted bilaterally, in which case, in the adult population, the possibility of systemic vasculitis or lymphoproliferative disease is raised. *Syn.* orbital pseudotumour.

**syndrome, overwear** Ocular pain which may be very intense, accompanied by corneal epithelium damage, conjunctival injection, lacrimation, blepharospasm, photophobia, and hazy vision following corneal hypoxia caused by overwear of contact lenses, principally the PMMA type. The symptoms usually begin to appear 2–3 hours after the lenses are removed and recovery usually occurs within 24 hours, although an antibiotic may be needed.
*See* **corneal abrasion; hypoxia; oedema; syndrome, corneal exhaustion.**

**syndrome, Parinaud's** Paralysis of the conjugate movements of the eyes either for elevation or depression, or both, and sometimes with paralysis of convergence, fixed pupils and lid retraction. This condition is due to a lesion at the level of the superior colliculi or in the subthalamic region. *Syn.* dorsal midbrain syndrome; tectal midbrain syndrome.
*See* **colliculi, superior; nystagmus, convergence-retraction; sign, Collier's.**

**syndrome, pigment dispersion** A degenerative process in the iris and ciliary body epithelium in which pigment granules are disseminated and deposited on the back surface of the cornea, the lens, the zonules and within the trabecular meshwork. On the corneal endothelium it may form a vertical spindle shape (called **Krukenberg's spindle**). Deposition of pigment in the trabecular meshwork may give rise to glaucoma (called **pigmentary glaucoma**).
*See* **glaucoma, open-angle; Krukenberg's spindle; line, Sampaolesi's; meshwork, trabecular.**

**syndrome, Posner–Schlossman** A condition characterized by recurrent episodes of high intraocular pressure (40–80 mmHg) associated with intraocular inflammation. Keratic precipitates commonly appear with each attack, especially on the trabecular meshwork. Patients are typically young adults. Main complaint is blurred vision, due to corneal oedema. The cause is unknown, although herpes simplex virus has been implicated. With repeated attacks chronic uveitis and open-angle glaucoma may develop. Treatment usually consists of topical steroids to control the inflammation and carbonic anhydrase inhibitors or beta-blockers to reduce the secretion of aqueous humour and decrease the intraocular pressure. *Syn.* glaucomatocyclitic crisis.

**syndrome, pseudoexfoliation** *See* **pseudoexfoliation.**

**syndrome, Reiter's** *See* **disease, Reiter's.**

**syndrome, retraction** *See* **syndrome, Duane's.**

**syndrome, Rieger's** A hereditary developmental anomaly of the cornea, iris and the angle of the anterior chamber. It is characterized by posterior embryotoxon, stromal hypoplasia of the iris, pupillary anomalies, adhesion of strands of iris tissue to the cornea at the angle of the anterior chamber and glaucoma in about half of the cases, as well as dental and skeletal abnormalities. *Syn.* mesodermal dysgenesis of the cornea and iris.
*See* **ring of Schwalbe, anterior limiting; syndrome, Axenfeld's.**

**syndrome, Riley–Day** A hereditary nervous disorder largely confined to Ashkenazic Jews. It is characterized by alacrima, corneal hypoaesthesia, exotropia, myopia and excessive sweating, vomiting, attacks of high fever, incoordination and lack of pain sensitivity. Few patients survive to adulthood as most die from pneumonia and cardiovascular collapse. *Syn.* familial autonomic dysfunction.
*See* **alacrima.**

**syndrome, rubella** Congenital defects in infants whose mothers contracted rubella in the first few months of pregnancy. The infant may have cardiac malformation, cataract, pigment epithelium disorders, deafness, microcephaly and mental handicap. *Syn.* Gregg syndrome.
*See* **deaf-blind.**

**syndrome, scotopic sensitivity** *See* **syndrome, Meares–Irlen.**

**syndrome, Sjögren's** A chronic connective tissue disease characterized by a failure of lacrimal secretion leading to keratoconjunctivitis sicca, with dryness of the mouth, of the upper respiratory tract and other mucous membranes and associated with rheumatoid arthritis. The condition occurs predominantly in women after menopause.
*See* **alacrima; keratitis sicca; syndrome, Mikulicz's; tears.**

**syndrome, Stevens–Johnson** An acute form of erythema exudativum multiforme involving the mucous membranes and large areas of the body. Some form of conjunctivitis occurs in most cases but **symblepharon** (an adhesion between the palpebral and bulbar conjunctiva) and keratoconjunctivitis sicca with corneal opacification and loss of vision may also occur. Common causes include reaction to some drugs (e.g. sulfonamides, penicillin, NSAIDS), secondary to an infection (herpes simplex virus, *Mycoplasma pneumoniae*).
*See* **conjunctivitis, pseudomembranous; erythema multiforme.**

**syndrome, Stilling–Turk–Duane** *See* **syndrome, Duane's.**

**syndrome, Sturge–Weber** A rare, congenital disease characterized by reddish pigmentation or 'port-wine' stains (**naevus flammeus**), usually on one side of the face in the area supplied by the trigeminal nerve. It is associated with an haemangioma of the choroid and high intraocular pressure which give rise to megalocornea or glaucoma. *Syn.* Sturge–Weber disease, encephalotrigeminal angiomatosis.

**syndrome, superior oblique sheath** *See* **syndrome, Brown's superior oblique tendon sheath.**

**syndrome, Swann's** An esotropia in which the angle of deviation is such that the retinal image of the fixation object in the deviated eye falls on the optic disc. *Syn.* blind spot esotropia; syndrome, blind spot.
*See* **disc, optic.**

**syndrome, Terson's** Subarachnoid haemorrhage followed by retinal haemorrhage (in about 30% of patients) which breaks through the inner limiting membrane of the retina into the vitreous. It is due to an acute rise in intracranial pressure. The condition often subsides spontaneously, otherwise treatment usually consists of vitrectomy.
*See* **haemorrhage, preretinal.**

**syndrome, tight lens** *See* **contact lens acute red eye.**

**syndrome, tilted disc** *See* **crescent, congenital scleral.**

**syndrome, trisomy 21** *See* **syndrome, Down's.**

**syndrome, Turner's** A disorder caused by the absence of, or sometimes defective, X chromosomes in females. It is characterized by shortness of stature, webbing of the skin and neck, congenital heart disease and genitourinary anomalies. The ocular manifestations include epicanthus, ptosis, strabismus, blue sclera, myopia, cataract and colour vision deficiencies.
*See* **inheritance.**

**syndrome, Usher's** A hereditary condition characterized by a degeneration of the retinal pigment epithelium, and accompanied by deafness.
*See* **deaf-blind.**

**syndrome, V** *See* **pattern, V.**

**syndrome, van der Hoeve's** *See* **sclera, blue.**

**syndrome, Vogt–Koyanagi–Harada (VKH)** A severe, multisystem disorder of unknown origin. It is characterized by various systemic features: alopecia, poliosis, vitiligo and/or hearing difficulties. The ocular manifestations, bilateral in nature, are: iridocyclitis which often leads to the formation of posterior synechia and secondary glaucoma, choroiditis and retinal detachment. Management includes antiinflammatory drugs. *Syn.* Vogt–Koyanagi–Harada disease.
*See* **disease, Harada's; iridocyclitis; poliosis; vitiligo.**

**syndrome, Wagner's** *See* **disease, Wagner's.**

**syndrome, Weber's** A syndrome caused by a lesion (usually vascular) in the cerebral peduncle of the brain. It is characterized by an ipsilateral third nerve paralysis associated with facial paralysis and contralateral hemiplegia.
*See* **paralysis of the third nerve; syndrome, Benedikt's.**

**syndrome, Weill–Marchesani** An autosomal dominant or recessive inherited connective tissue disorder characterized by spherophakia, lenticular myopia and glaucoma which results from lens subluxation and pupil block, associated with brachydactyly and short stature.
*See* **spherophakia; syndrome, Marfan's.**

**syndrome, Wernicke's** *See* **disease, Wernicke's.**

**synechia, annular** Adhesion of the entire pupillary margin of the iris to the capsule of the crystalline lens. *Note*: also spelt synechiae.
*See* **iris bombé; pupillary block.**

**synechia, anterior** Adhesion of the iris to the cornea.
*See* **glaucoma, angle-closure; gonioscopy, indentation; goniosynechia; iris, prolapse of the; Peter's anomaly; syndrome, Rieger's.**

**synechia, posterior** Adhesion of the iris to the capsule of the crystalline lens.
*See* **iris bombé; iritis; uveitis.**

**syneresis** A degenerative shrinkage of the vitreous humour in which the gel breaks into liquid-filled particles which coalesce and render it partially or completely fluid. It occurs in elderly individuals and may precede vitreous detachment.
*See* **synchisis scintillans; vitreous detachment.**

**synergist muscle** *See* **muscles, synergistic.**

**synaesthesia** Phenomenon in which the stimulation of one of the senses produces a response from another sensory modality. *Example*: seeing the colour red when a particular sound is heard.
*See* **modality.**

**synkinetic reflex, near** *See* **reflex, near.**

**Synoptiscope** *See* **amblyoscope, Worth.**

**Synoptophore** A type of major amblyoscope (Fig. S12).
*See* **amblyoscope, Worth.**

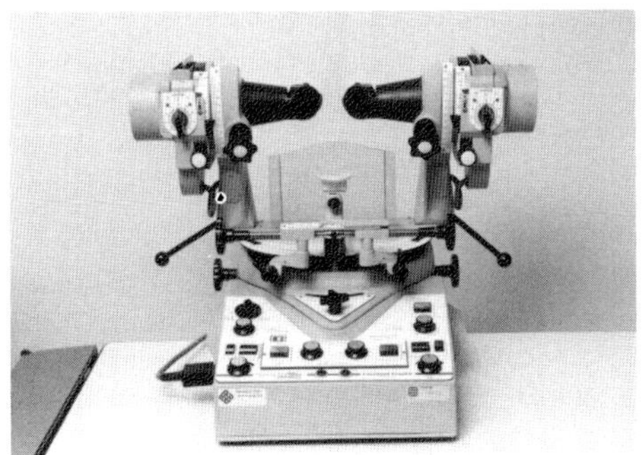

Fig. S12 Synoptophore (Clement Clarke)

**syphilis** *See* **anisocoria; conjunctivitis; dacryoadenitis; fundus, salt and pepper; keratitis, interstitial; luxation of the lens; pupil, Adie's; pupil, Argyll Robertson; sign, Hutchinson's; tabes dorsalis; uveitis.**

**system, boxing** A method of measurement of the eyesize of spectacle frames. It is based on a rectangle with its horizontal and vertical length tangential to the edges of the lens. The horizontal lens size is equal to the horizontal length of the rectangle. *Syn.* box system of lens measurement; boxing method.
*See* **centre, boxing; centre, standard optical position.**

**system, centred optical** *See* **system, optical.**

**system, compound optical** An optical system consisting of more than one lens.

**system, magnocellular visual** *See* **magnocellular visual system.**

**system, optical** A collection of lenses, prisms, mirrors, etc. which act together to produce an image of an external object. If the axes of all the components coincide, the system is called a **centred optical system**.
*See* **system, compound optical.**

**system, parvocellular visual** *See* **parvocellular visual system.**

**system, 'what'** *See* **parvocellular visual system.**

**system, 'where'** *See* **magnocellular visual system.**

# T

**tabes dorsalis** A degenerative disease of the posterior columns of the spinal cord, the posterior spinal roots and the peripheral nerves accompanied by a number of ocular signs and symptoms such as atrophy of the optic nerve, visual field defects, ptosis, Argyll Robertson pupil and paralysis of one or more of the extraocular muscles. The disease is a result of neurosyphilis.
*See* **pupil, Argyll Robertson.**

**TABO notation** *See* **axis notation, standard.**

**tachistoscope** An instrument which presents visual stimuli for a brief and variable period of time (usually less than 0.1 s).

**Talbot–Plateau law** *See* **law, Talbot–Plateau.**

**tamponade agent** A gas, pad or silicone oil used to plug a cavity, stop a haemorrhage or compress a part. In the eye it may be employed in vitreous surgery to fill the vitreous space with either gas or silicone, and in retinal detachment therapy.

**tangent scale** *See* **Maddox cross.**

**tangent screen** *See* **screen, tangent.**

**tangential focus** *See* **astigmatism, oblique.**

**tapetoretinal degeneration** *See* **degeneration, tapetoretinal.**

**tapetum lucidum** A reflecting pigment layer lying behind the visual receptors of the retina of certain mammals (e.g. cats, dogs), birds and fish which gives a shining appearance to the eyes when illuminated in the dark. The tapetum is located either in the pigment epithelium or in the choroid and covers either the whole fundus or more often only the upper and back portion. The role of the tapetum lucidum is to increase the probability of visual stimulation of the photoreceptors by reflecting light back after having already traversed them once, thus aiding vision in dim illumination. In some species the tapetum consists of guanine crystals.

**target** A pattern or an object of fixation such as a red dot or an optotype.
*See* **optotype.**

**tarsal** Pertaining to the tarsus.

**tarsal gland** *See* **glands, meibomian.**

**tarsal muscles** *See* **muscles, Müller's palpebral.**

**tarsal plate** *See* **tarsus.**

**tarsorrhaphy** A surgical procedure consisting of suturing the upper and lower eyelids together either partially or completely. It provides a temporary protection to the eye or forms part of the treatment of dry eyes.
*See* **alacrima; keratitis sicca.**

**tarsus** Thin flat plate of dense connective tissue, situated one in each eyelid, which gives it shape and firmness. Each tarsus extends from the orbital septum to the eyelid margin. The upper tarsal plate, shaped like the letter D placed on its side, is much larger than the lower. Its width is 11 mm in the centre whereas the corresponding measurement in the lower tarsus, which is somewhat oblong in form, is 5 mm. Each tarsus is about 29 mm long and 1 mm thick. Within each tarsus are the meibomian glands, approximately 25 in the upper and 20 in the lower. *Syn.* tarsal plate.
*See* **glands, meibomian; ligament, palpebral; orbital septum.**

**Tay's choroiditis** *See* **drusen, familial dominant.**

**Tay–Sachs disease** *See* **disease, Tay–Sachs.**

**tear duct** One of about a dozen ducts of the lacrimal gland. It originates in the orbital part of the gland, traverses the palpebral part of the gland and opens into the lateral superior fornix of the conjunctival sac. *Syn.* lacrimal duct.
*See* **gland, lacrimal; lacrimal apparatus.**

**tear exchange** *See* **lens, fenestrated.**

**tear film** *See* **film, precorneal.**

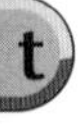

**tear film break-up test** *See* **test, break-up time.**

**tear film, prelens** Tear film found on the front surface of a contact lens on the eye. The oily layer of the film is slightly thinner with soft lenses than in the precorneal film and almost absent with rigid lenses. The aqueous layer is thinner with rigid lenses than in the precorneal film. The exact composition of the prelens tear film varies with the characteristics of the contact lens on the eye.
*See* **film, precorneal.**

**tear layer** *See* **film, precorneal.**

**tear meniscus** A thin strip of tear fluid with concave outer surface at the upper and lower lid margins. It contains most of the exposed tear volume. The absence of a tear meniscus is an indication of a dry eye. *Syn.* marginal tear strip; lacrimal prism; tear prism.
*See* **film, precorneal; lacrimal lake.**

**tear prism** *See* **tear meniscus.**

**tear pumping** The mechanism involving blinking which acts to bring fresh tears with oxygen and nutrients to the cornea behind a contact lens, and pumping stale tears containing carbon dioxide, lactic acid and other waste products from beneath the lens. It occurs most readily with hard contact lenses (between 14% and 20% of the tear volume is exchanged with each blink) and to a much smaller extent with soft lenses (between 1% and 5% of the tear volume is exchanged with each blink).
*See* **hypoxia; oxygen transmissibility.**

**tear, retinal** *See* **retinal tear.**

**tear secretion** There are two types of tear secretion: (1) **Basal tear secretion** which occurs normally without any stimulation and comes mainly from the accessory glands of Krause and Wolfring. It maintains the cornea and conjunctiva continuously moist, but is reduced in dry eyes (e.g. keratitis sicca) and in elderly individuals. (2) **Reflex tear secretion** which is produced mainly by the lacrimal gland in response to an irritant and also depends on psychological factors. The amount of tears secreted amounts to 14–33 grams per 24 hours or 0.5–2.2 microlitre/minute, being about 2 microlitre/minute at 15 years of age and less than 1 microlitre/minute at 65 years of age.
*See* **reflex tearing; test, basic secretion; test, Schirmer's.**

**tear stasis** The slowing down or stoppage of tear flow behind a contact lens. It can lead to **lens adherence** (or **lens binding**) to the cornea with the possible consequences of acute red eye, arcuate corneal staining, and, if severe, corneal ulceration. Fitting or refitting in such a way that some lens movement is maintained usually prevents this condition.
*See* **lens adherence; staining, fluorescein.**

**tear strip, marginal** *See* **tear meniscus.**

**tearing reflex** *See* **reflex, tearing.**

**tears** The clear watery fluid secreted by the lacrimal gland which, together with the secretions from the meibomian glands, the goblet cells, the gland of Zeis, as well as the accessory lacrimal glands of Krause and Wolfring, helps to maintain the conjunctiva and cornea moist and healthy. Periodic involuntary blinking spreads the tears over the cornea and conjunctiva and causes a pumping action of the lacrimal drainage

system, through the lacrimal puncta into the nasolacrimal duct. Approximately 25% of the tears is lost by evaporation, the remaining 75% is pumped into the nasal cavity and over 60% of the tear volume is drained through the lower canaliculus. Tears contain water (98.2%), salts, lipids (e.g wax esters, sterol esters, hydrocarbons, polar lipids, triglycerides and free fatty acids), proteins (e.g. lysozyme, lactoferrin, albumin, IgA, IgE, IgG, complement proteins C3, C4, C5 and C9, and beta-lysin), magnesium, potassium, sodium, calcium, chloride, bicarbonate, urea, ammonia, nitrogen, citric acid, ascorbic acid, and mucin. Tears have a pH varying between 7.3 and 7.7 (shifting to a slightly less alkaline value when the eye is closed) and the quantity secreted per hour is between 30 and 120 μl. *Syn.* lacrimal fluid.
*See* **alacrima; blink; epiphora; film, precorneal; gland, lacrimal; hyperlacrimation; lacrimal apparatus; lacrimal lake; lysozyme; mucin; staining, fluorescein; syndrome, Sjögren's; test, break-up time; test, non-invasive break-up time; test, phenol red cotton thread; test, Schirmer's.**

**tears, artificial** Any eye drop solution which can replace tears by approximating its consistency in terms of viscosity and tonicity and may contain many of the substances found in tears. The most common agents found in artificial tears are cellulose derivatives, such as methylcellulose, hydroxymethylcellulose, hydroxypropylcellulose, hydroxypropylmethylcellulose (or hypromellose), hydroxyethylcellulose and carboxymethycellulose, polyvinyl alcohol or polyacrylic acid, as well as a preservative and a substance to produce isotonicity (e.g. sodium chloride).
*See* **alacrima; antiseptic; hypromellose; keratitis sicca; methylcellulose; palsy, Bell's; wetting solution.**

**tears, crocodile** Copious secretion of tears occurring during eating in cases of abnormal regeneration of the seventh cranial nerve after recovery from Bell's palsy. *Syn.* paradoxic lacrimation.
*See* **palsy, Bell's.**

**Tearscope plus** Tradename of a hand-held instrument designed to view the tear film non-invasively. It uses a cold light source to minimize any drying of the tear film during the examination. It can be used directly in front of the eye or in conjunction with a slit-lamp biomicroscope to gain more magnification. Evaluation of the interference patterns of the anterior surface of the tear film lipid layer facilitates the diagnosis of the cause of dry eye symptoms, as well as screening patients for contact lens wear. The instrument also allows the measurement of the non-invasive break-up time.
*See* **film, precorneal; glands, meibomian; test, non-invasive break-up time.**

**technique** *See* **method** or **test.**

**tectal midbrain syndrome** *See* **syndrome, Parinaud's.**

**tectum of the mesencephalon** Structure comprising the plate of grey and white matter (called the **tectal lamina**) which forms the roof of the midbrain and from which project the inferior and superior colliculi. The area anterior to it is called the pretectal region. *Syn.* tectum of the midbrain; optic tectum. *Note*: The word tectum comes from the Latin and means roof. The word mesencephalon is made up of two parts which come from the Greek and means middle brain.
*See* **colliculi, inferior; colliculi, superior; fibres, pupillary; nystagmus, convergence-retraction; pathway, retinotectal.**

**tectum of the midbrain** *See* **tectum of the mesencephalon.**

**teichopsia** A transient, shimmering visual sensation. *Example*: the fortification spectrum of a scintillating scotoma.
*See* **scotoma, scintillating.**

**Telebinocular** A tradename for a stereoscope based on that of Brewster–Holmes and used to investigate distance and near visual functions such as acuity, stereopsis, etc.
*See* **stereoscope, Brewster's.**

**telecanthus** Excessive separation between the medial canthi of the eyelids. It may occur in isolation or form part of the blepharophimosis syndrome. Treatment consists in shortening and re-fixating the medial canthal tendons to the lacrimal crest.
*See* **syndrome, blepharophimosis.**

**telecentric** Pertains to an optical system in which its aperture stop is positioned so that the entrance pupil falls in the first focal plane, the exit pupil is at infinity, and the rays through the centre of the entrance pupil from all points on the object are parallel to the axis in the image space. Similarly, if the exit pupil lies in the second focal plane the entrance pupil will be at infinity, and the rays through the centre of the exit pupil will be parallel to the axis in the object space.

**teleopsia** Anomaly of visual perception in which objects appear to be much further away than they actually are. It may be due to vision in a hazy atmosphere, intoxication, neurosis, etc.
*See* **metamorphopsia.**

**telescope** An optical instrument for magnifying the apparent size of distant objects. It consists, in principle, of two lenses: (1) the objective, being a positive lens which forms a real inverted image of the distant object; (2) the eyepiece through which the observer views a magnified image of that formed by the objective. The eyepiece may be either positive (**astronomical** or **Kepler telescope**) or negative (**galilean telescope**). The magnification $M$ of a telescope is given by the following formula

$$M = \frac{f'_o}{f_e} = \frac{D_o}{D_e}$$

where $f'_o$ is the second focal length of the objective, $f_e$ the first focal length of the eyepiece, and $D_o$ and $D_e$ are the diameters of the entrance and exit pupils of the telescope (approximately equal to the diameters of the objective lens and the eyepiece). There are also some telescopes that do not use a lens (or lens system) as objective, as these are difficult to produce if large apertures and minimum aberrations are required. These telescopes use a concave mirror (usually parabolic) as the objective. They are called **reflecting telescopes**. Light from a distant object is collected by the large concave mirror and reflected onto a small mirror (positive in the **Cassegrain telescope** and negative in the **gregorian telescope**). This mirror is located on the optical axis and light is then transmitted through a central hole in the concave mirror onto the eyepiece. In the **newtonian telescope** the light collected by the large concave mirror is reflected onto a small plane mirror at a 45° angle to the optical axis, and transmitted to the eyepiece which is at right angles to the optical axis. (Fig.T1)
*See* **binoculars; eyepiece; objective.**

**telescope, astronomical** *See* **telescope.**

**telescope, bioptic** A system of lenses forming a galilean or Kepler telescope which is mounted high on a plastic spectacle or carrier lens with the distance correction, so as to allow the patient to look through either the telescope, or below, by moving his or her head. It is used to magnify distant objects for patients with low vision. *Syn.* bioptic position telescope.
*See* **vision, low.**

**telescope, Cassegrain** *See* **telescope.**

**telescope, Dutch** *See* **telescope, galilean.**

**telescope, galilean** A simple optical system which allows observation of far objects with a low magnification and without image inversion. It consists of a convex lens which acts as the objective and a concave lens as the eyepiece. Magnification of such a telescope rarely exceeds × 5. This optical system is used in opera glasses and as a low vision aid (Fig. T1). *Syn.* Dutch telescope.
*See* **binoculars; minification.**

**telescope, gregorian; Kepler; newtonian** *See* **telescope.**

**telescope, reflecting** A telescope which uses a concave mirror as the objective.

**telescope, refracting** A telescope which uses a positive lens system as the objective.

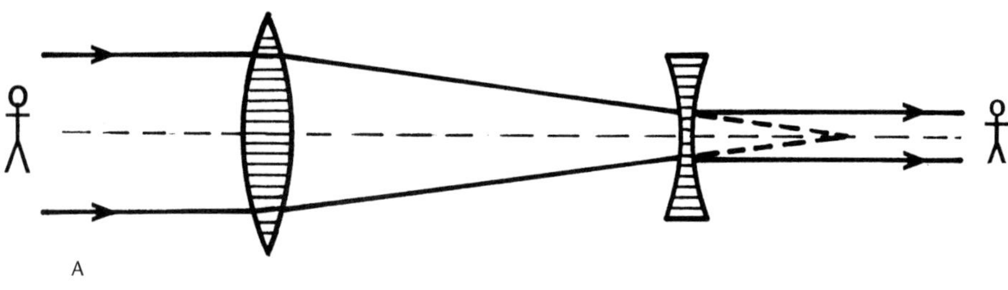


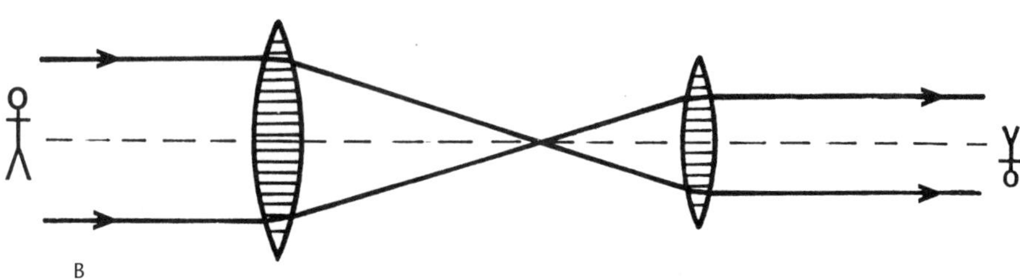


**Fig. T1** Telescopes: A, galilean; B, Kepler

**telescope, terrestrial** A telescope which provides an erect image of a distant object. The image is usually erected by means of a lens system placed between the objective and the eyepiece. It does, however, make the terrestrial telescope relatively longer than an astronomical telescope.
*See* **binoculars; erector.**

**telescopic spectacles** *See* **lens, telescopic.**

**telestereoscope, Helmholtz** Instrument designed to produce an exaggerated perception of depth by optically increasing the length of the base line of the viewer, using a system of mirrors or prisms (Fig. T2).

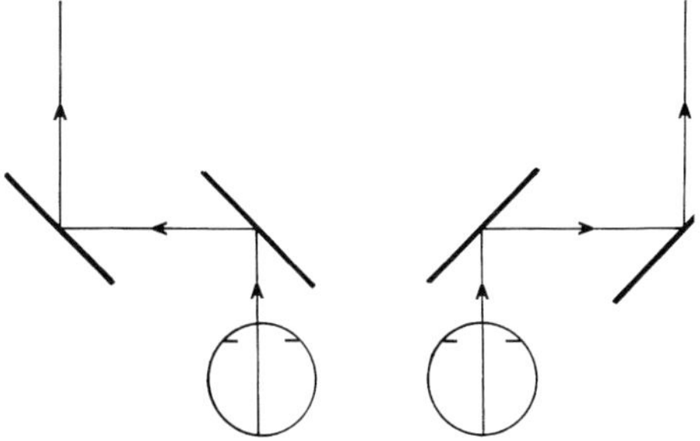

**Fig. T2** Optical principle of a telestereoscope

**Teller acuity cards** *See* **acuity cards, Teller.**

**temple 1.** *See* **side** of a spectacle frame. **2.** The lateral area of the human head between the outer canthi and the ears and above the zygomatic arch.

**temple, library** A straight side of a spectacle frame. *See* **spectacles, library.**

**temporal arteritis** *See* **arteritis, temporal.**

**temporal induction; summation** *See* under the nouns.

**tendon** *See* **muscles, extraocular.**

**tendon of Zinn** *See* **annulus of Zinn.**

**Tenon's capsule** The fibrous membrane which envelops the globe from the margin of the cornea to the optic nerve. Its inner surface is in close contact with the episclera to which it is connected by fine trabeculae. These trabeculae also attach it to the extraocular muscles. The posterior surface of the capsule is in contact with the orbital fat. Anteriorly, it becomes thinner and merges gradually into the subconjunctival connective tissue. *Syn.* Bonnet's capsule; capsule of the eyeball; fascia bulbi.
*See* **episclera; ligament of Lockwood.**

**tension, ocular** *See* **pressure, intraocular.**

**Terrien's disease** *See* **ectasia, corneal.**

**Terson's syndrome** *See* **syndrome, Terson's.**

**tertiary action** Term referring to the least effect of an extrocular muscle. The tertiary action of the inferior rectus is extorsion; of the superior rectus, intorsion; of the inferior and superior oblique, abduction. The medial and lateral recti muscles are regarded as having only a primary action, at least in the primary position.
*See* **primary action.**

**tertiary position** *See* **position, tertiary.**

**test 1.** A method of examination to determine a disease or a performance. **2.** To try; to prove. **3.** The equipment used to carry out the test.

**test, after-image** A subjective test used to determine the presence or absence of abnormal retinal correspondence (ARC). The subject is instructed to fixate the centre of a vertical light filament for some 15 s with one eye and then the centre of a horizontal light filament for some 15 s with the other eye. Looking at the after-images of the two filaments on a uniform surface (e.g. a wall) the subject sees either a cross, which indicates normal retinal correspondence or two separated filaments, indicating ARC. *Syn.* Hering's after-image test.
*See* **after-image; retinal correspondence, abnormal.**

**test, after-image transfer** Test aimed at detecting and measuring the angle of eccentric fixation in an amblyopic eye in a patient with normal retinal correspondence. The normal eye fixates an illuminated vertical line and is then occluded, while the amblyopic eye fixates a dot. If the after-image and the fixation point coincide the amblyopic eye has no eccentric fixation, otherwise the relative position of one to the other indicates the angle of eccentric fixation. *Syn.* Brock's after-image test.
*See* **fixation, eccentric; retinal corresponding points.**

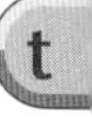


**test, Ammann's** *See* **test, neutral density filter.**

**test, Arden grating** A clinical test for contrast sensitivity. It consists of photographic plates, each with a sinusoidal grating of constant spatial frequency but of increasing contrast from top to bottom. There are seven plates, one being for demonstration. The other six, each with a different spatial frequency, are used for testing. The spatial frequencies are: 0.2, 0.4, 0.8, 1.6, 3.2 and 6.4 cycles per degree when viewed at a distance of 50 cm. Contrast levels are numbered from 1 to 20 on a vertical scale on the side of the plate. The testing procedure consists of slowly removing each plate from its folder until the

grating becomes visible to the patient, at which point the contrast level is noted. The testing is carried out monocularly with optical correction, if any. The procedure is repeated for each plate and all the contrast levels are added to arrive at a score which is compared to normal values provided in the instructions. *Syn.* Arden gratings; Arden plates.
*See* **chart, contrast sensitivity; sensitivity, contrast; Vistech.**

**test for astigmatism, cross-cylinder** A subjective test for measuring the axis and the amount of astigmatism using a cross-cylinder lens. Having obtained the best visual acuity with a spherical lens, the cross-cylinder lens is placed before the eye being tested with its axes at 45° to the cylinder axis determined by retinoscopy. The patient looks at a single circular target, often a letter (O or C or Verhoeff's circles), the cross-cylinder lens is then flipped and if one position provides a clearer image of the target, the axis of the correcting (minus) cylinder should be turned towards the minus axis of the cross-cylinder lens until vision is equally blurred in both positions of the cross-cylinder lens. That point indicates the correct axis of the correcting cylinder. The determination of the power of the correcting cylinder is carried out by placing the cross-cylinder lens with one of its axes parallel to the axis of the correcting cylinder. The cross-cylinder lens is flipped and the position which provides the clearer vision indicates whether to increase the cylinder power (when the minus axis of the cross-cylinder is parallel) or decrease cylinder power (when the plus axis is parallel). The proper amount of cylinder correction is obtained when the vision is equally blurred in both positions of the cross-cylinder lens. *Syn.* cross-cylinder method; cross-cylinder test; Jackson crossed cylinder test.
*See* **lens, cross-cylinder; Verhoeff's circles.**

**test, Bagolini's** *See* **glass, Bagolini's.**

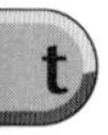

**test, balancing** A test designed to obtain equal focusing or equal accommodative states in the two eyes. This is accomplished either objectively (by retinoscopy) or, more commonly, subjectively using either the duochrome test, or comparing the visual acuity in the two eyes simultaneously or successively, or using prisms to present two images of a chart and ask the patient to compare these images, or using a binocular refraction technique (e.g. Turville infinity balance test). *Syn.* equalization test.
*See* **balance, binocular; method, Humphriss; test, duochrome; test, Turville infinity balance; vectogram.**

**test, bar reading** A test for determining the presence of binocular vision and also used in the management of amblyopia in which a narrow bar (or a pencil) is held vertically between the reader's eyes and a page of print. The bar occludes a vertical strip of print but the strip is different for the two eyes and if binocular vision is present the subject will experience no difficulty reading the text. *Syn.* Welland's test.

**test, basic secretion** Measurement of the basal tear secretion independently of reflex tear secretion. A filter paper strip (e.g. Whatman No. 41) is placed in the anaesthetized lower fornix and after 5 minutes the strip is removed and the amount of wetting measured from the folded end.
*See* **tear secretion, test, Schirmer's.**

**test, Bielschowsky's head tilt** A test to determine which of the inferior or superior extraocular muscles and of which eye is paretic. The test is based on the following fact: if the head is tilted to the right, the right intorters of the right eye (superior oblique and superior rectus muscles) contract as well as the extorters of the left eye (inferior oblique and inferior rectus muscles). If the head is tilted to the left, the inferior oblique and inferior rectus muscles of the right eye contract to cause extorsion while the superior oblique and superior rectus of the eye contract to cause intorsion. Thus, tilting the head towards one side will indicate the palsied muscle. For example, in the right superior rectus muscle palsy, when the head is tilted to the left there will be no change in the vertical deviation, since contraction of the right superior rectus muscle is not involved. However, when the head is tilted to the right there will be an increase in downward movement. This test is not reliable in an adult with congenital ocular palsy.
*See* **muscles, extraocular; test, forced duction; test, three-step.**

**test, blind** A method of testing in which the person receiving or recording the results of a treatment or test does not know its identity.
*See* **placebo; test, double-blind.**

**test, blue field entoptoscope** *See* **entoptoscope, blue field.**

**test, blur back** *See* **test, plus 1.00 D blur.**

**test, break-up time (BUT)** A test for assessing the precorneal tear film. Fluorescein is applied to the bulbar conjunctiva and the patient is asked to blink once or twice and then to refrain from blinking. The tear film is scanned through the slit-lamp using a cobalt blue filter with a wide beam, while the examiner counts or records the time between the last blink and the appearance of the first dry black spot which indicates that the tear film is breaking up. In normal subjects, break-up times vary between 15 and 35 s (in Caucasians). A BUT of 10 s or less is abnormal and may be due to mucin deficiency and is often considered to be a negative factor for success in contact lens wear, especially soft lenses. However, this test has been shown to be flawed, because fluorescein can disrupt the tear film. *See* **film, precorneal; lens, cobalt; mucin; test, non-invasive break-up time.**

**test, Brock's after-image** *See* **test, after-image transfer.**

**test, Brock's string** *See* **Brock's string.**

**test, Bruckner's** *See* **method, Bruckner's.**

**test, Cardiff acuity** A test for measuring the visual acuity of young children. It is composed of a series of cards, each with a different picture (either a car, a dog, a duck, a fish, a house or a train) drawn with a white band which is surrounded by a black line half the width of the white, on a neutral grey background. Thus the average luminance of the target is equal to that of the grey background. The picture is situated either in the top or bottom half of the card. The pictures remain of the same overall size on each card; only the width of the black and white bands decreases in size. There are 11 acuity levels ranging from 6/60 (or 20/200) to 6/6 (or 20/20) at a viewing distance of 1 metre, in 0.1 log steps. The acuity is given by the narrowest white band for which the picture is still recognizable, but the child's eye movements are also noted to confirm or establish recognition. This test is best used with toddlers and children with intellectual impairment. *See* **method, preferential looking.**

**test chart** *See* **chart, test.**

**test, colour vision** *See* **Edridge–Green lantern; plates, pseudoisochromatic; test, Farnsworth; test, wool.**

**test, confrontation** A rough method of determining the approximate extent of the visual field. The patient, with one eye occluded, faces the examiner at a distance of about 60 cm and fixates the opposite eye of the examiner. The test object is moved in a plane midway between the examiner and the patient, starting far in the periphery and moving it towards the patient and in various meridians until it is seen. *See* **field, visual.**

**test, contrast sensitivity** *See* **chart, contrast sensitivity; sensitivity, contrast; test, Arden grating; Vistech.**

**test, corneal reflex** *See* **method, Hirschberg's; method, Javal's; method, Krimsky's.**

**test, cotton thread** *See* **test, phenol red cotton thread.**

**test, cover (CT)** A test for determining the presence and the type of heterophoria or strabismus. The subject fixates a small letter or any fine detail at a given distance. Strabismus is usually tested first. The opaque cover or occluder is placed over one eye and then removed, while the examiner observes the other eye and then the same operation is repeated on the other eye (this is called the **unilateral cover test**). If neither uncovered eye moves the subject does not have strabismus. If the unoccluded eye moves when a cover is placed in front of the other, strabismus is present. In esotropia the unoccluded eye will move temporally to take up fixation, while in exotropia the unoccluded eye will move nasally, and an upward or downward movement indicates hypotropia or hypertropia, respectively. In alternating squint, in which either eye can take up fixation, the eye behind the cover will appear deviated when uncovered and will move as the cover is shifted to the other eye.
The type of heterophoria can be detected by observing the eye behind the cover. If there is no movement of the eye behind the cover, the subject is orthophoric. If the eye behind the cover moves inward, and outward when the cover is removed, the subject has esophoria. If the eye behind the cover moves outward, and inward when the cover is removed, the subject has exophoria. A similar procedure is used for hyperphoria and hypophoria. As it is difficult to view the eye behind the cover without allowing sufficient peripheral fusion to stop the eyes going to the phoria position, the observer usually watches for the recovery movement as the occluder is removed. By placing prisms of increasing power in front of one of the eyes until no movement is evoked, one can evaluate the approximate amount of the phoria. The cover test is the only objective method of measuring heterophoria. The determination of the magnitude of the deviation of the strabismus or heterophoria can also be done with the **alternate** (or **alternating**) **cover test** (ACT). The subject fixates a target and the cover is successively placed in front of one eye and then the other while watching the eye which has just been uncovered to see the direction of the deviation. The amount of deviation can be estimated by using prisms of appropriate strength and base direction until the movement of the eye is neutralized when the cover is alternated from one eye to the other (**prism cover test**).
Although these tests are objective, they are sometimes used subjectively, i.e. the patient indicates the apparent movement of the fixation object. The alternate cover test is the most appropriate test for subjective testing. An apparent movement of the fixation object in the same direction as the cover indicates exophoria, while an apparent movement of the fixation object in the

opposite direction to the cover indicates esophoria. An apparent downward movement of the fixation indicates hyperphoria of the eye from which the occluder is moved. Again prisms can be placed in front of the eyes until the apparent movement disappears, thus giving a measure of the heterophoria. This subjective perception of a movement of a stationary fixation object in people with heterophoria or strabismus is a particular example of the phi phenomenon. *Syn.* occlusion test; screen test.
*See* **heterophoria; strabismus.**

**test, cross-cylinder** *See* **test for astigmatism, cross-cylinder.**

**test, dark filter** *See* **test, neutral density filter.**

**test, dark room** *See* **test, provocative.**

**test, Denver Developmental Screening** *See* **test, developmental and perceptual screening.**

**test, development and perceptual screening** A test used to assess children's perceptual and processing skills, such as gross motor coordination, directionality, laterality, visual form perception, visual memory and visualization, visual–motor integration and auditory and language development. There are many such tests, each evaluating one or several of the above skills. The most common ones are: (1) The **Denver Developmental Screening Test** (DDST) which is used for children up to about 6 years of age. It is easy to administer and covers a wide range of skills which fall into four sectors: personal–social, fine motor–adaptive, language and gross motor. Treatment and/or referral will depend on the type of skills found to be abnormal. (2) The **Test of Visual Analysis Skills** (TVAS) assesses the child's visual perceptual skills. It consists of 18 squares containing dots and lines, each forming a different pattern and the child is given a pencil and a special test form on which to reproduce the visual stimuli. The test comes with an expected score for each grade up to grade 3 and failure to reach that score may indicate that the child has a perceptual skills disorder. (3) The **Gardner Reversal-Frequency Test** in which the child is asked to mark those letters and numbers which are printed backward. This test assesses the directionality skill.

**test, developmental eye movement (DEM)** An indirect test for saccadic eye movements in which the subject reads numbers placed in four vertical columns (total of 80 numbers) and 16 horizontal rows (total of 80 numbers). The lengths of time taken to perform the horizontal and the vertical subtests are measured independently and assessed as a ratio, as well as the number of errors (omissions, additions, transpositions, or substitutions). All results are compared to test norms for the age of the subject. The vertical array mainly gives an indication of visual-verbal number skills (automaticity), whereas the horizontal array provides additional information on oculomotor function.

**test, differential intraocular pressure** A test for differentiating between a muscle paresis and a mechanical restriction of the eye. The intraocular pressure is measured in the primary position and then again with the patient turning his or her eyes in the direction of action of the suspected paretic muscle. An increase in intraocular pressure of 6 mmHg or more indicates a mechanical restriction (e.g. a fracture of the orbital floor), whereas no change in pressure suggests a muscle paresis. This test produces less discomfort to the patient than the forced duction test.
*See* **pressure, intraocular; test, forced duction.**

**test, diplopia 1.** A test for measuring heterophoria in which the fusion reflex is prevented by displacing the retinal image of one eye with a prism as in the **von Graefe's test** in which the magnitude of the phoria is estimated by the amount of prism necessary to align the two images. To measure lateral phorias the images are displaced vertically and aligned one above the other, whereas to measure vertical phorias the images are displaced horizontally and realigned horizontally (if a phoria is present). *Syn.* displacement test; prism dissociation test. **2.** A test to investigate the integrity of the extraocular muscles in strabismus, in which the patient is required to view a light source in the dark with a red filter in front of one eye and a green filter in front of the other, to produce diplopia (prisms are sometimes necessary). The direction and extent of diplopia are evaluated relative to the size and direction of the angle measured with the cover test at the same distance.
*See* **dissociation; heterophoria; test, red-glass.**

**test, displacement** *See* **test, diplopia.**

**test, dissociating** Any test for measuring heterophoria in which fusion is dissociated.
*See* **dissociation; Maddox rod; test, diplopia.**

**test, distortion** A test for measuring heterophoria, in which the images presented to the two eyes are so unlike that they cannot be fused. The most common such test is the Maddox rod test.
*See* **test, Maddox rod.**

**test, Dolman's** *See* **test, hole in the card.**

**test, double-blind** A method of testing in which neither the person receiving or recording the results of a treatment or test, nor the person administering it, knows the identity of the treatment or test.
*See* **placebo; sampling; test, blind.**

**test, double prism** A test for determining the presence of cyclophoria, in which a double prism (a pair of prisms set base to base) with the base line horizontal is placed before one eye. The patient is requested to fixate a horizontal line (or row of letters) which through the double prism appears as two lines (or two rows) vertically separated. On uncovering the other eye, the patient sees three lines (or rows). If there is no cyclophoria, all three lines (or rows) will appear parallel, but lack of parallelism indicates cyclophoria. The double prism used in this test consists of two weak prisms (about 4 or 5 Δ): this clinical type of double prism is commonly called a Maddox double prism.
*See* **bi-prism, Fresnel's; cyclophoria; test, Maddox rod.**

**test, Dunlop** A test for determining motor ocular dominance. It consists in having the eyes fusing two slightly different targets in, for example, a synoptophore and diverging the targets until diplopia appears. Just beforehand, fixation disparity occurs in one eye. That eye is called the non-dominant or non-reference eye. The other eye is the dominant or reference eye.
*See* **dominance, ocular.**

**test, duochrome** A subjective refraction test in which the subject compares the sharpness of black targets (e.g. Landolt rings) of similar sizes, on a red background on one side and on a green background on the other side (blue is sometimes used) of a chart. In under-corrected myopia or overcorrected hyperopia, the letters on the red background will appear more distinct, while in overcorrected myopia or undercorrected hyperopia the letters on the green background will appear more distinct, and in emmetropia or corrected ametropia the letters should appear equally distinct on both sides. The test makes use of the chromatic aberration of the eye and assumes that when the eye is looking at distant objects it is focused on the yellow part of the visible spectrum. *Syn.* bichrome test; duochrome method.
*See* **aberration, chromatic; lens, cobalt; Verhoeff's circles.**

**test, dye dilution** A test for detecting a blockage in the lacrimal (or drainage) system. It consists of instilling a few drops of fluorescein (or a mixture of rose bengal and fluorescein) into the conjunctival sac and observing how long it takes before it dilutes which is shown by the change in colour. No change in colour indicates a blockage or a lack of tear production.
*See* **lacrimal apparatus; staining, fluorescein; test, Jones I.**

**test, 'E'** *See* **'E' game; chart, illiterate E.**

**test, equalization** *See* **test, balancing.**

**test, fan and block** A test for determining the axis and the amount of astigmatism of the eye. It consists of an astigmatic fan chart with an inner rotating central disc on which are printed an arrowhead forming an acute angle of typically 60° and two sets of mutually perpendicular lines or 'blocks'. The test follows the subjective determination of the best vision sphere which places the circle of least confusion on the retina. A positive spherical lens, of a power equal to half the estimated amount of astigmatism, is placed in front of the eye to create simple myopic astigmatism. The patient is asked to indicate the clearest line(s) on the chart and the arrowhead is rotated until its two sides appear equally blurred. The axis of the correcting negative cylindrical lens is then read on the fan chart. The amount of astigmatism is found when that cylindrical lens is of a power such that the two blocks appear equally clear. *Syn.* fan and block method.
*See* **chart, astigmatic fan; method, fogging.**

**test, Farnsworth** A colour vision test consisting of 85 small discs made up of Munsell colours of approximately equal chroma and value, but of different hue for normal observers. The examinee must place the discs so that they appear in a continuous and smooth series. Errors are scored and a diagnosis of the type and severity of the colour defect can be made. A smaller version of the Farnsworth test called the **Farnsworth D-15** exists (Figs T3 and T4). It consists of only 15 small discs and the procedure is the same but it is a more rapid test which does not give as much information as the large version. However, it has been found to be very valuable for detecting severe colour vision defects, including tritanopia. There exist also some versions of this test in which the colour samples are less saturated than the standard ones: (1) The **L'Anthony desaturated D-15 test** in which the colour samples are less saturated by 2 units of Munsell chroma but also lighter by 3 units of Munsell value than the standard D-15 test, and (2) the **Adams desaturated D-15 test** in which only the saturation (or chroma) has been reduced by 2 units. These desaturated D-15 tests are more effective in detecting mild colour vision deficiencies than the standard D-15 test. *Syn.* Farnsworth–Munsell 100 Hue test (or FM 100 Hue test).
*See* **colour vision, defective; lamp, Macbeth; Munsell colour system.**

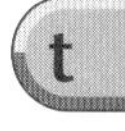


**test, Farnsworth–Munsell 100 Hue** *See* **test, Farnsworth.**

**test, fluorescein 1.** A test to assess the fit of hard contact lenses. Fluorescein is instilled between the cornea and the contact lens and under ultraviolet illumination areas where the lens touches the cornea appear purple or blue, whereas areas where there is a space between the lens and the

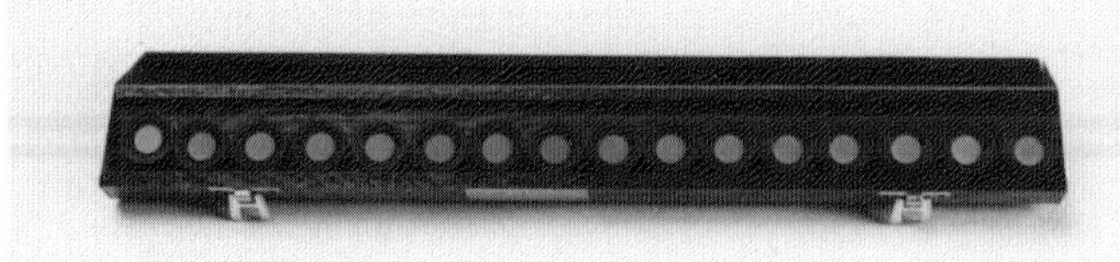

**Fig. T3** Farnsworth D-15 test

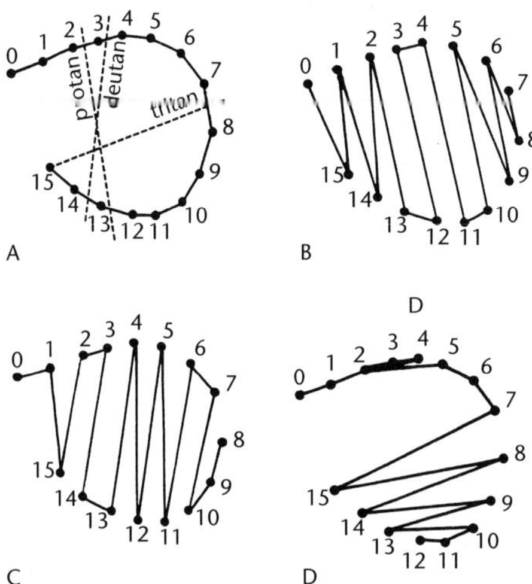


**Fig. T4** Score sheet of the Farnsworth D-15 colour test as arranged by a subject, A with normal colour vision, B with a protan defect, C with a deutan defect, and D with a tritan defect (0 is the fixed reference cap and 1–15 are the moveable caps which the subject must arrange in a logical sequence of colours)

cornea appear yellowish green. This appearance is often referred to as **fluorescein pattern**. **2.** Test using fluorescein and ultraviolet illumination to detect abrasions or other corneal epithelial defects which stain yellowish green.
*See* **bearing, apical; fluorescein; lamp, Burton; rose bengal; staining; test, Jones I; test, Jones II.**

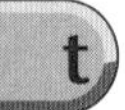

**test, fogging** *See* **method, fogging.**

**test, forced duction** A test for differentiating between a muscle paresis and a mechanical restriction of the eye. The eye in which the conjunctiva is anaesthetized is grasped with toothless forceps and passively rotated in the direction of action of the suspected paretic muscle. If the eye cannot be rotated further than the point where the patient can voluntarily rotate it, a mechanical restriction exists (e.g. a fracture of the orbital floor): if the examiner can passively rotate the eye to its full extent, the muscle is paretic. *Syn.* traction test.
*See* **paralysis of the third nerve; syndrome, Brown's superior oblique tendon sheath; test, Bielschowsky's head tilt; test, three-step.**

**test, four dot** *See* **test, Worth's four dot.**

**test, four prism dioptre base out** A test for the detection of microstrabismus and for the assessment of the suppression area. A 4 Δ BO is placed momentarily in front of the fixating eye (or the eye with the best acuity) and if the other eye moves outward but does not refixate inward it indicates suppression in that eye and a small angle strabismus. Microstrabismus is also indicated if, when the prism is placed BO in front of the eye which showed suppression, there is no movement of either eye. The extent of the suppression area can be assessed by momentarily placing prisms, of various powers and in various directions, in front of the affected eye until diplopia is noticed. The observation of the patient's eye movements is difficult because of the small angle of deviation and because of the variation in size of the suppression area. *Syn.* Irvine's prism displacement test.
*See* **microtropia; suppression.**

**test, FRIEND** A subjective test for simultaneous binocular vision in which the word FRIEND printed with the letters FIN in green and RED in red is viewed through red and green filters, one before each eye. People with simultaneous binocular vision see all the letters, whereas those with suppression see only some of the letters.
*See* **suppression; test, Worth's four dot.**

**test, Frisby stereo** *See* **stereotest, Frisby.**

**test, Gardner Reversal-Frequency** *See* **test, developmental and perceptual screening.**

**test, gradient** *See* **AC/A ratio.**

**test, von Graefe's** *See* **test, diplopia.**

**test, Hering after-image** *See* **test, after-image.**

**test, Hess–Lancaster** A test for measuring and classifying strabismus using the Hess screen.
*See* **screen, Hess.**

**test, Hirschberg's** *See* **method, Hirschberg's.**

**test, hole in the card** A test for determining which eye is dominant. It consists of a card with a hole in it, through which the patient views a spotlight (or a letter) on a distant test chart while holding the card with both hands. The eye that the patient uses to view the letter is the dominant eye. This is easily detected by having

the patient occlude each eye in turn and when the dominant eye is covered the spotlight can no longer be seen through the hole. *Syn.* Dolman's test.
*See* **dominance, ocular; manoptoscope.**

**test, hole in the hand** A test for binocular vision in which a distant object is viewed through a tube with one eye while a hand is placed against the tube at a distance of some 20–30 cm before the other eye. Subjects who see the object through an apparent hole in the hand have binocular vision, whereas seeing either the object through the tube only or the hand only indicates an absence of binocular vision. *Syn.* hole in the hand illusion.

**test, Holmgren's** *See* **test, wool.**

**test, Howard–Dolman** A test for measuring stereoscopic visual acuity consisting of two black vertical rods on a white background, viewed through an aperture from a distance of 6 m. By means of a double cord pulley arrangement, the subject manipulates one of the rods until it appears in the same plane as the fixed rod. The distance between the two rods is then measured, and calculations must be made to arrive at the acuity.
*See* **acuity, stereoscopic visual; test, three-needle; test, two-dimensional.**

**test, Humphriss immediate contrast** *See* **method, Humphriss.**

**test, infinity balance** *See* **test, Turville infinity balance.**

**test, Irvine's prism displacement** *See* **test, four prism dioptre base out.**

**test, Ishihara** *See* **plates, pseudoisochromatic.**

**test, Jackson crossed cylinder** *See* **test for astigmatism, cross-cylinder.**

**test, Jones I** A test to evaluate the tear drainage system. Fluorescein dye is instilled into the conjunctival sac. Over a period of 5 minutes at one-minute intervals, a cotton-tipped applicator is placed under the anaesthetized inferior nasal turbinate. Absence of dye suggests a blockage somewhere in the passage, the nasolacrimal duct being the most common site. Jones II test may then be performed. *Syn.* fluorescein instillation test; primary Jones test.

**test, Jones II** After Jones I test, fluorescein is washed out and physiological saline is injected into the anaesthetized lower canaliculus. If the fluid recovered from the nose is fluorescein-stained the test is positive indicating a partial obstruction in the nasolacrimal duct, otherwise there is a blockage in the punctum, canaliculus or common canaliculus or a defective pumping mechanism of the tears.
*See* **lacrimal apparatus; test, dye dilution.**

**test, Krimsky's** *See* **method, Krimsky's.**

**test, Lang** *See* **stereotest, Lang.**

**test, lantern** An occupational colour vision test used mainly to evaluate recognition of aviation and maritime signals. There are several such tests (e.g. Edridge–Green lantern, Giles–Archer lantern, Holmes–Wright lantern, Farnsworth lantern or Falant). The latter two show colours in pairs of which there are nine and the observer's task is to name the colours.
*See* **Edridge–Green lantern.**

**test, light-stress** *See* **test, photostress.**

**test, Maddox rod** **1.** *See* **Maddox rod**. **2.** A test for measuring cyclophoria in which a Maddox rod is placed in front of each eye, with axes parallel, while the subject views a spot light through a 10 to 15 Δ prism (to displace one image relative to the other). The subject will then see two streaks. If they appear parallel there is no cyclophoria. If not, one of the Maddox rods is rotated slowly until the subject reports that the two streaks are parallel. The angle of rotation as determined with a protractor scale indicates the amount of cyclophoria.
*See* **cyclophoria; Maddox rod; test, double-prism.**

**test, Maddox wing** *See* **Maddox wing.**

**test, Mallett** *See* **Mallett fixation disparity unit.**

**test, manoptoscope** *See* **manoptoscope.**

**test, motility** A test aimed at investigating the integrity of the extraocular muscles and their innervation. The most common method is to have the patient fixate a penlight, which is moved in eight meridians while keeping a still head: up, up and to the right, right, down and to the right, down, down and to the left, left, up and to the left, following a star pattern. The test can be done either binocularly or monocularly. Such movements will test the action of all six extraocular muscles of both eyes. If, for example, the penlight is moved up and to the right of the patient, any limitation in movement indicates a fault in either the right superior rectus or the left inferior oblique muscle. (Fig. T5)
*See* **cardinal positions of gaze; movement, pursuit; muscles, extraocular; muscles, yoke; positions of gaze, diagnostic; test, red-glass.**

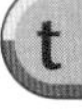


**test at near, cross-cylinder** A subjective test performed (monocularly or binocularly) at a distance of usually 40 cm with the patient wearing his or her subjectively determined lenses and cross-cylinder lenses with axes horizontal and vertical and viewing a test chart composed of parallel, horizontal and vertical black lines. Beginning with sufficient fogging lens power, the plus lens power is reduced until the patient reports that the vertical and horizontal lines are equally distinct. This finding represents an

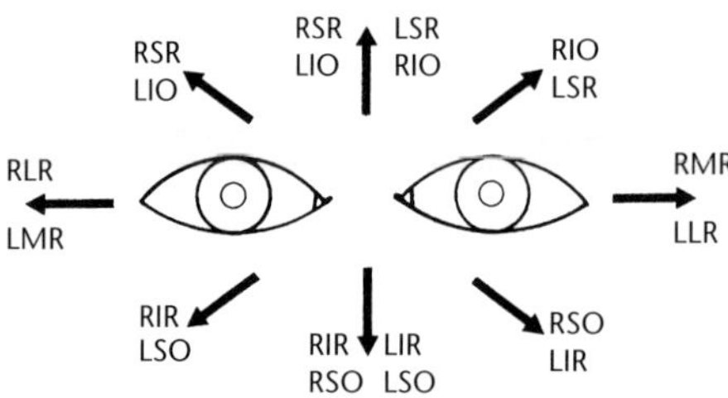


**Fig. T5** Diagnostic positions of gaze indicating the muscles which have maximum power to move the eyes in the direction of the arrows (RIO, LIO, right and left inferior oblique; RIR, LIR, right and left inferior rectus; RLR, LLR, right and left lateral rectus; RMR, LMR, right and left medial rectus; RSO, LSO, right and left superior oblique; RSR, LSR, right and left superior rectus)

additional method of determining the addition for near vision.
*See* **addition; method, fogging.**

**test, neutral density filter** A test to differentiate between functional and organic amblyopia by measuring visual acuity with or without a neutral density filter. If acuity is greatly reduced when looking through the filter, the amblyopia is organic (e.g. glaucoma, central retinal lesions), but if the acuity is unaffected or even slightly improved, the amblyopia is functional. The validity of this test has been questioned. *Syn.* Ammann's test; dark filter test.

**test, New Aniseikonia** A test for measuring aniseikonia. It consists of a booklet with pairs of half-moons, one green, the other red and of different sizes. The patient wears red and green filters and is asked to point to the set of half-moons that appear to have identical vertical diameters. If the sizes are actually equal the patient has no vertical aniseikonia; if the sizes are actually unequal the patient has vertical aniseikonia of a percentage amount indicated next to the target. The booklet is rotated to a horizontal position to measure the horizontal aniseikonia.

**test, non-invasive break-up time (NIBUT)** A test which does not require any interference with the eye used for assessing the stability of the precorneal tear film. The patient's head rests on a chin rest at the centre of a hemispherical bowl of 20 cm radius which is attached at the apex to a binocular microscope. A grid of white lines on a matt black background is inscribed on the inner surface of the bowl and the image of this grid pattern projected onto the open eye is observed. The subject fixates a hole in the centre of the grid pattern and refrains from blinking. The time taken for the appearance of the first randomly distributed distortion or discontinuity of some of the reflected grid lines is a measure of the precorneal tear film break-up. The values for normal subjects vary between 5 and 200 seconds with a mean of around 40 seconds. The instrument used to measure NIBUT is often referred to as a **toposcope.**
*See* **Tearscope plus; test, break-up time.**

**test, Norn's** A test for assessing tear secretion. It consists of instilling one drop of a mixture of 1% fluorescein and 1% rose bengal into the lower conjunctival sac. After 5 minutes a slit-lamp examination is made of the colour of the stain in the central portion of the tear meniscus along the lower lid. The colour may be compared either with known dilutions of the mixture in capillary tubes or simply classified into five colours: intense red, pale red, intense orange, weak orange and yellow. In normal eyes the colour is yellow or weak orange whereas in a dry eye it is red. *Syn.* tear dilution test.
*See* **eye, dry; keratitis sicca; test, break-up time; test, non-invasive break-up time; test, phenol red cotton thread; test, Schirmer's.**

**test object** *See* **test type.**

**test, optokinetic nystagmus (OKN)** A test for eliciting OKN. The subject sits in front of a rotating drum covered with uniform black and white vertical stripes parallel to the axis of rotation (this apparatus is called an **optokinetoscope** or **optokinetic drum**). When the eyes respond with a slow movement in the same direction as the drum lasting about 0.2 s, and a fast phase in the reverse direction of about 0.1 s, the OKN has been elicited and this fact provides evidence of vision. As finer and finer black and white stripes are used, this reflex response will cease to be elicited for a particular spatial frequency of the stripes corresponding to the **objective visual acuity** of the subject. (Fig. T6)
*See* **malingering; nystagmus.**

**test, Pepper** A test for assessing reading performance in low vision patients. It emphasizes the visual rather than the cognitive component of reading. Thus, each chart consists of unrelated letters and words, rather than continuous text. Each row contains either separate letters (at the top of the chart) or separate words (of increasing length in the lower portion of the chart), all of the same size. Missing the first or last half of the word indicates the position of the scotoma relative to the fixation point. The rows at the top of the chart are triple line spaced, they are double line spaced in the middle and single line spaced at the bottom, thus requiring more and more exacting saccadic eye movements. There are five charts, each of different sized print. A reading rate, such as the number of correct units read per minute, can be determined with this test. *Syn.* Pepper Visual Skills for Reading Test (VSRT).
*See* **vision, low.**

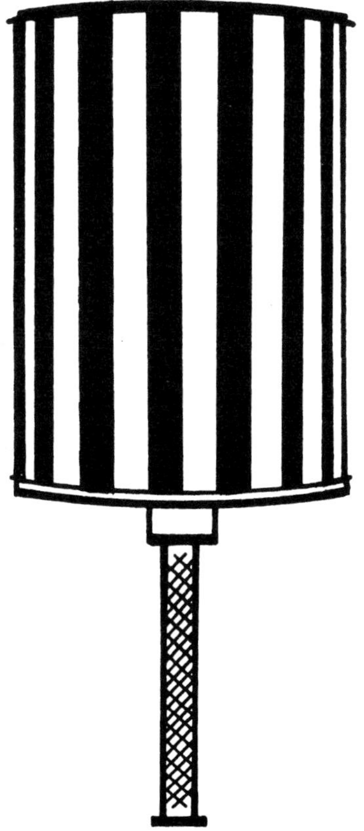

Fig. T6 Optokinetic drum

**test, phenol red cotton thread** A test for measuring tear secretion. It is accomplished by using a special cotton thread, impregnated with phenol red dye. The thread is inserted under the lower eyelid for 15 seconds, and both eyes are closed. The absorption of tears is determined by the length of thread that has turned from red to yellow (due to the pH of tears). The average length varies between 3 and 48 mm, and less than 9 mm is usually indicative of a dry eye. This test is much quicker and much less uncomfortable than Schirmer's test and has good reliability. However, questions have been raised as to whether it is the actual secretion rate which is being measured. There exist several **cotton thread tests** to measure tear secretion, using different cottons of different lengths and diameters and some are used without phenol red dye.
*See* **tear secretion; test, Norn's; test, Schirmer's.**

**test, phi phenomenon of Verhoeff** *See* **movement, phi.**

**test, photostress** A test to differentiate the cause of a reduced visual acuity in one eye, between a lesion in the optic nerve and a disease in the fundus of the eye. A bright light is directed into the eye with the best acuity, for 10 seconds, while the defective eye is covered. The light is then removed and the patient is instructed to read the line just above the best visual acuity line for that eye. The time taken until the patient can just read that line is recorded. The same procedure is then repeated with the defective eye. If the recovery time is about the same in both eyes, the cause of the reduced visual acuity is an optic nerve lesion (e.g. retrobulbar optic neuritis); if the recovery time is much longer for the defective eye the cause is in the fundus (e.g. retinal oedema, retinopathy, age-related maculopathy). The latter is attributed to a delay in the regeneration of visual pigments after being bleached with a bright light. *Syn.* light-stress test.

**test, pinhole** *See* **disc, pinhole.**

**test, plus 1.00 D blur** A check test used to verify a patient's spherical correction or to determine whether a person is hypermetropic. It consists of placing a +1.00 D lens in front of the eye: visual acuity should be reduced from 6/6 (20/20) to about 6/18 (20/60). If the patient can still read smaller letters than 6/18, the spherical prescription is incorrect or the patient is hypermetropic. This result could also be due to a much smaller pupil than average. This test is most helpful with young children as it helps relax accommodation. *Syn.* blur back test.
*See* **hypermetropia, absolute; method, fogging.**

**test, prism adaptation** A prognostic test in cases of esotropia, indicating whether surgical intervention is favourable or not. Prior to the intervention, the patient has to wear a BO prism, of an amount larger than the angle of deviation, for an hour or more. An increase in the angle of deviation is an unfavourable prognosis and no increase or a decrease is considered favourable.
*See* **strabismus, convergent.**

**test, prism dissociation** *See* **test, diplopia.**

**test, prism reflex** *See* **method, Krimsky's.**

**test, prone position** *See* **test, provocative.**

**test, provocative** A test performed to reproduce signs of a suspected disease in order to help in the diagnosis of that disease. A common provocative test for open-angle glaucoma is the **water-drinking test** in which a fasting patient has to drink one quart of water (or about 1 litre in a 70-kg adult) within 5 minutes. The IOP is measured before the water is taken and then at 15-minute intervals. An increase of 8 mmHg or more in 45 minutes is considered positive. Two common provocative tests for angle-closure glaucoma are: (1) The **dark room test** in which the patient is kept in a dark room for 1 hour and the IOP is measured before and after the test. An increase of 8 mmHg or more is generally considered positive. (2) The **prone position test** in which the patient lies in the prone position for 1 hour and if the IOP increases by 8 mmHg or more, compared to the value before the test, the result is considered positive. In open-angle glaucoma provocative tests have been found to be positive in less than half of the patients but that figure is higher in angle-closure glaucoma. *See* **glaucoma, angle-closure; glaucoma, open-angle; pressure, intraocular.**

**test, Purkinje tree** *See* **angioscotoma.**

**test, push-up 1.** *See* **method, push-up. 2.** A procedure used to ensure adequate lens movement of a soft contact lens. The lens is gently pushed upward by pressing on the patient's lower eyelid: it should move easily and return quickly to its original location.

**test, random-dot E** *See* **stereogram, random-dot.**

**test, Raubitschek** *See* **chart, Raubitschek.**

**test, red glass** A test for determining diplopia or suppression in which a bright target (e.g. a white light) is fixated while a red filter is held in front of one eye to interrupt fusion. The patient with diplopia will see a red light and a white light. The amount of deviation can be estimated by using a prism of an amount such that it eliminates the double image. The operation can be repeated in all the diagnostic positions of gaze to help identify a paretic extraocular muscle as the distance between the two images increases in the field of action of the paretic muscle. If only one light is seen it indicates suppression of one retinal image. *Syn.* red filter test.
*See* **primary action; suppression; test, diplopia; test, motility.**

**test, Scheiner's** A test for measuring the monocular near point of accommodation. It consists of using a Scheiner's disc in front of the eye which observes a small target such as a thin black line. The target is moved towards the eye until it is no longer seen single. That point represents the near point of accommodation.
*See* **accommodation, near point of; experiment, Scheiner's.**

**test, Schirmer's** A test for measuring tear secretion. It is accomplished by using a 35 × 5 mm strip of filter paper (e.g. Whatman No. 41). The filter strip is folded so that one end, about 5 mm long, is inserted at the mid-portion (or lateral portion) of the lower eyelid of a patient seated in a dimly lit room. Tear secretion is considered normal if 10 mm or more of the paper from the point of the fold becomes wet in a 4-minute period. More than 25 mm of wetting would indicate excessive tear secretion. Without any additional stimulation of any kind the test, called **Schirmer's test I**, measures mainly the basal tear production, but because the filter paper tends to irritate the conjunctiva, some of the reflex tear secretion may be also be measured as well. **Schirmer's test II** is aimed at measuring mainly reflex tear secretion. It is carried out with the filter paper inserted inside the lower lid of an eye with topical anaesthesia, while the contralateral half of the nasal mucosa is irritated by rubbing it with a dry cotton-tipped applicator. The amount of tear production is measured after 2 minutes. A value of more than 15 mm is considered to be normal and less than 15 mm may indicate a deficiency of reflex tear secretion. (Fig. T7)
*See* **alacrima; keratitis sicca; tear secretion; test, Norn's; test, phenol red cotton thread.**

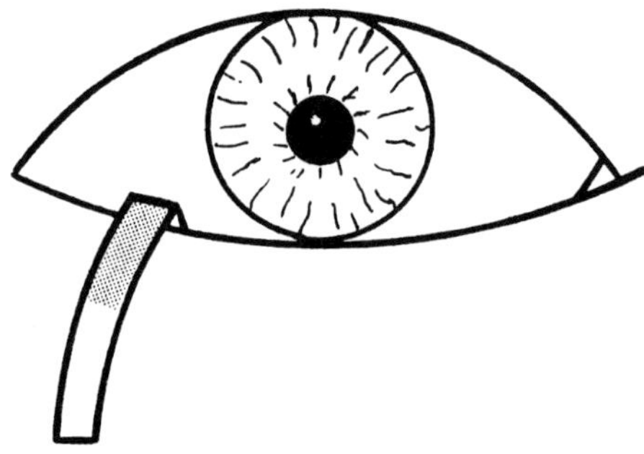

**Fig. T7** Schirmer's test

**test, screen** *See* **test, cover.**

**test, sessile drop** Measurement of the contact angle by observation of the formation of a drop of liquid on a solid surface. The image of the droplet may be photographed or projected.
*See* **angle, contact.**

**test, shadow 1.** A test which gives an approximate evaluation of the depth of the anterior chamber. It is carried out by placing a penlight on the temporal side of the eye at the level of the pupil and directing the beam of light horizontally towards the inner side of the eye. If the iris lies in a flat plane which usually indicates a deep anterior chamber the entire iris will be illuminated. If the iris is directed anteriorly, which usually indicates a narrow anterior chamber, the iris on the temporal side of the eye will be illuminated but the iris on the nasal side will be shadowed to varying degrees depending on the narrowness of the anterior chamber (Fig. T8). *Syn.* oblique illumination shadow test. **2.** *See* **retinoscopy. 3.** A test for the homogeneity of a lens (both material and surface quality) in which the light from a small, intense source of light

passes through the lens and falls on a screen. Any defects will show as shadows.
*See* **angle of the anterior chamber; glaucoma, angle-closure; glaucoma, open-angle; method, van Herick, Shaffer and Schwartz.**

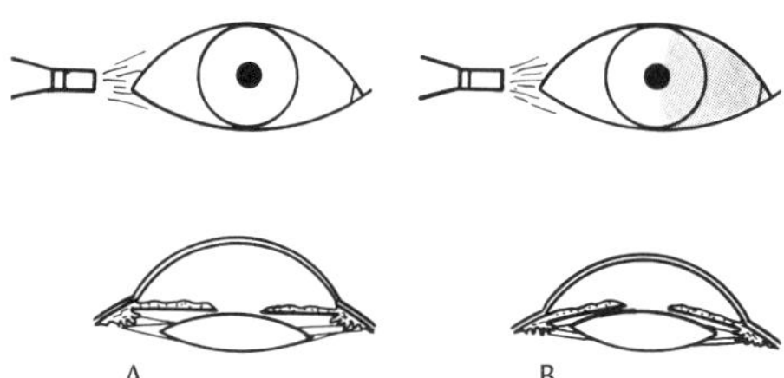


**Fig. T8** Two different widths of the angle of the anterior chamber. A, open angle associated with a deep anterior chamber. B, narrow angle associated with a narrow anterior chamber. Only the iris on the temporal side is illuminated, as shown in the upper diagram

**test, Sheridan–Gardiner** A visual acuity test consisting of a large card (called the key card) which is held by the patient who is asked to point to the letter on that key card that is the same as the letter shown on the distance (or near) chart. The test consists of several cards with single letters of various sizes. It is most useful for testing children and illiterates.

**test, Simultan** *See* **Simultantest.**

**test, stereotest** *See* **stereotest, Frisby; stereotest, Lang; vectogram.**

**test, swinging flashlight** *See* **pupil, Marcus Gunn.**

**test target** *See* **test type.**

**test, tear** *See* **test, basic secretion; test, break-up time; test, non-invasive break-up time; test, phenol red cotton thread; test, Schirmer's.**

**test, tear dilution** *See* **test, Norn's.**

**test, Thorington** A test for the measurement of heterophoria at near and at distance. It consists of a horizontal row of letters on one side of a light source and a horizontal row of numbers on the other side of that source. A Maddox rod, orientated horizontally, is placed in front of one eye and the patient who is fixating the light source is asked to report through which letter or number the vertical streak appears to pass, or to which it is closest. At 6 m the number of letters must be placed 6 cm apart to represent 1 Δ steps. If the Maddox rod is in front of the right eye, the numbers on the right side of the source and the letters on the left, each number represents 1 Δ of esophoria and each letter represents 1 Δ of exophoria. The Thorington test can also be used at near. At 40 cm, for example, the separation of the letters and numbers must be 0.4 cm to represent 1 Δ. It can also be placed vertically with the Maddox rod orientated vertically to measure vertical heterophoria.
*See* **heterophoria; Maddox rod.**

**test, three-dimensional** *See* **test, two-dimensional.**

**test, three-needle** A test for measuring stereoscopic visual acuity consisting of three fine rods placed vertically, two of them being fixed in the same plane, while the third one is movable in between. The subject views them through an aperture. The centre rod is placed in various positions backward and forward until the subject judges whether it is nearer or farther than the others (Fig. T9).
*See* **stereopsis; test, Howard–Dolman.**

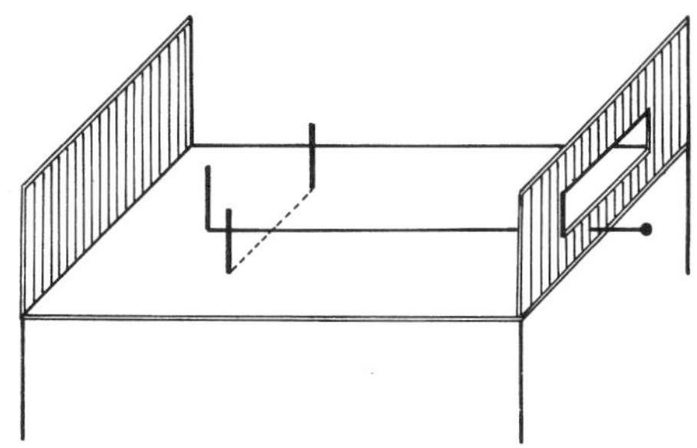

**Fig. T9** Three-needle test

**test, three-step** An objective test for determining which extraocular muscle is paretic in a patient with hypertropia. A three-step procedure is used: (1) to determine the type of hypertropia (right or left); (2) to determine the magnitude of the hypertropia (e.g. with prisms and cover test) when the patient fixates to the right and to the left; (3) to determine the magnitude of the hypertropia when the head is tilted towards each shoulder. Each step in this procedure reduces the number of possible muscles involved until it points to only one muscle of one eye. *Example*: paresis of the left superior oblique. Step (1) a left hypertropia points to a paresis of one of the following four muscles: left superior oblique, left inferior rectus, right inferior oblique or right superior rectus. Step (2) a hypertropia of the left eye increases when fixating to the right points to a paresis of either the left superior oblique or the right superior rectus. Step (3) a hypertropia of the left eye which increases when the head tilts to the left, points to a paresis of the left superior oblique.
*See* **test, Bielschowsky's head tilt; test, forced duction.**

**test, Titmus stereo** *See* **vectogram.**

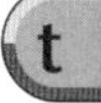

**test, Turville infinity balance (TIB)** A test for balancing the accommodative state of the eyes. It can also be used for detecting suppression, vertical and horizontal associated phorias and (with a target composed of two horizontal lines) aniseikonia in the vertical meridian. It consists of a 3 cm wide vertical septum placed in the centre of a mirror on which is reflected a reversed illuminated chart. Thus the patient can only see the right side of the chart with the right eye, and the left side with the left eye, which allows for simultaneous comparison of the chart seen by both eyes, while still retaining fusion for peripheral objects near the border of the chart. If the chart is projected onto a screen, the septum is placed halfway between patient and screen. The test is carried out after the conventional refractive procedures. *Syn.* infinity balance test.
*See* **balance, binocular; heterophoria, associated; suppression; test, balancing.**

**test, two-dimensional** A test for stereopsis consisting of two-dimensional objects as test material such as targets, cards, etc. as used in a stereoscope or a major amblyoscope (e.g. random-test stereogram; Titmus stereotest). Other tests for stereopsis are **three-dimensional** (3-D), the Howard–Dolman test being the most well known. Two-dimensional tests (2-D) are the most commonly used in clinical practice.
*See* **stereogram, random-dot; stereoscope; stereo-test; test, Howard–Dolman; vectogram.**

**test type** Any letter, figure or character used for vision testing. The term **test object** (*syn.* **test target**) is a more general term which encompasses any pattern or object (e.g. checkerboard, grating).
*See* **chart; grating; Jaeger test type; König bars; Landolt ring; optotype; pattern, checkerboard.**

**test, Verhoeff phi phenomenon** *See* **movement, phi.**

**test of Visual Analysis Skills** *See* **test, developmental and perceptual screening.**

**test, water-drinking** *See* **test, provocative.**

**test, Welland's** *See* **test, bar reading.**

**test, wool** A test for assessing colour vision deficiencies. It consists of a set of wool strands which are to be matched with loose wool strands of the same colour. The most well known of these is the **Holmgren's test**. *Syn.* colour wool test.

**test, Worth's four dot** A test for determining the presence of binocular vision. It consists of four illuminated discs: two green, one red and one white on a black background. The test is viewed at any distance by a subject wearing red and green filters such that one eye sees the red and the white discs, while the other eye sees the two green discs and the white disc. Subjects are asked to report how many dots they see: four dots indicates normal binocular vision; two dots, both red, indicates suppression of the image in the eye wearing the green filter; three dots, all green, indicates suppression of the image in the eye wearing the red filter; and five dots, two red and three green, indicates diplopia. *Syn.* four dot test.
*See* **suppression; test, FRIEND; vision, Worth's classification of binocular.**

**testing in parallel** Clinical test performed in such a way that different parameters are examined simultaneously. The effect of one parameter on another can be noticed and the final results appropriately altered. *Examples*: Parallel-Testing Infinity Balance test; Parallel-Testing Near Balance test; Turville Infinity Balance test.
*See* **testing in series.**

**testing in series** Clinical tests performed one after the other. Each parameter is measured and corrected and assumed to remain fixed afterward.
*See* **testing in parallel.**

**tetracaine hydrochloride (amethocaine)** A topical corneal anaesthetic, commonly used in 0.25–1% solution. It may be used to carry out tonometry, to remove a foreign body, etc.
*See* **benoxinate; cocaine; lidocaine; proxymetacaine.**

**tetrachromatic theory** *See* **theory, Hering's of colour vision.**

**tetracycline** *See* **antibiotic.**

**textural gradient** One of the monocular cues of depth perception produced by the change in the appearance of the grain of the structure of a surface, giving the impression that the thin, small details must be further away than the thick, large ones (Fig. T10).
*See* **perception, depth.**

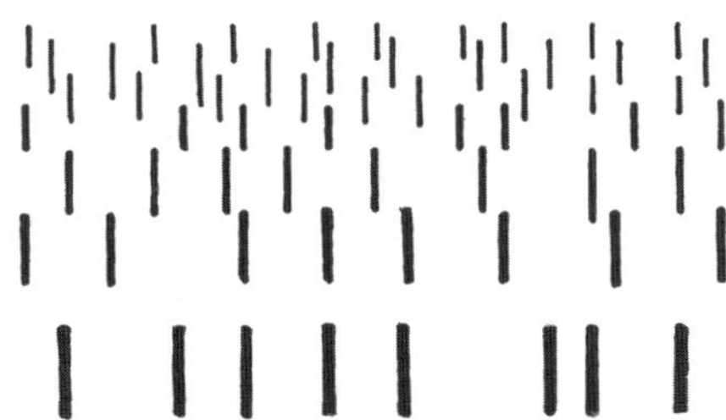

Fig. T10 An example of textural gradient

**thalamus** One of a pair of ovoid masses of grey substance which serves as a relay station for sensory stimuli to the cerebral cortex. It contains the lateral geniculate body, which is a continuation of the pulvinar and which is situated at the posterior end of the thalamus.
*See* **geniculate bodies, lateral.**

**theories of strabismus** Many theories have been presented to explain strabismus. They tend to fall into five categories: (1) Theories in which the cause of strabismus is a defect of motor fusion. This view was first developed by **Worth** who suggested a congenital absence or defect of the fusion faculty. **Chavasse** did not confine his view to a congenitally defective fusion mechanism, but held that strabismus could be the result of interference with the development of the binocular reflexes. Similarly, **Keiner** and **Zeeman** proposed that the causative factor in strabismus was a disturbance of the optomotor reflexes (or psycho-optical reflexes). Keiner believed that this disturbance was due to a delay in the process of myelination of nerve fibres in the visual pathway during the plastic stage of development. (2) Other theories have postulated that strabismus is due to mechanical factors such as anomalies of the ligaments, the muscles (or their insertions), and even of the orbit. Proponents of these theories were **Scobee**, **Nordlow**, **von Graefe**, **Landolt**, **Stilling**, etc. (3) The role of accommodation and refraction has also been proposed as a cause of strabismus, especially by **Donders**. He postulated that esotropia was due to uncorrected hypermetropia, and exotropia to uncorrected myopia. This is the best substantiated theory of the cause of certain types of strabismus. (4) Other authors suggested that strabismus was due to an anomaly in the brain and nerves (**Mackenzie**) and particularly to the innervation in the vergence systems (**Duane**, **Parinaud**, etc.). (5) Theories in which all the factors cited above contribute in varying degrees to the cause of strabismus (**Bielschowsky**, **van der Hoeve**, etc.).

**theory** An explanation of the manner in which a phenomenon occurs, has occurred, or will occur.

**theory, Bielschowsky's** *See* **theories of strabismus.**

**theory, biological–statistical** Theory of the development of refractive errors, based on the way in which the refractive components of the eye combine. It postulates a high correlation between the normally distributed refractive components to produce emmetropia. A breakdown of this correlation leads to ametropia. This theory depends essentially on hereditary factors.
*See* **myopia, physiological; theory, emmetropization; theory, use–abuse.**

**theory, Chavasse's** *See* **theories of strabismus.**

**theory, corpuscular** *See* **theory, Newton's.**

**theory, Donders'** *See* **theories of strabismus.**

**theory, Duane's** *See* **theories of strabismus.**

**theory, duplicity** The theory that vision is mediated by two independent photoreceptor systems in the retina: diurnal or photopic vision through the cones when the eyes see details and colours; and nocturnal or scotopic vision through the rods when the eyes see at very low levels of luminance.
*See* **cell, cone; cell, rod; interval, photochromatic; Purkinje shift; theory, two visual systems; vision, photopic; vision, scotopic.**

**theory, emission** *See* **theory, Newton's.**

**theory, emmetropization** A theory that explains the phenomenon of emmetropization on a biofeedback mechanism, involving cortical and subcortical control of the various components of the eye which contribute to its refractive power.
*See* **emmetropization.**

**theory, empiricist** Theory that certain aspects of behaviour, perception, development of ametropia, etc. depend on environmental experience and learning, and are not inherited.
*See* **empiricism; theory, nativist.**

**theory, Fincham's** Theory of accommodation which attributes the increased convexity of the front surface of the crystalline lens, when accommodating, to the elasticity of the capsule and to the fact that it is thinner in the pupillary area than near the periphery of the lens.
*See* **capsule; lens, crystalline; theory, Helmholtz's of accommodation.**

**theory, first order** *See* **theory, gaussian.**

**theory, gaussian** The theory that for tracing paraxial rays through an optical system, that system can be considered as having six cardinal planes: two principal planes, two nodal planes and two focal planes. The mathematical analysis can be carried out by the paraxial equation.
*Syn.* first order theory; paraxial theory.
*See* **Newton's formula; optics, paraxial; paraxial equation, fundamental; ray, paraxial.**

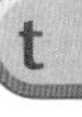


**theory, von Graefe's** *See* **theories of strabismus.**

**theory, Helmholtz's of accommodation** The theory that in accommodation the ciliary muscle contracts, relaxing the tension on the zonule of Zinn while the shape of the crystalline lens changes, resulting in increased convexity, especially of the anterior surface. Fincham's theory complements that of Helmholtz.

**Table T1** Main characteristics of the photopic and scotopic visual system

| | photopic vision | scotopic vision |
|---|---|---|
| type of vision | diurnal (above 10 cd/m$^2$) | nocturnal (below 10$^{-3}$ cd/m$^2$) |
| photoreceptor | cones | rods |
| max. receptor density | fovea | 20° from fovea |
| photopigment(s) (and max. absorption) | long-wave sensitive (560 nm)<br>middle-wave sensitive (530 nm)<br>short-wave sensitive (420 nm) | rhodopsin (507 nm) |
| colour vision | present | absent |
| light sensitivity | low | high |
| dark adaptation | | |
| time to cone threshold | about 10 min | |
| time to rod threshold (about 3 log units below) | | about 35 min |
| max. spectral sensitivity | 555 nm | 507 nm |
| spatial resolution (visual acuity) | excellent | poor |
| spatial summation | poor | excellent |
| temporal resolution (critical fusion frequency) | excellent | poor |
| temporal summation | poor | excellent |
| Stiles–Crawford effect | present | absent |

*See* **accommodation; muscle, ciliary; theory, Fincham's; Zinn, zonule of.**

**theory, Helmholtz's of colour vision** *See* **theory, Young–Helmholtz.**

**theory, Hering's of colour vision** Theory that colour vision results from the action of three independent mechanisms, each of which is made up of a mutually antagonistic pair of colour sensations: red-green, yellow-blue and white-black. The latter pair is supposed to be responsible for the brightness aspect of the sensation, whereas the former two would be responsible for the coloured aspect of the sensation. *Syn.* opponent-process theory; tetrachromatic theory.
*See* **cells, colour-opponent; theory, Young–Helmholtz.**

**theory, van der Hoeve's** *See* **theories of strabismus.**

**theory, Huygen's** *See* **theory, wave.**

**theory, Landolt's** *See* **theories of strabismus.**

**theory, lattice** *See* **theory, Maurice's.**

**theory, Luneburg's** A theory according to which the geometry of the visual space is described by a variable non-euclidean hyperbolic metric.

**theory, Mackenzie's** *See* **theories of strabismus.**

**theory, Maurice's** Theory that explains the transparency of the stroma of the cornea. It states that the stromal fibrils, which have a refractive index of about 1.55 in the dry state, are so arranged as to behave as a series of diffraction gratings permitting transmission through the liquid ground substance (refractive index 1.34). The fibrils are the grating elements that are arranged in a hexagonal lattice pattern of equal spacing and with the fibril interval being less than the wavelength of light. The diffraction gratings eliminate scattered light by destructive interference, except for the normally incident light rays. Light beams that are not normal to the cornea are also transmitted to the oblique lattice plane. However, recent work has demonstrated inconsistencies in lattice space and there is some modification to the original postulate of this theory. *Syn.* lattice theory.
*See* **diffraction.**

**theory, nativist** Theory that certain aspects of behaviour, perception, development of ametropia, etc. are inherited and independent of environmental experience.
*See* **nativism; theory, empiricist.**

**theory, Newton's** The theory that light consists of minute particles radiated from a light source at a very high velocity. *Syn.* corpuscular theory; emission theory.
*See* **theory, quantum; theory, wave.**

**theory, Nordlow's** *See* **theories of strabismus.**

**theory, opponent-colour** *See* **theory, Hering's of colour vision.**

**theory, paraxial** *See* **theory, gaussian.**

**theory, Parinaud's** *See* **theories of strabismus.**

**theory, Planck's** *See* **theory, quantum.**

**theory, quantum** Theory that radiant energy consists of intermittent and spasmodic, minute indivisible amounts called quanta (or photons). This is a somewhat modern version of the theory originally proposed by Newton. *Syn.* Planck's theory. *See* **photon; theory, Newton's; theory, wave.**

**theory, Scobee's** *See* **theories of strabismus.**

**theory of strabismus** *See* **theories of strabismus.**

**theory, three-component** *See* **theory, Young–Helmholtz.**

**theory, trichromatic** *See* **theory, Young–Helmholtz.**

**theory, two visual systems** The theory that there are two distinct modes of processing visual information: one pertaining to the identification (or 'what' system) and the other to localization (or 'where' system) of visual stimuli. The identification mode is concerned with resolution and pattern vision, and is associated with the foveal and parafoveal regions of the retina. It is subserved by primary cortical mechanisms. The localization mode is concerned with motion and orientation and is subserved by midbrain visual structures.
*See* **magnocellular visual system; parvocellular visual system; theory, duplicity.**

**theory, use–abuse** Theory which attributes the onset of myopia to an adaptation to the use or misuse of the eyes in prolonged close work. Environmental factors would be the main cause of myopia.
*See* **myopia; theory, biological–statistical.**

**theory, wave** Theory that light is propagated as continuous waves. This theory was quantified by the Maxwell equations. The wave theory of light can satisfactorily account for the observed facts of reflection, refraction, interference, diffraction and polarization. However, the interchange of energy between radiation and matter, absorption and the photoelectric effect are explained by the quantum theory. Both the wave and quantum theories of light were combined by the concept of quantum mechanics, and light is now considered to consist of quanta travelling in a manner that can be described by a wave form. *Syn.* Huygens' theory.
*See* **light; photon; theory, quantum; wavelength.**

**theory, Worth's** *See* **theories of strabismus.**

**theory, Young–Helmholtz** The theory that colour vision is due to a combination of the responses of three independent types of retinal receptors whose maximum sensitivities are situated in the blue, green and red regions of the visible spectrum. This theory has been shown to be correct, except that the pigment in the third receptor has a maximum sensitivity in the yellow and not in the red region of the spectrum. Hering's theory of colour vision, which explains phenomena at a level higher than that of the cone receptors, complements this theory. *Syn.* Helmholtz's theory of colour vision; three components theory; trichromatic theory.
*See* **pigment, visual; theory, Hering's of colour vision.**

**theoretical eye** *See* **eye, reduced; eye, schematic.**

**therapeutic soft contact lens** *See* **lens, therapeutic soft contact.**

**thimerosal** *See* **antiseptic.**

**third-degree fusion** *See* **stereopsis; vision, Worth's classification of binocular.**

**third cranial nerve** *See* **nerve, oculomotor.**

**third nerve paralysis** *See* **paralysis of the third nerve.**

**Thorington test** *See* **test, Thorington.**

**Thorpe four mirror fundus lens** *See* **slit-lamp.**

**three and nine o'clock staining** *See* **staining, 3 and 9 o'clock.**

**three dimension** *See* **perception, depth; stereopsis; stereoscopy.**

**three-needle test** *See* **test, three-needle.**

**threshold** The value of a stimulus that just produces a response. *Syn.* limen.

**threshold, absolute** The minimum luminance of a source that will produce a sensation of light. It varies with the state of dark adaptation, the retinal area stimulated, the wavelength of light, etc. *Syn.* light threshold.
*See* **interval, photochromatic.**

**threshold, contrast** *See* **threshold, differential.**

**threshold, differential** The smallest difference between two stimuli presented simultaneously that gives rise to a perceived difference in sensation. The difference may be related to brightness, but also to colour and specifically to either saturation (while hue is kept constant) or hue (while saturation is kept constant). The differential threshold of luminance is equal to about 1% in photopic vision. *Syn.* contrast threshold (if the difference is one of luminance); just noticeable difference (jnd).
*See* **law, Weber's; sensitivity, contrast.**

**threshold, light** *See* **threshold, absolute.**

**threshold, movement** **1.** The minimum motion of an object that can be perceived. **2.** The speed at which an object moving between two points just appears to be moving.
*See* **hyperacuity; movement, phi.**

**threshold, resolution** *See* **resolution, limit of.**

**threshold, stereo-** *See* **acuity, stereoscopic visual.**

**Thygeson's superficial punctate keratitis** *See* **keratitis, punctate epithelial.**

**thymoxamine (moxisylyte)** *See* **alpha-adrenergic antagonist.**

**thyroid eye disease** *See* **disease, Graves'; ophthalmopathy, thyroid.**

**tight junction** Refers to cells in which their membranes are fused rather than separated by a small extracellular space. The movement of substances through that space is restricted. *Syn.* zonulae occludentes.

**tilt, pantoscopic** *See* **angle, pantoscopic.**

**tilt, retroscopic** *See* **angle, retroscopic.**

**tilted optic disc** *See* **crescent, congenital.**

**timolol maleate** *See* **adrenergic receptors; beta-blocker.**

**tinted lens** *See* **lens, tinted.**

**Titmus stereo test** *See* **vectogram.**

**TNO test** *See* **stereogram, random-dot.**

**tobramycin** *See* **antibiotic.**

**tomography, computerized (CT)** A radiographic method of viewing a layer of body structures in which images indicate the X-ray absorption (called attenuation) of tissues (e.g. bones attenuate most, lungs attenuate least and blood vessels are in between). The X-rays are received by numerous gas or solid state detectors and computers are used to store, process and manipulate the information received from these detectors. The method yields far better differentiation of tissues than conventional radiography thus providing more precise diagnostic information. *Examples*: a tumour in the eye which is obscured by a cataract and a tumour of an extraocular muscle can be detected by this technique. *Syn.* computerized axial tomography (CAT); CAT scan; CT scan.
*See* **magnetic resonance imaging; radiology.**

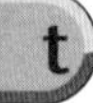

**tone, colour** Term often used in colorimetry, photography and industry to indicate hue.
*See* **hue.**

**tone, muscle** *See* **tonus.**

**tonic accommodation** *See* **accommodation, resting state of.**

**tonic convergence** *See* **vergence, tonic.**

**tonic pupil** *See* **pupil, Adie's.**

**tonic vergence** *See* **vergence, tonic.**

**tonicity** *See* **solution, hypertonic; solution, hypotonic; solution, isotonic.**

**tonography** Technique for measuring the facility of outflow of aqueous humour from the eye under the continuous pressure exerted by the weight of a tonometer over a given period of time. The instrument usually employed for tonography is an electronically recording Schiötz tonometer. In this technique, the pressure is continuously recorded over a four minute period and the outflow is deduced by utilizing a specifically designed diagram, called a **nomogram** (which is a graphical representation of one, or more, mathematical relationships whereby the desired value may be found without calculation by placing a straight edge across the diagram). The results of tonography can indicate the presence of established glaucoma, although the technique is not very reliable for borderline cases.
*See* **glaucoma; humour, aqueous.**

**tonometer** An instrument for estimating intraocular pressure. It measures either the degree of corneal deformation produced by a known force, or the force needed to produce a given degree of corneal deformation.
*See* **glaucoma; manometer; pressure, intraocular; rigidity, ocular.**

**tonometer, air-puff** *See* **tonometer, non-contact.**

**tonometer, applanation** A tonometer in which the intraocular pressure is estimated either by the force required to flatten a constant corneal area as, for example, in the **Goldmann** and **Perkins** (Fig. T11) tonometers, or by the area flattened by a constant force, as, for example, in the **Maklakov** and **Tonomat** tonometers. The Goldmann tonometer (Fig. T12) is used in conjunction with a slit-lamp and provides an accurate reading with which all other tonometers are usually compared. The Perkins tonometer is a hand-held instrument.
*See* **law, Imbert–Fick.**

**tonometer, electronic** Any tonometer with an electronic readout. These instruments act swiftly, the procedure usually being completed within a fraction of a second.

**tonometer, Goldmann** *See* **tonometer, applanation.**

**tonometer, impression** A tonometer in which the intraocular pressure is estimated by the degree of indentation of the cornea. The excursion of the plunger of the tonometer is read from a calibrated scale and converted into values of the intraocular pressure, often using appropriate tables. The most common such instrument is that of **Schiötz**. *Syn.* indentation tonometer.
*See* **rigidity, ocular.**

**tonometer, indentation** *See* **tonometer, impression.**

**tonometer, Mackay–Marg** An electronic tonometer in which a plunger in the centre of a flat footplate which applanates the cornea protrudes by a very small amount (5 μm). The intraocular pressure is related to the counter force required to resist displacement of this plunger when the cornea is flattened by the footplate. The result is read by interpretation of a graph on a strip chart.

**tonometer, Maklakov's** *See* **tonometer, applanation.**

**tonometer, non-contact (NCT)** A tonometer which does not require any contact to be made between the tonometer and the eye. Hence no anaesthesia is required with this instrument. It consists of sending a puff of air towards the cornea of sufficient strength to flatten a predetermined area of cornea. The time taken from the onset of the puff of air to the applanation of the cornea (which is monitored optically) is recorded electronically and is proportional to the intraocular pressure. A digital readout of pressure, in mmHg, appears within about 15 ms after the measurement is initiated. The same principle is applied in the hand-held **Pulsair** noncontact tonometer and in the **Reichert Non-Contact** tonometer. *Syn.* air-puff tonometer; pneumatic tonometer.

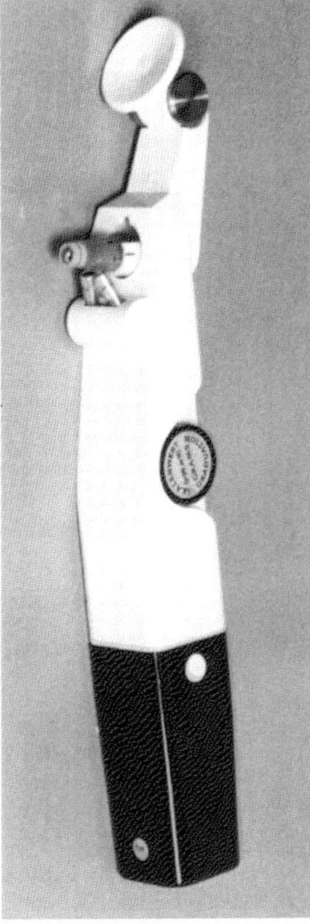

Fig. T11 Perkins tonometer

**tonometer, Perkins** *See* **tonometer, applanation.**

**tonometer, Pulsair noncontact** *See* **tonometer, non-contact.**

**tonometer, Reichert Non-Contact** *See* **tonometer, non-contact.**

**tonometer, Schiötz** *See* **tonometer, impression.**

**tonometer, Tonomat** *See* **tonometer, applanation.**

**tonometry** Measurement of intraocular pressure with a tonometer.
*See* **pressure, intraocular; tonometer.**

**Tonopen** A hand-held, compact, portable applanation tonometer based on the same principle as the Mackay–Marg tonometer. It is a very small instrument, 18 cm long by 2 cm in width weighing 56 g. It incorporates its own battery power supply and liquid crystal digital readout and provides both an intraocular pressure readout and an indicator of the reliability of the instrument. The results correlate well with the Goldmann tonometer, although it slightly overestimates low IOP's and underestimates high IOP's. It can take measurements in an eye with an irregular or oedematous cornea or through a soft contact lens and in a variety of clinical settings. (Fig. T13)
*See* **tonometer, applanation; tonometer, Mackay–Marg.**

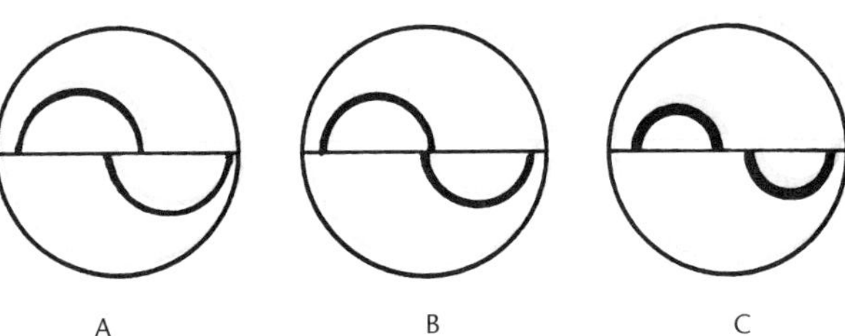


Fig. T12 Fluorescein pattern seen when the head of the Goldmann applanation tonometer rests against the anterior corneal surface. A, the dial reading is greater than the IOP. B, the dial reading is equal to the IOP and the applanated corneal area has a diameter of 3.06 mm. C, the dial reading is less than the IOP

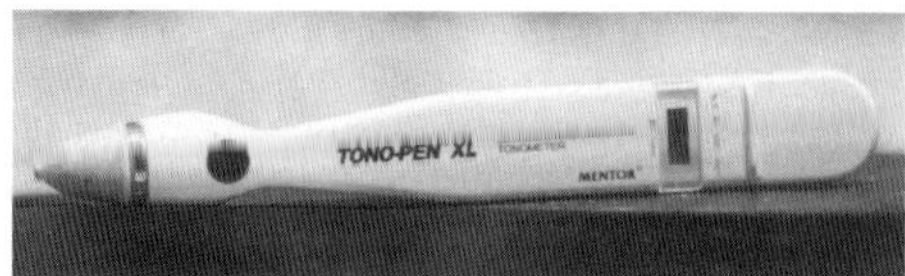


**Fig. T13** Tonopen

**tonus** A state of partial contraction present in a muscle in its passive state as, for example, when the eye is in the physiological position of rest. *Syn.* muscle tone.
*See* **accommodation, resting state of; position of rest, physiological; vergence, tonic.**

**Topogometer** A device attached to a keratometer that allows a measurement of the curvature of the cornea off the visual axis. It consists of an illuminated fixation light that can be moved along two axes, both of which are perpendicular to the axis of the keratometer. Scales are provided with the device to indicate, in millimetres, the amount of decentration of the visual axis from the optical axis of the keratometer at the corneal surface. This device helps in the fitting of contact lenses, by providing an estimation of the flattening of the peripheral cornea and of the position of the corneal apex. This instrument has been superseded by computerized instruments.
*See* **keratometer; videokeratoscope.**

**topography, corneal** A map of the variations in the curvature of the anterior surface of the cornea. It is typically done with a photokeratoscope or a videokeratoscope.
*See* **keratoscope; photokeratoscope; videokeratoscope.**

**Toposcope 1.** An instrument for measuring the curvature of the surfaces of a contact lens, based on moiré fringes. A bar pattern is reflected from the lens surface and the reflected image is viewed with a microscope that has a second bar pattern in the eyepiece. The two bar patterns superimposing each other at slightly different orientations create the **moiré patterns**. The magnification of the microscope is changed until the fringes are parallel to the central index line seen in the field and a dial monitoring this change in magnification indicates the radius of curvature in millimetres. **2.** *See* **test, non-invasive break-up time.**
*See* **optic zone radius, back; radiuscope.**

**toric lens** *See* **lens, toric.**

**toroidal surface** *See* **lens, toric.**

**torsion** Rotation of an eye about an anteroposterior axis. If the upper pole of the vertical meridian of the cornea appears to rotate inward, it is called **intorsion**, and outward, **extorsion**. If the eye rotates to the right it may be called **dextrotorsion** and if it rotates to the left it may be called **laevotorsion**. It may occur as a result of a head tilt, extraocular muscle weakness or rotation of the eye to a tertiary position. *Syn.* cycloduction; cyclorotation; torsional movement.
*See* **law, Donder's; position, tertiary; hemianopsia, incongruous.**

**torticollis** Head tilting usually accompanied by a twisting of the neck.

**tortoiseshell** Material used in the manufacture of spectacle frames. It is obtained from the shell plates of the hawksbill turtle.
*See* **spectacle frame, plastic; spectacles.**

**total astigmatism; diameter; reflection** *See* under the nouns.

**toughened glass** *See* **glass, safety.**

**tourmaline** *See* **polarizer.**

**toxic amblyopia** *See* **amblyopia, toxic.**

**toxoplasmosis** An infectious disease caused by the protozoan *Toxoplasma gondii*. It occurs either as a congenital or as an acquired type. The congenital type is characterized by bilateral retinochoroiditis in which the fovea is frequently destroyed, resulting in loss of central vision, hydrocephalus, convulsions and encephalomyelitis. The acquired type varies in severity and so does the ocular involvement, the more common lesion being a nonspecific intraocular inflammation involving either the anterior or posterior segment of the eye.

**trabecular meshwork** *See* **meshwork, trabecular.**

**trabeculectomy** A filtering operation for glaucoma, in which a portion of the trabecular meshwork is excised to increase the outflow of aqueous humour.

**trabeculoplasty, laser** A procedure aimed at improving the outflow of aqueous humour in open-angle glaucoma by producing a series of laser burns (usually with an argon laser) to the trabecular meshwork.
*See* **glaucoma, open-angle.**

**trachoma** A chronic, bilateral, contagious conjunctivitis caused by the serotypes A, Ba and C of *Chlamydia trachomatis*. The conjunctivitis results in conjunctival scarring (**Arlt's line**) and may lead to entropion and trichiasis and dry eyes. Follicles at the limbus may leave some sharply defined depressions (**Herbert's pits**). There is also keratitis with corneal infiltrates, pannus and vascularization. As the disease progresses there is corneal ulceration and opacification which may result in blindness. Trachoma is one of the main causes of blindness in the world. It is a disease most commonly encountered in hot regions of the globe where hygienic

conditions are poor. Treatment includes a course of tetracycline or erythromycin and surgical correction of entropion and trichiasis may be necessary. *Syn.* egyptian conjunctivitis; granular conjunctivitis.
*See* **alacrima; pannus.**

**tract 1.** A bundle of nerve fibres. **2.** A system of organs serving the same function, e.g. the respiratory tract.
*See* **tracts, optic.**

**tract, geniculocalcarine** *See* **radiations, optic.**

**traction retinal detachment** *See* **retinal detachment.**

**tracts, optic** Two cylindrical bands of nerve fibres carrying visual impulses. They run outward and backward from the posterolateral angle of the optic chiasma, then sweep laterally encircling the hypothalamus posteriorly on their way to the lateral geniculate bodies.
*See* **chiasma, optic; geniculate bodies, lateral; hemianopsia, incongruous; pathway, visual.**

**training, visual** Methods aimed at improving visual abilities, e.g. visual perception, spatial localization, heterophoria, hand/eye coordination, etc. to achieve optimal visual performance and comfort. These techniques represent an enlargement of the practice of orthoptics. *Syn.* vision therapy.
*See* **orthoptics.**

**transcleral illumination** *See* **transillumination.**

**transduction 1.** Generally, the conversion of one form of energy into another. **2.** *Example*: the transformation of light energy into receptor potentials in the photoreceptors of the retina (also called **phototransduction**). The absorption of light by the pigments of the photoreceptors triggers a cascade of biochemical events that leads to a change in ionic fluxes across the plasma membrane and to a change in resting potential from around −40 mV in the dark, to around −70 mV in light, that is a hyperpolarization of the cells.
*See* **potential, receptor; rhodopsin.**

**transillumination 1.** The shining of light through a translucent membrane. This is principally used to better visualize ocular tumours, cysts or haemorrhages within the eye. It is accomplished by directing a narrow intense beam of light on the side of the eye. *Example*: If a tumour is present in the eye some light will not be reflected and the pupil will appear partially or completely black, instead of bright red as when the healthy eye is thus illuminated. *Syn.* transcleral illumination. **2.** *See* **illumination, retro-.**

**transition of a scleral contact lens** The zone between the optic (or corneal) and haptic (or scleral) portions.
*See* **blending; lens, scleral contact.**

**translucent** Pertains to a medium or substance that transmits light but diffuses or scatters it on the way so that objects cannot be seen through it, e.g. paraffin wax, tracing paper, cloth, smoke, fog, ground glass, etc.
*See* **glass, ground; transparent.**

**transmission** Passage of radiations through a medium or a substance. Transmission can be either diffuse (light is scattered in all directions) or regular (i.e. without diffusion).
*See* **absorption; translucent; transmittance; transparent.**

**transmission curve** A graph in which the transmission of an optical medium is plotted against the wavelength.
*See* **lens, tinted.**

**transmission factor** *See* **factor, transmission.**

**transmittance** The measure of transmission expressed as the ratio of the transmitted luminous flux to the incident flux. *Syn.* transmission factor; total transmittance.
*See* **transmission.**

**transparent** Pertains to a medium or a substance which transmits light without scattering and with little absorption, so that objects can be seen through it. Optical lenses, prisms, etc. are made of such material.
*See* **opaque; translucent.**

**transplant, corneal** *See* **keratoplasty.**

**transport, active** A process by which particles (e.g. ions, molecules) are transported across cell membranes, against, in almost all instances, the concentration gradient. It requires energy which is provided by the metabolism of carbohydrates, proteins or lipids. It requires cellular energy which is obtained from splitting adenosine triphosphate (ATP). *Example*: the sodium/potassium pump that keeps sodium ions out of a cell and potassium ions in. When this process results in a compound being released, it is termed 'secretion'. This process is one of the mechanisms by which aqueous humour is produced in the ciliary body.
*See* **potential, action.**

**transposition 1.** The act of converting the prescription of an ophthalmic lens from a sphere with minus cylinder form to a sphere with plus cylinder form or vice versa. *Example*: −3 D sphere −2 D cylinder axis 180° transposes to −5 D sphere +2 D cylinder axis 90°. **2.** A surgical procedure used to correct muscle paralysis. In this procedure, adjacent muscles are transferred (transposed) to the paralysed muscle, allowing for partial movement in the field of action of the paretic muscle.
*See* **focimeter; lens, astigmatic; primary action.**

**Trantas' dots** *See* **conjunctivitis, vernal.**

**travoprost** *See* **prostaglandin analogues.**

**tremors** *See* **movements, fixation.**

**trial case** A case containing pairs of positive and negative spherical lenses, plano cylinders, thin prisms as well as discs, pinhole discs, etc. used in refraction with a trial frame. The contents of the case are referred to as a **trial set**.
*See* **refraction.**

**trial frame** Spectacle frame with variable adjustments for interpupillary distance, side length, etc. in which each lens rim is fitted with a number of cells into which trial lenses can be placed when testing vision (Fig.T14).
*See* **phoropter; refraction; Simultantest.**

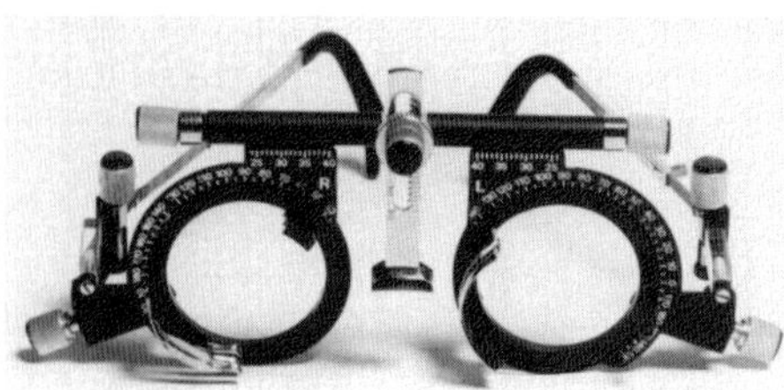

**Fig. T14** Trial frame

**trial lens** *See* **lens, trial.**

**trial lens clip** *See* **clipover.**

**trial set** A number of objects used to measure the refraction of the eye. It includes a trial case with various lenses, prisms, pinhole discs, Maddox rod, etc. and a trial frame.

**triamcinolone** *See* **antiinflammatory drug; chalazion.**

**triangle, colour** *See* **chromaticity diagram.**

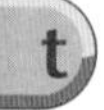

**triangulation, amplitude of** *See* **convergence, amplitude of.**

**triangulation, angle of** *See* **angle of convergence.**

**tricarboxylic acid cycle** *See* **cycle, Krebs.**

**trichiasis** A condition in which the eyelashes due to entropion, blepharitis or injury, are directed towards the globe and cause irritation of the cornea and conjunctiva. Temporary relief may be achieved with epilation but permanent treatment consists of cryotherapy or laser ablation or in severe cases surgical excision and replacement with a mucous membrane.
*See* **blepharitis; distichiasis; entropion; epilation; lens, therapeutic soft contact.**

**trichromatic theory** *See* **theory, Young–Helmholtz.**

**trichromatism** Colour vision characterized by the fact that any perceived hues can be matched by three independent primaries (e.g. red, green and blue). *Syn.* trichromacy; trichromatic vision.

**trichromatism, anomalous** A form of defective colour vision in which three primary colours are required for colour matching, but the proportion of each primary is not the same as those required by a normal trichromat. There are three types of anomalous trichromatism; deuteranomaly, protanomaly and tritanomaly. *Syn.* anomalous trichromacy; anomalous trichromatic vision.
*See* **colours, primary; colour vision, defective.**

**trifluorothymidine** *See* **antiviral agents.**

**trifocal lens** *See* **lens, trifocal.**

**trigeminal ganglion** *See* **ganglion, gasserian.**

**trigeminal nerve** *See* **nerve, trigeminal.**

**trimethoprim** *See* **antibiotic.**

**triplet** Lens system composed of three lenses as, for example, a convex crown glass lens cemented between two concave flint lenses. The aim of such a system is to minimize aberrations. (Fig. T15)
*See* **doublet; eyepiece, orthoscopic; glass, crown; glass, flint; lens, achromatizing.**

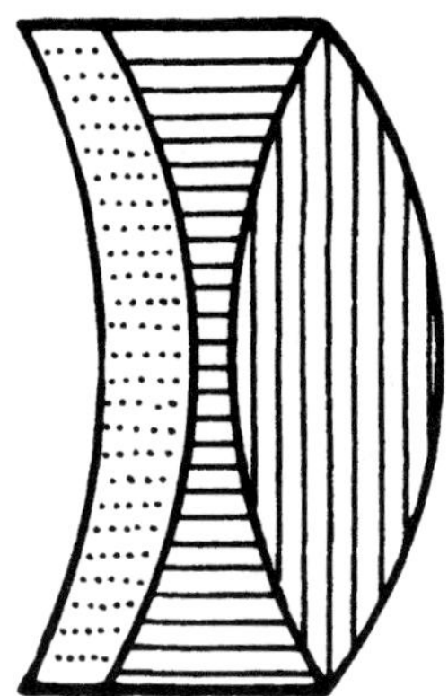

**Fig. T15** Triplet

**triplopia** Condition in which a subject sees three images of a single object. This condition may be the result of crystalline lens sclerosis, multiple pupils, etc.
*See* **diplopia; polyopia.**

**trisomy 21 syndrome** *See* **syndrome, Down's.**

**tritan** A person who has either tritanopia or tritanomaly.

**tritanomal** A person who has tritanomaly.

**tritanomaly** A type of anomalous trichromatism in which an abnormally high proportion of blue is needed when mixing blue and green to match a given blue-green stimulus. This condition is exceedingly rare: it is estimated at about one person in a million. *Syn.* tritanomalous trichromatism; tritanomalous vision.
*See* **anomaloscope; colour vision, defective; plates, pseudoisochromatic; trichromatism.**

**tritanope** A person who has tritanopia.

**tritanopia** A rare type of dichromatism in which blue and yellow are confused. The tritanope only sees two colours: reds on the long-wave side, and greens or bluish greens on the other side of his neutral point which is situated around 570 nm. Tritanopia occurs more often as an acquired type as a result of retinal disease or detachment, glaucoma, diabetes, retinitis pigmentosa, etc. Congenital tritanopia is very rare: it is estimated at about five males and three females in 100 000. *Syn.* blue blindness; blue-yellow blindness.
*See* **colour vision, defective; dichromatism; plates, pseudoisochromatic; test, Farnsworth.**

**trochlea** *See* **fossa, trochlear; muscle, superior oblique.**

**trochlear nerve** *See* **nerve, trochlear.**

**trochlear paralysis** *See* **paralysis of the fourth nerve.**

**troland** Unit of retinal illuminance equal to that produced when the luminance of the observed object is one candela per square metre seen through a pupil having an area of one square millimetre. *Syn.* photon (no longer used).
*See* **retinal illuminance.**

**tropia** *See* **strabismus.**

**tropicamide** *See* **acetylcholine; cycloplegia; mydriatic.**

**Troxler's phenomenon** *See* **phenomenon, Troxler's.**

**true image** *See* **image, true.**

**true negative** *See* **specificity.**

**true positive** *See* **sensitivity.**

**truncation** Removal of the peripheral part of a contact lens. The truncation is often undertaken at the base of a prism ballast lens.
*See* **ballast.**

**Tscherning ellipse** *See* **ellipse, Tscherning.**

**tubercle, lacrimal** A small bump on the frontal process of the maxilla situated near the lower orbital and the anterior lacrimal crest, to which the medial palpebral ligament attaches. *Syn.* papilla lacrimalis.
*See* **ligament, palpebral; lacrimal crest, anterior.**

**tubercle, lateral orbital** A small elevation on the orbital surface of the zygomatic bone just behind and within the orbital margin, about 11 mm below the frontozygomatic suture. It serves as an attachment for the check ligament of the lateral rectus muscle, the lateral palpebral ligament, the suspensory ligament of Lockwood and the levator palpebrae superioris muscle. *Syn.* Whitnall's tubercle.
*See* **ligament of Lockwood; ligament, palpebral; orbit.**

**tungsten-halogen lamp** *See* **lamp, halogen.**

**tunica vasculosa lentis** *See* **artery, hyaloid.**

**tunnel vision** *See* **vision, tunnel.**

**Turk's disease** *See* **syndrome, Duane's.**

**Turner's syndrome** *See* **syndrome, Turner's.**

**Turville infinity balance test** *See* **test, Turville infinity balance.**

**twilight vision** *See* **vision, mesopic.**

**two visual systems theory** *See* **theory, two visual systems.**

**Tyndall effect** *See* **effect, Tyndall.**

**typoscope** A reading shield made of black material in which there is a rectangular aperture allowing one or more lines of print to be seen. It reduces extraneous light reflected from the surface of the paper and assists in staying on the correct line (Fig. T16). It can be helpful for people with low vision who have, for example, media involvement. Recent models embody built-in lighting to provide even and controlled illumination. *Syn.* reading slit.
*See* **vision, low.**

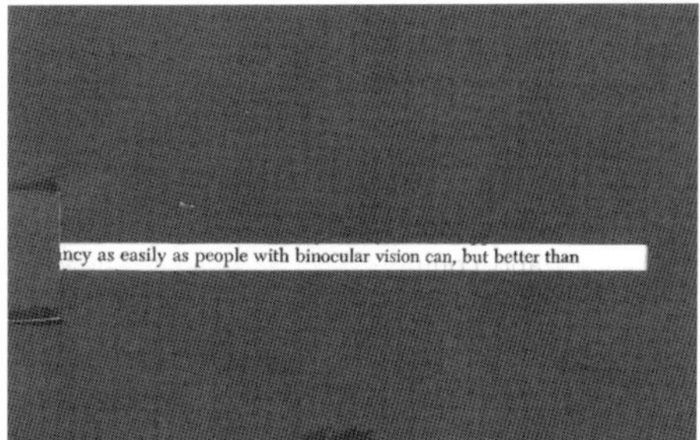


**Fig. T16** Typoscope

# U

**Uhthoff's symptom** Temporary blurring of vision occurring when there is an increase in body temperature (e.g. during or following exercise) in patients with multiple sclerosis, optic neuritis and other optic neuropathies. The symptom may also occur as a result of emotional stress, menstruation, increased illumination or a hot bath. Uhthoff's symptom is sometimes considered to be a prognostic indicator of multiple sclerosis in patients with idiopathic optic neuritis. *Syn.* Uhthoff's phenomenon; Uhthoff's sign; Uhthoff's syndrome.

**ulcer** A localized lesion of the skin or of a mucous layer in which the superficial epithelium is destroyed and deeper tissues are exposed.
*See* **abscess.**

**ulcer, corneal** A superficial loss of corneal tissue as a result of infection which has led to necrosis. It may be caused by a bacterium (e.g. *Pseudomonas aeruginosa, Streptococcus pneumoniae*), by a virus (e.g. herpesvirus), or by a fungus (e.g. *Candida, Aspergillus, Penicillium*). It causes pain and usually reduced visual acuity, especially if the ulcer occurs in the centre of the cornea. Corneal ulcers usually look dirty grey or white and are opaque areas of various sizes and a mucopurulent discharge may be present. If induced by contact lenses, especially extended wear lenses, patients must cease wearing their lenses immediately, and the appropriate therapy instituted: antibacterial, antifungal or antiviral agent.
*See* **facet; keratitis, dendritic; keratitis, hypopyon; keratitis, rosacea; keratitis, ulcerative; keratocele; keratomycosis; leukoma.**

**ulcer, dendritic** *See* **keratitis, dendritic.**

**ulcer, marginal corneal** Benign condition due to a hypersensitivity reaction to bacterial conjunctivitis, particularly staphylococcal blepharoconjunctivitis. It is characterized by infiltration of the peripheral cornea by white cells and by ocular irritation. The condition is usually self-limiting but painful. Treatment includes frequent cleaning of the eyelid margin with a cotton-tipped applicator or face cloth or cotton ball with baby shampoo, warm compresses, antibiotic ointment and occasionally topical corticosteroids.

**ulcer, Mooren's** A rare, superficial ulcer of the cornea of unknown origin. It starts near the limbus as an overhanging advancing edge that in severe cases spreads over the entire cornea and may even invade the sclera. The patient complains of pain and blurred vision. There are two types: a self-limiting form, usually unilateral, affecting old people, and a progressive form, bilateral, affecting young people. The condition is difficult to treat and this may include topical and systemic steroids or conjunctival excision.

**ulcer, serpiginous** *See* **keratitis, hypopyon.**

**ulcer, shield** A localized corneal ulcer noted in severe cases of vernal conjunctivitis. The lesion is usually oval or pentagonal resembling a warrior's shield. It is located in the upper portion of the cornea as a result of irritation from the large papillae on the palpebral surface of the overlying eyelid.

**ulcer, von Hippel's internal** A depression noted in the posterior surface of the cornea. This lesion resembles posterior lenticonus, except that it is thought to be due to an infection or inflammation. The lesion can be differentiated from Peter's anomaly by the presence of endothelium and Descemet's membrane in the former. Due to its posterior location, the lesion does not usually disturb visual function.
*See* **Peter's anomaly.**

**ulcerative keratitis** *See* **keratitis, ulcerative.**

**ultrafiltration** One of the mechanisms which produce aqueous humour from blood plasma in the ciliary processes. This mechanism takes advantage of the natural pressure gradient between the capillary vascular pressure and intraocular aqueous pressure, to drive fluid into the eye. Ultrafiltration is one of three physiological processes that create aqueous fluid.
*See* **humour aqueous.**

**ultrasonography** A technique utilizing high frequency ultrasound waves (greater than 18 000 Hz) emitted by a transducer placed near the eye. The silicone probe, which rests on the eye, is separated from the transducer by a water column to segregate the noise from the transducer. The technique is used to make biometric measurements such as the axial length of the eye, the depth of the anterior chamber, the thickness of the lens, the distance between the back of the lens and the retina and the thickness of the cornea. The ultrasound wave is reflected back when it encounters a change in density (or elasticity) of the medium through which it is passing. The reflected vibration is called an **echo.** Echoes from the interfaces between the various media of the eye are converted into an electrical potential by a piezoelectrical crystal and can be displayed as deflections or spikes on a cathode-ray oscilloscope. Two types of ultrasonographic measurements are used: (1) The time-amplitude or **A-scan** which measures the time or distance from the transducer to the interface and back. Thus echoes from surfaces deeper within the eye take longer to return to the transducer for conversion into electrical potential and so they appear further along the time base on the oscilloscope display. The A-scan is more useful for the study of the biometric measurements, as well as measurements of intraocular tumour size (e.g. choroidal melanoma) (Fig. U1). (2) The intensity-modulated or **B-scan** in which various scans are taken through the pupillary area and any change in acoustic impedance is shown as a dot on the oscilloscope screen, and these join up as the transducer moves across a meridian. The B-scan is useful to indicate the position of a retinal or vitreous detachment, or of an intraocular foreign body, and for the examination of the orbit. The B-scan is especially useful in the examination of the posterior structures of the eye when opacities prevent ophthalmoscopic examination (e.g. cataract, corneal oedema). *Syn.* echography. *See* **length of the eye, axial.**

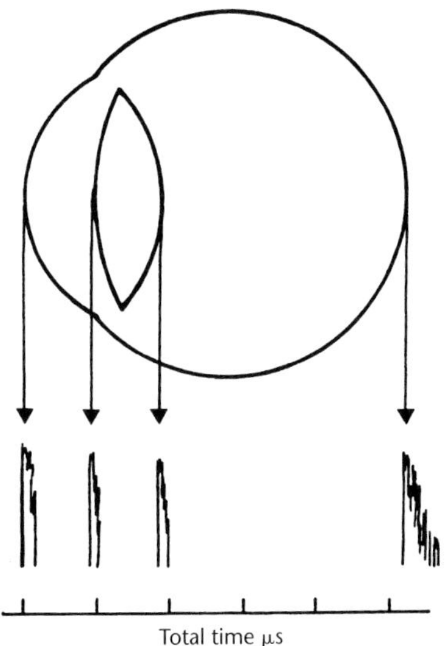


**Fig. U1** Histogram of ultrasound reflections (or echoes) in the eye. Echoes from the various boundaries are given against total time, i.e. the time interval from the cornea to the boundary and back to the cornea. The velocity of the ultrasound waves in the eye is approximately 1550 m/s (it is 1641 m/s in the lens and 1532 m/s in the humours). In the above diagram the total time between the cornea and the retina is 32 μs. The length is then equal to $32/2 \times 10^{-6} \times 1550 \times 10^{3} = 24.80$ mm

**ultraviolet (UV)** Radiant energy of wavelengths smaller than those of the violet end of the visible spectrum and longer than about 1 nm. The wave band comprising radiations between 315 and 380 nm is referred to as **UV-A**. Excessive exposure to these radiations can cause cataract. The wave band comprising radiations between 280 and 315 nm is referred to as **UV-B**. Excessive exposure to all these radiations can cause photokeratitis and corneal opacity, while radiations between 295 and 315 nm can cause cataract. The wave band comprising radiations between 200 and 280 nm is referred to as **UV-C**. Excessive exposure to these radiations can cause photokeratitis and corneal opacity.
*See* **blepharospasm; cataract; keratoconjunctivitis, actinic; laser, excimer; lens, absorptive; light; nanometre; pinguecula; wavelength.**

**Table U1** Divisions of the ultraviolet spectrum

| | |
|---|---|
| UV-A (near) | 380–315 nm |
| UV-B (middle) | 315–280 nm |
| UV-C (far) | 280–200 nm |

**umbra** *See* **penumbra.**

**unaided vision; visual acuity** *See* **acuity, unaided visual.**

**uncompensated heterophoria** *See* **heterophoria, uncompensated.**

**uncrossed diplopia** *See* **diplopia, homonymous.**

**uncut lens** *See* **lens, uncut.**

**undercorrected spherical aberration** *See* **aberration, spherical.**

**unharmonious retinal correspondence** *See* **retinal correspondence, abnormal.**

**uniocular** *See* **monocular.**

**unoprostone isopropyl** *See* **prostaglandin analogues.**

**upbeat nystagmus** *See* **nystagmus.**

**upgaze** Movement of the eyes upward with the head in the straight-ahead position.
*See* **elevation of the eye.**

**urea** *See* **hyperosmotic agent.**

**use–abuse theory** *See* **theory, use–abuse.**

**Usher's syndrome** *See* **syndrome, Usher's.**

**uvea** The vascular tunic of the eye, consisting of the choroid, ciliary body and the iris. The last

two structures are usually considered to form the **anterior uvea.** The uvea contains most of the blood supply. (Fig. U2) *Syn.* uveal tract; vascular tunic of the eye.
*See* **uveitis; vein, vortex.**

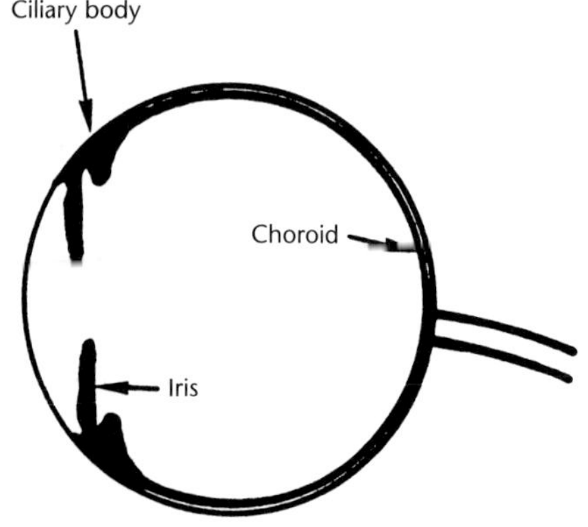


**Fig. U2** The uvea

**uveal meshwork** *See* **meshwork, trabecular.**

**uveal tract** *See* **uvea.**

**uveitis** Inflammation of the uvea. All three tissues of the uvea tend to be involved to some extent in the same inflammatory process because of their common blood supply. However, the most severe reaction may affect one tissue more than the others as in iritis, cyclitis or choroiditis or sometimes two tissues, e.g. iridocyclitis. The symptoms also vary depending upon which part of the tract is affected. **Anterior uveitis** will be accompanied by pain, photophobia and lacrimation and some loss of vision because of exudation of cells (aqueous flare), protein-rich fluid and fibrin into either the anterior chamber or vitreous body, as well as ciliary injection, adhesion between the iris and lens (posterior synechia) and keratic precipitates. The condition is often associated with ankylosing spondylitis, rheumatoid arthritis, sarcoidosis or syphilis. Treatment includes corticosteroids (e.g. prednisolone) and mydriatics (e.g. homatropine) to reduce the risk of posterior synechia and to relieve a spasm of the ciliary muscle.
*See* **aqueous flare; cataract, cuneiform; choroiditis; cyclitis; hypopyon; injection, ciliary; iridocyclitis; iritis; keratic precipitates; Koeppe's nodules; mydriatics; phthisis bulbi; synchisis scintillans; synechia, posterior.**

**uveitis, posterior** A uveitis involving the posterior segment of the eye. Symptoms include floaters and visual loss if the choroiditis involves the macular area. Ophthalmoscopically there is an accumulation of debris in the vitreous and choroidal lesions appear as yellow-white areas of infiltrates surrounded by normal fundus. Retinitis is also present in most cases, as well as retinal vasculitis. Posterior uveitis may be associated with AIDS, Behçet's disease, Lyme disease, histoplasmosis, sarcoidosis, toxoplasmosis, syphilis, tuberculosis, Vogt–Koyanagi–Harada syndrome, sympathetic ophthalmia, etc.

# V

**v gauge** A device used to measure the total diameter of a rigid contact lens. It consists of a channel cut into a long rectangle of plastic or metal. The channel increases in width from 6.0 to 12.50 mm and a scale is printed beside it. The lens is placed with its concave surface down at the widest end of the channel and that end of the gauge is raised so that the lens slides down the channel until it stops. The diameter is then read from the scale where the lens touches the side of the channel. *Syn.* v-channel gauge.
*See* **diameter, total.**

**V pattern** *See* **pattern, V.**

**validity** The extent to which a measurement correctly measures what it is supposed to measure or to which extent the findings of an investigation reflect the truth. In health sciences validity is commonly assessed by determining the sensitivity and specificity factors.
*See* **reliability; sensitivity; specificity.**

**value f** *See* **f number.**

**value, Munsell** *See* **Munsell colour system.**

**value, V-** *See* **constringence.**

**valve of Hasner** A fold of mucous membrane at the lower end of the nasolacrimal duct. If well developed, it generally prevents air from being blown back from the nose into the lacrimal sac. *Syn.* plica lacrimalis; valve of Bianchi.
*See* **lacrimal apparatus.**

**valve of Krause** A fold of mucous membrane at the junction of the lacrimal sac and the nasolacrimal duct. *Syn.* valve of Beraud.
*See* **lacrimal apparatus.**

**valve of Rosenmuller** A fold of mucous membrane found at the junction between the common canaliculus and the lacrimal sac. It is not strictly a valve because fluids can be blown back to emerge at the puncta. It is not always fully developed.
*See* **lacrimal apparatus.**

**van Herick, Shaffer and Schwartz method** *See* **method, van Herick, Shaffer and Schwartz.**

**vancomycin** *See* **antibiotic.**

**varicella-zoster** *See* **herpes zoster.**

**varifocal lens** *See* **lens, progressive.**

**vasa hyaloidea propria** *See* **artery, hyaloid.**

**vascularization** *See* **pannus.**

**vase, Rubin's** An ambiguous drawing which may be perceived either as a vase or as two human profiles facing each other (Fig. V1).
*See* **figure, Blivet; Necker cube; Schroeder's staircase.**

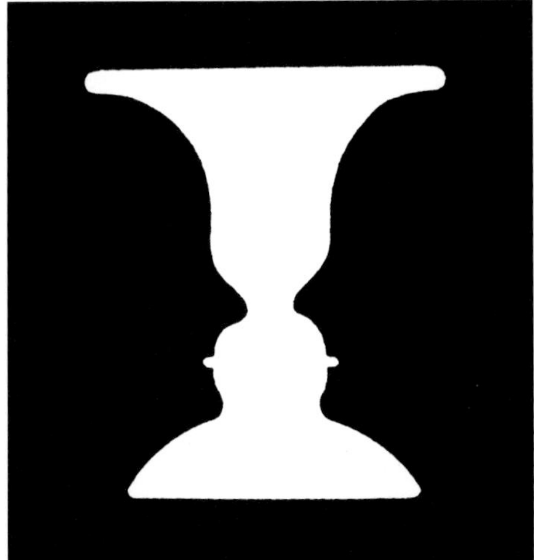

**Fig. V1** Rubin's vase

**vectogram** A polarized stereogram consisting of two polarized images at right angles to each other. When viewed through polarizing filters it presents one image to one eye and another image to the other eye. The Vectograph is a chart based on this principle in which almost one half of a chart is seen by one eye and almost the other half by the other eye while some lines, letters or numbers are seen binocularly to lock fusion. The **Vectograph** is useful for balancing refraction and to detect suppression and fixation disparity. The **Titmus stereotest** (Fig. V2) consists of various vectograms, including one with a stereoscopic pattern representing a **housefly**, to establish whether the patient has gross stereopsis (it produces approximately 3000 seconds of arc of retinal disparity at 40 cm). Children are often tested by asking them to hold one of the wings of the fly, which they will do above the plate if it is seen stereoscopically. The other vectograms of the test provide finer tests for stereoscopic acuity.
*See* **acuity, stereoscopic visual; disparity, retinal; stereogram, random-dot; suppression; test, balancing; test, two-dimensional.**

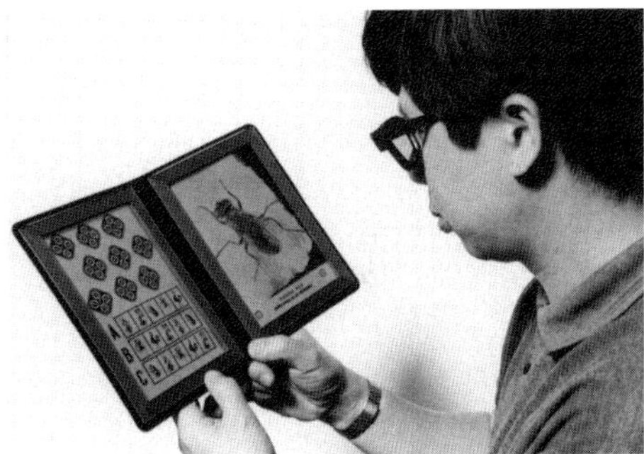

**Fig. V2** Titmus stereotest

**veiling glare** *See* **glare, veiling.**

**vein** A tubular vessel which carries blood towards the heart.
*See* **artery.**

**vein, anterior ciliary** One of many veins which drains the ciliary body, the deep and superficial plexuses, the anterior conjunctival veins and the episcleral veins to empty into the vortex veins.

**vein, anterior facial** Vein branching from the angular vein at the side of the nose and running obliquely downward and backward across the face. It crosses the mandible and joins the posterior facial vein to form the common facial vein which opens into the internal jugular. The anterior facial vein drains the part of the eyelids anterior to the tarsus.

**vein, aqueous** One of several veins serving as exit channels for the aqueous humour which they

carry from the canal of Schlemm to the episcleral, conjunctival and subconjunctival veins. *See* **canal, Schlemm's; humour, aqueous.**

**vein, central retinal** A vein formed by the junction of the superior and inferior retinal veins at about the level of the lamina cribrosa on the temporal side of the central retinal artery. After a short course within the optic nerve, it empties into the cavernous sinus, the superior ophthalmic vein and sometimes into the inferior ophthalmic vein. *See* **artery, central retinal; retinal vein occlusion.**

**vein, conjunctival** One of many veins which drains the tarsal conjunctiva, the fornix, and the major portion of the bulbar conjunctiva.

**vein, inferior ophthalmic** Vein which commences as a plexus near the floor of the orbit, runs backward on the inferior rectus muscles and divides into two branches, one which runs to the pterygoid venous plexus and the other which joins the cavernous sinus, usually via the superior ophthalmic vein. The inferior ophthalmic vein receives tributaries from the lower and lateral ocular muscles, the conjunctiva, the lacrimal sac and the two inferior vortex veins.

**vein, palpebral** One of the veins of the upper or lower eyelid which empties for the most part into the anterior facial vein as well as into the angular, supraorbital, superior and inferior ophthalmic, the lacrimal and the superficial temporal veins.

**vein, posterior ciliary** *See* **vein, vortex.**

**vein, superior ophthalmic** Vein which is formed near the root of the nose by a communication from the angular vein soon after it has been joined by the supraorbital vein. It passes into the orbit above the medial palpebral ligament, runs backward to the sphenoidal fissure where it usually meets the inferior ophthalmic vein, and drains into the cavernous sinus. It has many tributaries: the inferior ophthalmic vein, the anterior and posterior ethmoidal veins, the muscular vein, the lacrimal vein, the central retinal vein, the anterior ciliary vein and two of the posterior ciliary veins (the superior ones).

**vein, vortex** One of usually four (two superior and two inferior) veins which pierce the sclera obliquely on either side of the superior and inferior recti muscles, some 6 mm behind the equator of the globe. The two superior ones open into the superior ophthalmic vein and the two inferior open into the inferior ophthalmic vein. These veins drain the posterior uveal tract. *Syn.* posterior ciliary vein; vena vorticosa.
*See* **vein, anterior ciliary; vein, inferior ophthalmic.**

**velocity of light** *See* **light, speed of.**

**velonoskiascopy** A subjective method of detecting ametropia in which a thin rod held near the eye is moved across the pupil while the subject fixates a distant light source. The rod casts a shadow on the retina if the eye is ametropic. This shadow will appear to move with the rod in myopia and opposite to the movement of the rod in hypermetropia. By moving the rod across the pupil in different meridians, astigmatism can be explored. No shadow is seen in emmetropia. *See* **ametropia; refractive error.**

**vena vorticosa** *See* **vein, vortex.**

**venous-stasis retinopathy** *See* **retinal vein occlusion.**

**vergence** **1.** Denotes divergence of light travelling from, or convergence of light travelling from, or to an object or image. The **object vergence** at a refracting surface is equal to

$$L = \frac{n}{l}$$

where $n$ is the index of refraction of the first medium and $l$ the distance between the object plane and the refracting surface in metres. The **image vergence** at a refracting surface is equal to

$$L' = \frac{n'}{l'}$$

where $n'$ is the index of refraction of the second medium and $l'$ the distance between the image plane and the refracting surface in metres. The unit of vergence is the dioptre. **2.** Disjunctive movements of the eyes such as convergence, divergence, cyclovergence, infravergence or supravergence.
*See* **distance, image; distance, object; duction; movements, disjunctive; paraxial equation, fundamental; power, refractive.**

**vergence accommodation** *See* **accommodation, convergence.**

**vergence accommodative** *See* **convergence, accommodative.**

**vergence, disparity** *See* **fusion, motor.**

**vergence facility** Ability of the eyes to make fusional vergence movements in a given period of time. Clinically, this is measured by introducing a relatively large prism in front of one or both eyes of a patient fixating a target until it appears single. The operation is repeated many times and the results are commonly presented in cycles per minute (one cycle indicates that single vision was reported both with the prism and after removing the prism).
*See* **convergence, fusional; fusion, motor; lens flippers.**

**vergence formula** *See* **paraxial equation, fundamental.**

**vergence, fusional** *See* **convergence, relative.**

**vergence power** *See* **power, refractive.**

**vergence, proximal** *See* **convergence, proximal.**

**vergence reflex** *See* **reflex, vergence.**

**vergence, relative** *See* **convergence, relative.**

**vergence, tonic** The passive state of vergence of the eyes in the absence of a stimulus, i.e. when the eyes are in total darkness or when looking at a bright empty field. This position is maintained by the tonus of the extraocular muscles. Only at death or when paralysed do the eyes return to their anatomical position of rest and tonic vergence disappears. *Syn.* dark vergence; tonic convergence.
*See* **accommodation, resting state of; position of rest, physiological; tonus.**

**vergence, vertical fusional** Movement of the eyes upward until an object which was imaged on slightly disparate vertical parts of the retina falls on corresponding retinal points.

**Verhoeff phi phenomenon test** *See* **movement, phi.**

**Verhoeff's circles** Two black concentric circles designed for use with the duochrome test and as a target for the cross-cylinder method. The thickness and overall diameter of the inner ring are equivalent to a 6/6 (or 20/20) Snellen letter while the thickness and overall diameter of the outer ring are equivalent to a 6/15 (or 20/50) Snellen letter. *Syn.* Verhoeff's rings.
*See* **chart, Snellen; test for astigmatism, cross-cylinder; test, duochrome.**

**Verhoeff's rings** *See* **Verhoeff's circles.**

**vernal catarrh; conjunctivitis** *See* **conjunctivitis, vernal.**

**vernier visual acuity** *See* **acuity, vernier visual.**

**version** Conjugate movements of the two eyes in the same direction, such as **dextroversion**, both eyes rotate to the right; **laevoversion** (or **levoversion**), both eyes rotate to the left; **supraversion** (or **sursumversion**), both eyes rotate upward; **infraversion** (or **deorsumversion**), both eyes rotate downward: these versions bring the eyes into the **secondary positions of gaze**. Movements of the eyes up and to the right are called **dextroelevation**, up and to the left, **laevoelevation**, down and to the right, **dextrodepression** and down and to the left, **laevodepression**: these versions bring the eye into the **tertiary positions of gaze**. Version eye movements are performed by yoke muscles (Fig. V3). *Syn.* conjugate eye movements.
*See* **cardinal positions of gaze; deviation, conjugate; muscles, yoke; test, motility.**

**version prisms** *See* **prisms, yoke.**

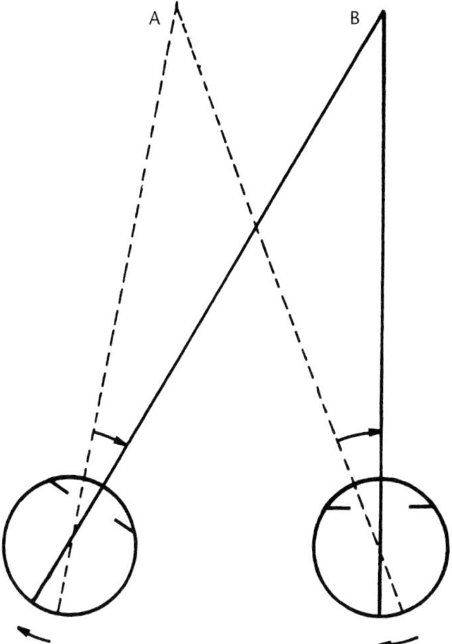


**Fig. V3** Version movements of the eyes from A to B

**vertex** The point where the optical axis intersects a reflecting or refracting surface. In a spectacle lens the back vertex is the point of intersection of the optical axis with the surface nearest to the eye, the other being the front vertex. *Plural*: vertices.

**vertex depth** Distance between the posterior pole of a spectacle lens and the plane containing the posterior edge of the lens. The vertex depth *s* is given by the following formula

$$s = r - \sqrt{(r^2 - y^2)}$$

where *r* is the radius of curvature of the surface of the spectacle lens and *y* is the semi-diameter at the edge of the surface (Fig. V4). *Syn.* sag.
*See* **clearance, apical; lens measure.**

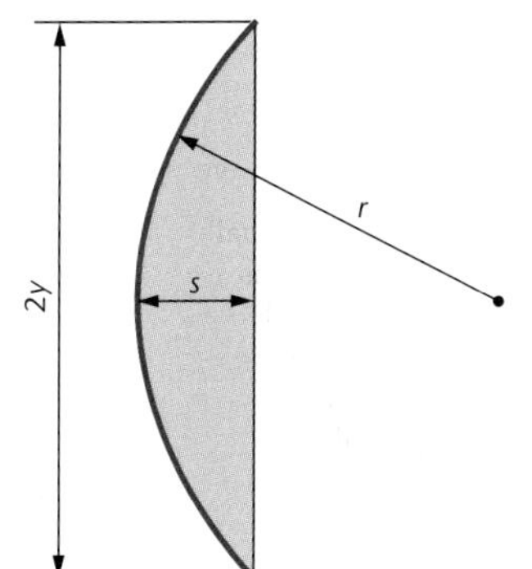


**Fig. V4** Vertex depth (or sagittal depth) *s* of a spherical surface (*r*, radius of curvature; 2*y*, diameter of the surface)

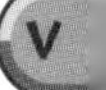

**Table V1** Vertex depths of various spherical surfaces. They also represent the centre thickness of a planoconvex lens with a front surface of radius of curvature *r* and diameter 2*y*, with an edge thickness of zero. Index of refraction of the lens 1.49

| surface power (D) | radius *r* (mm) | lens diameter 2*y* (mm) | | | |
|---|---|---|---|---|---|
| | | 40 | 50 | 60 | 70 |
| 1 | 490 | 0.41 | 0.64 | 0.92 | 1.25 |
| 2 | 245 | 0.82 | 1.28 | 1.84 | 2.51 |
| 3 | 163.3 | 1.23 | 1.92 | 2.78 | 3.79 |
| 4 | 122.5 | 1.61 | 2.58 | 3.73 | 5.11 |
| 5 | 98 | 2.06 | 3.24 | 4.70 | 6.46 |
| 6 | 81.7 | 2.49 | 3.92 | 5.71 | 7.88 |
| 7 | 70 | 2.92 | 4.62 | 6.75 | 9.38 |
| 8 | 61.3 | 3.38 | 5.33 | 7.85 | 10.99 |
| 9 | 54.4 | 3.81 | 6.08 | 9.01 | 12.74 |
| 10 | 49 | 4.27 | 6.86 | 10.26 | 14.71 |
| 12 | 40.8 | 5.23 | 8.55 | 13.13 | 19.80 |
| 14 | 35 | 6.28 | 10.51 | 16.97 | 35.00 |
| 16 | 30.6 | 7.43 | 12.94 | 24.47 | |
| 18 | 27.2 | 8.75 | 16.45 | | |
| 20 | 24.5 | 10.35 | | | |

**vertex distance** Distance along the line of sight between the apex of the cornea and the posterior surface of a spectacle lens. This distance normally varies between 11 mm and 15 mm.
*See* **clearance, apical; plane, spectacle.**

**vertex focal length** The linear distance separating the principal focal point (or focus) of an optical system or lens from the front or back vertices. They are called the **front vertex focal length** ($f_v$) and the **back vertex focal length** ($f'_v$), respectively. In the case of a biconcave or biconvex lens the front and back vertex focal lengths are equal. In the case of a positive meniscus lens, the back vertex focal length is shorter than the front vertex focal length and vice versa in the case of a negative meniscus lens.
*See* **power, back vertex; power, front vertex.**

**vertex power** *See* **power, back vertex; power, front vertex.**

**vertexometer** **1.** Synonym of focimeter. **2.** Synonym of distometer.
*See* **distometer; focimeter.**

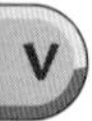

**vertical fusional vergence** *See* **vergence, vertical fusional.**

**vertigo** The sensation of irregular movement in space of either oneself or of external objects. It can be experienced after vestibular stimulation.

**vesicle, optic** A hollow, spherical outgrowth from the lateral aspect of the forebrain, derived from the optic pit after closure of the embryonic neural groove. It subsequently invaginates to form the optic cup. *Syn* primary optic vesicle.
*See* **anophthalmia; cup, optic; pit, optic.**

**vestibular nystagmus** *See* **nystagmus.**

**vestibulo-ocular reflex** *See* **reflex, vestibulo-ocular.**

**vial** A very small bottle. It may contain a soft contact lens, medicine or perfume.

**vidarabine** *See* **antiviral agents.**

**videokeratoscope** An electro-optical instrument for measuring the corneal topography. It produces a colour coded three-dimensional map of the shape of the cornea and of the dioptric power of the different corneal regions. These instruments are computer-assisted providing rapid, on-line analysis of the image and most of them are based on the corneal reflection of the Placido pattern. They are used to evaluate keratoconus, irregular corneal shape, contact lens fitting, monitor the cornea after keratoplasty or refractive surgery, etc. There are many commercial models (e.g. EyeSys, Tomey, Humphrey, Dicon, Orbscan II). The latter, which incorporates a scanning slit measurement system, simultaneously measures both corneal surfaces enabling a diagnosis of anterior and posterior keratoconus.
*See* **keratoconus, posterior; photokeratoscope; Topogometer.**

**Vieth–Müller circle** *See* **horopter, Vieth–Müller.**

**viewing angle** *See* **angle, visual.**

**viewing, eccentric** Fixation in which the eye moves so as to place the image of an object outside the fovea. The object is perceived by the patient as looking 'past' it and not directly at it as in eccentric fixation. Eccentric viewing is often applied by people with low vision suffering from macular degeneration to improve reading a letter or a word by looking slightly above, below or to the side of it.
*See* **fixation, eccentric; vision, low.**

**vignetting** **1.** A graduated reduction in retinal illuminance due to light reaching the pupil at very oblique angles. **2.** The difference in absorption between the two portions of photochromic fused bifocal lenses when the segment is not made of photochromic glass.
*See* **lens, photochromic; retinal illuminance.**

**violet** One of the hues of the visible spectrum evoked by stimulation of the retina by wavelengths shorter than 450 nm and somewhat longer than 380 nm.
*See* **colour; light.**

**virtual image; object** *See* under the nouns.

**viscosity agents** *See* **methylcellulose; wetting solution.**

**visibility 1.** The property of being visible to the eye. **2.** The range of vision through different densities of atmosphere.

**visible spectrum** *See* **light.**

**vision (V) 1.** The appreciation of differences in the external world, such as form, colour, position, etc. resulting from the stimulation of the retina by light. **2.** *See* **acuity, unaided visual.**

**vision, achromatic** *See* **achromatopsia.**

**vision, alternating** *See* **lens, contact.**

**vision, ambient** Vision mediated primarily by the peripheral retina and involved in spatial orientation and recognition of motion.
*See* **vision, focal.**

**vision, anomalous trichromatic** *See* **trichromatism, anomalous.**

**vision, binocular (BV)** Condition in which both eyes contribute towards producing a percept which may or may not be fused into a single impression.
*See* **fusion, sensory; monoblepsia; test, bar reading; test, FRIEND; test, hole in the hand; test, Worth's four dot; vision, Worth's classification of binocular; zone of clear, single, binocular vision.**

**vision, binocular single** *See* **vision, single binocular.**

**vision, blue** *See* **chromatopsia.**

**vision, blurred** Vision characterized by poor visual acuity or in which the edges of objects are indistinct. It may be due to uncorrected or poorly corrected ametropia or presbyopia, anomalies of the ocular media (e.g. cataract, corneal opacity, haemorrhage in the vitreous), amblyopia, excess lacrimation, spasm of accommodation, optic neuritis, angle-closure glaucoma, diabetes, multiple sclerosis, migraine, etc.

**vision, central** Vision of objects formed on the foveola or the macula.
*See* **foveola; fusion, sensory; macula.**

**vision, chromatic** *See* **vision, colour.**

**vision, colour (CV)** Vision in which the colour sense is experienced. *Syn.* chromatic vision.
*See* **theory, Young–Helmholtz.**

**vision, daylight** *See* **vision, photopic.**

**vision, defective colour** *See* **colour vision, defective.**

**vision, deuteranomalous** *See* **deuteranomaly.**

**vision, dichromatic** *See* **dichromatism.**

**vision, distance (DV)** Vision of objects situated either at infinity or more usually at some 5 or 6 m.
*See* **chart, Snellen; vision, near.**

**vision, diurnal** *See* **vision, photopic.**

**vision, double** *See* **diplopia.**

**vision, eccentric** *See* **fixation, eccentric; vision, peripheral.**

**vision, entoptic** *See* **image, entoptic.**

**vision, extrafoveal** *See* **vision, peripheral.**

**vision, field of** *See* **field, visual.**

**vision, focal** Vision mediated by, primarily, the macular area of the retina and involved in the examination and identification of objects.
*See* **vision, ambient.**

**vision, green** *See* **chromatopsia.**

**vision, gun barrel** *See* **vision, tunnel.**

**vision, haploscopic** Vision as obtained by looking in a haploscope.
*See* **haploscope.**

**vision, indirect** *See* **vision, peripheral.**

**vision, industrial** The branch of optometry concerned with vision and perception by the individual at work, the evaluation of visual performance in a given occupation, the prescribing of protective ocular devices and the determination of the optimum environment (e.g. illumination) to accomplish a visual task efficiently.

**vision, intermediate** Vision of objects situated beyond 40 cm from the eye but closer than say, 1.5 m.
*See* **vision, distance; vision, near.**

**vision, low** Vision below normal even after correction by conventional lenses, resulting from either congenital anomalies or ocular diseases such as cataract, glaucoma, age-related maculopathy, pathological myopia, etc. The correction and rehabilitation of patients with subnormal vision is achieved by special aids called **low vision aids** (LVA) such as a telescopic lens, and appropriate counselling (e.g. about illumination and reading distance). The criteria which the health authorities normally use to classify a person as having partial sight take into consideration not only the corrected visual acuity but also the extent of visual field loss, if any. *Syn.* partial sight; subnormal vision.
*See* **aids, low vision; bracketing; chart, Bailey–Lovie; chart, contrast sensitivity; clipover; deaf-blind; lamp, halogen; lens, cross-cylinder; lens, telescopic; maculopathy, age-related;**

**magnification, apparent; magnification, relative distance; magnification, relative size; magnifier; rule, Kestenbaum's; spectacles, magnifying; spectacles, pinhole; telescope, galilean; test, Pepper; typoscope; viewing, eccentric.**

**vision, mesopic** Vision at intermediate levels between photopic and scotopic vision, and corresponding to luminances ranging from about $10^{-3}$ to 10 cd/m². *Syn.* twilight vision.

**vision, monochromatic** Synonym of monochromatism.
*See* **monochromat.**

**vision, monocular** Vision of one eye only.

**vision, multiple** *See* **polyopia.**

**vision, near (NV)** Vision of objects situated 25–50 cm from either the eye, or more commonly the spectacle plane.
*See* **Jaeger test types; vision, distance.**

**vision, night; nocturnal** *See* **vision, scotopic.**

**vision, panoramic** Vision of some animals whose eyes are located laterally so that the two visual fields overlap only slightly or are adjacent, thus providing vision over a much larger region of the environment than if the two lines of sight were aimed in the same direction.

**vision, peripheral** Vision resulting from stimulation of the retina outside the fovea or macula. *Syn.* eccentric vision; extrafoveal vision; indirect vision.
*See* **fusion, sensory; vision, central.**

**vision, photopic** Vision at high levels of luminance (above 10 cd/m²) and resulting from the functioning of the cones. *Syn.* daylight vision; diurnal vision.
*See* **cell, cone; theory, duplicity; threshold, differential.**

**vision, protanomalous** *See* **protanomaly.**

**vision, red** *See* **chromatopsia.**

**vision science** The scientific study of how the visual system contributes to an understanding of the environment by processing and interpreting the light stimulation to the eye. Various disciplines contribute to vision science including anatomy, biology, optics, physiology and psychology.

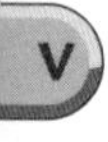

**vision, scotopic** Vision at low levels of luminance, below about $10^{-3}$ cd/m² and resulting from the functioning of the rods. *Syn.* night vision; nocturnal vision; scotopia.
*See* **cell, rod; theory, duplicity.**

**vision, simultaneous** *See* **lens, contact.**

**vision, single binocular (SBV)** Condition in which both eyes contribute towards producing a single fused percept.
*See* **fusion, sensory.**

**vision, spatial** *See* **perception, depth.**

**vision, stereoscopic** *See* **stereopsis.**

**vision, subnormal** *See* **vision, low.**

**vision, telescopic** *See* **vision, tunnel.**

**vision therapy; training** *See* **training, visual**

**vision, tritanomalous** *See* **tritanomaly.**

**vision, tunnel** Vision limited to the central part of the visual field as though one were looking through a hollow tube. It may be a symptom of hysteria, malingering, the final stage of either open-angle glaucoma or retinitis pigmentosa, etc. *Syn.* gun barrel vision; telescopic vision.
*See* **amblyopia, hysterical; glaucoma, open-angle; malingering; retinitis pigmentosa.**

**vision, twilight** *See* **vision, mesopic.**

**vision, Worth's classification of binocular** For the purpose of visual rehabilitation, binocular vision is often classified into three grades: (1) simultaneous binocular vision (or first-degree fusion or superimposition); (2) fusion (or sensory fusion or second-degree fusion or flat fusion); (3) stereopsis (or third-degree fusion).
*See* **fusion, sensory; superimposition.**

**vision, yellow** *See* **xanthopsia.**

**Vistech** A clinical test for contrast sensitivity. It consists of a chart containing five horizontal rows, each with nine circular patches of sinusoidal gratings. The gratings are either vertical or 15° to the right or to the left. Each row has a different spatial frequency, starting from the top of the chart: 1.5, 3.0, 6.0, 12.0 and 18.0 cycles per degrees when viewed at a distance of 40 cm. The contrast level of each of the nine gratings decreases from 33% to 0% from left to right in approximately 0.2 log unit steps. The patient is asked to look along each row, identifying the orientation of the grating. The testing is carried out monocularly with optical correction, if any. The last grating of each row which is incorrectly identified is noted on an evaluation form which is provided with the test. The end points of each of the five rows are connected to form a contrast sensitivity curve for each patient. It is then compared with normal values indicated on the form. There is also a version for testing at distance. *Syn.* Vision Contrast Test System (VCTS).
*See* **chart, contrast sensitivity; sensitivity, contrast; test, Arden grating.**

**visual** Relating to vision.

**visual acuity** *See* **acuity, visual.**

**Table V2** Relationship between visual acuity and the Snell–Sterling visual efficiency scale (in percentage round figures)

| visual acuity (m) | (ft) | efficiency (in %) | loss of vision (in %) |
|---|---|---|---|
| 6/6 | 20/20 | 100 | 0 |
| 6/7.5 | 20/25 | 96 | 4 |
| 6/9 | 20/30 | 91 | 9 |
| 6/12 | 20/40 | 84 | 16 |
| 6/15 | 20/50 | 77 | 23 |
| 6/18 | 20/60 | 70 | 30 |
| 6/24 | 20/80 | 59 | 41 |
| 6/30 | 20/100 | 49 | 51 |
| 6/48 | 20/160 | 29 | 71 |
| 6/60 | 20/200 | 20 | 80 |
| 6/90 | 20/300 | 8 | 92 |
| 6/120 | 20/400 | 3 | 97 |
| 6/150 | 20/500 | 1.5 | 98.5 |

**visual agnosia** *See* **agnosia.**

**visual agraphia** *See* **agraphia.**

**Visual Analysis Skills Test** *See* **test, developmental and perceptual screening.**

**visual angle; area; association areas; axis; centre; cliff** *See* under the nouns.

**visual cortex** *See* **area, visual.**

**visual deprivation** *See* **deprivation, visual.**

**visual direction** *See* **line of direction.**

**visual display unit (VDU)** The visual image appearing on the screen of a cathode ray tube. *See* **syndrome, computer vision.**

**visual efficiency scale, Snell–Sterling** A representation of visual efficiency as a function of visual acuity, in which are taken into account other factors such as perception, experience, etc. in estimating how much vision a person has for a given visual acuity.

**visual evoked cortical potential** *See* **potential, visual evoked cortical.**

**visual extinction** *See* **phenomenon, extinction.**

**visual fatigue; field** *See* under the nouns.

**visual field, binocular** *See* **field, binocular visual.**

**visual field analyser** *See* **analyser, Friedmann visual field.**

**visual field screener** *See* **screener, Harrington–Flocks visual field.**

**visual hallucination** *See* **hallucination, visual.**

**visual illusion** *See* **illusion.**

**visual integration** Term referring to the integration occurring in the brain to give us a final percept, presumably in the prefrontal cortex. Information from the dorsal (or parietal or medial temporal) stream dealing with localization or movement is integrated with information from the ventral (or inferotemporal) stream dealing with colour or form, so that, for example, one can see a red car moving towards us.

**visual line of direction** *See* **line of direction.**

**visual neglect** A rare phenomenon in which a patient can see all of the visual field binocularly but somehow ignores objects on one side (e.g. patient may draw a diagram omitting one side or shave only one side of the face). It is due to a lesion of the brain (e.g. a stroke), most often in the right cortex and the patient, although conscious of objects in the left visual field does not pay attention to them. A confrontation visual field test in which objects are presented to both sides simultaneously often facilitates detection of the condition.
*See* **phenomenon, extinction.**

**visual optics; pathway; pigment; plane; point** *See* under the nouns.

**visual perseveration** *See* **palinopsia.**

**visual purple** *See* **rhodopsin.**

**visual system, magnocellular** *See* **magnocellular visual system.**

**visual system, parvocellular** *See* **parvocellular visual system.**

**visual system, sustained** *See* **parvocellular visual system.**

**visual system, transient** *See* **magnocellular visual system.**

**visual training** *See* **training, visual.**

**visualization** **1.** The ability to form a mental image of an object not present in the field of view. **2.** Synonym for imagery. *Example*: visualizing the face of a person speaking on the radio.
*See* **imagery.**

**visus** Vision.

**Visuscope** A modified ophthalmoscope containing a small graticule target for the measurement of eccentric fixation. The examiner projects a shadow of the target on the patient's retina. The patient is asked to look at the centre of the target. The position of the foveal reflex relative to the centre of the graticule target indicates whether the patient has eccentric fixation and in which direction and by how much. A modified version is the **Euthyscope** in which the graticule

target consists of black spots rather than a star and concentric circles as in the Visuscope. The Euthyscope is used more for eccentric fixation therapy.
*See* **fixation, eccentric; pleoptics.**

**vitamin A deficiency** A deficiency of vitamin A (also called retinol) leads to interference with growth, atrophy of epithelial tissues resulting in keratomalacia, corneal ulcerations, xerophthalmia with Bitot's spots, reduced resistance to infection of mucous membranes, and abnormal production and regeneration of rhodopsin resulting in night blindness. Management includes a balanced diet and may require large vitamin A supplement with a topical antibiotic to prevent secondary infections.
*See* **Bitot's spot; carotene; hemeralopia; keratomalacia; rhodopsin; xerophthalmia.**

**vitamin B** *See* **neuritis, optic.**

**vitelliform degeneration; macular dystrophy** *See* **disease, Best's.**

**vitiligo** A disease of the skin characterized by areas of depigmentation of various sizes and shapes. In the eye, it can be seen in the choroid or iris. It is often associated with syphilis or tuberculosis and forms part of the **Vogt–Koyanagi–Harada syndrome.**
*See* **poliosis; syndrome, Vogt–Koyanagi– Harada.**

**vitrectomy** Removal of the whole or a portion of the vitreous humour and replacement by saline or, more commonly, silicone oil. Indications for this surgical intervention include persistent vitreous opacities (usually as a result of unabsorbed haemorrhage), severe penetrating trauma, luxation of the lens, retention of some foreign bodies which cannot be removed with a magnet, endophthalmitis, and especially advanced diabetic eye disease such as proliferative retinopathy to prevent retinal detachment because the fibrovascular network of the retina tends otherwise to adhere to the vitreous body.
*See* **endophthalmitis; retinopathy, proliferative.**

**vitreoretinal degeneration** *See* **disease, Wagner's.**

**vitreous base** A dense, broad-band (2 mm wide) of vitreous attachement to the peripheral retina near the ora serrata. Collagen vitreous fibrils blend anteriorly with the basal lamina of the non-pigmented epithelium of the pars plana ciliaris of the ciliary body and posteriorly with the internal limiting membrane of the retina.

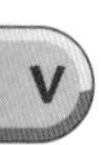

**vitreous body** *See* **humour, vitreous.**

**vitreous chamber** *See* **chamber, vitreous.**

**vitreous detachment** Separation of the vitreous body from the internal limiting membrane of the retina due to shrinkage from degenerative or inflammatory conditions, trauma, progressive myopia, old age, diabetes and in aphakic eyes in which the lens extraction was intracapsular. The most common cases are elderly individuals in whom the posterior part of the vitreous, which becomes liquid, detaches from the internal limiting membrane (called **posterior vitreous detachment (PVD)**). Symptoms are floaters and photopsia because as the eye moves the vitreous body comes into contact with the retina. The condition is sometimes associated with retinal tears and retinal detachment.
*See* **floaters; myopia, pathological; photopsia; retinal detachment; retinal tear; syneresis.**

**vitreous floaters** *See* **floaters.**

**vitreous haemorrhage** *See* **haemorrhage, preretinal; retinopathy, diabetic.**

**vitreous humour** *See* **humour, vitreous.**

**vitreous, persistent hyperplastic primary (PHPV)** A congenital, abnormal vitreous development characterized by a retrolental mass formed by remnants of the hyaloid system and tunica vasculosa lentis. The eye presents with leukocoria and there may also be cataract and congenital glaucoma. Treatment should begin as early in life as possible to avoid the risk of damage to the globe and amblyopia.
*See* **artery, hyaloid; hyaloid remnant.**

**Vogt's striae** *See* **striae, Vogt's.**

**Vogt, palisades of** *See* **palisades of Vogt.**

**Volk lens** *See* **slit-lamp.**

**von Graefe's sign** *See* **disease, Graves'; sign, von Graefe's.**

**von Graefe's test** *See* **test, diplopia.**

**von Hippel's disease** *See* **disease, von Hippel's.**

**von Hippel–Lindau disease** *See* **disease, von Hippel–Lindau.**

**von Recklinghausen's disease** *See* **disease, von Recklinghausen's.**

**vortex vein** *See* **vein, vortex.**

**V-pattern** *See* **pattern, V.**

**V syndrome** *See* **pattern, V.**

**V-value** *See* **constringence.**

# W

**W cell** *See* **cell, W.**

**wafer** A very thin lens to be cemented on a larger lens to make a bifocal lens.
*See* **lens, bifocal.**

**Wagner's disease** *See* **disease, Wagner's.**

**wall eye** *See* **eye, wall.**

**water content** Water in a contact lens expressed as a percentage of the total mass of the lens in its hydrated state under equilibrium conditions with physiological saline solution containing 9 g/l sodium chloride at a temperature of 20 ± 0.5°C and with a stated pH value.

$$\text{Water content} = \frac{M - m}{M} \times 100$$

where $M$ is the mass of hydrated lens, $m$ is the mass of dry lens.
The FDA has categorized hydrogel contact lenses into four groups according to their water content and their surface reactivity (referred to as ionic if it contains more than 0.2% ionic material, and nonionic otherwise). Group 1: water content less than 50% and non-ionic. Group 2: water content greater than 50% and non-ionic. Group 3: water content less than 50% and ionic. Group 4: water content greater than 50% and ionic.
*See* **lens, high water content; lens, low water content; lens, mid water content.**

**water-drinking test** *See* **test, provocative.**

**waterfall after-effect; illusion** *See* **after-effect, waterfall.**

**watery eye** *See* **epiphora.**

**wave, alpha** *See* **alpha waves.**

**wave number** *See* **wavelength.**

**wave theory** *See* **theory, wave.**

**wavefront** A virtual surface emanating from an object or an optical system, perpendicular throughout to a bundle of rays.
*See* **aberration, wavefront.**

**wavelength** Distance in the direction of propagation of a periodic wave between two successive points at the same position in the wave (e.g. the distance between two crests). *Symbol*:λ. *Note 1*: The wavelength in a medium is equal to the wavelength in vacuum divided by the refractive index of the medium. Unless otherwise stated, values of wavelength are generally those in air. The refractive index of standard air (15°C, 101 325 N/m²) lies between 1.000 27 and 1.000 29 for visible radiations. *Note 2*: The reciprocal of the wavelength is called the **wave number**. *Note 3*: The wavelength is longer for red light than for blue light. Wavelength λ is equal to

$$\lambda = \frac{c}{v}$$

where $c$ is the velocity of light and $v$ is the frequency of light. (Fig. W1)
*See* **fluorescence; index of refraction; infrared; interferometer; light; phase; phenomenon, Bezold–Brücke; spectrum, electromagnetic; ultraviolet; theory, wave.**

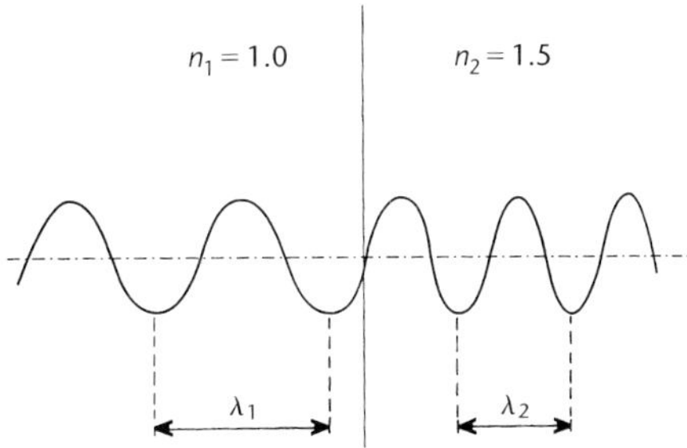


**Fig. W1** Wavelength of light in air and in a medium of refractive index $n_1$ and $n_2$, respectively ($\lambda_2 = \lambda_1/n_2$)

**wavelength, complementary** *See* **colour, complementary.**

**wavelength, dominant (of a colour stimulus, not purple)** Wavelength of the monochromatic light stimulus that, when combined in suitable proportions with the specified achromatic light stimulus, yields a match with the colour stimulus considered. *Note*: When the dominant wavelength cannot be given (this applies to purples), its place is taken by the complementary wavelength (CIE).
*See* **colour, complementary.**

**Weber's fraction; law** *See* **law, Weber's.**

**Weber's syndrome** *See* **syndrome, Weber's.**

**Weber–Fechner law** *See* **law, Weber's.**

**wedge, optical** A filter in which the transmittance varies continuously along a path (straight or curved) on its surface. If the filter transmits all the wavelengths more or less equally, it is called a **neutral wedge**.
*See* **filter; phenomenon, Bielschowsky's.**

**weeping** Excessive lacrimation.
*See* **epiphora; lacrimal apparatus; lacrimation.**

**weeping reflex** *See* **reflex, lacrimal.**

**Weill–Marchesani syndrome** *See* **syndrome, Weill–Marchesani.**

**Welland's test** *See* **test, bar reading.**

**Wernicke's disease** *See* **disease, Wernicke's.**

**Wernicke's hemianopic pupil; pupillary reaction; pupillary reflex; sign** *See* **reflex, hemianopic pupillary.**

**Wessley ring** *See* **ring, Wessley.**

**Wesson Fixation Disparity Card** *See* **disparity, retinal.**

**wettability** *See* **angle, contact.**

**wetting angle** *See* **angle, contact.**

**wetting solution** A solution which (1) transforms a hydrophobic surface into a hydrophilic one; (2) acts as a lubricant; (3) helps to clean the surface; (4) helps to prevent contamination of the lens while being inserted. It is spread on both surfaces of a rigid contact lens prior to insertion. However, the effect of a wetting solution only lasts a short time because it is quickly removed by the tear layer. A common wetting agent is **polyvinyl alcohol** which also has viscosity building properties.
*See* **enzyme; tears, artificial.**

**'what' system** *See* **parvocellular visual system.**

**Wheatstone amblyopia** *See* **amblyoscope, Wheatstone.**

**'where' system** *See* **magnocellular visual system.**

**white** *See* **colour, achromatic; colour, complementary; light, white.**

**white body** *See* **body, white.**

**white pupil; pupillary reflex** *See* **leukocoria.**

**Whitnall's tubercle** *See* **tubercle, lateral orbital.**

**wide-angle lens** *See* **lens, wide-angle.**

**Wieger, ligament of** *See* **ligament of Wieger.**

**Wilbrand's knee** That portion of the decussating optic nerve fibres from the inferior nasal retina which loop forward into the contralateral optic nerve for a distance of up to 3 mm from the anterior part of the optic chiasma and then pass backward into the optic tract. The existence of Wilbrand's knee in normal subjects has been questioned.
*See* **scotoma, junction.**

**Willis, circle of** *See* **circle of Willis.**

**Wilson's disease** *See* **disease, Wilson's.**

**Wilson three mirror fundus lens** *See* **slit-lamp.**

**wing cells** *See* **corneal epithelium.**

**wink** The rapid, voluntary closure and opening of one eye.
*See* **blink.**

**with movement** *See* **retinoscope.**

**with the rule astigmatism** *See* **astigmatism, with the rule.**

**Wolfring, glands of** *See* **glands of Wolfring.**

**Wollaston ellipse** *See* **ellipse, Tscherning.**

**Wollaston lens** *See* **lens, Wollaston.**

**Wollaston polarizer; prism** *See* **prism, Wollaston.**

**Wood's light** *See* **light, Wood's.**

**word blindness** *See* **alexia.**

**working distance** *See* **distance, working.**

**Worth amblyoscope** *See* **amblyoscope, Worth.**

**Worth's classification of binocular vision** *See* **vision, Worth's classification of binocular.**

**Worth's four dot test** *See* **test, Worth's four dot.**

**Wundt's visual illusion** *See* **illusion, Wundt's visual.**

**X cell** *See* **cell, X.**

**xanthelasma** A cutaneous deposition of lipid material which appears in the skin of the eyelids, most commonly near the inner canthi. It appears as a yellowish, slightly elevated area. It is a benign and chronic condition that occurs primarily in the elderly. It may be associated with raised blood cholesterol, high-density lipoprotein and triglyceride levels, leading to heart disease or diabetes. *Syn.* xanthoma; xanthelasma palpebrarum; xanthoma palpebrarum.
*See* **arcus, corneal; diabetes; eyelids; plaque, Hollenhorst's.**

**xanthogranuloma, juvenile (JXG)** A benign proliferation of single or multiple, small yellowish-brown papules or nodules in the skin and the anterior uvea, especially the iris. The condition mainly appears in young children, although it may occur in adults. The lesions consist of dermal infiltration by histiocytes, lymphocytes, eosinophils and Touton giant cells. The skin lesions increase in size and number but eventually regress spontaneously into an atrophic scar, otherwise they may need to be treated by excision or corticosteroid injection. In the eye it is commonly associated with hyphaemia (in the anterior chamber), uveitis and secondary glaucoma with visual loss. Therapy includes topical and systemic corticosteroids. *Syn.* juvenile nevoxanthoendothelioma.

**xanthoma** *See* **xanthelasma.**

**xanthopsia** A condition in which all objects appear of a yellow colour. It may occur as a result of picric acid and santonin poisoning, or jaundice. *Syn.* yellow vision.
*See* **chromatopsia.**

**x-axis** *See* **axis, transverse.**

**X-Chrom lens** *See* **lens, X-Chrom.**

**xeroderma pigmentosum** An autosomal recessive inherited disease in which there is progressive pigmentary degeneration of the skin, especially in sun-exposed areas. It results from a deficient enzyme used in the repair of DNA damaged by ultraviolet light. The condition begins in infancy and is characterized by the appearance of numerous pigmented spots resembling freckles and telangiectases. Eventually atrophic patches appear as well as wart-like excrescence and often squamous cell carcinoma. Patients are photophobic and the eyelids are frequently affected with atrophy and ectropion which may be accompanied with conjunctival inflammation and corneal ulceration. Protection of the eyes and skin is essential as well as surgical removal of the carcinomatous tumours, but many patients eventually succumb to metastases.

**xeroma** *See* **xerophthalmia.**

**xerophthalmia** Extreme dryness of the conjunctiva and cornea due to a failure of the secretory activity of the mucin-secreting goblet cells of the conjunctiva. The conjunctiva and cornea lose their lustre and become skin-like in appearance. The condition may even propagate to the cornea and give rise to keratoconjunctivitis sicca and, if severe, keratomalacia. Xerophthalmia may be due to trauma, exposure or systematic deficiency of vitamin A, etc. *Syn.* xeroma; xerosis of the conjunctiva (if the cornea is not involved).
*See* **Bitot's spot; cell, goblet; keratitis sicca; keratomalacia; mucin.**

**xerosis** *See* **xerophthalmia.**

**X-linked inheritance** *See* **inheritance.**

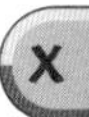

# Y

**Y cell** *See* **cell, Y.**

**y-axis** *See* **axis, anteroposterior.**

**y sutures of the lens** *See* **suture, lens.**

**yag laser** *See* **laser, neodymium-yag.**

**yellow** One of the hues of the visible spectrum evoked by stimulation of the retina by wavelengths situated in a narrow region between about 560 and 590 nm, i.e. between red and green. The complementary colours to yellow are blues. *See* **colour, complementary; light.**

**yellow spot** *See* **macula lutea.**

**yellow vision** *See* **xanthopsia.**

**yoke muscles** *See* **muscles, yoke.**

**yoke prisms** *See* **prisms, yoke.**

**Young's experiment** *See* **experiment, Young's.**

**Young's modulus of elasticity** *See* **modulus of elasticity.**

**Young's optometer** *See* **optometer, Young's.**

**Young–Helmholtz theory** *See* **theory, Young–Helmholtz.**

# Z

**z-axis** *See* **axis, vertical.**

**Zeis, glands of** *See* **glands of Zeis.**

**Zeiss lens** *See* **lens, Zeiss.**

**zinc sulphate** An astringent and antiseptic agent sometimes used topically in solution 0.2% or 0.25%, to clear mucous from the outer surface of the eye (by precipitating proteins), to give temporary relief of minor eye infections, and to treat some types of bacterial conjunctivitis.

**Zinn, annulus of** *See* **annulus of Zinn.**

**Zinn, circle of** *See* **circle of Zinn.**

**Zinn, zonule of** A series of fibres passing from the ciliary body to the capsule of the lens at or near its equator, holding the lens in position and enabling the ciliary muscles to act upon it. The lens and zonule form a diaphragm that divides the eye into a small anterior area which contains aqueous humour, and a larger posterior area which contains vitreous humour. The zonule forms a ring that is roughly triangular in a meridional section. It is made up of fibres that are transparent and straight for the most part. The tension of these fibres varies with the state of contraction of the ciliary muscle and thus affects the convexity of the lens. The zonule of Zinn is made up of many non-cellular fibres, the fibrils of which consist of a cysteine-rich microfibrillar component of the elastic system, fibrillin. The fibres have been classified as follows: (1) The **hyaloid zonule** (or **orbiculo-posterior capsular fibres**) which originate from the pars plana of the ciliary body and insert into the capsule just posterior to the equator at the edge of the patellar fossa. (2) The **anterior zonule** (or **orbiculo-anterior capsular fibres** or **anterior zonular sheet**), which originate from the pars plana of the ciliary body and insert into the capsule just anterior to the equator. These are the strongest and thickest of the zonular fibres. (3) The **posterior zonule** (or **cilio-posterior capsular fibres** or **posterior zonular sheet**), which originate from the pars plicata of the ciliary body and insert into the lens capsule posterior to the equator. These are the most numerous. (4) The **equatorial zonule** (or **cilio-equatorial fibres**) which originate from the pars plicata of the ciliary body

and insert into the lens capsule at the equator. *Syn.* suspensory apparatus of the lens; suspensory ligament; zonular fibres.
*See* **canal, Hannover's; canal of Petit; ciliary body; ciliary processes; ora serrata.**

**Zollner's visual illusion** *See* **illusion, Zollner's visual.**

**zone, ciliary** *See* **iris.**

**zone of comfort** *See* **criterion, Percival.**

**zone of the cornea, optical** *See* **optical zone of the cornea.**

**zone, optic** *See* **optic zone.**

**zone, pupillary** *See* **iris.**

**zone, scleral** *See* **scleral zone.**

**zone of clear, single, binocular vision** In Donders' diagram it is the region determined by the extremes of accommodation and convergence that can be evoked while retaining a clear, single image. Clinically, this is determined by measuring the limits of negative and positive relative convergence by using base-in and base-out prisms to blur, or by measuring relative accommodation by binocularly adding concave or convex lenses, for various binocularly fixated distances. (Fig. Z1)
*See* **accommodation, relative amplitude of; convergence, relative; Donders' diagram; prism bar; prism, rotary; vision, binocular.**

**zonula occludentes** *See* **tight junction.**

**zonular cataract** *See* **cataract, zonular.**

**zonular fibres** *See* **Zinn, zonule of.**

**zonule of Zinn** *See* **Zinn, zonule of.**

**zoom lens** *See* **lens, zoom.**

**zoster, herpes** *See* **herpes zoster ophthalmicus.**

**zygomatic bone** *See* **orbit.**

**zygomycosis** *See* **phycomycosis.**

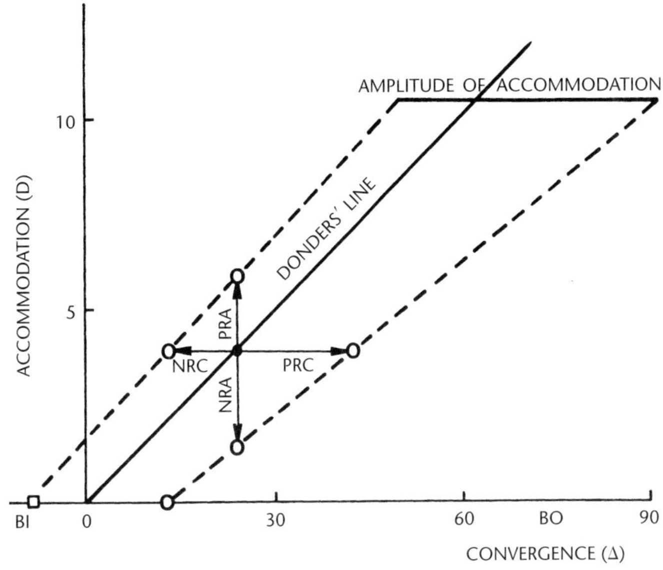


**Fig. Z1** Zone of clear, single, binocular vision (NRC, negative relative convergence; PRC, positive relative convergence; NRA, negative relative accommodation; PRA, positive relative accommodation; BI, base-in prism; BO, base-out prism)

Z